Traditional Herbal Therapy for the Human Immune System

Exploring Medicinal Plants

Series Editor
Azamal Husen
Wolaita Sodo University, Ethiopia

Medicinal plants render a rich source of bioactive compounds used in drug formulation and development; they play a key role in traditional or indigenous health systems. As the demand for herbal medicines increases worldwide, supply is declining as most of the harvest is derived from naturally growing vegetation. Considering global interests and covering several important aspects associated with medicinal plants, the Exploring Medicinal Plants series comprises volumes valuable to academia, practitioners, and researchers interested in medicinal plants. Topics provide information on a range of subjects including diversity, conservation, propagation, cultivation, physiology, molecular biology, growth response under extreme environment, handling, storage, bioactive compounds, secondary metabolites, extraction, therapeutics, mode of action, and healthcare practices.

Led by Azamal Husen, PhD, this series is directed to a broad range of researchers and professionals consisting of topical books exploring information related to medicinal plants. It includes edited volumes, references, and textbooks available for individual print and electronic purchases.

Traditional Herbal Therapy for the Human Immune System

Edited by
Azamal Husen
Wolaita Sodo University, Wolaita, Ethiopia

CRC Press
Taylor & Francis Group
Boca Raton London New York

CRC Press is an imprint of the
Taylor & Francis Group, an **informa** business

First edition published 2022
by CRC Press
6000 Broken Sound Parkway NW, Suite 300, Boca Raton, FL 33487-2742

and by CRC Press
2 Park Square, Milton Park, Abingdon, Oxon, OX14 4RN

ISBN: 9780367685256 (hbk)
ISBN: 9781032109121 (pbk)
ISBN: 9781003137955 (ebk)

DOI: 10.1201/9781003137955

Typeset in Times
by Deanta Global Publishing Services, Chennai, India

Dedication

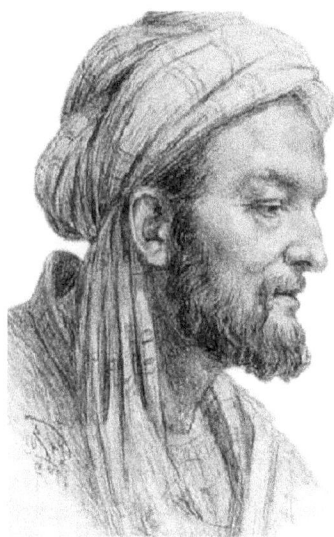

Abu Ali Ibn Sina (980–1037 AD)

(A great physician, astronomer, thinker, and writer of the Islamic Golden Age, and the father of early modern medicine)

Contents

Preface

The goal of this book is to provide a review, as thorough and up-to-date as possible, of the state-of-the-art herbal therapy for strong human immune systems and research-based information on medicinal plants used for this purpose. A large number of people around the world suffer from daily inconvenience and unpleasantness of a deficient immune system. Tiredness, frequent colds, infections, allergies, mood swings, and premature ageing are all common manifestations of a weakened immunity. The human immune system is an invisible bodyguard, fighting off invasion and working tirelessly around the clock to keep the human body fit and healthy. The immune system is responsible for responding when anyone is exposed to viruses, bacteria, or other microbes, has a cut or a broken bone, or when cells begin to change in an abnormal way, as in the early stages of cancer. The immune system also plays the vital role of differentiating the live materials belonging to the body from those coming from outside, and quickly eliminating the foreign proteins from bacteria, virus, or other microbes. It is also responsible for inflammation, the natural process that occurs in response to injury and is incredibly important to initiate healing, although too much of it can be detrimental and is linked to heart disease, diabetes, cancer, and many other illnesses.

In this connection, medicinal plants and their products are able to affect the immune system and act as immunomodulators. Numerous medicinal plants are popularly used in folk medicine to increase resistance of the body; they strengthen the human immune defence and improve body reactions against infectious agents or exogenous injuries, suppressing the abnormal immune response occurring in immune disorders. Many herbs, shrubs, climbers, or trees, such as *Allium fistulosum, Allium sativum, Aloe vera, Andrographis paniculata, Calendula officinalis, Camellia sinensis, Catharanthus roseus, Cinnamomum camphora, Curcuma longa, Echinacea purpurea, Echinacea angustifolia, Elettaria cardamomum, Emblica officinalis, Eucalyptus* spp., *Glycyrrhiza glabra, Hypericum perforatum, Mentha piperita, Nigella sativa, Origanum vulgare, Ocimum sanctum, Ocimum basilicum, Panax ginseng, Salvia officinalis, Sambucus nigra, Taraxacum officinale, Thymus vulgaris, Withania somnifera, Zingiber officinale,* etc., have shown success in strengthening immunity against the H1N1 virus, influenza, hepatitis and swine flu-virus, among others. These plants and their products have some specific properties to reduce stress and anxiety, absorb odours and mould, eliminate headaches, improve mood and brain function, enhance blood and oxygen circulation, increase energy levels, boost healing processes, maintain blood pressure, act as a source of vitamins and improve a number of bodily functions. Moreover, these plants have acted as an antiviral and antibacterial agent; and boosted the immune system against cancer, HIV, and COVID-19. This book addresses these issues and many more. In the future, medicinal plant-based products are likely to be in higher demand to facilitate and strengthen the human immune system against infections, allergies, and related ailments. Taken together, this book aims to cover both the indigenous and scientific knowledge about medicinal plants, and the protective and therapeutic potential and mode of action of plant-based drinks, supplements, nutraceuticals, synergy foods, superfoods, and other products. I hope that this book will be a useful resource to stimulate further research interest in plant-derived medications and will inspire students, industrialists, and policy makers.

With great pleasure, I extend my sincere thanks to all contributors for their timely response, and the excellent, up-to-date contributions. I am extremely thankful to Ms. Randy Brehm, Dr Julia Tanner, and all associates at Taylor & Francis Group, LLC/ CRC Press for their sustained cooperation. I shall be happy receiving comments and criticism, if any, from subject experts and general readers of this book.

Azamal Husen
Wolaita, Ethiopia

About the Editor

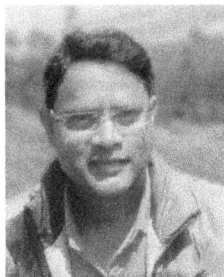

Professor Azamal Husen (BSc from Shri Murli Manohar Town Post Graduate College, Ballia, UP, MSc from Hamdard University, New Delhi, and PhD from Forest Research Institute, Dehra Dun, India) is a Foreign Delegate at Wolaita Sodo University, Wolaita, Ethiopia. He has served the University of Gondar, Ethiopia, as a Full Professor of Biology, and also worked as the Coordinator of the MSc Program and as the Head, Department of Biology. He was a Visiting Faculty of the Forest Research Institute, and the Doon College of Agriculture and Forest at Dehra Dun, India. He has more than 20 years' experience of teaching, research, and administration.

Dr Husen specializes in biogenic nanomaterial fabrication and their application, plant responses to nanomaterials, plant production and adaptation to harsh environments at the physiological, biochemical, and molecular levels, herbal medicine, and clonal propagation and improvement of tree species. He has conducted several research projects sponsored by various funding agencies, including the World Bank, the Indian Council of Agriculture Research (ICAR), the Indian Council of Forest Research Education (ICFRE); and the Japan Bank for International Cooperation (JBIC).

He has published over 150 research papers, review articles and book chapters, edited books of international repute, presented papers in several conferences, and produced over a dozen manuals and monographs. Dr Husen received four fellowships from India and a recognition award from the University of Gondar, Ethiopia, for excellent teaching, research, and community service. An active organizer of seminars/conferences and an efficient evaluator of research projects and book proposals, Dr Husen has been on the Editorial board and the panel of reviewers of several reputed journals published by Elsevier, Frontiers Media SA, Taylor & Francis, Springer Nature, RSC, Oxford University Press, Sciendo, The Royal Society, CSIRO, PLOS, and John Wiley & Sons. He is on the advisory board of Cambridge Scholars Publishing, UK. He is a Fellow of the Plantae group of the American Society of Plant Biologists, and a Member of the International Society of Root Research, Asian Council of Science Editors, ISDS, and INPST. In addition, he is Editor-in-Chief of the American Journal of Plant Physiology; and a Series Editor of 'Exploring Medicinal Plants', published by Taylor & Francis Group, USA.

Contributors

Limenew Abate
Department of Industrial Chemistry
College of Applied Sciences
Addis Ababa Science and Technology
University
Addis Ababa, Ethiopia

Swati Agarwal
Department of Bioscience and
Biotechnology
Banasthali University
P.O. Banasthali Vidyapith
Rajasthan, India

Mohd Ahmad
S.R. Institute of Management and
Technology
Lucknow, India

Jamal Akhtar
Central Council for Research in Unani
Medicine
Institutional Area
New Delhi, India

Atul Arya
Medicinal Plant Research Laboratory
Department of Botany
Ramjas College
University of Delhi
Delhi, India

Archana Bachheti
Department of Environment Science
Graphic Era University, Dehra Dun
Uttarakhand, India

Rakesh Kumar Bachheti
Centre of Excellence in Nanotechnology
Addis Ababa Science and Technology
University
Addis Ababa, Ethiopia

**Solma Lúcia Souto Maior
de Araújo Baltar**
Department of Biological Sciences
Campus Arapiraca
Federal University of Alagoas
Brazil

Fouzia Bashir
Central Council for Research in Unani
Medicine
Institutional Area
New Delhi, India

Maria Lusia de Morais Belo Bezerra
Department of Biological Sciences
Campus Arapiraca
Federal University of Alagoas
Brazil

Callistus Bvenura
Cape Peninsula University of
Technology
Horticultural Sciences Department
Cape Town, South Africa

Anuj Choudhary
Department of Botany
Punjab Agricultural University
Ludhiana, India

Mani Divya
Biomaterials and Biotechnology in
    Animal Health Lab
Nanobiosciences and
    Nanopharmacology Division
Department of Animal Health and
    Management
Alagappa University
Karaikudi, India

Anywar Godwin
Department of Plant Sciences
Microbiology & Biotechnology
Makerere University
Kampala, Uganda

Azamal Husen
Wolaita Sodo University
Wolaita, Ethiopia

Muhammad Iqbal
Department of Botany
Faculty of Science
Hamdard University
New Delhi, India

Learnmore Kambizi
Cape Peninsula University of
    Technology
Horticultural Sciences Department
Cape Town, South Africa

Harmanjot Kaur
Department of Botany
Punjab Agricultural University
Ludhiana, India

Amrendra Kumar
Division of Livestock Production
Indian Council of Agricultural
    Research
Research Complex for North Eastern
    Hill Region
Meghalaya, India

Antul Kumar
Department of Botany
Punjab Agricultural University
Ludhiana, India

Deepak Kumar Verma
Centre for Health Research and
    Innovation (CHRI)
Lucknow, India

Madan Kumar P
Department of Biochemistry
CSIR-Central Food Technological
    Research Institute
Mysore, India

and

Academy of Scientific and Innovative
    Research (AcSIR)
Ghaziabad, India

Rakesh Kumar
Vijay Singh Pathik Government Post
    Graduate College
Kairana, India

Sahil Mehta
International Centre for Genetic
    Engineering and Biotechnology
Aruna Asaf Ali Marg
New Delhi, India

Vinod Kumar Mishra
S.R. Institute of Management and
    Technology
Lucknow, India

Sanjeev Kumar Singh
Department of Bioinformatics
Alagappa University
Karaikudi, India

Sonu Kumari
Department of Bioscience and
  Biotechnology
Banasthali University
P.O. Banasthali Vidyapith Rajasthan
Rajasthan, India

Asish Kumar Padhy
National Institute of Plant Genome
  Research
Aruna Asaf Ali Marg
New Delhi, India

Saumya Pandey
School of Agriculture
Uttaranchal University
Uttarakhand, India

Chandrabose Selvaraj
Department of Bioinformatics
Alagappa University
Karaikudi, India

José Crisólogo de Sales Silva
Department of Animal Science
Campus Santana do Ipanema
State University of Alagoas
Brazil

Baljinder Singh
National Institute of Plant Genome
  Research
Aruna Asaf Ali Marg
New Delhi, India

Yashdeep Srivastava
S.R. Institute of Management and
  Technology
Lucknow, India

Kirubel Teshome Tadele
Chemistry Department
Natural Sciences College
Jimma University
Jimma, Ethiopia

Swati Upadhyay
S.R. Institute of Management and
  Technology
Lucknow, India

Sekar Vijayakumar
Marine College
Shandong University
Weihai, P.R. China

Vani V
Department of Biochemistry
CSIR-Central Food Technological
  Research Institute
Mysore, India

and

Academy of Scientific and Innovative
  Research (AcSIR)
Ghaziabad, India

Venkateish V P
Department of Biochemistry
CSIR-Central Food Technological
  Research Institute
Mysore, India

and

Academy of Scientific and Innovative
  Research (AcSIR)
Ghaziabad, India

Nivya V
Department of Biochemistry
CSIR-Central Food Technological
  Research Institute
Mysore, India

and

Academy of Scientific and Innovative
  Research (AcSIR)
Ghaziabad, India

Baskaran V
Department of Biochemistry
CSIR-Central Food Technological
    Research Institute
Mysore, India

and

Academy of Scientific and Innovative
    Research (AcSIR)
Ghaziabad, India

Chandrabose Yogeswari
Vetri Siddha Medical College
    Hospital & Research Institute
Madurai, India

Gebeyanesh Worku Zerssa
Natural Resource Management
    Department
College of Agriculture and Veterinary
    Medicine
Jimma University
Jimma, Ethiopia

Disclaimer

The author and the publishers of this work have checked the sources and believe that the given information presented is genuine. This is only a reference book, not intending to offer any nutritional or medical advice. The information on the role and uses of medicinal plants does not constitute any recommendation. The author and publishers are not responsible if any reader uses these plants for a nutritional or therapeutic purpose.

1 Plant-based Potential Nutraceuticals for Improving the Human Immune System

Azamal Husen and Muhammad Iqbal

CONTENTS

1.1 INTRODUCTION

Our immune system uses our body's own defence mechanisms to guard against damage, disease, and infections. Composed of various tissues, cells, and proteins, the immune system is a highly complex and multifaceted system, forming an intricate network of cells and proteins that moves throughout the human body *via* the lymph stream and blood stream. A healthy immune system is able to distinguish between body cells (self) and foreign materials (non-self), eliminating the latter. It can also recognize and destroy abnormal cells derived from host tissues. In an autoimmune reaction, however, antibodies and immune cells target the body's own healthy tissues by mistake, signalling the body to attack them (Terrie, 2017). Undernourishment or deficiency of zinc, selenium, iron, copper, or vitamins A, C, E, B_6, or B_9 (folic acid) significantly influence immune system responses. On the other hand, overeating and being overweight or obese may also hamper the immune response. Moreover, chronic stress, lack of sleep, specific medical conditions, prolonged use of corticosteroids or immunosuppressive agents, or immune-mediated diseases damage our immune system (Terrie, 2017). Immunity decreases and morbidity increases with increasing age due to deficiencies of vitamins C, D, E, B_6, B_9, and elements such as zinc, and/or selenium. (Ritz et al., 2009). Use of vitamin D supplements strengthens the physical barrier against viruses, stimulates production of antimicrobial peptides, and attenuates formation of inflammatory cytokines, whereas selenium improves the function of cytotoxic effector cells and helps in maintaining T-cell functions and the production of T-cell-dependent antibodies. Vitamin C enhances production of antiviral cytokines and free radicals, thus reducing the virus yield, and also inhibits excessive inflammatory responses and/or hyperactivation of immune cells (Bae and Kim, 2020). Use of nutraceuticals supports restoration of the immune system, particularly in the elderly.

Immunomodulators influence the immune system efficiently. These agents strengthen the immune defences, improve the body's reaction against microbial infections and/or injuries, and suppress irregular immune responses. Nutraceuticals (chemicals from food with health benefits in excess of their nutritional value) are bioactive compounds naturally present in foods, dietary supplements, and plant products/extracts, which have acknowledged potential health applications (Figure 1.1). They play a vital role in maintaining a healthy body by providing necessary supplements required for various metabolic processes in order to regulate bodily functions.

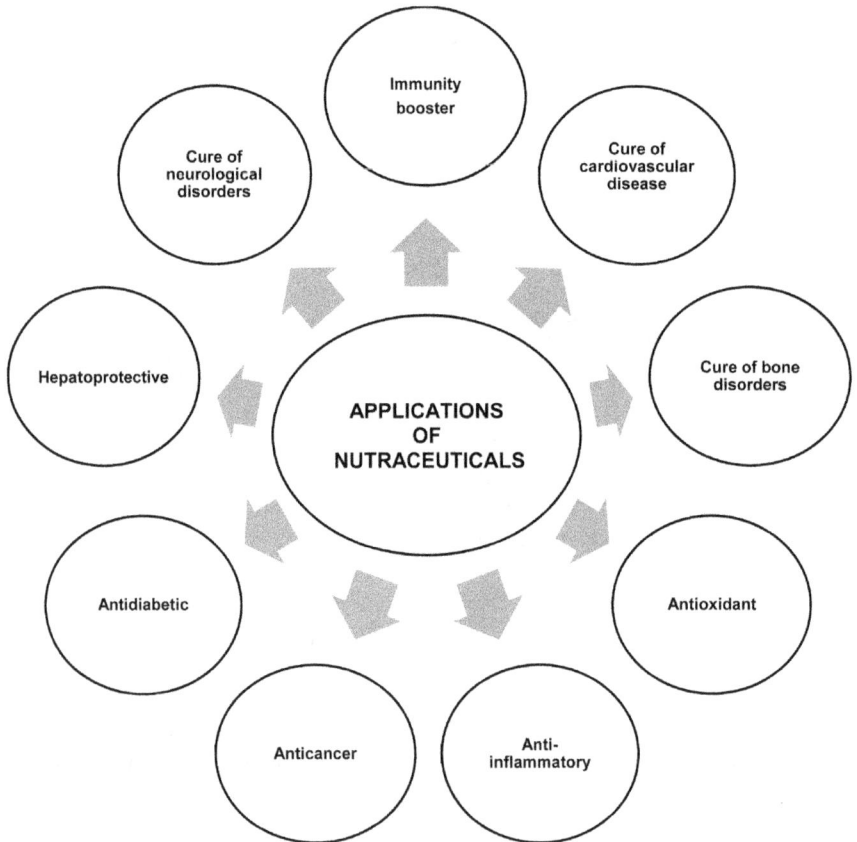

FIGURE 1.1   Various potential applications of nutraceuticals.

Herbs or herbal products may not act as precisely as antibiotics but have proven to be antibacterial (even antiviral) by boosting our body's own defence mechanisms (Nasri et al., 2014; Chanda et al., 2019). Nutraceuticals obtained from plants act as the probable immunomodulating agents in such products. Phytochemicals (flavonoids, folate, polyamines, alkaloids, terpenoids, etc.) and other, essential nutrients (mainly carbohydrates, proteins, fatty acids, minerals, and vitamins) play an important role in maintaining a balance between health and disease (Parveen et al., 2020b). Thus, nutrition is a crucial factor in modulating immune homoeostasis. Protein–energy malnutrition or even subclinical deficiencies of a single micronutrient may impair immune responses (Bhaskaram, 2001). Calder et al. (2020) elucidated the significance of optimal nutritional status to resist against viral infections, asserting the roles of vitamins (such as A, B_6, B_{12}, C, D, E, and folate), trace elements (such as zinc, iron, selenium, magnesium, and copper) and the omega-3 fatty acids (such as eicosapentaenoic acid and docosahexaenoic acid) in supporting the immune system. Vitamins A and D have a potential benefit, especially in vitamin-deficient populations, while the micronutrients selenium and zinc give favourable immunomodulatory effects during viral respiratory infections, and many nutraceuticals and probiotics facilitate immune functions (Jayawardena et al., 2020). While proposing nutritional strategies to reduce damage to lungs from coronavirus and other infections, Wu and Zha (2020) asserted that the most promising, fact-acting treatments are herbal formulations, which probably address lung, heart, liver, and kidney functions simultaneously. Rathaur et al. (2020) and Parveen et al. (2020a, 2020b) have described the usefulness of single and compound herbal drugs used in the Ayurvedic and Unani systems of Indian medicine, respectively.

Various food components have the ability to modulate cellular processes and stimulate the immune system. For instance, peppermint (*Mentha × piperita*) and oils obtained from this plant are used as antispasmodic, aromatic, and antiseptic agents and are used for treating cancers, colds, cramps, indigestion, nausea, sore throat, and toothaches (Briggs, 1993). Yellow turmeric powder, a product of *Curcuma longa*, is very active against a range of bacteria, fungi, and viruses, as well as parasites (Moghadamtousi et al., 2014; Prasad and Tyagi, 2015). *Panax ginseng* (Asian ginseng) is used as a tonic, is known to promote immunity (Kang and Min, 2012), and has protective effects for the treatment of neurological disorders (Ong et al., 2015). *Astragalus membranaceus* (commonly known as Mongolian milkvetch) is rich in polysaccharides, flavonoids, and saponins (Auyeung et al., 2016), and exhibits powerful immunity-enhancing, antioxidant, hepatoprotective, antidiabetic, and anticancer activities (Zhao et al., 1990; Auyeung et al., 2016; Wu et al., 2017). The most common and widely used herbal plants, such *Allium sativum* (garlic), *Allium cepa* (onion), and *Zingiber officinale* (ginger), are the basis of all healing herbal products, and can be categorized as food and spice, as well as medicine. In many remote areas, various plants and their products are used as ethnomedicines for treatment of all physical ailments of the local populations (Anis and Iqbal, 1994; Anis et al., 2000; Beigh et al., 2014). We intend to briefly discuss in this chapter some plant-based nutraceuticals and their role in improving the human immune system to ensure and maintain a high quality of life.

1.2 IMMUNOMODULATORY PHYTOCHEMICALS AND ASSOCIATED RESPONSES

Phytochemicals, mainly alkaloids, phenolics, glycoproteins and saponins, can exhibit anti-inflammatory and immunomodulatory features. Additionally, terpenoids, polysaccharides, fatty acids, minerals, vitamins, etc. also play an important role as immunomodulatory agents and help in disease prevention. Polysaccharides from plants have shown low toxicity in comparison with immunomodulatory bacterial polysaccharides and many synthetic compounds (Albuquerque et al., 2020). Therefore, they are the ideal alternative agents to achieve immunomodulation. Since ancient times, it has been recognized that plants, plant parts, or their products and extracts are the sources of medicinally active compounds (Figure 1.2). For instance, alkaloids from plants are utilized as antimalarial agents (quinine), anticancer agents (vinblastine, vincristine, and taxol), and to regulate blood circulation, especially in the brain (vincamine). The terpenoid steroidal saponins obtained from plants, including *Solanum aethiopicum* (Ethiopian eggplant), *Capsicum annuum* (capsicum peppers), *Panax ginseng* (ginseng), and *Yucca schidigera* (Mojave yucca) (Hussain et al., 2015), have shown hypoglycaemic, antioxidant, antifungal, neurotrophic, neuroprotective, and viricidal effects. Such saponins are also involved in the reduction of low-density lipoprotein (LDL)-cholesterol and serum cholesterol levels, inhibition of cancer cell proliferation, and fortification of the cell-mediated immune system (Ding et al., 2019). Reports have also suggested that carotenoids, another class of terpenoids, significantly decrease the risk of prostate, lung, and breast cancers (Mills et al., 1989; Ziegler et al., 1996; Zhang et al., 1997) and provide protection against eye diseases (Yeum et al., 1995).

Many plants, such as vegetables (broccoli, green bell pepper, kale, onion, spinach, and tomato), fruits and herbs, mainly *Citrus grandis*, *Hypericum perforatum*, and *Sophora japonica*, are a rich source of flavonoids (a subclass of plant phenolics). Flavonoids play a defensive role in coronary heart diseases, and exhibit antiviral, anti-allergenic, anti-cholinesterase, anticancer, and antioxidant activities (Ren et al. 2003; Ullah et al. 2020). Quercetin, a plant flavonol from the flavonoid group of

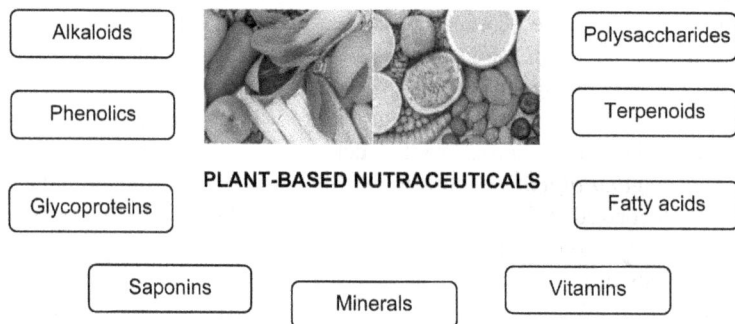

Alkaloids		Polysaccharides
Phenolics		Terpenoids
Glycoproteins	**PLANT-BASED NUTRACEUTICALS**	Fatty acids
Saponins	Minerals	Vitamins

FIGURE 1.2   Major plant-based nutraceuticals.

polyphenols, is an effective antioxidant, and plays a significant role against cardio-vascular disease (Finotti and Di Majo, 2003), diabetes, and HIV (Li et al., 2000). Likewise, tannins (water-soluble polyphenol derivatives), which are naturally syn-thesized and accumulated in various plant parts, are a secondary metabolic product exhibiting numerous useful healthy properties, showing anti-inflammatory, antimi-crobial, antileishmanial, immunomodulatory, analgesic, anti-lymphocytic, neuro-protective, antidiarrhoeal, and antihypertensive activities (Uritu et al., 2018). Garlic is rich in sulphur compounds, which stimulate the immune system and decrease atherogenesis, platelet stickiness, and cancer (Arreola et al., 2015; Shang et al., 2019). Sulphoraphane (an antioxidant and stimulator of natural detoxifying enzymes, abundantly found in *Brassica oleracea* var *italica* (broccoli), is an effective phase 2 enzyme inducer, and produces D-glucarolactone, which is an important breast can-cer inhibitor (Ghazanfari et al., 2002). Some common plant-based nutraceuticals and their roles in stimulating the immune system are listed in Table 1.1.

1.3 SYNERGISTIC EFFECT OF HERBAL AND OTHER PLANT PRODUCTS

Many nutraceuticals act together synergistically, exhibiting superior performances when co-delivered (Leena et al., 2020). For instance, the interactive herbal combina-tion, known as Triphala ("three fruits"), is prepared by mixing *Terminalia bellirica*, *Terminalia chebula*, and *Emblica officinalis* together for use as a nutritive tonic. This herbal preparation, based on synergy, benefits almost all organs/systems of the human body, most specifically skin, liver, eyes, and the digestive and respiratory systems. It is therapeutically useful in terms of immunomodulation, and as an anti-bacterial and antimutagenic product (Belapurkar et al., 2014; Peterson et al., 2017). Phytochemicals from tomatoes (*Solanum lycopersicum*) and olive oil from *Olea europaea* also have synergistic effect, as tomatoes contain carotenoids (principally lycopene), which are fat-soluble and their absorption into the bloodstream is higher in a lipid medium, such as olive oil. Lycopene, with its powerful antioxidant nature, minimizes the risk of cardiovascular diseases by improving the serum lipid profile in a high-fat diet. Lycopene bioavailability increases between five- and six-fold fol-lowing cooking of tomatoes, compared with eating them raw (Fielding et al., 2005; Ahuja et al., 2006; Story et al., 2010). Black grapes are rich in catechins, polyphenol antioxidants that can reduce the risk of obesity, cardiovascular disorders, cancer, and neurological problems. In combination with onion, consumption of black grapes causes a synergistic anti-proliferative effect, compared with consuming onions or grapes alone. The combination inhibits blood clots, improves blood circulation, and boosts cardiovascular health (Wang et al., 2013). Foods like green tea and black pep-per also work in a synergistic way, with black pepper increasing the bioavailability of epigallocatechin-3-gallate (EGCG), a useful component of green tea. Piperine, a major alkaloid present in black pepper, inhibits the glucouronidation of EGCG, thereby lowering the transit rate of EGCG in the gastrointestinal (GI) tract and thus increasing its residence time, which ensures maximum absorption. The high catechin content of green tea improves immunotolerance, thereby reducing the possibility of

TABLE 1.1
Examples of Plants Commonly Used as Nutraceuticals, Their Important Phytochemical Constituents, and Their Immune System Functions

Plant Name	Family	Phytochemical Constituents	Immune System Functions
Acacia catechu Willd.	Fabaceae	Flavonoids, phenolic acids, catechins	Immunoadjuvant and anti-inflammatory activity
Aloe vera (L.) Burman	Asphodelaceae	Acemannan, dihydrocoumarins	Immunostimulant
Andrographis paniculata (Burm. f.) Nees	Acanthaceae	Diterpene lactones (andrographolide)	Immunomodulant/immunosuppressor
Artocarpus tonkinensis A. Chev. ex Gagnep	Moraceae	Auronol glycosides (maesopsin 4-*O*-glucoside and alphitonin-4-*O*-glucoside)	Inhibits humoral and cellular adaptive immunity/immunosuppressor
Astragalus membranaceus (Fisch.) Bge.	Fabaceae	Polysaccharides	Stimulate cellular immunity/immunostimulant
Boswellia serrata Roxb. ex Colebr.	Burseraceae	Boswellic acid	Anti-anaphylactic and mast cell stabilization/immunosuppressor
Camellia sinensis (L.) Kuntze	Theaceae	Polysaccharides	Immunomodulant/immunostimulant
Centella asiatica (L.) Urban	Apiaceae	Madecassoside	Regulates the abnormal humoral and cellular immunity/immunosuppressor
Curcuma longa L.	Zingiberaceae	Curcuminoids	Anti-inflammatory and immunosuppressive activity/immunosuppressor
Echinacea purpurea (L.) Moench	Asteraceae	Alkylamides, glycoproteins, polysaccharides	Anti-inflammatory, immunomodulator and antiviral
Glycyrrhiza glabra L.	Fabaceae	Triterpene saponins (glycyrrhizin)	Anti-inflammatory activity/immunostimulant
Hypoxis rooperi T. Moore	Hypoxidaceae	Phenolic glucosides (hypoxoside)	Immunoadjuvant and anti-inflammatory activity
Ocimum sanctum L.	Lamiaceae	Monoterpenes (eugenol and methyl eugenol), sesquiterpenes (β-caryophyllene)	Immunostimulant
Panax ginseng C.A. Meyer	Araliaceae	Ginsenosides and panaxosides	Immunostimulant
Syzigium aromaticum (L.) Merr. and L.M. Perry	Myrtaceae	Monoterpenes (eugenol), sesquiterpenes (β-caryophyllene)	Immunostimulant
Tinospora cordifolia (Thunb.) Miers	Menispermaceae	Arabinogalactan	Immunostimulant
Withania somnifera (L.) Dunal	Solanaceae	Steroidal lactones (withaferin A)	Immunostimulant
Zingiber officinalis Roscoe	Zingiberaceae	Phenolics (gingerols)	Immunostimulant

cancer incidence, cardiovascular disease, and elevated cholesterol (Lambert et al., 2004). Similarly, lemon juice, consumed with green tea, enhances the absorption of EGCG ten-fold, as compared with the absorption when green tea is taken alone (Tewari et al., 2000). Furthermore, ascorbic acid (vitamin C), present at high concentrations in lemon, acts synergistically with catechins to stimulate the absorption and utilization of the antioxidant components of green tea five-fold, in comparison with green tea taken alone (Majchrzak et al., 2004; Intra and Kuo, 2007). All these combinations of nutraceuticals boost our immune system in one way or another and enable our body to fight against diseases and disorders.

Honey and garlic each have remarkable antibacterial properties, stimulating the immune system and exhibiting antibacterial activity, while acting synergistically to reduce bacterial growth, an effect which is further enhanced by the presence of phenolics and fatty acids (Natarajan et al., 2019). The combination of honey and garlic is also well known for lowering blood cholesterol and triglyceride levels and providing relief of cardiovascular problems (Shoba et al., 1998). Garlic increases the production of gastric juices and helps in increasing iron absorption (Shoba et al., 1998). Chen et al. (2005) reported that the flavonoids from almond skin acted synergistically with vitamins C and E to protect LDL-cholesterol oxidation. Similarly, a combination of green leafy vegetables and lemon is effective at increasing haemoglobin concentration in iron-deficient anaemic patients, as vitamin C accelerates the dietary absorption of non-haem iron (Hallberg et al., 1989). Furthermore, Fernandez and Marette (2017) suggested that bananas energize growth of beneficial bacteria in yoghurt, with the combination increasing immunity and regulating digestion. Inulins, prebiotic polysaccharides in a number of plants, are present in bananas, promoting the growth of probiotic (good) bacteria in yoghurt, which improves immunity and help in regulating our digestion. This banana–yoghurt combination also increases the level of calcium in our body. Studies on the interaction between turmeric and fish revealed that curcumin, the active component in turmeric, acts synergistically with the polyunsaturated fatty acids (PUFA), docosahexaenoic acid or eicosapentaenoic acid, in fish, decreasing the production of inflammatory eicosanoids and reactive oxygen species (ROS) to relieve oxidative stress (Saw et al., 2010). Piperine, the hot and active component of black pepper, increases the bioavailability of curcumin 1000-fold when added to turmeric or turmeric-based foods (Shoba et al., 1998). Piperine inhibits the metabolic breakdown of curcumin compounds in the gut and liver, thus promoting the bioavailability of curcumin compounds in the body.

In-vitro and *in-vivo* animal studies have shown that ginger (*Z. officinale*) has excellent anti-inflammatory, antioxidant, anti-platelet, hypotensive, and hypolipidaemic effects. Human trials with low ginger doses have demonstrated significant anti-platelet activity (Nicoll and Henein, 2007), although some recent studies have emphasized the need for more clinical trials (Marx et al., 2015). Evidence from animal studies suggests that ginger may help prevent ischaemia–reperfusion injury (IRI) in the heart. Hasanvand et al. (2019) have reported that the use of ginger reduced chest pain during coronary angioplasty, but its effect on the release of biochemical markers of myocardial damage was unclear. Pharmaceutical industries dealing in herb-based Ayurvedic and Unani medicines have developed several combinations of garlic juice, ginger juice, lemon juice, honey, and apple cider vinegar for managing cardiovascular ailments and maintaining the overall physical and physiological health of the patient. Lipikyure, from Ekyure Herbals in India, is one such preparation with markedly positive results in lowering cholesterol and triglyceride levels, reducing body weight, improving blood circulation, and preventing cardiovascular disorders (e-Kyure, 2021). In addition, Lipikyure also strengthens the digestive system, lowers blood sugar, and ensures skin health due to the inclusion of apple cider vinegar as one of its components.

Recently, Jampilek and Kralova (2020) have suggested a special kind of food supplemented with various types of nanoparticles (nanonutraceuticals) for greater stability, bioavailability, and efficacy. However, it is important to make sure that all these combinations are safe, and do not have any adverse side-effects.

1.4 CONCLUSION

Nutraceuticals are foods based on plants and/or their products/extracts that have an established positive effect on human health. Plants are rich in bioactive constituents (phenolics, alkaloids, terpenoids, folates, polyamines, etc.) and other, essential nutrients (carbohydrates, proteins, fatty acids, minerals, and vitamins), which play a significant role in maintaining the balance between health and disease. Upgrading food products with nutraceuticals is highly desirable to reload the missing vitamins and other health-promoting substances in foodstuffs. Furthermore, the concept of food component synergy is beneficial as an immunity booster for disease control and other health benefits. However, due to limited information, more intensive research on this subject is both highly desirable and of vital importance. Additionally, the concept and practice of using synergistic food combinations for specific health benefits also require thorough investigation.

REFERENCES

Ahuja, K.D., Pittaway, J.K. & Ball, M.J. 2006. Effects of olive oil and tomato lycopene combination on serum lycopene, lipid profile, and lipid oxidation. *Nutrition* 22: 259–265.

Albuquerque, P., de Oliveira, W.F., Dos Santos Silva, P.M., Dos Santos Correia, M.T., Kennedy, J.F. & Coelho, L. 2020. Epiphanies of well-known and newly discovered macromolecular carbohydrates - A review. *International Journal of Biological Macromolecules* 156: 51–66.

Anis, M. & Iqbal, M. 1994. Medicinal plantlore of Aligarh, India. *International Journal of Pharmacognosy* 32: 59–64.

Anis, M., Sharma, M.P. & Iqbal, M. 2000. Herbal ethnomedicine of the Gwalior forest division in Madhya Pradesh, India. *Pharmaceutical Biology* 38: 241–253.

Arreola, R., Quintero-Fabián, S., López-Roa, R.I., Flores-Gutiérrez, E.O., Reyes-Grajeda, J.P., Carrera-Quintanar, L. & Ortuño-Sahagún, D. 2015. Immunomodulation and anti-inflammatory effects of garlic compounds. *Journal of Immunology Research* 2015: 401630.

Auyeung, K.K., Han, Q.B. & Ko, J.K. 2016. *Astragalus membranaceus*: a review of its protection against inflammation and gastrointestinal cancers. *The American Journal of Chinese Medicine* 44: 1–22.

Bae, M. & Kim, H. 2020. The Role of vitamin C, vitamin D, and selenium in immune system against COVID-19. *Molecules* 25(22): 5346.

Beigh, S.Y., Nawchoo, I.A., Sharma, M.P. & Iqbal, M. 2014. Traditional herbal therapy in the Kashmir Himalaya. In: Iqbal, M. & Ahmad, A. (eds) *Current Trends in Medicinal Botany*: 1–15, I.K. International, New Delhi.

Belapurkar, P., Goyal, P. & Tiwari-Barua. P. 2014. Immunomodulatory effects of triphala and its individual constituents: a review. *Indian Journal of Pharmaceutical Sciences* 76: 467–475.

Bhaskaram, P. 2001. Immunobiology of mild micronutrient deficiencies. *British Journal of Nutrition* 85(Suppl 2): S75–S80.

Briggs, C. 1993. Peppermint: medicinal herb and flavouring agent. *Canadian Pharmacists Journal* 126: 89–92.

Calder, P.C., Carr, A.C., Gombart, A.F. & Eggersdorfer, M. 2020. Optimal nutritional status for a well-functioning immune system is an important factor to protect against viral infections. *Nutrients* 12: 1181.

Chanda, S., Tiwari, R.K., Kumar, A. & Singh, K. 2019. Nutraceuticals Inspiring the Current Therapy for Lifestyle Diseases. *Advances in Pharmacological and Pharmaceutical Sciences* 2019: 6908716 (doi: org/10.1155/2019/6908716)

Chen, C.Y., Milbury, P.E., Lapsley, K. & Blumberg, J.B. 2005. Flavonoids from almond skins are bioavailable and act synergistically with vitamins C and E to enhance hamster and human LDL resistance to oxidation. *The Journal of Nutrition* 135: 1366–1373.

Ding, X., Zhang, W., Li, S. & Yang, H. 2019. The role of cholesterol metabolism in cancer. *American Journal of Cancer Research* 9: 219–227.

e-Kyure, 2021. Welcome to eKyure Herbals: Lipikyure. www.ekyureherbals.com; www.healthmug.com.

Fernandez, M.A. & Marette, A. 2017. Potential health benefits of combining yogurt and fruits based on their probiotic and prebiotic properties. *Advances in Nutrition* 8: 155S–164S.

Fielding, J.M., Rowley, K.G., Cooper, P. & O'Dea, K. 2005. Increases in plasma lycopene concentration after consumption of tomatoes cooked with olive oil. *Asia Pacific Journal of Clinical Nutrition* 14: 131–136.

Finotti, E. & Di Majo, D. 2003. Influence of solvents on the antioxidant property of flavonoids. *Die Nahrung* 47: 186–187.

Ghazanfari, T., Hassan Z.M. & Ebrahimi M. 2002. Immunomodulatory activity of a protein isolated from garlic extract on delayed type hypersensitivity. *International Immunopharmacology* 2: 1541–1549.

Hallberg, L., Brune, M. & Rossander, L. 1989. The role of vitamin C in iron absorption. *International Journal for Vitamin and Nutrition Research Supplement* 30: 103–108.

Hasanvand, A., Yahya Ebrahimi, Y., Asghar Mohamadi, A. & Afshin Nazari, A. 2019. *Zingiber officinale* Roscoe reduces chest pain on patients undergoing coronary angioplasty: a clinical trial. *Journal of Herbmed Pharmacoogy* 8(1): 47–50.

Hussain, S.A., Panjagari, N.R., Singh, R.R. & Patil, G.R. 2015. Potential herbs and herbal nutraceuticals: food applications and their interactions with food components. *Critical Reviews in Food Science and Nutrition* 55: 94–122.

Intra, J. & Kuo, S.M. 2007. Physiological levels of tea catechins increase cellular lipid antioxidant activity of vitamin C and vitamin E in human intestinal caco-2 cells. *Chemico-Biological Interactions* 169: 91–99.

Jampilek, J. & Kralova, K. 2020. Potential of Nanonutraceuticals in Increasing Immunity. *Nanomaterials (Basel, Switzerland)* 10: 2224.

Jayawardena, R., Sooriyaarachchi, P., Chourdakis, M., Jeewandara, C. & Ranasinghe, P. 2020. Enhancing immunity in viral infections, with special emphasis on COVID-19: a review. *Diabetes & Metabolic Syndrome* 14(4): 367–382.

Kang, S. & Min, H. 2012. Ginseng, the 'immunity boost': the effects of Panax ginseng on immune system. *Journal of Ginseng Research* 36: 354–368.

Lambert, J.D., Hong, J., Kim, D.H., Mishin, V.M. & Yang, C.S. 2004. Piperine enhances the bioavailability of the tea polyphenol (–)-epigallocatechin-3-gallate in mice. *Journal of Nutrition* 134(8): 1948–1952.

Leena, M.M., Silvia, M.G., Vinitha, K., Moses, J.A. & Anandharamakrishnan, C. 2020. Synergistic potential of nutraceuticals: mechanisms and prospects for futuristic medicine. *Food & Function*, 11: 9317–9337.

Li, B.Q., Fu, T., Dongyan, Y., Mikovits, J.A., Ruscetti, F.W. & Wang, J.M. 2000. Flavonoid baicalin inhibits HIV-1 infection at the level of viral entry. *Biochemical and Biophysical Research Communications* 276: 534–538.

Majchrzak, D., Mitter S. & Elmadfa, I. 2004. The effect of ascorbic acid on total antioxidant activity of black and green teas. *Food Chemistry* 88: 447–451.

Marx, W., McKavanagh, D., McCarthy, A.L. & Isenring, E. 2015. The effect of ginger (*Zingiber officinale*) on platelet aggregation: a systematic literature review. *PLoS ONE* 10(10): e0141119.

Mills, P.K., Beeson, W.L., Phillips, R.L. & Fraser, G.E. 1989. Cohort study of diet, lifestyle, and prostate cancer in Adventist men. *Cancer* 64: 598–604.

Moghadamtousi, S.Z., Kadir, H.A., Hassandarvish, P., Tajik, H., Abubakar, S. & Zandi, K. 2014. A review on antibacterial, antiviral, and antifungal activity of curcumin. *BioMed Research International* 2014: 186864.

Nasri, H., Baradaran, A., Shirzad, H. & Rafieian-Kopaei, M. 2014. New concepts in nutraceuticals as alternative for pharmaceuticals. *International Journal of Preventive Medicine* 5: 1487–1499.

Natarajan, T.D., Ramasamy, J.R. & Palanisamy, K. 2019. Nutraceutical potentials of synergic foods: a systematic review. *Journal of Ethnic Foods* 6: 27.

Nicoll, R. & Henein, M.Y. 2007. Ginger (*Zingiber officinale* Roscoe): a hot remedy for cardiovascular disease? *International Journal of Cardiology* 131(3): 408–409.

Ong, W.Y., Farooqui, T., Koh, H.L., Farooqui, A.A. & Ling, E.A. 2015. Protective effects of ginseng on neurological disorders. *Frontiers in Aging Neuroscience* 7: 129.

Parveen, A., Parveen, R., Akhatar, A., Parveen, B., Siddiqui, K.M. & Iqbal, M. 2020a. Concepts and quality considerations in Unani system of medicine. *Journal of AOAC International* 103: 609–633.

Parveen, B., Parveen, A., Parveen, R., Ahmad, S., Ahmad, M. & Iqbal, M. 2020b. Challenges and opportunities for traditional herbal medicine today, with special reference to its status in India. *Annals of Phytomedicine* 9(2): 97–112.

Peterson, C.T., Denniston, K. & Chopra, D. 2017. Therapeutic uses of Triphala in Ayurvedic medicine. *Journal of Alternative and Complementary Medicine* 23: 607–614.

Prasad, S. & Tyagi, A.K. 2015. Curcumin and its analogues: a potential natural compound against HIV infection and AIDS. *Food & Function* 6: 3412–3419.

Rathaur, V.K., Pathania, M., Bhardwaj, P., Pathania, N. & Amisha. 2020. A review on exploring evidence-based approach to harnessing the immune system in times of corona virus pandemic: best of modern and traditional Indian system of medicine. *Journal of Family Medicine and Primary Care* 9: 3826–3837.

Ren, W., Qiao, Z., Wang, H., Zhu, L. & Zhang, L. 2003. Flavonoids: promising anticancer agents. *Medicinal Research Reviews* 23: 519–534.

Ritz, B.W. & Gardner, E.M. 2009. Nutraceuticals and immune restoration in the elderly. In: Fulop T., Franceschi C., Hirokawa K., Pawelec G. (eds) *Handbook on Immunosenescence.* Springer, Dordrecht. (doi.org/10.1007/978-1-4020-9063-9_75)

Saw, C.L., Huang, Y. & Kong, A.N. 2010. Synergistic anti-inflammatory effects of low doses of curcumin in combination with polyunsaturated fatty acids: docosahexaenoic acid or eicosapentaenoic acid. *Biochemical Pharmacology* 79: 421–430.

Shang, A., Cao, S.Y., Xu, X.Y., Gan, R.Y., Tang, G.Y., Corke, H., Mavumengwana, V. & Li, H.B. 2019. Bioactive compounds and biological functions of garlic (*Allium sativum* L.). *Foods (Basel, Switzerland)* 8: 246.

Shoba, G., Joy, D., Joseph, T., Majeed, M., Rajendran, R. & Srinivas, P.S. 1998. Influence of piperine on the pharmacokinetics of curcumin in animals and human volunteers. *Planta Medica* 64: 353–356.

Story, E.N., Kopec, R.E., Schwartz, S.J. & Harris, G.K. 2010. An update on the health effects of tomato lycopene. *Annual Review of Food Science and Technology* 1: 189–210.

Terrie, Y.C. 2017. Nutritional supplements marketed to boost the immune system. *Pharmacy Times* (www.pharmacytimes.com/publications/issue/2017/September2017/nutritional -supplements-marketed-to-boost-the-immune-system).

Tewari, S., Gupta, V. & Bhattacharya, S. 2000. Comparative study of antioxidant potential of tea with and without additives. *Indian Journal of Physiology and Pharmacology* 44: 215–219.

Ullah, A., Munir, S., Badshah, S.L., Khan, N., Ghani, L., Poulson, B.G., Emwas, A.H. & Jaremko, M. 2020. Important Flavonoids and Their Role as a Therapeutic Agent. *Molecules (Basel, Switzerland)* 25: 5243.

Uritu, C.M., Mihai, C.T., Stanciu, G.D., Dodi, G., Alexa-Stratulat, T., Luca, A., Leon-Constantin, M.M., Stefanescu, R., Bild, V., Melnic, S. & Tamba, B.I. 2018. Medicinal plants of the family Lamiaceae in pain therapy: a review. *Pain Research & Management* 2018: 7801543.

Wang, S., Zhu, F., Meckling, K.A. & Marcone, M.F. 2013. Antioxidant capacity of food mixtures is not correlated with their antiproliferative activity against MCF-7 breast cancer cells. *Journal of Medicinal Food* 16(12): 1138–1145.

Wu, C.Y., Ke, Y., Zeng, Y.F., Zhang, Y.W. & Yu, H.J. 2017. Anticancer activity of *Astragalus* polysaccharide in human non-small cell lung cancer cells. *Cancer Cell International* 17: 115.

Wu, J. & Zha, P. 2020. Treatment strategies for reducing damages to lungs in patients with coronavirus and other infections. *Preprints* 2020020116.

Yeum, K.J., Taylor, A., Tang, G. & Russell, R.M. 1995. Measurement of carotenoids, retinoids, and tocopherols in human lenses. *Investigative Ophthalmology & Visual Science* 36: 2756–2761.

Zhang, S., Tang, G., Russell, R.M., Mayzel, K.A., Stampfer, M.J., Willett, W.C. & Hunter, D.J. 1997. Measurement of retinoids and carotenoids in breast adipose tissue and a comparison of concentrations in breast cancer cases and control subjects. *The American Journal of Clinical Nutrition* 66: 626–632.

Zhao, K.S., Mancini, C. & Doria, G. 1990. Enhancement of the immune response in mice by *Astragalus membranaceus* extracts. *Immunopharmacology* 20: 225–233.

Ziegler, R.G., Mayne, S.T. & Swanson, C.A. 1996. Nutrition and lung cancer. *Cancer Causes Control* 7: 157–177.

2 Antibacterial Properties of Medicinal Plants

Recent Trends, Progress, and Challenges

Limenew Abate, Archana Bachheti,
Rakesh Kumar Bachheti, and Azamal Husen

CONTENTS

DOI: 10.1201/9781003137955-2

2.1 INTRODUCTION

There are various types of disease-causing microorganisms in nature which can cause infectious diseases in human beings. The main cause of morbidity and mortality is still microbial contagious diseases and microbial disease remains a dominant threat to the world (Cos et al. 2006). According to the World Health Organization (WHO, 2014), microbial infections are responsible for approximately half of the deaths each year, occurring mostly in developing and tropical countries worldwide (Fankam et al. 2011). The occurrence of drug-resistant bacterial pathogens leaves many bacterial infectious disease cases untreated and causes a major health problem in the world, resulting in morbidity and morbidity due to such failures of treatment (Levy and Marshall 2004; Ghosh and Haldar 2015). Inappropriate use of antibiotics is the main cause for the development of multidrug- resistant (MDR) pathogens (Bologa et al. 2013). The occurrence of MDR bacteria throughout the world results in ineffective treatment (Djeussi et al. 2013). This has an overwhelming effect on patients suffering from MDR bacterial infections, with the increased treatment cost also making it difficult to afford, as well as causing long-lasting illness and even death (World Health Organization 2014). Some infections diseases, such as cholera, diphtheria, gonorrhoea, meningitis, syphilis, tetanus, and tuberculosis, cause large numbers of deaths annually, especially in developing countries, as a result of antibiotic resistance problems (Wang et al. 2008). Some research has indicated that, by 2050, the annual number of deaths annually due to MDR bacteria will increase to ten million each year, at a cost of one hundred trillion dollars (Anand et al. 2019). Reports on the significance of drug-resistant bacteria causing untreatable infections showed that the requirement for the development of new antibacterial therapies is more pressing than ever (Cushnie et al. 2014). To alleviate this problem, the use of natural active ingredients obtained from medicinal plants is one of the alternatives (Dhama et al. 2014). Recently, the interest in and awareness of medicinal plants as an alternative source of bioactive compounds against drug-resistant microorganisms have been growing (Uche-Okereafor et al. 2019). For instance, the bioactive compound berberine, extracted from *Berberis vulgaris*, is active against bacteria and protozoa, and piperine, isolated from *Piper nigrum*, is active against some fungi and bacteria, such as *Lactobacillus* spp., *Micrococcus* spp., *Escherichia coli*, and *Enterococcus faecalis*. Moreover, some infectious diseases caused by bacteria, fungi, and viruses can be treated by using tannins isolated from *Rhamnus purshiana* (Khameneh et al. 2019) (Figure 2.1). Bioactive compounds isolated from *Dorstenia* spp., such as amentoflavone and prenyl flavones, showed marked antibacterial activities against *Bacillus cereus* with minimum inhibitory concentration (MIC) values of 3 and 2.4 µg/ml, respectively (Kuete et al. 2007; Mbaveng et al. 2008) and, from flower extracts of *Retama raetam*, bioactive flavonoids called licoflavones also showed antibacterial activities against *E. coli*, with a MIC value of 7.81 µg/ml *via* the formation of complexes with soluble and extracellular proteins (Edziri et al. 2012). The alkaloids isolated by ethanol extraction of *Datura stramonium* tissue showed *in vitro*-antibacterial activities against some bacterial species, such as *Klebsiella pneumoniae*, *Proteus mirabilis*, *Staphylococcus aureus*, *E. coli*, and *Pseudomonas aeruginosa*, using the agar well diffusion method. The *Datura*

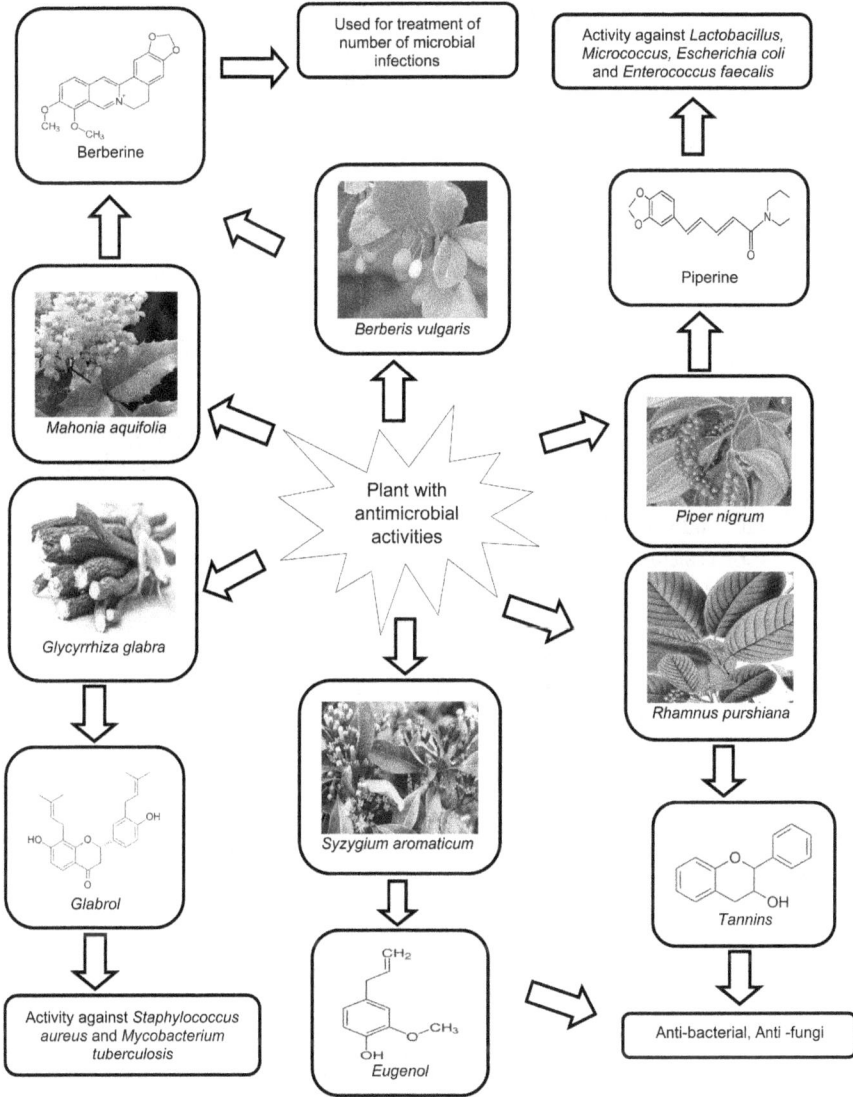

FIGURE 2.1 Antimicrobial activity of some plants and their extracts.

extract showed greater antibacterial effect than that achieved by standard antibiotics (Altameme et al. 2015). Adukwu et al. (2016) indicated that the components of essential oils (EOs) obtained from *Cymbopogon citratus* reduced the growth of *S. aureus* and *Acinetobacter baumannii*. According to Lahmar et al. (2017), synergistic antibacterial activity was achieved by mixing antibiotics and different EO components derived from *Thryptomene calycina*, *Clausena anisata*, *Callitris glaucophylla*, *Melaleuca alternifolia*, and *Eucalyptus* spp. The results showed a marked inhibitory effect against *Alcaligenes faecalis, E. coli, Salmonella typhimurium, S. aureus* and *Ps. aeruginosa.* Nanoparticles synthesized from plant have been used for antibacterial activities, especially MDR bacteria (Alavi and Rai 2019). Nowadays, because of the presence and growing impact of antibiotic-resistant bacteria and the failure of conventional chemotherapy to treat infectious disease, the burden of bacterial infectious diseases is increasing. The behaviour of only a few phytochemicals from medicinal plants has been studied and the possible modes of action are not fully understood. The aim of this chapter is to provide up-to-date information on the use of medicinal plants as antibacterial agents and the challenges associated with this approach.

2.2 COMMON BACTERIAL DISEASES AND THEIR PATHOGENESIS

Bacteria are single-celled microbes (Bilombele 2019), coming in different sizes and shapes, and being very diverse (Yang et al. 2016). Bacteria can exist in any environment, such as in or on our bodies, in water, or in soil (Seiler and Berendonk 2012). Worldwide, they are the main cause of human morbidity and mortality. The inappropriate and excessive use of antibacterial and antibiotic drugs has caused the emergence of resistance in bacterial populations, which results in increases in the risks of health problems, such as the inability to treat illnesses caused by antibiotic-resistant bacteria (Asadi et al. 2019). Some examples of bacterial diseases include Legionnaires' pneumonia, bacterial vaginosis, gonorrhoea, chlamydia, syphilis, anthrax, tetanus, botulism, cholera, Lyme disease, bacterial meningitis, pneumococcal pneumonia, whooping cough, tuberculosis, listeriosis, etc. (Centers for Disease Control and Prevention 1997).

Different types of disease are associated with, if not definitively caused by, bacteria. For instance, Lyme disease and its complications by the tick-borne bacterium *Borrelia burgdorferi* (Diuk-Wasser et al. 2012), atherosclerosis is associated with *Chlamydia pneumoniae* (Watson and Alp 2008), Sudden Infant Death Syndrome (SIDS) with *Clostridium perfringens* (Deixler 2009), and bloodstream infections with *Klebsiella pneumonia* (Trecarichi et al. 2016). Additionally, *Parachlamydia acanthamoebae* in the human lung acts as an agent of pneumonia causing inflammation of the air sacs (Casson et al. 2008).

Another bacterial disease is cholera, caused by consuming drinking water or eating food contaminated with the bacterium *Vibrio cholerae.* It is an acute diarrhoeal infection, which induces disease exclusively in humans (Moore et al. 2014). Pelvic inflammatory disease (PID) is another bacterial disease that commonly occurs in females aged under 24 years of age. It is caused by bacterial vaginosis and results in infection and inflammation of the female genital tract, which can result in ectopic pregnancy, infertility, and serious reproductive morbidity (Kamwendo et al. 2000; Taylor et al. 2013). The common sexually transmitted disease (STD) gonorrhoea is caused by the bacterium *Neisseria gonorrhoeae.* This disease is transmitted from one person to another person *via* contact with contaminated clothes or bedsheets, or by sexual intercourse (Torpy et al. 2013). Some other common bacterial diseases are listed in Table 2.1.

TABLE 2.1
Common Diseases Caused by or Associated with Different Bacterial Species

Bacterium	Disease	Reference
Bartonella henselae	Cat-scratch fever	Florin et al. (2008)
Borrelia burgdorferi	Lyme disease and its complications	Diuk-Wasser et al. (2012)
Campylobacter jejuni	Gastroenteritis	Sails et al. (2003)
Chlamydia pneumoniae	Atherosclerosis	Watson and Alp (2008)
Clostridium perfringens	Sudden Infant Death Syndrome (SIDS)	Deixler (2009)
Clostridium difficile	Antibiotic-induced diarrhoea and pseudomembranous colitis	Wilcox (2003)
Corynebacterium amycolatum	Hospital-acquired endocarditis	Knox and Holmes (2002)
Escherichia coli	Haemorrhagic colitis and haemolytic uraemic syndrome	Ameer et al. (2020)
Ehrlichia chaffeensis	Human ehrlichiosis	Mogg et al. (2020)
Helicobacter pylori	Duodenal and gastric ulcers	Ahmed and Belayneh (2019)
Klebsiella pneumoniae	Blood stream infections	Trecarichi et al. (2016)
Legionella pneumophila	Legionnaires' pneumonia	Edelstein et al. (2020)
Enterococcus faecalis	Nosocomial infections	Noskin et al. (1995)
Listeria monocytogenes	Listeriosis	Todd and Notermans (2011)
Methicillin-resistant *Staphylococcus aureus* (MRSA)	Nosocomial and community-associated infections	Alvarez et al. (2010)
Salmonella enterica	Salmonellosis	Dallap Schaer et al. (2010)
Staphylococcus aureus	Toxic shock syndrome	Tang et al. (2006)
Streptococcus pyogenes	Necrotizing and streptococcal toxic shock syndrome	Tang et al. (2006)
Vibrio cholerae	Epidemic cholera	Moore et al. (2014)
Vibrio vulnificus	Wound infection, septicaemia, and gastrointestinal disease	Tacket et al. (1984)

2.3 ORIGIN-BASED CLASSIFICATION OF MEDICINAL PLANTS FOR TREATMENT OF BACTERIAL DISEASES, AND THEIR IMPORTANT PHYTOCONSTITUENTS

2.3.1 AFRICAN MEDICINAL PLANTS

Approximately 80% of people in Africa cannot afford conventional drugs for treatment of bacterial infections. Nowadays, considerable attention is paid to finding new antibacterial drugs from local medicinal plants (Sieberi et al. 2020). In South Africa, the bioactive compounds from *Teucrium trifidum*, like phenolic compounds such as tannins and flavonoids, showed antibacterial activity against *Bacillus subtilis, Streptococcus pyogenes, K. pneumoniae, P. aeruginosa, B. cereus, S. aureus* and *V. cholerae* (Mazhangara et al. 2020). In Ethiopia, the antibacterial activity of *Jasminum floribundum, Euphorbia hirta, Euphorbia abyssinica, Sarcophy tepiriei* or *Commiphora myrrha* extracts are used in traditional treatment of infections of common human wounds by *E. coli, Ps. aeruginosa, S. aureus, S. pyogenes, P. mirabilis*, and *K. pneumoniae*. The results confirmed that the extracts exhibited growth inhibition zones on bacterial plates ranging from (mean ± standard deviation) 10 ± 2 mm to 24.9 ± 0.9 mm in diameter (Mahammed et al. 2020). Phytochemicals such as glycosides (6.29 mg/g), flavonoids (6.51 mg/g), tannin (9.14 mg/g), saponins (10.54 mg/g), terpenoids (19.72 mg/g), and alkaloids (30.63 mg/g) were isolated from *Dacryodes edulis* leaf extracts, which showed antibacterial activities (Hassan-Olajokun et al. 2020). The polyphenols derived from four medicinal plants from Burkina Faso, namely *Sida acuta, Pterocarpus erinaceus, Khaya senegalensis,* and *Combretum micranthum,* were tested for their antibacterial activities against pathogenic bacteria such as *Klebsiella ozenae, S. aureus, Salmonella paratyphi*, and *Shigella dysenteriae*. The results showed antibacterial activities with MIC values in the range of 20–2000 mg/ml (Karou et al. 2005). Phytochemicals that were extracted in Kenya from *Centella asiatica*, such as terpenoids, flavonoids, tannins, saponins, cardiac glycosides, and alkaloids, showed antibacterial properties. For instance, flavonoids like catechins inhibited the growth of *Streptococcus mutans* and *V. cholerae* (Tapas et al., 2008), whereas quercetin caused growth reduction of *S. aureus* (Zwenger and Basu 2008). Alkaloids extracted from *Aspidosperma ramiflovum* were found to be significantly inhibitory toward *E. faecalis* and *S. aureus* (Tanaka et al. 2006), whereas those from *Sida acuta* showed antibacterial activity against *E. coli, E. faecalis, B. cereus, S. dysenteriae*, and *S. aureus* (Oyekunle et al. 2006). Tannins from extracts also showed inhibition against *Bacillus subtilis* and *S. aureus* (Kumar and Pandey 2013). Saponins from *Sorghum bicolor* were reported to be active against *S. aureus* (Anantharaman et al. 2010). In Nigeria, extracts of some plants, like *Acanthus montanus, Carica papaya, Acalypha fimbriata, Bauhinia variegata, Azadirachta indica*, and *Berlinia grandiflora*, have been used to treat syphilis (Abd El-Ghani 2016).

2.3.2 MEDICINAL PLANTS FROM THE AMERICAS

In the Americas, 20% of deaths annually are due to infectious diseases caused by bacteria. Approximately 2,600 species of vascular plants have been used as traditional medicines by people from North and South America (Mahady 2005). In Belize in central America, methanol, chloroform or hexane extracts of herbal plants were tested for the treatment of skin infections. Extracts of bark of *Bursera simaruba*, leaves and bark of *Syngonium podophyllum* and *Aristolochia trilobata*, leaves of *Hamelia patens*, and bark of *Guazuma ulmifolia* were tested against the bacteria *E. faecalis, S. aureus* and *Ps. aeruginosa* (Camporese et al. 2003). In New York state in the USA, the Haudenosaunee peoples used the medicinal plants *Solidago canadensis, Hieracium pilosella, Ipomoea pandurata*, and *Achillea millefolium* for the treatment of diseases caused by different bacterial species. The result of a study showed that aqueous leaf extracts were strong enough to inhibit some species of bacteria, such as *E. coli* and *S. typhimurium*, with predicted MIC values in the range of 1 μg/ml to10 μg/ml. However, the value was 100–1000 μg/ml against *Lactococcus lactis* and *S. aureus* (Frey and Meyers 2010). Medicinal herbs in North America, such as *Allium sativum, Hyptis suaveolens, Syzygium aromaticum, Artemisia absinthium, Murraya koenigii, Datura metel, Lippia alba,* and *Chrysopogon zizanioides,* were used to treat Lyme disease and other tick-borne infections (Yarnell 2016).

2.3.3 CHINESE MEDICINAL PLANTS

Currently, the uses of Chinese herbal medicinal plants is receiving great attention. These herbal medicines are used in traditional Chinese medicine (TCM) to treat different infectious bacterial diseases (Wang et al. 2018). In Northwest Yunnan, China, some traditional medicinal plants, such as *Potentilla fulgens, Geranium strictipes, Elsholtzia blanda,* and *Elsholtzia rugulosa,* exhibited inhibition of *S. aureus* (Zuoa et al. 2008). McMurray et al. (2020) described the antibacterial activities of some Chinese medicinal plants, such as *Iris domestica, Anemone chinensis, Smilax glabra,* and *Agrimonia pilosa,* against *E. coli* and *L. monocytogenes.* The results showed MIC values in the range between 7.81 and 125 mg/l, compared with ampicillin. However, ampicillin MIC range was between 0.25 and 8 mg/l. Ginsenosides, bioactive compounds extracted from *Panax ginseng,* a common plant important in traditional Chinese medicine, also show a good antibacterial effect against *L. monocytogenes, Ps. aeruginosa,* and *Helicobacter pylori* (Kim et al. 2017), while flavonol glycosides extracted from another Chinese medicinal plant, *Ginkgo biloba,* indicated antibacterial activities against *E. coli* and *C. perfringens* (Lee and Kim 2002). Twelve A-type proanthocyanidins, isolated from *Ephedra sinica* using ethanol as the solvent, exhibited high bacterial inhibition (MIC values in the range 0.00515–1.38 mmol/l) against bacterial species, such as *S. aureus* and *Ps. aeruginosa* (Zang et al. 2013). Phenolic compounds isolated from the TCM plant *E. sinica* also showed considerable antibacterial activity against Gram-positive (*S. aureus*) and Gram-negative bacteria *(Ps. aeruginosa)* (Khan et al. 2017). Janovska et al. (2003) examined the antibacterial activities of ethanolic extracts of *Tussilago farfara, Salvia officinalis,* and *Chelidonium majus,* which are all TCM plants, the extracts showing very high activity against the bacteria *B. cereus, E. coli, S. aureus,* and *Ps. aeruginosa,* and the fungus *Candida albicans.*

2.3.4 INDIAN MEDICINAL PLANTS

The antibacterial activities of some Indian medicinal plants have been investigated. For instance, extracts of the plants *Woodfordia fruticosa, Mesua ferrea,* and *Manilkara hexandra* exhibited significant antibacterial activity against several *Staphylococcus* species (Hasan et al. 2013). Bioactive chemicals, like flavonoids, steroids, saponins, and/or tannins, from leaf extracts of *Cassia auriculata* exhibited strong antibacterial activities against five bacterial species, namely *P. mirabilis, S. aureus, P. aeruginosa, K. pneumoniae* and *E. coli* (Murugan et al. 2013). Shihabudeen et al. (2010) reported the antimicrobial effects of methanol extracts of *C. auriculata* or *Eugenia jambolana*, containing phytochemicals, such as steroids, saponins, tannins, phenols, glycosides, coumarins, and flavonoids. The results revealed the greatest toxicity against the bacteria *E. coli, Staphylococcus epidermidis, Ps. aeruginosa, K. pneumoniae,* and *S. aureus,* and the fungi *C. albicans* and *Aspergillus niger,* using the disc diffusion method. South Indian traditional medicinal plants, like *Adhatoda vasica, Aegle marmelos, Ocimum gratissimum,* and *Ocimum sanctum,* were examined for their antibacterial activities against *K. pneumoniae, S. paratyphi, S. typhi, S. aureus,* and *E. coli.* The methanolic extract of some of those plants, such as *O. sanctum* and *O. gratissimum.* indicated antibacterial effects, with maximum zone of inhibition diameters of 25.5 mm and 30.0 mm diameter, respectively, against *S. typhi* (Prasannabalaji et al. 2012).

Swain and Rautray (2021) examined the antibacterial activities of regularly consumed Indian medicinal plants. The greatest antibacterial activities were observed in methanol extracts of turmeric (*Curcuma longa*) tested against *Ps. aeruginosa, K. pneumoniae,* and *S. aureus,* whereas some inhibition zone was observed in response to extracts of ginger (*Zingiber officinale*) against the same bacteria. Some Indian plants that had not previously been shown to be medicinal plants, such as *Pterygota alata, Murraya paniculata, Holigarna caustica, Acacia pennata, Elaeocarpus serratus, Bischofia javanica, Trema orientalis, Syzygium praecox, Smilax zeylanica,* and *Cinnamomum glaucescens,* have been used to control the formation of *S. aureus* biofilms (Panda et al. 2020).

2.3.5 EUROPEAN MEDICINAL PLANTS

Different plants have been studied in European countries for treatment of bacterial diseases (Toth et al. 2011). In a review of well-known medicinal plants in Italy used between 1850s to 1950s to treat bacterial skin diseases, some bioactive compounds, such as phenolics extracted from the root of *Beta vulgaris,* sulphides from the essential oil of garlic cloves (*A. sativum*), and alkaloids from the methanolic extract of the leaves of lettuce (*Lactuca sativa*) were used to treat skin infections caused by bacteria such as *E. coli, S. typhimurium* and *Providencia stuartii* (Mazzei et al. 2020). Aqueous and alcoholic extracts of aerial parts of *Achillea millefolium,* which grows in Europe, showed antibacterial activity against *E. faecalis, Micrococcus luteus, Salmonella enterica, S. aureus, Shigella flexneri,* and *Ps. aeruginosa,* although the aqueous extract exhibited low inhibition against *M. luteus* and *Ps. aeruginosa.* The greatest inhibitory effect of the alcoholic extract was against *M. luteus, S. aureus,* and *Ps. aeruginosa* (Hasson 2011). In another study, which was carried out on medicinal plants grown in the warmer part of southern Europe, the aqueous, chloroform or ethanolic extracts of *Tribulus terrestris* showed a marked inhibition of bacterial growth (Al-Bayati and Al-Mola 2008). The fruit of the plant had significant antibacterial activity towards *Bacillus subtilis, Corynebacterium diphtheriae,* and *S. aureus,* with effective MIC values of 0.15, 0.31, and 0.62 mg/ml, respectively (Al-Bayati and Al-Mola, 2008). In Poland, aqueous extracts of members of the Rosaceae family, such as *Rosa canina, Fragaria vesca, Rubus fruticosus, Rubus idaeus,* and *Agrimonia eupatoria,* have been widely used to neutralize the cholera toxin (Komiazyk et al. 2019) (Table 2.2).

TABLE 2.2

Ethnobotanical Data on the Medicinal Plants Identified as Active Against Various Bacterial Diseases

Bacteria	Antibacterial Plant	Antibacterial Active Compound(s)	Plant Parts	Extraction Solvent/ Analytical Method	Mechanism of Action	References
Bacillus subtilis	Dracocephalum foetidum	Limonene, n-menthol, and 8-dien-10-al	Aerial part	Hydrodistillation	Initiates changes in integrity or permeability of the cell membrane	Lee et al. (2007)
Bacillus subtilis	Aloe secundiflora	Quercetin 3, 3', 4'-trimethyl ether	Aerial part	Methanol and acetone	Inhibits the activities of β-galactosidase and phosphatase, elevates extracellular, reduces the activities of GrYB protein and ATPase activity	Ahmadu et al. (2011)
Corynebacterium ulcerans	Pachygrapsus crassipes	Quercetin-3-O-rutinoside	Leaf	Aqueous	Inhibit ATPase activity, GrYB protein, elevates extracellular phosphatase and β-galactosidase activities	Bello et al. (2011)
Campylobacter jejuni and Escherichia coli	Allium sativum	Ajoene	Bulb		Sulphydryl-dependent enzyme inhibitor	Rehman and Mairaj (2013)
Escherichia coli	Ipomoea muricata	Chanoclavine	Seed	Fast centrifugal partition chromatography	Efflux pump inhibitor	Dwivedi et al. (2019)
Escherichia coli	Diplotaxis harra	Sulphoraphane	Needles	Water	Protein and DNA synthesis inhibitor, ATP synthase inhibitor, and destruction of bacterial membrane	Wu et al. (2012)

(Continued)

TABLE 2.2 (CONTINUED)

Ethnobotanical Data on the Medicinal Plants Identified as Active Against Various Bacterial Diseases

Bacteria	Antibacterial Plant	Antibacterial Active Compound(s)	Plant Parts	Extraction Solvent/ Analytical Method	Mechanism of Action	References
Enterococcus faecalis	*Polymnia fruticosa*	Naringenin	—	—	β-Ketoacyl acyl carrier protein synthase (KAS) III	Jeong et al. (2009)
Escherichia coli	*Citrus aurantifolia*	Flavonoid	Fruits	Methanol	Complex with bacterial cell walls and ability to complex with soluble and extracellular proteins	Lee et al. (2014)
Escherichia coli	*Pancratium illyricum*	Berberine	Bulbs	Methanol	Inhibition of DNA and protein, as well as cell division	Zorić et al. (2017); Boberek et al. (2010)
Haemophilus influenzae	*Achillea clavennae*	Geranyl acetate, linalool, camphor, myrcene, β-caryophyllene, and 1,8-cineole	Leaves and flowers	GC–MS analysis	Initiate changes in integrity or permeability of the cell membrane	Skocibusic et al. (2004)
Klebsiella pneumoniae	*Achillea clavennae*	Geranyl acetate, linalool, camphor, myrcene, β-caryophyllene, and 1,8-cineole	Leaves and flowers	GC–MS analysis	Initiate changes in the integrity or permeability of the cell membrane	Skocibusic et al. (2004)
Listeria monocytogenes	*Cyperus longus*	B-Himachalene, α-humulene, and γ-himachalene	Aerial parts	GC–MS analysis	Initiate changes in the integrity or permeability of the cell membrane	Ait-Ouazzou et al. (2012)

(Continued)

TABLE 2.2 (CONTINUED)

Ethnobotanical Data on the Medicinal Plants Identified as Active Against Various Bacterial Diseases

Bacteria	Antibacterial Plant	Antibacterial Active Compound(s)	Plant Parts	Extraction Solvent/ Analytical Method	Mechanism of Action	References
Mycobacterium smegmatis	—	Formononetin	—	—	Efflux pump inhibitor	Lechner et al. (2008)
Mycobacterium smegmatis, Methicillin-resistant *Staphylococcus aureus* (MRSA) and *Candida albicans*	*Scutellaria baicalensis*, *Scutellaria lateriflora*, *Thymus vulgaris*	Baicalein	Root	Methanol	Efflux pump inhibitor	Lechner et al. (2008); Chan et al.(2011)
Mycobacterium tuberculosis	*Terminalia chebula*	Chebulinic acid	—	Water	DNA gyrase	Patel et al. (2015)
Methicillin-resistant *Staphylococcus aureus* (MRSA) and *Staphylococcus aureus*	*Piper nigrum* and *Piper longum*	Piperine	—	Distilled water	Efflux pump inhibitor	Khameneh et al. (2015b)
Micrococcus luteus	*Dracocephalum foetidum*	Limonene, *n*-menthol, and 8-dien-10-al	Leaves	Hydrodistillation	Changes the integrity or permeability of the cell membrane	Lee et al. (2007)
MRSA and *Candida albicans*	*Alpinia calcarata*	Kaempferol	Rhizomes	Soxhlet extraction with ethyl acetate and methanol	Efflux pump inhibitor	Randhawa et al. (2016); Shao et al. (2016)

(Continued)

TABLE 2.2 (CONTINUED)
Ethnobotanical Data on the Medicinal Plants Identified as Active Against Various Bacterial Diseases

Bacteria	Antibacterial Plant	Antibacterial Active Compound(s)	Plant Parts	Extraction Solvent/ Analytical Method	Mechanism of Action	References
Mycobacterium smegmatis and Campylobacter jejuni	—	Resveratrol	Seed	Aqueous methanol	Efflux pump inhibitor	Klancnik et al. (2017)
Neisseria gonorrhoeae	Pavetta crassipes	Quercetin-3-O-rutinoside	Leaf	Aqueous	Complexes with bacterial cell walls, inhibits ability to complex with soluble proteins and extracellular proteins	Bello et al. (2011)
Pseudomonas aeruginosa	Struchium sparganophora	β-caryophyllene, germacrene D, humulene, caryophyllene oxide, and 1,8-cineole	Aerial parts, stem, and leaf	Hydrodistillation	Changes the integrity or permeability of the cell membrane	Anyanwu and Okoye (2017)
Pseudomonas aeruginosa	Pavetta crassipes	Quercetin-3-O-rutinoside	Leaf	Aqueous	Complexes with bacterial cell walls and affects ability to complex with soluble proteins and extracellular proteins	Bello et al. (2011)
Pseudomonas aeroginosa	Achillea clavennae	Camphor, myrcene, cineole, β-caryophyllene, linalool, and geranyl acetate	Leaves and flowers	GC-MS	Changes the integrity or permeability of the cell membrane	Skocibusic et al. (2004)

(Continued)

TABLE 2.2 (CONTINUED)
Ethnobotanical Data on the Medicinal Plants Identified as Active Against Various Bacterial Diseases

Bacteria	Antibacterial Plant	Antibacterial Active Compound(s)	Plant Parts	Extraction Solvent/ Analytical Method	Mechanism of Action	References
Pseudomonas aeroginosa	Holarrhena antidysenterica	Conessine		Dimethyl sulphoxide (DMSO) and diatrizoic acid (DTA)	Efflux pump inhibitor	Siriyong et al. (2017)
Pseudomonas aeruginosa	Cyperus longus	B-Himachalene, α-humulene, and γ-himachalene	Aerial parts		Changes the integrity or permeability of the cell membrane	Ait-Ouazzou et al. (2012)
Salmonella enterica	Cyperus longus	β-Himachalene, α-humulene, and γ-himachalene	Aerial parts	GC-MS	Changes the integrity or permeability of the cell membrane	Ait-Ouazzou et al. (2012)
Salmonella typhimurium	Cuminum cyminum	Cuminaldehyde, β-pinene, γ-terpinene, and terpin-7-al	Leaves	GC-MS	Changes the integrity or permeability of the cell membrane	Bisht et al. (2014)
Salmonella typhimurium	Struchium sparganophora	β-caryophyllene, germacrene D, humulene, caryophyllene oxide, and 1,8-cineole	Aerial, stem, leaf	Hydrodistillation	Changes the integrity or permeability of the cell membrane	Anyanwu and Okoye (2017)
Staphylococcus aureus	Artemisia annua	Chrysosplenol-D	Leaves	Chromatography	Efflux pump inhibitor	Stermitz et al. (2003)
Staphylococcus aureus	Artimisia frigida	1,8-cineole, methyl chavicol, and camphor	Aerial parts	GC-MS	Changes the integrity or permeability of the cell membrane	Lopes-Lutz et al. (2008)
Staphylococcus aureus	Cedrus deodara	3-p-trans-coumaroyl-2-hydroxyquinic acid	—	—	Damage to the cytoplasmic membrane	Wu et al. (2016)

(Continued)

TABLE 2.2 (CONTINUED)
Ethnobotanical Data on the Medicinal Plants Identified as Active Against Various Bacterial Diseases

Bacteria	Antibacterial Plant	Antibacterial Active Compound(s)	Plant Parts	Extraction Solvent/ Analytical Method	Mechanism of Action	References
Staphylococcus aureus	Cymbopogon citratus	Limonene, n-menthol, 8-dien-10-al	Leaves	Hydrodistillation	Changes the integrity or permeability of the cell membrane	Lee et al. (2007)
Staphylococcus aureus	Cyperus longus	β-Himachalene, α-humulene, γ-himachalene	Aerial parts	GC-MS	Changes the integrity or permeability of the cell membrane	Ait-Ouazzou et al. (2012)
Staphylococcus aureus	Maytenus buchananii	Epicatechin, kaempferol, epigallocatechin, quercetin-3-O-β-D-glucopyanoside, quercetin-3-O-α-L-arabinopyranoside, and quercetin	Leaves	Methanol	Ability to complex with bacterial cell walls and soluble proteins and extracellular proteins, and to complex, disrupt membranes of bacteria	Tebou et al. (2017)
Staphylococcus aureus	Momordica charantia	Cis-dihydrocarvacol, trans nerolidol, and germacrene D	Seed	GC-MS	Changes the integrity or permeability of the cell membrane	Braca et al. (2008)
Staphylococcus aureus	Persea lingue	Kaempferol rhamnoside	Leaves	Ethanol	Efflux pump inhibitor	Holler et al. (2012)
Staphylococcus epidermidis	Artimisia frigida	1,8 cineole, methyl chavicol, and camphor	Aerial parts	GC-MS	Changes to integrity or permeability of the cell membrane	Lopes-Lutz et al. (2008)
Staphylococcus epidermidis	Eugenia caryophyllata	Thymol, eugenol, carvacrol, and cinnamaldehyde	Flower buds	GC-MS	Changes the integrity or permeability of the cell membrane	Santos et al. (2015)

(Continued)

TABLE 2.2 (CONTINUED)
Ethnobotanical Data on the Medicinal Plants Identified as Active Against Various Bacterial Diseases

Bacteria	Antibacterial Plant	Antibacterial Active Compound(s)	Plant Parts	Extraction Solvent/ Analytical Method	Mechanism of Action	References
Staphylococcus epidermidis	Eremanthus erythropapps	Viridiflorol, p-cymene, germacrene D, and γ-terpinene (Z)-caryophyllene	Leaves	GC-MS	Changes the integrity or permeability of the cell membrane	Chaieb et al. (2007)
Staphylococcus epidermidis	Plectranthus amboinicus	P-cymene (Z)-caryophyllene, germacrene D, viridiflorol, and γ-terpinene	Leave	GC-MS	Changes the integrity or permeability of the cell membrane	Arumugam et al. (2016)
Streptococcus sp. and Micrococcus sp	Rauwolfia serpentina	Reserpine	Root	Methanol	Efflux pump inhibitor	Sridevi et al. (2017)
Vibrio cholerae	Graptophyllum grandulosum	Chrysoeriol-7-O-β-D-xyloside, luteolin-7-O-β-D-apiofuranosyl, β-D- xylopyranoside, chrysoeriol-7-O-α-L rhamnopyranosyl-glucopyranoside, and isorhamnetin-3-O-α-L rhamnopyranosyl	Aerial parts	n-Butanol	High capacity for disruption of plasma membrane and disruption of the permeability barrier of bacterial membrane structures	Tagousop et al. (2018)
Vibrio parahaemolyticus	Eleutherine bulbosa	Fatty acid esters, isoquinolines, naphthalenes, phenolics, and E- (7-hydroxy-1,2-dimethoxy xanthone)	Bulb	Ethanol	Inhibition of cell division, targeting RNA polymerase, and DNA intercalation	Munaeni et al. (2019)

2.4 RECENT PROGRESS IN BACTERIAL ACTIVITIES OF MEDICINAL PLANTS

2.4.1 Medicinal Plants for Treating Bacterial Pneumonia

Bacterial pneumonia is an infectious disease characterized by lung inflammation. It is not a single disease but can be caused by many species of bacteria, such as *Streptococcus pneumoniae, S. aureus, P aeruginosa, Moraxella catarrhalis, K. pneumoniae* and *Haemophilus influenzae* (Brooks, 2020; Cock and Van Vuuren 2020). Different medicinal plants and parts which have been used for the treatment of bacterial pneumonia include the root of *Abutilon angulatum, Combretum platypetalum, Rhynchosia caribaea,* and *Terminalia sericea,* leaves of *Acacia eriloba, Dodonaea viscosa,* and *Trichilia emetica,* essential oils from the wood of *Cinnamomum camphora,* tubers of *Pelargonium sidoides,* branches of *Rhamnus prinoides,* the bark of *Urtica urens,* twigs of *Dodonaea viscosa,* and whole plants of *Oncosiphon suffruticosum* (Cock and Van Vuuren 2020). Bioactive compounds isolated from peel waste of *Opuntia ficus-indica* fruits, like isorhamnetin, isorhamnetin 3-*O*-glucoside, quercetin 5,4'-dimethyl ether, and flavonols, were shown to be the most potent active fractions against pneumonia pathogens (Elkadya et al. 2020). In the Himalayan region, the plant families most commonly used for the treatment of pneumonia are the Fabaceae, Bignoniaceae, and Asteraceae, of which *Justicia adhatoda, Punica granatum,* and *Curcuma longa* exhibited the greatest inhibitory potential (Adnana et al. 2019).

2.4.2 Medicinal Plants for Treating Cholera

Cholera is an infectious bacterial disease of the intestine. The disease is caused by the bacterium *V. cholerae* (Sousaa et al. 2020). In developing countries, it is an acute, diarrhoeal illness, although it is rare in the developed world. The distribution of the disease globally shows that it still occurs in Africa, South America, and Eastern Asia, with the incidence increasing since 2005 (Mandal et al. 2011). The WHO has encouraged the investigation of medicinal plants as alternative strategies for the control of various diarrhoeal diseases, including cholera (Laloo and Hemalatha 2011). Flavonoids extracted from the leaves of *Maytenus buchananii* using methanol showed a potential anticholera chemotherapeutic agent (Tebou et al. 2017). Kayira and Nakanoa (2020) showed that cholera can be treated using methanol extracts of *Syzygium aromaticum, Corymbia citriodora, Glycyrrhiza glabra, Salvia rosmarinus, Salvia officinalis,* or *Thymus praecox.* Their results indicated significant activity against *V. cholerae* with diameters of inhibitory zone of between 11.3 mm and 25 mm. The antibacterial activity was in the order *S. aromaticum > S. officinalis > T. praecox > C. citriodora > G. glabra.* Jose et al. (2017) also showed that methanolic extracts obtained from the plants *Holarrhena antidysenterica, Camellia sinensis, Elephantopus scaber,* or *Centella asiatica* exhibited promising antibiofilm activity against *V. cholerae.* In some studies, aqueous extracts of members of the Rosaceae family, such as *Rosa canina, Fragaria vesca, Rubus fruticosus, Rubus idaeus,* and *Agrimonia eupatoria,* have been widely used to neutralize the cholera toxin (Komiazyk et al. 2019).

2.4.3 MEDICINAL PLANTS FOR TREATING DIPHTHERIA

Diphtheria is another bacterial infectious disease that can result in mortality. Among infected people, 5–10 % of cases result in death. The mortality rate in people with ages of 40 years old and above and 5 years old and below is approximately 20% (Holy et al. 2017). In developed countries, because of advances in medical treatment, outbreaks of diphtheria are rare, although they are more common in continents like Africa and South America (Truelove et al. 2019). The disease is caused by the bacterium *Cornyebacterium diphtheriae* (Dover et al. 2004). Parts of different plant species, such as leaves of *Carissa edulis, Artemisia afra, Dodonaea viscosa, Eucalyptus globulus, Carpobrotus edulis, Ficus carica, Mentha longifolia,* and *Olea europea,* the sap of *Astridia velutina,* the roots of *Carissa edulis, Ficus carica, Mentha longifolia,* twigs of *Dodonaea viscosa,* stems of *Mentha longifolia,* and fruit of *Vitis vinifera,* have been used to prevent diphtheria (Cock and Van Vuuren 2020).

2.4.4 MEDICINAL PLANTS FOR TREATING GONORRHOEA

Gonorrhoea is the second most common sexually transmitted infectious disease (Chinsembu 2016), and is caused by the bacterium *Neisseria gonorrhoeae* (Rice et al. 2017). In the work of Silva et al. (2020), some traditional medicinal plants, such as *Prunus serotina* (bark), *Rhodiola rosea* (root), *Terminalia macroptera* (root and leaves), *Senna podocarpa* (root), *Guiera senegalensis* (leaves), and *Bersama engleriana* (bark) were shown to be the most active in preventing gonorrhoea infection. In different countries, medicinal plants *Adenia gummifera, Agave sisalana, Anredera cordifolia, Jacaranda mimosifolia, Lantana camara, Opuntia stricta, Senna didymobotrya,* and *Solanum mauritianum* in South Africa (Maema and Potgieter 2019), *Abelmoschus moschatus, Abroma augustum, Acacia farnesiana, Acalypha hispida, Aegle marmelos, Alternanthera sessilis, Arachis hypogaea, Asparagus racemosus, Benincasa hispida, Boerhavia diffusa, Caesalpinia bonducella,* and *Calophyllum inophyllum* in Bangladesh (Rahmatullah et al. 2011), and *Centella asiatica, Curculigo orchioides, Gloriosa superba, Grewia subinaequalis, Ocimum gratissimum, Pedalium murex, Phyllanthus fraternus, Pouzolzia zeylanica, Premna arborea,* and *Scoparia dulcis* in India (Das et al. 2013) have been used for gonorrhoea treatment. In Tanzania, for treatment of the disease, a decoction made from roots of *Achyranthes aspera* is given to a patient, whereas, in the Philippines, a decoction of the whole plant of *Centella coriacea* and or roots of *Amaranthus spinosus* is given. In addition, *Centella asiatica* is very important for treatment of gonorrhoea in the folk medicine of South Africa. The plant *Grewia asiatica* is also used in the Himalayan traditional medicinal system of India to treat gonorrhoea (Hossan et al. 2010).

2.4.5 MEDICINAL PLANTS FOR TREATING LYME DISEASE

Lyme disease is a well-known tick-borne bacterial disease in humans. In the United States, about 300,000 new cases of Lyme disease occur each year (Alinia-Ahandani et al. 2020). In most cases of Lyme disease, a bacterium, such as *Borrelia burgdorferi*, *Borrelia afzelii*, or *Borrelia garinii*, are responsible (Aguero-Rosenfeld et al. 2005). Essential oils from several common herbs and medicinal plants show strong activity against the bacterium that causes Lyme disease (Feng et al. 2018). Essential oils from cloves of *Allium sativum*, berries of *Pimenta officinalis*, seed of *Cuminum cyminum*, resin of *Commiphora myrrha*, flowers of *Hedychium spicatum*, wood of *Amyris balsamifera*, leaves of *Eucalyptus citriodora* or *Thymus vulgaris,* and fruit of *Litsea cubeba* have shown potent activities against *Borrelia burgdorferi* (Feng et al. 2018). In some studies, medicinal herbs such as *Hyptis suaveolens*, *Lippia alba*, *Allium sativum*, *Syzygium aromaticum*, *Artemisia absinthium*, *Murraya koenigii*, *Datura metel*, and *Chrysopogon zizanioides* have been used to treat Lyme disease and other tick-borne infections (Yarnell 2016).

2.4.6 MEDICINAL PLANTS FOR TREATING BACTERIAL MENINGITIS

Meningitis is an acute inflammation of the protective membranes covering the brain and neural structure. The inflammation can be caused by infection with bacteria, viruses, or other microorganisms (Priya et al. 2019). Tijani et al. (2019) studied the potential medicinal values of *Allium sativum* on bacterial meningitis pathogens such as *K. pneumoniae*, *E. coli*, *S. pneumoniae*, *Neisseria meningitidis*, and *Haemophilus influenzae*. Their results showed that the plant extracts reduced bacterial growth, with MIC values in the range 0.04–1.56 mg/ml. In the work of Akpo et al. (2020), the antibacterial activity of *Alchornea cordifolia* and *Moringa oleifera* against four meningitis-causing bacteria, namely *E. coli*, *Micrococcus* spp., *B. subtilis*, and *S. aureus* were examined. The results indicated that an aqueous extract of *A. cordifolia* inhibited all the bacteria tested, with a range of zones of inhibition from 7.0 mm to 17.5 mm in diameter, whereas the ethanolic extract of *M. oleifera* inhibited *S. aureus* and *B. subtilis*, with zones of inhibition in the range of 3.0–9.0 mm diameter.

2.4.7 MEDICINAL PLANTS FOR TREATING SYPHILIS

Syphilis is a common disease caused by the bacterium *Treponema pallidum*. The disease can be transmitted *via* sexual activities or by contact with an infected person (Santacroce et al. 2020). The disease can be treated using different medicinal plants, such as *Streblus asper* (leaves, roots, and stems) or *Plumbago indica* (leaves and stems). A tincture of the roots of *Plumbago indica* is also used to treat secondary syphilis in India (Hossan et al. 2010). In Nigeria, parts of traditional medicinal plants, such as leaves of *Acanthus montanus*, *Carica papaya*, *Acalypha fimbriata*, *Bauhinia variegata*, or *Azadirachta indica*, the root of *Bauhinia variegata* or *Berlinia grandiflora*, the bark of *B. variegata*, *B. grandiflora*, and *A. indica*, seed of *Carica papaya* or *A. indica*, the stem of *B. grandiflora* or *A. indica*, fruits of *Carica papaya*, and the whole plant of *Ambrosia maritima*, *Centaurea perrottetii*, or *Adenia venenata*, have been used to treat syphilis (Abd El-Ghani 2016). In Jharkhand state in India, some of the traditional medicinal plants used for the treatment of syphilis are *Cynodon dactylon* (whole plant), *Benincasa hispido* (fruit), *Benincasa hispida*, and *Fumaria parviflora* (aerial parts) (Pandey et al. 2020). An ethnomedicinal survey of plants used by Abagusii traditional healers of Southwest Kenya indicated that the root of *Agave americana* and *Tabernaemontana stapfiana*, whole plants of *Achyranthes aspera*, leaves of *Cassia didymobotrya*, and stems of *Cassia floribunda* are used for treatment of syphilis (Charles and Bonareri 2020).

2.4.8 MEDICINAL PLANTS FOR TREATING TETANUS

Tetanus is a serious, life-threatening infectious disease caused by a bacterial toxin that affects the nervous system, leading to painful muscle contractions; if not diagnosed and treated at an early stage, it can result in death (Lakonawa et al. 2020). In the developing world, tetanus has a high mortality rate but, in the developed world, the disease is rare (Cook et al. 2001). Indian medicinal plants, such as *Lantana camara*, are used to treat tetanus infections, possibly due to the presence of phytochemicals like saponins, flavonoids, alkaloids, tannins, anthocyanins, flavones, isoflavones, coumarins, lignans, catechins, carotenoids, carbohydrates, proteins, glycosides, and steroids in the plant extract (Poddar et al. 2020). *Hymenocardia acida* extract is used to treat tetanus in Benin (Novotna et al. 2020) and *Aristolochia esperanzae*, *Copaifera langsdorffii*, *Capsicum frutescens*, and *Nicotiana tabacum* are also used for treatment of the disease in Brazil (Ribeiro et al. 2017).

2.4.9 MEDICINAL PLANTS FOR TREATING TUBERCULOSIS

Tuberculosis (TB) is one of the most serious infectious bacterial diseases of the respiratory system, caused by the bacterium *Mycobacterium tuberculosis* (Floyd et al. 2018). It is one of the top ten diseases in terms of number of deaths caused. Nowadays, it is very difficult to control the disease, with the evolution of drug-resistant bacteria making ineffective the use of medications previously used to control the bacterium. This has resulted in an urgent search for new medicines from local traditional medicinal plants (Tabuti et al. 2010). Flowers, leaves, roots, and the whole plant of *Taraxacum officinale* can be used to treat TB. Furthermore, bark extracts of *Cryptocarya latifolia*, *Acacia xanthophloea*, *Berchemia discolor*, *Bridelia micrantha*, *Cassia petersiana*, and *Cassine papillosa*, and leaf extracts of *Artemisia afra*, *Bauhinia petersiana*, *Chaetachme aristata*, *Clerodendrum glabrum*, *Combretum molle*, and *Conyza scabrida* have been used to treat TB (Cock and van Vuuren 2020). *Acalypha indica* has proved to be important in treatment against *M. tuberculosis*. Various phytochemicals, like gallic acid, myricetin, quercetin, piperine, vasicine, curcumin, and ascorbic acid, obtained from *A. indica* have been shown to exhibit antibacterial activities (Adnana et al. 2019). In addition, aqueous extracts of pure gel from *Aloe vera* leaves, cloves of *Allium sativum,* bulbs of *Allium cepa*, *Adhatoda vasica*, and *Acalypha indica* were examined *in vitro* for their potential activity against multidrug-resistant *M. tuberculosis*. Extracts of all five species exhibited anti-tuberculosis activity with inhibition of 95, 32, 37, 72, and 32%, respectively (Gupta et al. 2010).

2.4.10 MEDICINAL PLANTS FOR TREATING TYPHOID

Typhoid is an infectious disease of concern throughout developing countries around the world (Khadka et al. 2020). It is a systemic infection caused by the bacterium *Salmonella enterica* ssp. *enterica* serotype *typhi*, by ingestion of contaminated water or food (Iroha et al. 2010). Different solvent extracts of the bark of *Azadirachta indica*, leaves of *Crinum purpurascens*, *Bidens pilosa*, *Carica papaya*, *Cymbopogon citratus*, *Mangifera indica*, *Momordica charantia*, and *Psidium guajava*, and fruit of *Aegel marmelous*, *Punica granatum*, *Myristica fragrans*, and *Solanum lycopersicum* have been used to treat typhoid (Syarif et al. 2020). Traditional medicine practitioners have described that the root of *Vitex doniana*, the leaf of *Cassia tora*, the bark of *Alstonia boonei*, and the leaf of *Stachytarpheta jamaicensis* and *Carica papaya* are also beneficial for effective treatment against typhoid fever (Abbas and Ain, 2020). Roger et al. (2015) described *Bidens pilosa* antibacterial activity as being effective against *Salmonella*. *B. pilosa* contains many phytochemicals, such as porphyrins, flavonols, chalcones, phenols, acetylenic hydrocarbons, aliphatic carboxylic acids, saturated carbohydrates, tannins, triterpenoids, steroids, alkaloids, phenylacetylenes, and flavonoids. According to Iroha et al. (2010), typhoid can also be prevented by using medicinal plant extracts such as both crude cold and hot water extracts and ethanol extracts of *Carica papaya* (leaf), *Stachytarpheta jamaicensis* (leaf), *Alstonia boonei* (bark), *Cassia tora* (leaf), and *Vitex doniana* (root). More frequently used medicinal plants to treat typhoid and the associated fever are *Aconitum gammiei*, *Neopicrorhiza scrophulariiflora*, *Abelmoschus manihot*, *Mussaenda frondosa*, *Asparagus racemosus*, *Rubus ellipticus*, *Iris domestica*, *Begonia picta*, and *Achyranthes bidentata* (Khadka et al., 2020).

2.5 SIGNIFICANCE OF ANTIBACTERIAL DRUGS FROM NATURAL SOURCES

Antibacterial drugs may be naturally derived from living organisms, such as plants, actinomycetes, and fungi, and prepared semi-synthetically or synthetically in the laboratory. Natural antibacterial drugs exhibit some remarkable properties, such as the low possibility of the evolution of bacterial resistance, long-lasting antibacterial effects, low cost, high solubility in the bodily fluids, nontoxicity to the human body, and long shelf life (Moellering 1981). Over the past ten years, the development of antimicrobial resistance (AMR), which started after the widespread use of antibiotics, has focused attention on the sustainability of current modern medical practices in the global arena (Moloney 2016). Each year, approximately 8,000 people die from antibiotic-resistant infections; synthetic antibiotics or drugs could make a significant contribution to reducing these deaths. Because of increasing resistance to man-made antibiotics, there is a vital need to change the focus to naturally occurring plant-derived antibacterial products because their vast chemical diversity not only possesses a potent therapeutic effect but also makes the microbes unable to adapt to them to achieve resistance (Naqvi et al. 2019). Natural occurring antibacterial drugs will be used to supplement the body's natural ability to fight off bacterial infections in the future. Unlike pharmaceutical antibiotics, with a single, specific point of action, plant-derived antibacterial drugs have multiple points of action, so that drug resistance does not develop in the target bacteria (Naqvi et al. 2019). Also, they will not kill beneficial bacterial species that exist in our gut microbiome to help break down the food we eat (Corrêa et al. 2020), to benefit our immune system and to improve other aspects of our physiological and mental health. The effectiveness of traditional medicines is becoming widely accepted because of their fewer side effects, better cultural acceptability, and greater compatibility with the human body (Mustafa et al. 2017).

2.6   MECHANISM AND MODE OF ACTION OF PLANT-BASED ANTIBACTERIAL DRUGS

In many countries, synthetic antibacterial drugs have been widely used, but the importance of plant-derived drugs is increasingly attracting the attention of many researchers (Khameneh et al. 2015). In nature, plants are rich in phytochemicals. These plant-derived chemical compounds have advantages for controlling bacteria through their antibacterial properties (Barbieri et al. 2017). Some of the bioactive compounds in plants used as antibacterials are glucosinolates, lignans, tannins, essential oils, terpenoids, flavonoids, alkaloids, phenolics, quinines, and other secondary metabolites (Chandra et al. 2017). Plant-based constituents may affect bacterial cells in many ways (Figure 2.2), such as inhibiting bacterial enzymes involved in the synthesis of essential structural bacterial components or in the production of cellular energy, or by increasing the permeability of the cell, resulting in the loss of cellular constituents (Kotzekidou et al. 2008), interrupting the communication between normal cells, inducing the coagulation of cytoplasmic constituents, affecting RNA/DNA function, interrupting cell component synthesis, disrupting the structure and function of membranes, and interfering with intermediary metabolism (Radulovic et al. 2013), plus synergistic effects (Wagner and Ulrich-Merzenich 2009).

In general, the mode of action of antibacterial phytochemicals is considered to involve the coagulation of cell components, disturbance of active transport mechanisms and electron flow, and disruption of the proton motive force and the cytoplasmic membrane function (Kotzekidou et al. 2008). Phytochemicals affect the stability and structure of the phospholipid bilayer of the membrane, increasing its permeability to ions as a result of damage or disturbed membrane integrity. The effect also alters the electrochemical potential of membranes and membrane-associated enzyme activities. Some phytochemicals can also affect the transfer of protons across the membrane of the cell by interrupting the synthesis of ATP, inhibiting anabolism/catabolism and respiration, and decreasing active transport (Radulovi et al. 2013).

Different phytochemicals vary in their mechanism of action (Omojate Godstime et al. 2014). For instance, flavonoids have the following modes of action against

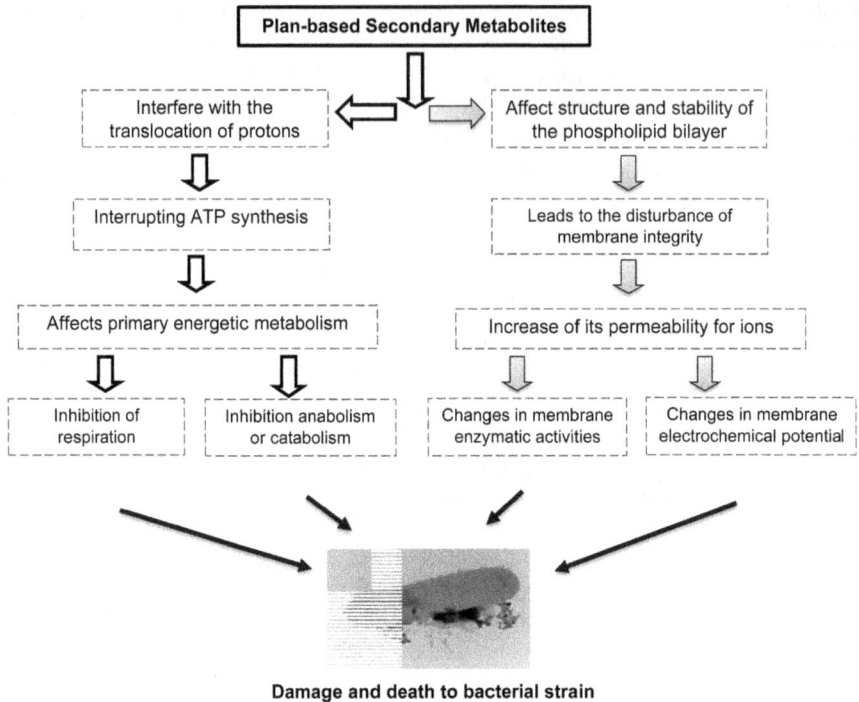

FIGURE 2.2 Possible mode of action of plant-based metabolic products on bacterial cell growth, damage, or death.

bacteria: attenuation of pathogenicity, change in membrane permeability, inhibition of nucleic acid synthesis, reduction in cell attachment and biofilm formation, inhibition of energy metabolism, and change in the function of the cytoplasmic membrane (Farhadi et al. 2019). Flavonoids like epigallocatechin, myricetin, and robinetin (Figure 2.3) exhibit antibacterial activities against *Proteus vulgaris* due to inhibition of DNA synthesis, by the formation of hydrogen bonds between the B-ring of flavonoids and nucleic acid bases, preventing the synthesis of bacterial DNA (Mori et al. 1987; Cushnie and Lamb, 2005). Sophoraflavanone G and naringenin (Figure 3) exhibit considerable antibacterial activity against methicillin-resistant *Staphylococcus aureus* (MRSA) and streptococci. A change of membrane fluidity in the region of hydrophobic and hydrophilic may be attributed to flavonoids, decreasing the fluidity of the inner and outer components of membranes (Cushnie and Lamb 2005). Anthraquinones from *Cassia italica* showed antibacterial activities against *Burkholderia pseudomallei*, *P aeruginosa*, *Corynebacterium pseudodiphthericum*, and *Bacillus anthracis* because of their ability to make a complex between the bacterial cell wall and extracellular soluble proteins (Al-AlSheikh et al. 2020). Quercetin flavonoids, derived from the skin of yellow onion, reduced the effect on antibiotic-resistant *Helicobacter pylori* by obstructing the DNA supercoils from achieving DNA scission by forming the gyrase DNA-quercetin cleavable

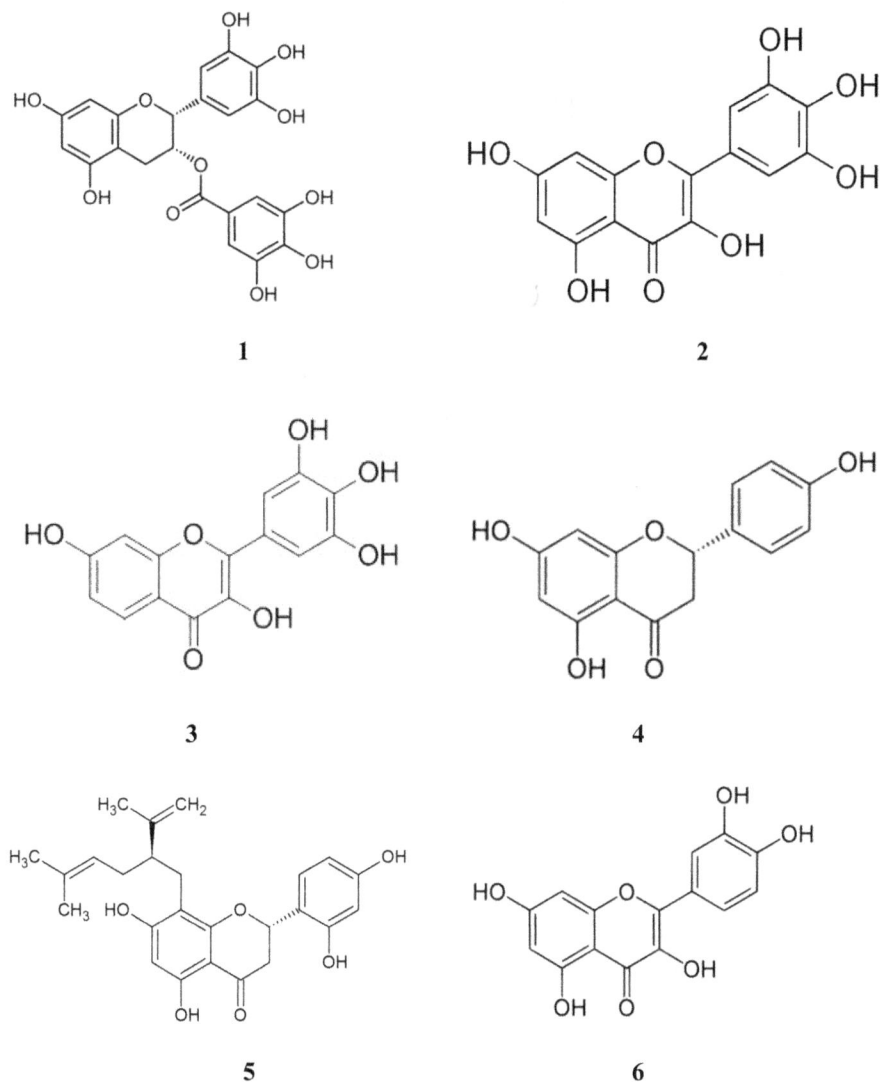

FIGURE 2.3 Structures of epigallocatechin (1), myricetin (2), robinetin (3), naringenin (4), sophoraflavanone G (5), and quercetin (6).

complex. Other flavonoids, such as kaempferol, daidzein, and apigenin, act to reduce the growth of some bacteria, like *Vibrio harveyi*, *E. coli*, and *B. subtilis*, by imposing drastic effects on bacterial RNA and DNA synthesis (Naqvi et al. 2019).

Alkaloids also have different mechanisms in different classes of alkaloids, such as polyamines, agelasine, quinolone, isoquinoline, and indolizidine alkaloids. A class of phenanthroindolizidine alkaloids, including tylophorinidine and pergularinine (Figure 2.4), operate by inhibiting the enzyme dihydrofolate reductase and

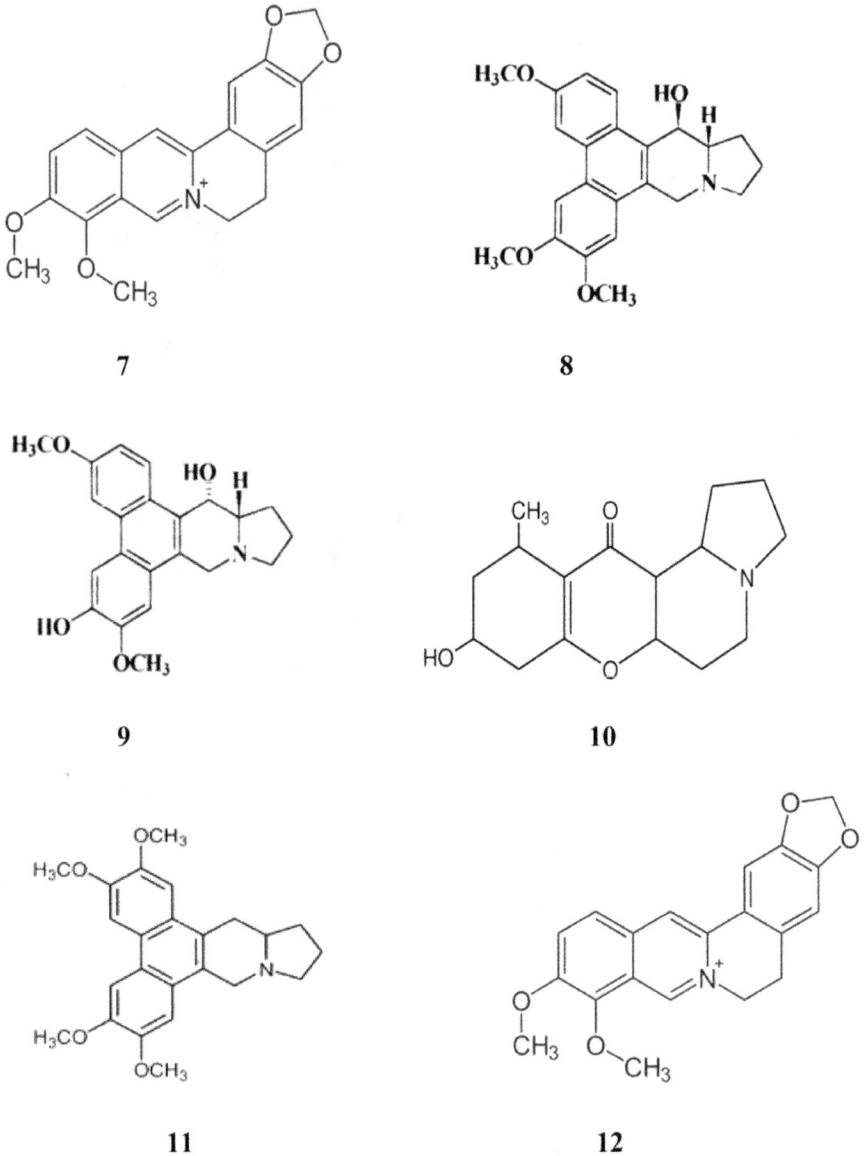

FIGURE 2.4   Structures of the alkaloids berberine (7), pergularinine (8), tylophorinidine (9), indolizidine (10), tylophorinidine (11), and protoberberine (12).

blocking nucleic acid synthesis (Cushnie et al. 2014), whereas a class of isoquino-line alkaloids, including isoquinolines, protoberberine, and benzophenanthridine (Figure 2.4), reduce the growth of bacteria by inhibiting cell division and by per-turbing the Z ring at the site of cell division (Cushnie et al. 2014). In another study, berberine (Figure 2.4), which is obtained from plants like *Rhizoma coptidis* and

Cortex phellodendri, showed antibacterial activity against *Streptococcus agalactiae* by increasing the membrane permeability of the bacteria, by intercalating with DNA (Chandra et al. 2017). Antibacterial activity was also exhibited by alkyl methyl quinolone alkaloids against *Helicobacter pylori* through a respiratory inhibitory effect (Tominaga et al. 2002). Moreover, squalamine, a polyamine alkaloid, has the same mode of action as a detergent. It depolarizes Gram-positive bacteria membranes, leading, in Gram-negative bacteria, to the disruption of their outer membranes (Alhanout et al. 2010).

Essential oils in different extracts from various plants have been used by exploiting their antibacterial activities (Akthar et al. 2014). The chemical structure of an essential oil enables it to have antibacterial activity against different bacteria. Essential oils, like thymol, eugenol, and carvacrol, originating from various plants, are highly active against many microorganisms (Saad et al. 2013). The hydroxide group present in essential oils shows strong antibacterial activity (Guimaraes et al. 2019). Ultee et al. (2002) explained that the carvacrol phenolic hydroxyl group was responsible for its antibacterial activities against *Bacillus cereus* by enhancing membrane fluidity and reducing the pH gradient across the cytoplasmic membrane, causing bacterial cell death by the resulting collapse of the proton motive force and depletion of the ATP pool. Essential oils result in bacteria cell death by increasing cell membrane permeability for K^+ and depleting intracellular ATP. A study on the mechanism of antibacterial activity towards *E. coli* by thymol and carvacrol (Figure 2.5) showed the leakage of protons and potassium ions, increased membrane permeability, and the disruption of membrane integrity (Xu et al. 2008). Some essential oil components, like terpenoids and terpenes, exhibit a particular mechanism to kill bacterial cells. The passage of lipophilic compounds through the cell wall and disruption of cytoplasmic membranes are part of the mechanism. Permeabilization is also involved in the mechanism of bacterial cell death by initiating a cascade of reactions as a result of a collapse of proton pumps and depletion of the ATP pool, reduction of the membrane potential, and damage to the cell wall and membrane, resulting in leakage of macromolecules and subsequent cell lysis (Oussalah et al. 2006). Diterpenoid essential oils, like aethiopinone and salvipisone (Figure 2.5), obtained from the roots of *Salvia sclarea*, kill bacterial cells, in combination with betalactam antibiotics, as a result of increased cell surface hydrophobicity or greater cell wall permeability (Walencka et al. 2007).

2.7 MEDICINAL PLANT-BASED ANTIBACTERIAL CHEMICALS

Plant-based antibacterial chemicals, either alone or in combination with antibiotics, can be used to solve the problem of controlling infectious bacterial disease caused by antibiotic resistance. A chemical compound obtained from saffron crocus (*Crocus sativus*) has been studied by Carradori et al. (2016). The result indicated that the plant extracts exhibited antibacterial activity to control multidrug-resistant *S. aureus*. Also, the diverse effects of clinical isolates of MRSA in Kolkata, India were resolved by using ethanolic extract of the stem bark of *Cinnamomum verum* (Mandal et al. 2011). The result concluded that the plant can be used for the preparation of

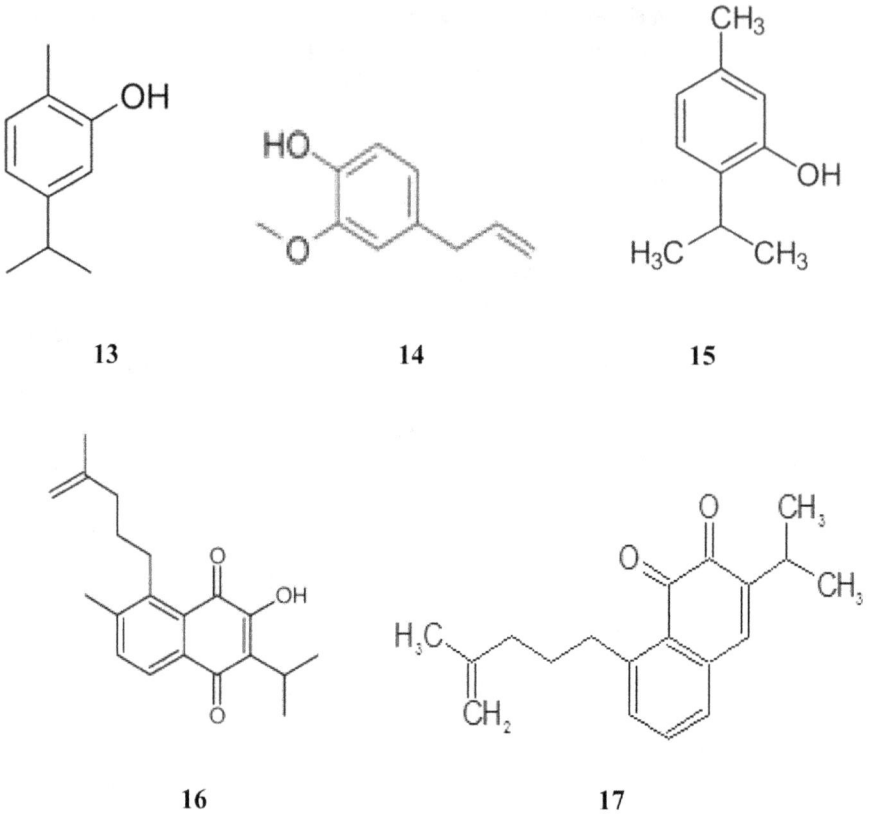

FIGURE 2.5   Structure of the essential oil chemicals carvacrol (13), eugenol (14), thymol (15), salvipisone (16), and aethiopinone (17).

potential antibacterial agents against MRSA. Pandaa et al. (2020) prepared a novel antibiotic drug from Indian plant extracts, such as those of *Beilschmiedia roxburghiana* and *Mikania micrantha*. The bacterium *Porphyromonas gingivalis* is the key-stone pathogen of periodontitis, a chronic inflammatory disease that results in the deterioration of gingival tissues and causes tooth loss (Hajishengallis et al. 2012). Carrol et al. (2020) showed that, to maintain oral hygiene and to prevent tooth loss and deterioration, extracts of some plants, such as *Sassafras albidum, Morella cerifera, Zanthoxylum armatum, Citrus sinensis, Juglans regia, Carya alba,* and *Vicia faba,* can be used as antibacterial agents. Their results indicated a promising collection of resources of natural products that could be further explored for use for the development of oral hygiene care products and for pharmaceutical development.

The work of Fadhel et al. (2012) investigated, for the first time, the antibacterial effects of leaf extracts of *Eucalyptus cinerea* and *Eucalyptus odorata*, applied on wool or woven cotton fabrics, against *E. coli* and *S. aureus*. The results indicated that the *E. odorata* extract showed good antibacterial activity when applied to a piece of wool fabric. These effects remained without change until the wool was washed ten times, although loss of antibacterial activity occurred after only three washes of the cotton fibre.

The antibacterial activities of some phytochemicals are very important for food preservation and cosmetics. For instance, the bioactive compounds cinnamaldehyde and eugenol eliminate or reduce bacterial degradation and decrease the incidence of infection of cosmetics and food (Nabavi et al. 2015). Plant-based antibacterial products also showed their importance in cleaning products, such as hand lotions, disinfectants, toothpaste, cleaning cloths, soaps and detergents, and rubbish bags and plastic wrap (Lewis and Elvin-Lewis 2003) (Figure 2.6). The antibacterial properties of extracts of different plant species can also be used for improved oral health against *P. gingivalis*. For example, *Syzygium aromaticum* essential oil (mouthwash) and *Salvadora persica* twigs (toothbrush) are very important for oral hygiene in Africa and the Middle East. Also twigs of *Azadirachta indica* are used as toothbrushes, tongue cleaner, toothache reliever, and oral deodorant in Asia (Carrol et al. 2020). In India, *Zanthoxylum armatum* and *Juglans regia* bark and wood are used as chewing sticks to control *P. gingivalis* bacteria, and, in the Americas, *Sassafras albidum* is also used as a chewing stick (Lewis and Elvin-Lewis 2003).

2.8 PLANT-BASED NANOPARTICLES FOR ANTIBACTERIAL ACTIVITY

The emergence of MDR bacteria and other drug-resistant pathogenic bacteria has become a global health concern because of the inability to treat infectious diseases caused by these bacteria (Tomasz 1994). Treatment of the illness using the available antibiotics is insufficient to arrest the increasing incidence of multidrug-resistant bacteria (Olaitan et al. 2014). Combined with plant-derived antibacterial drugs, the development of nanotechnology offers an alternative means for treating and curing an infectious disease caused by these bacteria (Yuan et al. 2018). Various metal and metal-oxide nanoparticles (NPs) with different morphological features have been synthesized (Siddiqi and Husen 2016, 2017; Siddiqi et al. 2016; 2020). They have shown several uses, including antibacterial activities against a number of Gram-positive and Gram-negative bacteria (Husen et al. 2019; Bachheti et al. 2019; Siddiqi et al. 2019, 2020; Bachheti et al. 2020a, 2020b, 2020c; Husen 2020a, 2020b, 2020c). NPs are designed at the atomic or molecular level, and as extremely small-sized nanospheres. Hence, they can move more freely in the human body in comparison to larger materials. Silver nanoparticles (AgNPs) exhibiting antibacterial activities against Gram-negative and Gram-positive bacteria in combination with different plant extracts were investigated by Mohanta et al. (2020). According to their results, AgNPs prepared by using a leaf extract of *Glochidion lanceolarium* exhibited MIC (IC_{50}) values of 43.94 mg/ml, 68.6 mg/ml, and 44.02 mg/ml against *S. aureus*, *Ps. aeruginosa*, and *E. coli*, respectively, whereas AgNPs prepared from extracts of *Semecarpus anacardium* showed corresponding MIC values of 33.77 mg/ml, 12.9 mg/ml, and 23.49 mg/ml. Moreover, AgNPs synthesized with an extract of *Breynia retusa* also showed significant antibacterial activities towards the test pathogens, with MIC values of 43.94 mg/ml, 12.90 mg/ml, and

64.13 mg/ml for *E. coli*, *Ps. aeruginosa*, and *S. aureus*, respectively. In another study, a preparation of zinc oxide NPs (ZnONPs) with aqueous *Prosopis juliflora* extract was carried out by a straightforward green synthetic approach by Mydeen et al. (2020), according to which the synthesized nanoparticles exhibited significant MIC values against four different bacterial species, namely *E. coli*, *V. cholerae*, *B. subtilis*, and *Rhodococcus rhodochrous*. A study on the green synthesis of chromium oxide (Cr_2O_3) nanoparticles, using *Abutilon indicum* leaf extract as a capping and reducing agent, showed significant antibacterial activities against *B. subtilis*, *S. aureus*, *E. coli*, and *Bordetella bronchiseptica*, using the agar well diffusion assay (Khan et al. 2021). In addition, the preparation of AgNPs, using an extract of *Allium giganteum*, *exhibited* higher antibacterial activity than AgNPs without the extract towards pathogenic bacteria such as *Ps. aeruginosa*, *E. coli*, *B. subtilis*, and *S. aureus* (Taghavizadeh et al. 2019). Mubarak Ali et al. (2011) examined plant extract-mediated synthesis of AgNPs and AuNPs and their antibacterial properties towards clinically isolated pathogens, such as *E. coli* and *S. aureus*. The results showed very strong antibacterial activities. Cavallo et al. (2021) examined the antibacterial activities of polylactic acid (PLA) and PLA nanocomposite films containing 3 % wt of lipid nanoparticles (LNPs) against *E. coli* and *Micrococcus luteus*. The results indicated that, for either bacterium, PLA/LNPs caused a decrease in the growth of the microorganism, compared with PLA alone. In addition, the LNPs, which were delivered by linen fabrics, using ultrasonic treatment, also exhibited antibacterial characteristics for bacteria, such as *Ps. aeruginosa*, *E. coli*, *K. pneumoniae*, *S. aureus*, *Staphylococcus haemolyticus*, *Micrococcus flavus*, *Bacillus licheniformis*, and *Corynebacterium xerosis* (Zimniewska et al. 2008). The biological synthesis of gold nanoparticles (AuNPs) with essential oils (EOs) from *Nigella sativa* (*Ns*EO-AuNPs) exhibited antibacterial activities against Gram-positive bacteria, like *S. aureus*, and Gram-negative bacteria by reducing the hydrophobicity index by 46% and 78%, respectively (Manju et al. 2016). In an alloy nanoparticle antibacterial study against *S. aureus* and *E. coli* conducted using the agar well diffusion assay, the bactericidal effect of the alloy nanoparticles has been shown to be prominent against *E. coli* with an inhibition zone diameter of 28 mm at a concentration of 150 µl (Vilas et al. 2016).

2.9   CONCLUSION AND FUTURE PERSPECTIVE

Worldwide, especially in developing countries, the occurrence of human illness due to different bacterial pathogens has become a great burden, resulting in huge economic loss and social losses. For many years, the development and mass production of chemically synthesized antibiotics have been very important in improving health by controlling different bacterial pathogens in different parts of the world. The evolution of drug-resistant bacteria due to the overuse and abuse of synthetic antibiotics has increased the burden on people and society to treat bacterial diseases. The presence of MDR bacteria is a global problem with respect to different bacteria infectious diseases, such as pneumonia, cholera, diphtheria, gonorrhoea, meningitis, syphilis, tetanus, tuberculosis, etc. MDR bacteria are continuously challenging the scientific community, especially in the developing world, and particularly in African countries. The reduction in efficacy of synthetic drugs is aggravating the problem and has forced researchers to look towards plant-derived bioactive antibacterial drugs to alleviate the effects of diseases caused by bacteria, because plant-derived products are safer, have fewer side effects, are cheap, offer new or alternative modes of action, improve the body's natural ability to fight off bacterial disease, and do not select for resistant bacteria. For instance, berberine, which is extracted from *Berberis vulgaris*, is active against bacteria and protozoa, and piperine, isolated from *Piper nigrum*, is active against some bacteria, like *Micrococcus* spp. and *E. coli*. Alkaloids isolated from *Datura stramonium* are active against *E. coli, Ps. aeruginosa, S. aureus, P. mirabilis*, and *K. pneumoniae*. The antibacterial activities of nanoparticles, combined with extracts of medicinal plants, also show great potential for addressing the problem of MDR bacteria. However, only small numbers of combinations of phytochemicals from medicinal plants and nanoparticles have been investigated and the modes of action of different bioactive compounds have still not been widely investigated. Great attention must be paid to evaluating and exploring molecular characterization of the potential bioactive compounds found in plants to identify less toxic and more effective drugs that will benefit the global population.

REFERENCES

Abbas, S. & W. Ain. 2020. A review paper on medicinal plants for Typhoid. *Journal of Natural Sciences* 8: 98–103.

Abd El-Ghani, M.M. 2016. Traditional medicinal plants of Nigeria: an overview. *Agriculture and Biology Journal of North America* 7: 220–47.

Adnana, M., S. Alib, K. Sheikh & R. Amber. 2019. Review on antibacterial activity of Himalayan medicinal plants traditionally used to treat pneumonia and tuberculosis. *Journal of Pharmacy and Pharmacology* 71(11): 1599–1625.

Adukwu, E.C., M. Bowles, V. Edwards-Jones & H. Bone. 2016. Antimicrobial activity, cytotoxicity and chemical analysis of lemongrass essential oil (*Cymbopogon flexuosus*) and pure citral. *Applied Microbiology Biotechnology* 100(22): 9619–9627.

Aguero-Rosenfeld, M., G. Wang, I. Schwartz & G. Wormser. 2005. Diagnosis of lyme borreliosis. *Clinical Microbiology Reviews* 18: 484–509.

Ahmadu, A., A. Onanuga & B. Ebeshi. 2011. Isolation of antibacterial flavonoids from the aerial parts of *Indigofera secundiflora*. *Pharmacognosy Journal* 3(19): 25–28.

Ahmed, S. & Y.M. Belayneh. 2019. *Helicobacter pylori* and duodenal ulcer: systematic review of controversies in causation. *Clinical Experimental Gastroenterology* 12: 441.

Ait-Ouazzou, A., S. Lorán, A. Arakrak, A. Laglaoui, C. Rota, A. Herrera, R. Pagán & P. Conchello. 2012. Evaluation of the chemical composition and antimicrobial activity of *Mentha pulegium, Juniperus phoenicea*, and *Cyperus longus* essential oils from Morocco. *Food Research International* 45(1): 313–319.

Akpo, C.O., O.E. Okolosi-Patani & M.O. Uzama. 2020. Activities of stem barks of *Alchornea cordifolia* (Schumach. & Thonn.) Müll. Arg. and *Moringa oleifera* Lam. on some Meningitis-causing Bacteria. *Nigerian Journal of Pharmaceutical Applied Science Research* 9(3): 30–34.

Akthar, M.S., B. Degaga & T.Azam. 2014. Antimicrobial activity of essential oils extracted from medicinal plants against the pathogenic microorganisms: a review. *Issues in Biological Sciences and Pharmaceutical Research* 2(1): 1–7.

Al-AlSheikh, H., I. Sultan, V. Kumar, I. Rather, H. Al-Sheikh, A. Jan & Q. Haq. 2020. Plant-based phytochemicals as possible alternative to antibiotics in combating bacterial drug resistance. *Antibiotics* 9(480): 1–23.

Al-Bayati, F. & H. Al-Mola. 2008. Antibacterial and antifungal activities of different parts of *Tribulus terrestris* L. growing in Iraq. *Journal of Zhejiang University Science B* 9(2), 154–159.

Alhanout, K., S. Malesinki, N. Vidal, V. Peyrot, J. Rolain & J. Brunel. 2010. New insights into the antibacterial mechanism of action of squalamine. *Journal of Antimicrobial Chemotherapy* 65(8): 1688–1693.

Alinia-Ahandani, E., Z. Alizadeh-Terepoei, M. Sheydaei & Res. 2020. Some pointed medicinal plants to treat the tick-borne disease. *Open Access Journal of Biomedical Engineering and Biosciences* 1(5): 1–3.

Altameme, H., I. Hameed & M. Kareem. 2015. Analysis of alkaloid phytochemical compounds in the ethanolic extract of *Datura stramonium* and evaluation of antimicrobial activity. *African Journal of Biotechnology*, 14(19): 1668–1674.

Alvarez, C.A., N. Yomayusa, A.L. Leal, J. Moreno, S. Mendez-Alvarez, M. Ibañez & N. Vanegas. 2010. Nosocomial infections caused by community-associated methicillin-resistant *Staphylococcus aureus* in Colombia. *American Journal of Infection Control* 38(4): 315–318.

Alavi, M. & M. Rai. 2019. Recent advances in antibacterial applications of metal nanoparticles (MNPs) and metal nanocomposites (MNCs) against multidrug-resistant (MDR) bacteria. *Expert Review of Antiinfective therapy* 17(6): 419–428.

Ameer, M.A., A. Wasey & P. Salen. 2020. *Escherichia Coli* (E Coli 0157 H7). *StatPearls*.

Anand, U., N. Jacobo-Herrera, A. Altemimi & N. Lakhssassi. 2019. A comprehensive review on medicinal plants as antimicrobial therapeutics: potential avenues of biocompatible drug discovery. *Metabolites* 9(11): 1–13.

Anantharaman, A., M. Rizvi & D. Sahal. 2010. Synergy with rifampin and kanamycin enhances potency, kill kinetics, and selectivity of de novo-designed antimicrobial peptides. *Antimicrobial Agents and Chemotherapy* 54(5): 1693–1699.

Anyanwu, M.U. & R.C. Okoye. 2017. Antimicrobial activity of Nigerian medicinal plants. *Journal of Intercultural Ethnopharmacology* 6(2): 240–259.

Arumugam, G., M.K. Swamy & U.R. Sinniah. 2016. *Plectranthus amboinicus* (Lour.) Spreng: botanical, phytochemical, pharmacological and nutritional significance. *Molecules* 21(4): 1–26.

Asadi, A., S. Razavi, M. Talebi & M. Gholami. 2019. A review on anti-adhesion therapies of bacterial diseases. *Infection* 47(1): 13–23.

Barbieri, R., E. Coppo, A. Marchese, M. Daglia, E. Sobarzo-Sanchez & S. Nabavi. 2017. Phytochemicals for human disease: an update on plant-derived compounds antibacterial activity. *Microbiological Research*, 196: 44–68.

Bachheti, R.K., Konwarh, R., Gupta, V., Husen, A., Joshi, A. 2019. Green synthesis of iron oxide nanoparticles: cutting edge technology and multifaceted applications. In: Husen, A., Iqbal, M. (Eds.), *Nanomaterials and Plant Potential*. Springer Int. Publishing AG, Gewerbestrasse 11, 6330 Cham, pp. 239–259.

Bachheti, R.K., Fikadu, A., Bachheti, A. and Husen, A. 2020. Biogenic fabrication of nanomaterials from flower-based chemical compounds, characterization and their various applications: a review. *Saudi Journal of Biological Sciences* 27(10): 2551.

Bachheti, R.K., Godebo, Y., Bachheti, A., Yassin, M.O. and Husen, A., 2020b. Root-based fabricationof metal and or metal-oxide nanomaterials and their various applications. In: Husen, A., Jawaid, M. (Eds.), *Nanomaterials for Agriculture and Forestry Applications*. Elsevier Inc., 50 Hampshire St., 5th Floor, Cambridge, MA 02139, USA, pp. 135–166.

Bachheti, R.K., Sharma, A., Bachheti, A., Husen, A., Shanka, G.M. and Pandey, D.P. 2020c. Nanomaterials from various forest tree species and their biomedical applications. In: Husen, A., Jawaid, M. (Eds.), *Nanomaterials for Agriculture and Forestry Applications*. Elsevier Inc., 50 Hampshire St., 5th Floor, Cambridge, MA 02139, USA, pp. 81–106.

Bello, I.A., G.I. Ndukwe, O.T. Audu & J.D. Habila. 2011. A bioactive flavonoid from *Pavetta crassipes* K. Schum. *Organic Medicinal Chemistry Letters* 1(1): 1–5.

Bilombele, M. 2019. Searching for antibiotic producing bacteria. *JCC Science and Maths Poster Symposium*. 3-5-2019.

Bisht, D.S., K. Menon & M.K. Singhal. 2014. Comparative antimicrobial activity of essential oils of *Cuminum cyminum* L. and *Foeniculum vulgare* Mill. seeds against *Salmonella typhimurium* and *Escherichia coli. Journal of Essential Oil Bearing Plants* 17(4): 617–622.

Boberek, J.M., J. Stach & L.J.P.O. Good. 2010. Genetic evidence for inhibition of bacterial division protein FtsZ by berberine. *Public Library of Science* 5(10): 1–9.

Bologa, C.G., O. Ursu, T.I. Oprea, C.E. Melançon III & G.P. Tegos. 2013. Emerging trends in the discovery of natural product antibacterials. *Current Opinion in Pharmacology* 13(5): 678–687.

Braca, A., T. Siciliano, M. D'Arrigo & M.P. Germanò. 2008. Chemical composition and antimicrobial activity of *Momordica charantia* seed essential oil. *Fitoterapia* 79(2): 123–125.

Brooks, W. 2020. Bacterial pneumonia. In: *Hunter's Tropical Medicine and Emerging Infectious Diseases*. tenth ed. Elsevier, Amsterdakm, Netherlands, pp. 446–453.

Camporese, A., M. Balick, R. Arvigo, R. Esposito, N. Morsellino, F. De Simone & A. Tubaro. 2003. Screening of anti-bacterial activity of medicinal plants from Belize (Central America). *Journal of Ethnopharmacology* 87: 103–107.

Carradori, S., P. Chimenti, M. Fazzari, A. Granese & L. Angiolella. 2016. Antimicrobial activity, synergism and inhibition of germ tube formation by *Crocus sativus*-derived compounds against Candida spp. *Journal of Enzyme Inhibition and Medicinal Chemistry* 31: 189–193.

Carrol, D.H., F. Chassagne, M. Dettweiler & C.L. Quave. 2020. Antibacterial activity of plant species used for oral health against *Porphyromonas gingivalis. Public Library of Science* 15(10): 1–22.

Casson, N., J.M. Entenza, N. Borel, A. Pospischil & G. Greub. 2008. Murine model of pneumonia caused by *Parachlamydia acanthamoebae. Microbial Pathogenesis* 45(2): 92–97.

Cavallo, E., X. He, F. Luzi, F. Dominici, P. Cerrutti, C. Bernal, M. Foresti, L. Torre & D. Puglia. 2021. UV protective, antioxidant, antibacterial and compostable polylactic acid composites containing pristine and chemically Modified lignin nanoparticles. *Molecules* 26(1): 1–20.

CDCP. 1997. Case definitions for infectious conditions under public health surveillance. Centers for Disease Control and Prevention. *MMWR Recommendations and Reports* 1997 May 2, 46(RR-10): 1–55.

Chaieb, K., H. Hajlaoui, T. Zmantar, A.B. Kahla-Nakbi, M. Rouabhia, K. Mahdouani & A. Bakhrouf. 2007. The chemical composition and biological activity of clove essential oil, *Eugenia caryophyllata* (*Syzigium aromaticum* L. Myrtaceae). *Phytotherapy Research: An International Journal Devoted to Pharmacological Toxicological Evaluation of Natural Product Derivatives* 21(6): 501–506.

Chan, B.C., M. Ip, C. Lau, S. Lui, C. Jolivalt, C. Ganem-Elbaz, M. Litaudon, N.E. Reiner, H. Gong & R.H. See. 2011. Synergistic effects of baicalein with ciprofloxacin against NorA over-expressed methicillin-resistant *Staphylococcus aureus* (MRSA) and inhibition of MRSA pyruvate kinase. *Journal of ethnopharmacology* 137(1): 767–773.

Chandra, H., P. Bishnoi, A. Yadav, B. Patni, A. Mishra & A. Nautiyal. 2017. Antimicrobial resistance and the alternative resources with special emphasis on plant-based antimicrobials—A review. *Plants* 6(16): 1–11.

Charles, N.N. & N.L. Bonareri. 2020. Ethnomedicinal survey of plants used by Abagusii traditional healers of South West Kenya in the treatment of sexually transmitted diseases. *International Journal of Advanced Research* 6(9): 260–265.

Chinsembu, K. 2016. Ethnobotanical study of medicinal flora utilised by traditional healers in the management of sexually transmitted infections in Sesheke District, Western Province, Zambia, Brazilian. *International Journal of Pharmacognosy and Phytochemical Research* 26: 268–274.

Cock, I. & S. Van Vuuren. 2020. The traditional use of southern African medicinal plants for the treatment of bacterial respiratory diseases: a review of the ethnobotany and scientific evaluations. *Journal of Ethnopharmacology* 263: 1–26.

Cook, M., R. Protheroe & J. Handel. 2001. Tetanus: a review of the literature. *British Journal of Anaesthesia* 87(3): 477–487.

Correa, R.C., S.A. Heleno, M.J. Alves & I.C. Ferreira. 2020. Bacterial resistance: antibiotics of last generation used in clinical practice and the arise of natural products as new therapeutic alternatives. *Current Pharmaceutical Design* 26(8): 815–837.

Cos, P., A.J. Vlietinck, D.V. Berghe & L. Maes. 2006. Anti-infective potential of natural products: how to develop a stronger in vitro 'proof-of-concept'. *Journal of Ethnopharmacology* 106(3): 290–302.

Cushnie, T.T., B. Cushnie & A.J. Lamb. 2014. Alkaloids: an overview of their antibacterial, antibiotic-enhancing and antivirulence activities. *International Journal of Antimicrobial Agents* 44(5): 377–386.

Cushnie, T.T. & A.J. Lamb. 2005. Antimicrobial activity of flavonoids. *International Journal of Antimicrobial Agents* 26(5): 343–356.

Dallap Schaer, B., H. Aceto & S. Rankin. 2010. Outbreak of salmonellosis caused by *Salmonella enterica* serovar Newport MDR-AmpC in a large animal veterinary teaching hospital. *Journal of Veterinary Internal Medicine* 24(5): 1138–1146.

Das, D., N. Sinha & J. Chattopadhyay. 2013. The use of medicinal plants for the treatment of gonorrhoea and syphilis in West Bengal of India. *International Journal of Phytomedicine* 5: 14–17.

Deixler, E. 2009. Sudden infant death syndrome (SIDS) caused by ATP-depletion following hyperventilation, tissue-hypoxia and hypermetabolism--a hypothesis. *Zeitschrift Fur Geburtshilfe und Neonatologie* 213(4): 122–134.

Dhama, K., R. Tiwari, S. Chakraborty, M. Saminathan, A. Kumar, K. Karthik, M.Y. Wani, S.S. Amarpal & A. Rahal. 2014. Evidence based antibacterial potentials of medicinal plants and herbs countering bacterial pathogens especially in the era of emerging drug resistance: an integrated update. *International Journal of Pharmacology* 10(1): 1–43.

Diuk-Wasser, M.A., A.G. Hoen, P. Cislo, R. Brinkerhoff, S.A. Hamer, M. Rowland, R. Cortinas, G. Vourc'h, F. Melton & G.J. Hickling. 2012. Human risk of infection with *Borrelia burgdorferi*, the Lyme disease agent, in eastern United States. *The American Journal of Tropical Medicine Hygiene* 86(2): 320–327.

Djeussi, D.E., J.A. Noumedem, J.A. Seukep, A.G. Fankam, I.K. Voukeng, S.B. Tankeo, A.H. Nkuete & V. Kuete. 2013. Antibacterial activities of selected edible plants extracts against multidrug-resistant Gram-negative bacteria. *BMC Complementary Alternative Medicine* 13(1): 1–8.

Dover, L.G., A.M. Cerdeno-Tárraga, M.J. Pallen, J. Parkhill & G.S. Besra. 2004. Comparative cell wall core biosynthesis in the mycolated pathogens, *Mycobacterium tuberculosis* and *Corynebacterium diphtheriae*. *FEMS Microbiology Reviews* 28(2): 225–250.

Dwivedi, G.R., A. Maurya, D.K. Yadav, V. Singh, F. Khan, M.K. Gupta, M. Singh, M.P. Darokar & S.K. Srivastava. 2019. Synergy of clavine alkaloid 'chanoclavine' with tetracycline against multi-drug-resistant *E. coli*. *Journal of Biomolecular Structure Dynamics* 37(5): 1307–1325.

Edelstein, P.H., C.S. Jorgensen & L.A. Wolf. 2020. Performance of the ImmuView and BinaxNOW assays for the detection of urine and cerebrospinal fluid *Streptococcus pneumoniae* and *Legionella pneumophila* serogroup 1 antigen in patients with Legionnaires' disease or *pneumococcal pneumonia* and meningitis. *Public Library of Science* 15(8): 1–13.

Edziri, H., M. Mastouri, M.A. Mahjoub, Z. Mighri, A. Mahjoub & L. Verschaeve. 2012. Antibacterial, antifungal and cytotoxic activities of two flavonoids from *Retama raetam* flowers. *Molecules* 17(6): 7284–7293.

Elkadya, W., M. Bishr, M. Abdel-Azizc & O. Salamaa. 2020. Identification and isolation of anti-pneumonia bioactive compounds from *Opuntia ficus-indica*, fruits waste peels. *Food & Function* DOI: 10.1039/D0FO00817F.

Fadhel, B., A. Aissi, N. Ladhari, M. Deghrigue, R. Chemli & J.P.J. Joly. 2012. Antibacterial effects of two Tunisian *Eucalyptus* leaf extracts on wool and cotton fabrics. *Journal of The Textile Institute* 103(11): 1197–1204.

Fankam, A.G., V. Kuete, I.K. Voukeng, J.R. Kuiate & J.M. Pages. 2011. Antibacterial activities of selected Cameroonian spices and their synergistic effects with antibiotics against multidrug-resistant phenotypes. *BMC Complementary Alternative Medicine* 11(1): 1–11.

Farhadi, F., B. Khameneh, M. Iranshahi & M. Iranshahy. 2019. Antibacterial activity of flavonoids and their structure–activity relationship: an update review. *Phytotherapy Research* 33: 13–40.

Feng, J., W. Shi, J. Miklossy, G.M. Tauxe, C.J. McMeniman & Y. Zhang. 2018. Identification of essential oils with strong activity against stationary phase *Borrelia burgdorferi*. *Antibiotics (Basel, Switzerland)* 7(4): 89

Florin, T.A., T.E. Zaoutis & L.B. Zaoutis. 2008. Beyond cat scratch disease: widening spectrum of *Bartonella henselae* infection. *Pediatrics* 121(5): 1413–1425.

Floyd, K., P. Glaziou, A. Zumla & M. Raviglione. 2018. The global tuberculosis epidemic and progress in care, prevention, and research: an overview in year 3 of the end TB era. *Lancet Respiratory Medicine* 6(4): 299–314.

Frey, F. & R. Meyers. 2010. Antibacterial activity of traditional medicinal plants used by Haudenosaunee peoples of New York State. *BMC Complementary and Alternative Medicine* 10: 1–10.

Ghosh, C. & J.Haldar. 2015. Membrane-active small molecules: designs inspired by antimicrobial peptides. *ChemMed Chem* 10(10): 1606–1624.

Guimaraes, A.C., L.M. Meireles, M.F. Lemos, M.C.C. Guimarães, D.C. Endringer, M. Fronza & R.M. Scherer. 2019. Antibacterial activity of terpenes and terpenoids present in essential oils. *Molecules* 24: 1–12.

Gupta, R., B. Thakur, P. Singh, H. Singh, V. Sharma, V. Katoch & S. Chauhan. 2010. Anti-tuberculosis activity of selected medicinal plants against multi-drug resistant *Mycobacterium tuberculosis* isolates. *Indian Journal of Medical Research* 131(6): 809–813.

Hajishengallis, G., R.P. Darveau & M.A. Curtis. 2012. The keystone-pathogen hypothesis. *Nature Reviews Microbiology* 10(10): 717–725.

Hasan, R.N., M. Ali, S.M. Shakier, A.M. Khudhair, M.S. Hussin, Y.A. Kadum, A.I. Mohammed & A.A. Abbas. 2013. Antibacterial activity of aqueous and alcoholic extracts of *Capsella bursa* against selected pathogenic bacteria. *American Journal of BioScience* 1(1): 6–10.

Hassan-Olajokun, R., A. Deji-Agboola, O. Olasunkanmi, T. Banjo & O. Olaniran. 2020. Antimicrobial activity of fractioned components from *Dacryodes edulis: invitro* study. *European Journal of Medicinal Plants* 31: 71–82.

Hasson, R. 2011. Antibacterial activity of water and alcoholic crude extract of flower *Achillea millefolium*. *Rafidain Journal of Science* 22: 11–20.

Holler, J.G., S.B. Christensen, H.-C. Slotved, H.B. Rasmussen, A. Gúzman, C.E. Olsen, B. Petersen & P. Molgaard. 2012. Novel inhibitory activity of the *Staphylococcus aureus* NorA efflux pump by a kaempferol rhamnoside isolated from *Persea lingue* Nees. *Journal of Antimicrobial Chemotherapy* 67(5): 1138–1144.

Holy, O., J. Vlckova, L. Janouskova & I. Matouskova. 2017. Prevalence of diphtheria, tetanus and pertussis in the world. Klinicka Mikrobiol. *A Infekcni Lekarství* 23(1): 10–16.

Hossan, S., B. Agarwala, S. Sarwar, M. Karim, R. Jahan & M. Rahmatullah. 2010. Traditional use of medicinal plants in Bangladesh to treat urinary tract infections and sexually transmitted diseases. *Ethnobotany Research Applications* 8: 061–074.

Husen, A., Rahman, Q.I., Iqbal, M., Yassin, M.O. and Bachheti, R.K. 2019. Plant-mediated fabrication of gold nanoparticles and their applications. In: Husen, A., Iqbal, M. (Eds.), *Nanomaterials and Plant Potential*. Springer Int. Publishing AG, Gewerbestrasse 11, 6330 Cham, pp. 71–110.

Husen, A. 2020a. Carbon-based nanomaterials and their interactions with agricultural crops. In: Husen Jawaid, A. (Ed.), *Nanomaterials for Agriculture and Forestry Applications*. Elsevier Inc., 50 Hampshire St., 5th Floor, Cambridge, MA 02139, USA, pp. 199–218.

Husen, A. 2020b. Interactions of metal and metal-oxide nanomaterials with agricultural crops: an overview. In: Husen Jawaid, A. (Ed.), *Nanomaterials for Agriculture and Forestry Applications*. Elsevier Inc., 50 Hampshire St., 5th Floor, Cambridge, MA 02139, USA, pp. 1–14.

Husen, A. 2020c. Introduction and techniques in nanomaterials formulation. In: Husen, A., Jawaid, M. (Eds.), *Nanomaterials for Agriculture and Forestry Applications*. Elsevier Inc., 50 Hampshire St., 5th Floor, Cambridge, MA 02139, USA, pp. 1–14.

Iroha, I., D. ILang, T. Ayogu, A. Oji & E. Ugbo. 2010. Screening for anti-typhoid activity of some medicinal plants used in traditional medicine in Ebonyi state, Nigeria. *African Journal of Pharmacy and Pharmacology* 4(12): 860–864.

Janovska, D., K. Kubikova & L. Kokoska. 2003. Screening for antimicrobial activity of some medicinal plants species of traditional Chinese medicine. *Czech Journal of Food Sciences* 21(3): 107–110.

Jeong, K.-W., J.-Y. Lee, D.I. Kang, J.-U. Lee, S.Y. Shin & Y. Kim. 2009. Screening of flavonoids as candidate antibiotics against *Enterococcus faecalis*. *Journal of Natural Products* 72(4): 719–724.

Jose, D., N. Lekshmi, A. Goel, R.A. Kumar & S. Thomas. 2017. Development of a novel herbal formulation to inhibit biofilm formation in toxigenic *Vibrio cholerae*. *Journal of Food Protection* 80(11): 1933–1940.

Kamwendo, F., L. Forslin, L. Bodin & D. Danielsson. 2000. Epidemiology of ectopic pregnancy during a 28 year period and the role of pelvic inflammatory disease. *Sexually Transmitted Infections* 76(1): 28–32.

Karou, D., M. Dicko, J. Simpore & A. Traore. 2005. Antioxidant and antibacterial activities of polyphenols from ethnomedicinal plants of Burkina Faso. *African Journal of Biotechnology* 4: 823–828.

Kayira, T. & H. Nakanoa. 2020. Antibacterial effects of plant extracts with hurdle technology against Vibrio cholerae. *FEMS Microbiology Letters* 367(16): 119.

Khadka, B., M. Panthi & S. Rimal. 2020. Folklore medicinal plants used against typhoid and fever in Lwangghalel, Kaski District, Central Nepal. *Journal of Plant Resources* 18(1): 258–266.

Khadka, B., M. Panthi & S. Rimal. 2020. Folklore medicinal plants used against typhoid and fever in Lwangghalel, kaski district, Central Nepal. *Journal of Plant Research* 18(1): 258–256.

Khameneh, B., V. Halimi, M.R. Jaafari & S. Golmohammadzadeh. 2015. Safranal-loaded solid lipid nanoparticles: evaluation of sunscreen and moisturizing potential for topical applications. *Iranian Journal of Basic Medical Sciences* 18(1): 58–63.

Khameneh, B., M. Iranshahy, V. Soheili & B. Bazzaz. 2019. Review on plant antimicrobials: a mechanistic viewpoint. *Antimicrobial Resistance and Infection Control* 8(118): 1–28.

Khameneh, B., M. gIranshahy, M. Ghandadi, D. Ghoochi Atashbeyk, B.S. Fazly Bazzaz, M.J.D.D. Iranshahi & I. Pharmacy. 2015. Investigation of the antibacterial activity and efflux pump inhibitory effect of co-loaded piperine and gentamicin nanoliposomes in methicillin-resistant *Staphylococcus aureus*. *Drug Development and Industrial Pharmacy*, 41(6): 989–994.

Khan, A., G. Jan, A. Khan, F. Gul Jan, A. Bahadur & M. Danish. 2017. In vitro antioxidant and antimicrobial activities of *Ephedra gerardiana* (root and stem) crude extract and fractions. *Evidence-Based Complementary Alternative Medicine* https://doi.org/10.1155/2017/4040254

Khan, S.A., S. Shahid, S. Hanif, H.S. Almoallim, S.A. Alharbi & H. Sellami. 2021. Green synthesis of chromium oxide nanoparticles for antibacterial, antioxidant anticancer, and biocompatibility activities. *International Journal of Molecular Sciences* 22(2): 1–17.

Kim, J.H., Y.-S. Yi, M.-Y. Kim & J.Y. Cho. 2017. Role of ginsenosides, the main active components of *Panax ginseng*, in inflammatory responses and diseases. *Journal of Ginseng Research* 41(4): 435–443.

Klancnik, A., M. Sikic Pogacar, K. Trost, M. Tusek Znidaric, B. Mozetic Vodopivec & S. Smole Možina. 2017. Anti-Campylobacter activity of resveratrol and an extract from waste Pinot noir grape skins and seeds, and resistance of Camp. jejuni planktonic and biofilm cells, mediated via the Cme ABC efflux pump. *Journal of Applied Microbiology* 122(1): 65–77.

Knox, K.L. & A.H. Holmes. 2002. Nosocomial endocarditis caused by Corynebacterium amycolatum and other nondiphtheriae corynebacteria. *Emerging Infectious Diseases* 8(1): 97–99.

Komiazyk, M., M. Palczewska, I. Sitkiewicz, S. Pikula& P. Groves. 2019. Neutralization of cholera toxin by Rosaceae family plant extracts. *BMC Complementary Alternative Medicine* 19(1): 1–14.

Kotzekidou, P., P. Giannakidis & A. Boulamatsis. 2008. Antimicrobial activity of some plant extracts and essential oils against foodborne pathogens *in vitro* and on the fate of inoculated pathogens in chocolate. *LWT - Food Science and Technology* 41(1): 119–127.

Kuete, V., I.K. Simo, B. Ngameni, J.D. Bigoga, J. Watchueng, R.N. Kapguep, F.-X. Etoa, B.N. Tchaleu & V.P. Beng. 2007. Antimicrobial activity of the methanolic extract, fractions and four flavonoids from the twigs of *Dorstenia angusticornis* Engl.(Moraceae). *Journal of Ethnopharmacology* 112(2): 271–277.

Kumar, S. & A.K. Pandey. 2013. Chemistry and biological activities of flavonoids: an overview. *The Scientific World Journal* 2013: 162750.

Lahmar, A., A. Bedoui, I. Mokdad-Bzeouich, Z. Dhaouifi, Z. Kalboussi, I. Cheraif, K. Ghedira & L. Chekir-Ghedira. 2017. Reversal of resistance in bacteria underlies synergistic effect of essential oils with conventional antibiotics. *Microbial Pathogenesis* 106: 50–59.

Lakonawa, K.Y., I.M. Utama & I.W. Gustawan. 2020. Generalized tetanus in an 8-years-old boy: a case report. *American Journal of Pediatric* 6(4): 428–432.

Laloo, D. & S. Hemalatha. 2011. Ethnomedicinal plants used for diarrhea by tribals of Meghalaya, Northeast India. *Pharmacogn* 5: 147–154.

Lechner, D., S. Gibbons & F. Bucar. 2008. Plant phenolic compounds as ethidium bromide efflux inhibitors in *Mycobacterium smegmatis*. *Journal of Antimicrobial Chemotherapy* 62(2): 345–348.

Lee, H.-S. & M.-J. Kim 2002. Selective responses of three *Ginkgo biloba* leaf-derived constituents on human intestinal bacteria. *Journal of Agricultural Food Chemistry* 50(7): 1840–1844.

Lee, J., S. Cho, H. Paik, C. Choi, K. Nam, S. Hwang & S. Kim. 2014. Investigation on antibacterial and antioxidant activities, phenolic and flavonoid contents of some thai edible plants as an alternative for antibiotics. *Asian Australas. Journal of Animal Science* 27(10): 1461–1468.

Lee, S.B., K.H. Cha, S.N. Kim, S. Altantsetseg, S. Shatar, O. Sarangerel & C.W. Nho. 2007. The antimicrobial activity of essential oil from *Dracocephalum foetidum* against pathogenic microorganisms. *Journal of Microbiology* 45(1): 53–57.

Levy, S.B. & B. Marshall. 2004. Antibacterial resistance worldwide: causes, challenges and responses. *Nature Medicine* 10(12) Supplement: S122–S129.

Lewis, W.H. & M.P. Elvin-Lewis. 2003. *Medical Botany: Plants Affecting Human Health*. John Wiley & Sons.

Lopes-Lutz, D., D.S. Alviano, C.S. Alviano & P.P. Kolodziejczyk. 2008. Screening of chemical composition, antimicrobial and antioxidant activities of *Artemisia* essential oils. *Phytochemistry* 69(8): 1732–1738.

Maema, L. & M. Potgieter. 2019. A. Samie, Ethnobotanical survey of invasive alien plant species used in the treatment of sexually transmitted infections in Waterberg district, south Africa. *South African Journal of Botany*122: 391–400.

Mahady, G. 2005. Medicinal plants for the prevention and treatment of bacterial infections. *Current Pharmaceutical Design* 11: 2405–2427.

Mahammed, A., H. Mitiku & J. Mohammed. 2020. In vitro antibacterial activity of selected medicinal plants extract used in traditional treatment of common human wound infection in Fafan zone, Somali region, Ethiopia. *International Journal of Herbal Medicine* 8: 6–11.

Mandal, S., M. DebMandal, K. Saha & N.K. Pal. 2011. In vitro antibacterial activity of three Indian spices against methicillin-resistant Staphylococcus aureus. *Oman Medical Journal* 26(5): 319–323.

Mandal, S., M. Mandal & N. Pal. 2011. Cholera: a great global concern. *Asian Pacific Journal of Tropical Medicine* 4: 573–580.

Manju, S., B. Malaikozhundan, S. Vijayakumar, S. Shanthi, A. Jaishabanu, P. Ekambaram & B. Vaseeharan. 2016. Antibacterial, antibiofilm and cytotoxic effects of *Nigella sativa* essential oil coated gold nanoparticles. *Microbial Pathogenesis* doi: 10.1016/j.micpath.2015.11.021.

Mazhangara, I., E. Idamokoro, E. Chivandi & A. Afolayan. 2020. Phytochemical screening and in vitro evaluation of antioxidant and antibacterial activities of *Teucrium trifidum* crude extracts. *Heliyon* 6: 1–8.

Mazzei, R., M. Leonti, S. Spadafora, A. Patitucci & G. Tagarelli. 2020. A review of the antimicrobial potential of herbal drugs used in popular Italian medicine (1850s–1950s) to treat bacterial skin diseases. *Journal of Ethnopharmacology* 250: 112443.

Mbaveng, A.T., B. Ngameni, V. Kuete, I.K. Simo, P. Ambassa, R. Roy, M. Bezabih, F.-X. Etoa, B.T. Ngadjui & B.M. Abegaz. 2008. Antimicrobial activity of the crude extracts and five flavonoids from the twigs of *Dorstenia barteri* (Moraceae). *Journal of Ethnopharmacology* 116(3): 483–489.

McMurray, R., M. Ball, M. Tunney, N. Corcionivoschi & C. Situ. 2020. Antibacterial activity of four plant extracts extracted from traditional chinese medicinal plants against *Listeria monocytogenes*, *Escherichia coli*, and *Salmonella enterica* subsp. enterica serovar Enteritidis. *Microorganisms* 8(962): 1–12.

Moellering, R. 1981. Essential characteristics of antibiotics for the treatment of seriously ill patients. *Clinical Therapeutics* 4 Supplement A: 1–7.

Mogg, M., H.-H. Wang, A. Baker, Z. Derouen, J. Borski & W.E. Grant. 2020. Increased incidence of *Ehrlichia chaffeensis* infections in the United States, 2012 through 2016. Vector-borne zoonotic diseases.

Mohanta, Y.K., K. Biswas, S.K. Jena, A. Hashem, E.F. Abd-Allah & T.K. Mohanta. 2020. Anti-biofilm and antibacterial activities of silver nanoparticles synthesized by the reducing activity of phytoconstituents present in the Indian medicinal plants. *Frontiers in Microbiology* 11: 1–15.

Moloney, M.G. 2016. Natural products as a source for novel antibiotics. *Trends in Pharmacological Sciences* 37(8): 689–701.

Moore, S., N. Thomson, A. Mutreja, R. Piarroux & Infection. 2014. Widespread epidemic cholera caused by a restricted subset of *Vibrio cholerae* clones. *Clinical Microbiology* 20(5): 373–379.

Mori, A., C. Nishino, N. Enoki & S. Tawata. 1987. Antibacterial activity and mode of action of plant flavonoids against *Proteus vulgaris* and *Staphylococcus aureus*. *Phytochemistry* 26(8): 2231–2234.

MubarakAli, D., N. Thajuddin, K. Jeganathan & M. Gunasekaran. 2011. Plant extract mediated synthesis of silver and gold nanoparticles and its antibacterial activity against clinically isolated pathogens. *Colloids Surfaces B: Biointerfaces* 85(2): 360–365.

Munaeni, W., M. Yuhana, M. Setiawati & A. Wahyudi. 2019. Phytochemical analysis and antibacterial activities of *Eleutherine bulbosa* (Mill.) Urb. extract against *Vibrio parahaemolyticus*. *Asian Pacific Journal of Tropical Biomedicine* 9: 397–404.

Murugan, T., J.A. Wins & M. Murugan. 2013. Antimicrobial activity and phytochemical constituents of leaf extracts of *Cassia auriculata*. *Indian Journal of Pharmaceutical Sciences* 75(1): 122–125.

Mustafa, G., R. Arif, A. Atta, S. Sharif & A. Jamil. 2017. Bioactive compounds from medicinal plants and their importance in drug discovery in Pakistan. *Matrix Science Pharma* 1(1): 17–26.

Mydeen, S.S., R.R. Kumar, M. Kottaisamy & V. Vasantha. 2020. Biosynthesis of ZnO nanoparticles through extract from *Prosopis juliflora* plant leaf: antibacterial activities and a new approach by rust-induced photocatalysis. *Journal of Saudi Chemical Society*, 24(5): 393–406.

Nabavi, S.F., A. Di Lorenzo, M. Izadi, E. Sobarzo-Sánchez, M. Daglia & S.M. Nabavi. 2015. Antibacterial effects of cinnamon: from farm to food, cosmetic and pharmaceutical industries. *Nutrients* 7(9): 7729–7748.

Naqvi, S.A.R., S. Nadeem, S. Komal, S.A.A. Naqvi, M.S. Mubarik, S.Y. Qureshi, S. Ahmad, A. Abbas, S.S. Raza & N. Aslam. 2019. Antioxidants: natural antibiotics. In *Antioxidants*. IntechOpen, pp. 351–405.

Noskin, G.A., L.R. Peterson & J.R. Warren. 1995. *Enterococcus faecium* and *Enterococcus faecalis* bacteremia: acquisition and outcome. *Clinical Infectious Diseases* 20(2): 296–301.

Novotna, B., Z. Polesny, M.F. Pinto-Basto, P. Van Damme, P. Pudil, J. Mazancova & M.C. Duarte. 2020. Medicinal plants used by 'root doctors', local traditional healers in Bié province, Angola. *Journal of Ethnopharmacology* 260: 1–27.

Olaitan, A.O., S. Morand & J.-M. Rolain. 2014. Mechanisms of polymyxin resistance: acquired and intrinsic resistance in bacteria. *Frontiers in microbiology* 5: 1–18.

Omojate Godstime, C., O. Enwa Felix, O. Jewo Augustina & O. Eze Christopher. 2014. Mechanisms of antimicrobial actions of phytochemicals against enteric pathogens– a review. *Journal of Pharmaceutical, Chemical and Biological Sciences* 2(2): 77–85.

Oussalah, M., S. Caillet & M. Lacroix. 2006. Mechanism of action of Spanish oregano, Chinese cinnamon, and savory essential oils against cell membranes and walls of *Escherichia coli* O157: H7 and *Listeria monocytogenes*. *Journal of Food Protection* 69(5): 1046–1055.

Oyekunle, M., O. Aiyelaagbe & M. Fafunso. 2006. Evaluation of the antimicrobial activity of saponins extract of *Sorghum bicolor* L. Moench. *African Journal of Biotechnolog* 5(23): 31–39.

Panda, S.K., R. Das, R. Lavigne & W. Luyten. 2020. Indian medicinal plant extracts to control multidrug-resistant *S. aureus*, including in biofilms. *South African Journal of Botany* 128: 283–291.

Pandey, K., A. Sinha & Z. Perween. 2020. Important medicinal plants with their medicinal uses from Jharkhand State. *International Journal of Research in Engineering, Science Management* 3(8): 532–542.

Patel, K., C. Tyagi, S. Goyal, S. Jamal, D. Wahi, R. Jain, N. Bharadvaja & A. Grover. 2015. Identification of chebulinic acid as potent natural inhibitor of *M. tuberculosis* DNA gyrase and molecular insights into its binding mode of action. *Computational Biology Chemistry* 59: 37–47.

Poddar, S., T. Sarkar, S. Choudhury, S. Chatterjee & P. Ghosh. 2020. Indian traditional medicinal plants: a concise review. *International Journal of Botany Studies* 5(5): 174–190.

Prasannabalaji, N., G. Muralitharan, R. Sivanandan, S. Kumaran & S. Pugazhvendan. 2012. Antibacterial activities of some Indian traditional plant extracts. *Asian Pacific Journal of Tropical Disease* 2: S291–S295.

Priya, C., M. Venkataswamy, G. Harshini, P. Pravalika, S. Mandadi & J. Bandla. 2019. Medicinal plants used for the treatment of bacterial Meningitis. *Research Journal of Pharmaceutical Dosage Forms and Technology* 11(3): 239–244.

Radulovi, N., P. Blagojevi, Z. StojanoviRadi & N. Stojanovi. 2013. Antimicrobial plant metabolites: structural diversity and mechanism of action. *Current Medicinal Chemistry* 20: 932–952.

Rahmatullah, M., R. Jahan, S. Seraj, F. Islam, F. Jahan, Z. Khatun, S. Sanam, M. Monalisa, T.T. Khan & K.K.R. Biswas. 2011. Medicinal plants used by folk medicinal practitioners in three randomly surveyed. *American-Eurasian Journal of Sustainable Agriculture* 5: 226–232.

Randhawa, H.K., K.K. Hundal, P.N. Ahirrao, S.M. Jachak & H.S. Nandanwar. 2016. Efflux pump inhibitory activity of flavonoids isolated from *Alpinia calcarata* against methicillin-resistant *Staphylococcus aureus*. *Biologia* 71(5): 484–493.

Rehman, F. & S. Mairaj. 2013. Antimicrobial studies of allicin and ajoene. *International Journal of Pharma and Bio Sciences* 4(2): 1095–1105.

Ribeiro, R.V., I.G.C. Bieski, S.O. Balogun & D.T. Oliveira. 2017. Ethnobotanical study of medicinal plants used by Ribeirinhos in the North Araguaia microregion, Mato Grosso, Brazil. *Journal of Ethnopharmacology* 205: 69–102.

Rice, P., W. Shafer, S. Ram & A. Jerse. 2017. Annual review of microbiology *Neisseria gonorrhoeae*: drug resistance, mouse models, and vaccine development. *Annual Review of Microbiology* 71: 665–686.

Roger, T., M. Pierre-Marie, V. Igor & V. Patrick. 2015. Phytochemical screening and antibacterial activity of medicinal plants used to treat typhoid fever in Bamboutos division, West Cameroon. *Journal of Applied Pharmaceutical Science* 5(6): 34–49.

Saad, N.Y., C.D. Muller & A. Lobstein. 2013. Major bioactivities and mechanism of action of essential oils and their components. *Flavour Fragrance Journal* 28(5): 269–279.

Sails, A.D., B. Swaminathan & P.I. Fields. 2003. Utility of multilocus sequence typing as an epidemiological tool for investigation of outbreaks of gastroenteritis caused by *Campylobacter jejuni*. *Journal of Clinical Microbiology* 41(10): 4733–4739.

Santacroce, L., L. Bottalico, S. Topi, F. Castellaneta & I.A. Charitos. 2020. The "Scourge of the Renaissance". A short review about *Treponema pallidum* infection. *Endocrine, Metabolic Immune Disorders-Drug Targets* 20(3): 335–343.

Santos, N.O.D., B. Mariane, J.H.G. Lago, P. Sartorelli, W. Rosa, M.G. Soares, A.M. Da Silva, H. Lorenzi, M.A. Vallim & R.C.J.M. Pascon. 2015. Assessing the chemical composition and antimicrobial activity of essential oils from Brazilian plants—*Eremanthus erythropappus* (Asteraceae), *Plectrantuns barbatus*, and *P. amboinicus* (Lamiaceae). *Molecules* 20(5): 8440–8452.

Seiler, C. & T.U. Berendonk. 2012. Heavy metal driven co-selection of antibiotic resistance in soil and water bodies impacted by agriculture and aquaculture. *Frontiers in Microbiology* 3: 1–10.

Shao, J., M. Zhang, T. Wang, Y. Li & C. Wang. 2016. The roles of CDR1, CDR2, and MDR1 in kaempferol-induced suppression with fluconazole-resistant *Candida albicans*. *Pharmaceutical Biology* 54(6): 984–992.

Shihabudeen, M., H. Priscilla & K. Thirumurugan. 2010. Antimicrobial activity and phytochemical analysis of selected Indian folk medicinal plants. *International Journal of Pharma Sciences and Research* 1(10): 430–434.

Siddiqi, K.S. & A. Husen. 2016. Green synthesis, characterization and uses of palladium/platinum nanoparticles. *Nanoscale Research Letters* 11(1): 1–13.

Siddiqi, K.S. & A. Husen. 2017. Recent advances in plant-mediated engineered gold nanoparticles and their application in biological system. *Journal of Trace Elements in Medicine and Biology* 40: 10–23.

Siddiqi, K.S. & A. Husen. 2020. Current status of plant metabolite-based fabrication of copper/copper oxide nanoparticles and their applications: a review. *Biomaterials Research* 24: 1–15.

Siddiqi, K.S., A. Rahman, & A. Husen. 2016. Biogenic fabrication of iron/iron oxide nanoparticles and their application. *Nanoscale Research Letters* 11(1): 1–13.

Siddiqi, K.S., M Rashid, A. Rahman, A. Husen, & S. Rehman. 2020. Green synthesis, characterization, antibacterial and photocatalytic activity of black cupric oxide nanoparticles. *Agriculture and Food Security* 9(1): 1–15.

Siddiqi, K.S., M. Rashid, A. Husen, & S. Rehman. 2019. Biofabrication of silver nanoparticles from *Diospyros montana*, their characterization and activity against some clinical isolates. *BioNanoScience* 9(2): 302–312.

Sieberi, B., G. Omwenga, R. Wambua, J. Samoei & M. Ngugi. 2020. Screening of the Dichloromethane: methanolic extract of *Centella asiatica* for antibacterial activities against *Salmonella typhi*, *Escherichia coli*, *Shigella sonnei*, *Bacillus subtilis*, and *Staphylococcus aureus*. *The Scientific World Journal* 2020: 6378712.

Silva, O., G. Caldeira & R. Serrano. 2020. A review of the role of medicinal plants on *Neisseria gonorrhoeae* infection. *European Journal of Integrative Medicine* 39: 1–19.

Siriyong, T., P. Srimanote, S. Chusri, B.E. Yingyongnarongkul, C. Suaisom, V. Tipmanee & S.P. Voravuthikunchai. 2017. Conessine as a novel inhibitor of multidrug efflux pump systems in *Pseudomonas aeruginosa*. *BMC Complementary Alternative Medicine* 17(1): 1–7.

Skocibusic, M., N. Bezić, V. Dunkić & A. Radonic. 2004. Antibacterial activity of *Achillea clavennae* essential oil against respiratory tract pathogens. *Fitoterapia* 75(7–8): 733–736.

Sousaa, F., I. Noleto, L. Chavesa, G. Pachecoa, A. Oliveiraa, M. Fonsecad & J. Medeirosa. 2020. A comprehensive review of therapeutic approaches available for the treatment of cholera. *Journal of Pharmacy and Pharmacology* doi: 10.1111/jphp.13344.

Sridevi, D., C. Shankar, P. Prakash, J.H. Park & K. Thamaraiselvi. 2017. Inhibitory effects of reserpine against efflux pump activity of antibiotic resistance bacteria. *Chemical Biology Letters* 4(2): 69–72.

Stermitz, F.R., K.K. Cashman, K.M. Halligan, C. Morel, G.P. Tegos & K. Lewis. 2003. Polyacylated neohesperidosides from *Geranium caespitosum*: bacterial multidrug resistance pump inhibitors. *Bioorganic Medicinal Chemistry Letters* 13(11): 1915–1918.

Swain, S. & T.R. Rautray. 2021. Estimation of trace elements, antioxidants, and antibacterial agents of regularly consumed Indian medicinal plants. *Biological Trace Element Research* 199: 1185–1193.

Syarif, L., A. Junita, M. Hatta, R. Dwiyanti, C. Kaelan, M. Sabir, R. Noviyanthi, M. Primaguna & N. Purnamasari. 2020. A mini review: medicinal plants for typhoid fever in Indonesia. *Journal Systematic Reviews in Pharmacy* 11(6): 1171–1180.

Tabuti, J.R., C.B. Kukunda & P.J. Waako. 2010. Medicinal plants used by traditional medicine practitioners in the treatment of tuberculosis and related ailments in Uganda. *Journal of Ethnopharmacology* 127(1): 130–136.

Tacket, C.O., F. Brenner & P.A.S. Blake. 1984. Clinical features and an epidemiological study of *Vibrio vulnificus* infections. *Journal of Infectious Disease* 149(4): 558–561.

Taghavizadeh Yazdi, M.E., A. Hamidi, M.S. Amiri, R. Kazemi Oskuee, H.A. Hosseini, A. Hashemzadeh & M. Darroudi. 2019. Eco-friendly and plant-based synthesis of silver nanoparticles using Allium giganteum and investigation of its bactericidal, cytotoxicity, and photocatalytic effects. *Materials Technology* 34(8): 490–497.

Tagousop, C., J. Tamokou, S. Ekom, D. Ngnokam & L. Voutquenne-Nazabadioko. 2018. Antimicrobial activities of flavonoid glycosides from *Graptophyllum grandulosum* and their mechanism of antibacterial action. *BMC Complementary and Alternative Medicine* 18(252): 1–10.

Tanaka, J., C. Da Silva, A. De Oliveira, C. Nakamura & B. Dias Filho. 2006. Antibacterial activity of indole alkaloids from *Aspidosperma ramiflorum*. *Brazilian Journal of Medical Biological Research* 39(3): 387–391.

Tang, J., C. Wang, Y. Feng, W. Yang, H. Song, Z. Chen, H. Yu, X. Pan, X. Zhou & H. Wang. 2006. Streptococcal toxic shock syndrome caused by Streptococcus suis serotype 2. *Public Library of Science Medicine* 3(5): 668–676.

Tapas, A.R., D. Sakarkar & R. Kakde. 2008. Flavonoids as nutraceuticals: a review. *Tropical Journal of Pharmaceutical Research* 7(3): 1089–1099.

Taylor, B.D., T. Darville & C.L. Haggerty. 2013. Does bacterial vaginosis cause pelvic inflammatory disease? *Sexually Transmitted Diseases* 40(2): 117–122.

Tebou, P., J. Tamokou, D. Ngnokama, L. Voutquenne-Nazabadioko, J. Kuiate & P. Bag. 2017. Flavonoids from Maytenus buchananii as potential cholera chemotherapeutic agents. *South African Journal of Botany* 109: 58–65.

Tijani, K.B., A.A. Alfa & A.A. Sezor. 2019. Studies on phytochemical, nutraceutical profiles and potential medicinal values of *Allium sativum* Linn (Lilliaceae) on Bacterial Meningitis. *International Neuropsychiatric Disease Journal* 13(2): 1–15.

Todd, E. & S. Notermans. 2011. Surveillance of listeriosis and its causative pathogen, Listeria monocytogenes. *Food Control* 22(9) 1484–1490.

Tomasz, A.N.E. 1994. Multiple-Antibiotic-Resistant Pathogenic Bacteria--A Report on the Rockefeller university workshop. *New England Journal of Medicine* 330(17): 1247–1251.

Tominaga, K., K. Higuchi, N. Hamasaki, M. Hamaguchi, T. Takashima, T. Tanigawa & S. Kadota. 2002. In vivo action of novel alkyl methyl quinolone alkaloids against *Helicobacter pylori*. *Journal of Antimicrobial Chemotherapy* 50(4): 547–552.

Torpy, J.M., C. Lynm & R.M. Golub. 2013. Gonorrhea. *Journal of the American Medical Association* 309(2): 196–196.

Toth, I., J. Van Der Wolf, G. Saddler, E. LOjkowska, V. Helias, M. Pirhonen, L. Tsror & J. Elphinstone. 2011. Dickeya species: an emerging problem for potato production in Europe. *Plant Pathology* 60: 385–399.

Trecarichi, E.M., L. Pagano, B. Martino, A. Candoni, R. Di Blasi, G. Nadali, L. Fianchi, M. Delia, S. Sica & V. Perriello. 2016. Bloodstream infections caused by Klebsiella pneumoniae in onco-hematological patients: clinical impact of carbapenem resistance in a multicentre prospective survey. *American Journal of Hematology* 91(11): 1076–1081.

Truelove, S., L. Keegan, W. Moss, L. Chaisson, E. Macher, A. Azman & J. Lessler. 2019. Clinical and epidemiological aspects of diphtheria: a systematic review and pooled analysis. *Clinical Infectious Diseases* https://doi.org/10.1093/cid/ciz808.

Uche-Okereafor, N., T. Sebola, K. Tapfuma, L. Mekuto, E. Green, V. Mavumengwana & p. health. 2019. Antibacterial activities of crude secondary metabolite extracts from Pantoea species obtained from the stem of *Solanum mauritianum* and their effects on two cancer cell lines. *International Journal of Environmental Research* 16(4): 1–12.

Ultee, A., M. Bennik & R. Moezelaar. 2002. The phenolic hydroxyl group of carvacrol is essential for action against the food-borne pathogen *Bacillus cereus*. *Applied Environmental Microbiology* 68(4): 1561–1568.

Vilas, V., D. Philip & J. Mathewb. 2016. Biosynthesis of Au and Au/Ag alloy nanoparticles using *Coleus aromaticus* essential oil and evaluation of their catalytic, antibacterial and antiradical activities. *Journal of Molecular Liquids* 221: 179–189.

Wagner, H. & G. Ulrich-Merzenich. 2009. Synergy research: approaching a new generation of phytopharmaceuticals. *Phytomedicine* 16(2–3): 97–110.

Walencka, E., S. Rozalska, H. Wysokinska, M. Rozalski, L. Kuzma & B. Rozalska. 2007. Salvipisone and aethiopinone from *Salvia sclarea* hairy roots modulate staphylococcal antibiotic resistance and express anti-biofilm activity. *Planta Medica* 73: 545–551.

Wang, D., K. Xie, D. Zou, M. Meng & M. Xie. 2018. Inhibitory effects of silybin on the efflux pump of methicillinresistant *Staphylococcus aureus*. *Molecular Medicine Reports* 18(1): 827–833.

Wang, L., Y. Wang, S. Jin, Z. Wu, D.P. Chin, J.P. Koplan & M.E. Wilson. 2008. Emergence and control of infectious diseases in China. *The Lancet* 372(9649): 1598–1605.

Watson, C. & N. Alp. 2008. Role of *Chlamydia pneumoniae* in atherosclerosis. *Clinical Science* 114(8): 509–531.

WHO 2014. Antimicrobial resistance global report on surveillance: 2014 summary. World Health Organization.

Wilcox, M.H. 2003. Gastrointestinal disorders and the critically ill. *Clostridium difficile* infection and pseudomembranous colitis. Best Practice Research. *Clinical Gastroenterology* 17(3): 475–493.

Wu, H.Z., H.J. Fei, Y. Zhao, X. Liu, Y. Huang & S. Wu. 2012. Antibacterial mechanism of sulforaphane on Escherichia coli. *Sichuan da xue xue bao. Yi xue ban= Journal of Sichuan University. Medical Science Edition* 43(3): 386–390.

Wu, Y., J. Bai, K. Zhong, Y. Huang, H. Qi, Y. Jiang & H. Gao. 2016. Antibacterial activity and membrane-disruptive mechanism of 3-p-trans-coumaroyl-2-hydroxyquinic acid, a novel phenolic compound from pine needles of *Cedrus deodara*, against *Staphylococcus aureus*. *Molecules* 21(8): 1–12.

Xu, J., F. Zhou, B.P. Ji, R.S. Pei & N. Xu. 2008. The antibacterial mechanism of carvacrol and thymol against *Escherichia coli*. *Letters in Applied Microbiology* 47(3): 174–179.

Yang, D.C., K.M. Blair & N.R. Salama. 2016. Staying in shape: the impact of cell shape on bacterial survival in diverse environments. *Microbiology Molecular Biology Reviews* 80(1): 187–203.

Yarnell, E. 2016. Herbal Medicine for Lyme disease and other tick-borne infections. *Alternative Complementary Therapies* 22(6): 257–265.

Yuan, P., X. Ding, Y.Y. Yang & Q.H. Xu. 2018. Metal nanoparticles for diagnosis and therapy of bacterial infection. *Advanced Healthcare Materials* 7, 1–17.

Zang, X., M. Shang, F. Xu, J. Liang, X. Wang, M. Mikage & S. Cai. 2013. A-type proanthocyanidins from the stems of *Ephedra sinica* (Ephedraceae) and their antimicrobial activities. *Molecules* 18(5): 5172–5189.

Zimniewska, M., R. Kozłowski & J. Batog. 2008. Nanolignin modified linen fabric as a multifunctional product. *Molecular Crystals and Liquid Crystals* 484(1): 484, 409.

Zorić, N., I. Kosalec, S. Tomić, I. Bobnjarić, M. Jug, T. Vlainić & J. Vlainic. 2017. Membrane of *Candida albicans* as a target of berberine. *BMC Complementary Alternative Medicine* 17(1): 1–10.

Zuoa, G., G. Wanga, Y. Zhaoa, G. Xua, X. Hao, J. Hanc & Q. Zhaoc. 2008. Screening of Chinese medicinal plants for inhibition against clinical isolates of methicillin-resistant *Staphylococcus aureus* (MRSA). *Journal of Ethnopharmacology* 120: 287–290.

Zwenger, S. & C. Basu. 2008. Plant terpenoids: applications and future potentials. *Biotechnology Molecular Biology Reviews* 3(1): 1–7.

3 Antiviral Activity of Medicinal Plants

Current Understanding, Prospects, and Challenges

Venkateish V P, Nivya V, Vani V,
Baskaran V, and Madan Kumar P

CONTENTS

3.1 INTRODUCTION

Viruses are extremely small, infectious organisms surrounded by a protein coat, composed of either DNA or RNA as the genetic material, and requiring a host for multiplication (Wasik et al., 2019). Compared with bacteria, fungi, and parasites, viruses are not individual, autonomous organisms and need to replicate within living cells. Therefore, most replication processes require specific cellular host metabolic pathways, making it almost impossible to design a therapy that directly targets the

DOI: 10.1201/9781003137955-3

virion or inhibits it with no associated harmful effects on the injured host cells. Numerous medicinal plants have shown inhibition of the herpes simplex virus (HSV), hepatitis B virus (HBV), hepatitis C virus (HCV), human immunodeficiency virus (HIV), poxvirus, or severe acute respiratory syndrome coronavirus (SARS-CoV) (Chen, 2020). Certain viruses can replicate and contribute to host cell lysis and then further infect and propagate the condition, while others integrate into a host chromosome and stay latent for years. A shortage of specific treatments and the minimal clinical effectiveness of most medications for viral diseases have contributed to a reliance on vaccination as a viral disease prevention treatment. Viral diseases are usually handled with various antiviral drugs, but the development of resistance to such drugs by certain infectious viruses intensifies the situation, with these drugs also often having undesirable effects on patients (Nathanson, 2008).

Viral pathogens continue to evolve new methods of evading the host immune system. These are the challenges that researchers developing antiviral treatments face, since it is challenging to identify specific biochemical properties of viruses that can be selectively targeted. Much information is needed to understand plant anti-virus remedial qualities from the available knowledge of conventional Indian, Chinese, and other ethnic plant-derived medicines that can be evaluated as possible drugs for different viral diseases (Boukhatem and Setzer, 2020). However, improved knowledge of the molecular occurrence of virus infections has ensured that potential antiviral medications can be scanned for particular targets more rationally. Because of the overall burden of virus-related diseases, novel and more efficient antiviral drugs are desperately required. At present, medicinal plants and their bioactive metabolites are of particular importance, which may provide desirable medical options for citizens in developing countries where the bulk of the population cannot afford expensive Western therapeutics (Boukhatem and Setzer, 2020).

The term "antiviral agent/drug" is generally defined as 'substances, other than attenuated viruses or virus-containing vaccines, or unique antimicrobial antibodies, which offer protective or therapeutic effect to the virus-infected host". Plants possess tremendous biosynthetic capabilities, synthesizing a rich collection of natural compounds that are commonly employed as promising phytotherapeutics in human viral disease control. Medicinal plants have been directly employed for years as therapeutic agents in various traditional medicine practices. The recent development of sophisticated analytical instruments has rendered medicinal plants an invaluable resource for modern drug exploration (Saklani and Kutty, 2008). Plant-based antiviral medicines offer a stable worldwide market and antiviral medicinal plants tend to be an important source of new medications and lead compounds. Global commerce in the plant-derived antiviral chemicals is a growing market. The worldwide market is estimated to trade in approximately 2000 species of medicinal plants (Ma and Yao, 2020). This chapter intends to report on the antiviral medicinal plants and their metabolites commonly employed as safer alternatives to conventional antiviral drugs, mainly due to their limited side effects and their substantial overall therapeutic effect.

3.2 COMMON HUMAN VIRAL DISEASES AND THEIR PATHOGENESIS

Viruses (sizes in the range 100–1000 nm) cause diseases and spread from one individual to another. They have distinct characteristics which differentiate them from other pathogens. Using the host's own cell machinery, viruses synthesize proteins and nucleic acids to produce new virus particles. Based on the genome type, viruses are broadly classified into two types, namely RNA viruses and DNA viruses. Examples of RNA viruses include dengue virus, while DNA viruses include HSV and poxvirus (Payne, 2017). The most important RNA viruses that cause diseases in humans include influenza, rotavirus, arbovirus, HCV, SARS, Nipah virus, Hendra virus, and Ebola virus (Virgin, 2014).

Although the pathogenesis of each virus is unique, they all share common steps during their life cycle (Nathanson, 2008). The virus's entry into the host depends on its interaction with specific molecules or receptors on the host cell's surface. Virus interaction with the host cell receptor is crucial because it determines the cell or tissue tropism of the viruses and the efficiency of the virus to cause disease (Rossmann et al., 2002; Spear, 2004). Viruses interact with the host cell's different cell surface structures; for example, rhinoviruses bind to ICAM-1 to promote entry, whereas HSV interacts with heparin sulphate to achieve infection. Infection of HIV into a host cell depends on CD4 and CCR5, which allow virus interaction with viral gp120. CD4 is a protein expressed in a subset of T cells within the host and its expression is limited in other cell types, like macrophages. In addition to the binding of gp120 to the CD4 molecule, HIV binding to CCR5/4 is also essential for viral fusion. Some individuals have a non-functional form of CCR5, so are HIV resistant (Vicenzi et al., 2007; Akram et al., 2018). Zoonotic viruses interact with humans only if they have conserved receptors that can be recognized in humans. Also, the zoonotic viruses need to mutate to effectively interact with cell receptors in humans (Rose et al., 2011). SARS-CoV, a zoonotic virus typically seen in bats, infects human cells through their spike proteins, interacting with angiotensin-converting enzyme 2 (ACE2) receptors. Studies show that a mutation in this virus receptor-binding domain leads to its infection of humans (Hamming et al., 2004).

The target tissue of infection of any virus also depends on other factors, such as proviral factors. Proviral factors are molecules in the host system that help to achieve efficient viral replication. HCV infection provides an example of the importance of virus-specific proviral factors that interact with the host microRNA, miR-122. HCV is a single-stranded RNA virus that infects the liver, resulting in organ failure and liver cancer. The specificity of HCV in causing infection in the liver and its ability to replicate in the hepatocyte depends on the host miR-122. miR-122 is expressed explicitly in the hepatocytes, increasing the levels of HCV RNA in the liver. Lanford et al. (2010) showed that administration of an antagonist specific to miR-122 led to decreased HCV viral load in the liver and a reduction in the incidence of associated diseases.

During a viral infection, the host system also executes several defence mechanisms to prevent the virus from entering and causing infection. One such defence mechanism is provided by host restriction endonucleases that actively inhibit virus replication. A restriction endonuclease from Rhesus macaque, TRIM-5α, is known to interact with HIV to prevent its replication and subsequent disease progression (McNab et al., 2011). The host immune system is another factor that prevents the virus from infecting the host. Like the type 1 interferons (IFN) and CD8-positive T cells, the innate immune system prevents the virus from replicating within the host and clears the virus particles from the host. Therefore, for successful infection, replication, and dissemination, within-host infecting viruses should have the ability to invade the host and evade the immune system. Numerous viruses can inhibit the host immune system. For example, the SARS-CoV inhibits the host type 1 IFN through nucleocapsid proteins present on the SARS-CoV (García-Sastre et al., 1998; Lanford et al., 2010).

Once a virus enters a cell, the type of cell or tissue it affects and its impact on the tissue determines the type of disease it causes. Some viruses kill the target host cell after infection, while others do not. Examples of viruses that directly kill the host cell upon infection and replication are the Venezuelan equine encephalitis virus (VEE) and the Sindbis virus. Both these viruses directly infect the neuron, replicating, causing neuron cell death and inhibiting neuron functions (Kimura and Griffin, 2003; Spear, 2004). As mentioned above, some viruses are not cytopathic, where they cause diseases associated with a viral infection. Examples include HBV, which cause acute and chronic inflammation in hepatocytes in infected humans. This is because of the over-expressed target host immune system for clearing the viruses, where the immune system becomes less effective and leads to the viral disease (Chisari et al., 2010). HCV infection induces immune reactions, where complexes of viruses and antibodies precipitate in small blood vessels, leading to inflammation (Mutz et al., 2018).

3.3   ORIGIN-BASED CLASSIFICATION OF ANTIVIRAL MEDICINAL PLANTS

3.3.1   EUROPEAN MEDICINAL PLANTS WITH ANTIVIRAL ACTIVITY

Practically every culture around the world relies on the use of medicinal plants for therapeutic purposes. Numerous medicinal plants are reported to have antiviral activity and are widely used to treat humans and animals suffering from viral diseases. In Europe, research into antiviral agents began after World War II. Two hundred and eighty-eight plant species were screened for their antiviral activity against the influenza A virus by the Boots drug company in Nottingham, England, finding that 12 showed antiviral potential (Chantrill et al., 1952). *Veronica persica,* a plant native to Eurasia, was reported to exhibit antiviral activity against HSV-1 and HSV-2 viral strains in Vero cells (Sharifi-Rad et al., 2018). *Sambucus nigra*, also known as a black elder, is a shrub or small tree native to Europe and North America and is approved by USFDA as Generally Recognized as Safe (GRAS) for use as a flavouring agent. It has been reported to exhibit antiviral activity against influenza viral infections (Porter and Bode, 2017). *Verbascum thapsus*, native to Europe and North Africa and naturalized in North America, showed antiviral effect against HSV-1 (McCutcheon et al., 1995; Jassim and Naji, 2003).

3.3.2 CHINESE MEDICINAL PLANTS WITH ANTIVIRAL ACTIVITY

Traditional Chinese medicine includes numerous herbal medicines, as well as acupuncture, nutritional therapy, and massage techniques, which are based on more than 2000 years of historical usage. Aqueous extracts of *Morus alba* and *Dryopteris crassirhizoma* exhibited anti-dengue potential with a half-maximal inhibitory concentration (IC_{50}) values of 130 and 221 µg/ml, respectively (Maryam et al., 2020). In a study conducted against RSV, 27 Chinese herbs were among the 44 which exhibited the greatest antiviral activity. Other important Chinese herbal plants that have shown antiviral activity are *Sophora flavescens* and *Scutellaria baicalensis*, containing active ingredients, such as anagyrine, sophoranol, oxymatrine, wogonin, and oroxylin A (Ma et al., 2002). Extracts of *Agrimonia pilosa*, *Pithecellobium clypearia*, and *Punica granatum* from China exhibited inhibitory activity against HSV-1. Extracts of *Blumea laciniata*, *Elephantopus scaber*, *Laggera pterodonta*, *Mussaenda pubescens*, *Schefflera octophylla, and Scutellaria indica* showed anti-RSV activity with IC_{50} values ranging from 12.5 to 32 µg/ml (Li et al., 2004). Plants of the *Aglaia* genus, which typically grow in Southeast Asia, are widely used in traditional Chinese medicine, containing phytochemicals known as flavaglines. Flavaglines exhibit activity against several viral diseases, such as coronavirus, Ebola, dengue, and chikungunya (Nebigil et al., 2020). *Illicium verum*, a medicinal plant from China, exhibited dose-dependent antiviral activity against iridovirus infection (Liu et al., 2020).

3.3.3 MEDICINAL PLANTS FROM THE AMERICAS WITH ANTIVIRAL ACTIVITY

Ethanol extracts of *Heisteria acuminata* and aqueous extracts of *Eupatorium articulatum* displayed antiviral activity against vesicular stomatitis virus (VSV) and HSV-1. Aqueous extracts of *Tagetes pusilla* (native to Venezuela), *Baccharis teindalensis* (Ecuador) and *Eupatorium glutinosum* also prevented VSV replication (Abad et al., 1999). Other plants from South America such as *Limonium brasiliense*, *Psidium guajava*, and *Phyllanthus niruri* were reported to exhibit antiviral activity against HSV-1 with IC_{50} values of 185, 118, and 60 µg/ml, respectively (Faral-Tello et al., 2012). In another study, the antiviral activity of 100 medicinal plant species from British Columbia, Canada, were screened against seven viruses. Extracts from *Rosa nutkana* (Canada) and *Amelanchier alnifolia* (North America) were found to be potent against coronavirus. Extracts of *Potentilla arguta* root and *Sambucus racemosa* branch tips inhibited infection from the respiratory syncytial virus (RSV) whereas *Ipomopsis aggregata* inhibited infection by parainfluenza virus type 3 infection. Proliferation of rotavirus was prevented by root extract from *Lomatium dissectum* from North America. *Cardamine angulata, Lysichiton americanum, Polypodium glycyrrhiza, Conocephalum conicum* (all native to North America), and

Verbascum thapsus (native to Europe but naturalized in North America) showed antiviral effect against HSV-1 (McCutcheon et al., 1995; Jassim and Naji, 2003).

3.3.4 INDIAN AYURVEDIC PLANTS WITH ANTIVIRAL ACTIVITY

Ayurveda is a product of India's rich tradition of herbal knowledge, with the term meaning "the experience of life". Many medicinal plants are used in Ayurveda to treat viral diseases, and now research has been initiated to develop a scientific validation for the antiviral activity of these medicinal herbs (Kalyani, 2013). Aqueous extracts and freeze-dried powder of *Punica granatum* displayed antiviral activity against HSV infections and demonstrated the highest selectivity index (the ratio between antiviral activity and cytotoxicity) of 14 and 12.5, respectively (Jadhav et al., 2012). Aqueous extract of leaves and stem of *Swertia chirata* showed antiviral activity against HSV, confirmed by the plaque reduction assay and the time kinetics of the HSV-1 antigen expression assays (Verma et al., 2008). Balasubramanian et al. (2007) surveyed the viral white spot syndrome in shrimp and screened 20 medicinal plants for antiviral activity, finding that *Aegle marmelos, Cynodon dactylon, Lantana camara, Momordica charantia*, and *Phyllanthus amarus* exhibited potent activity. A study on the antiviral activity of medicinal plants from southern India found that several, such as *Sphaeranthus indicus, Cassia alata, Indigofera tinctoria, Vitex trifolia, Clerodendrum inerme, Leucas aspera*, and *Clitoria ternatea*, showed antiviral activity against mouse coronavirus and HSV infections (Vimalanathan et al., 2009). In addition to these plant extracts, many individual active phytochemicals, such as andrographolide from *Andrographis paniculata* and curcumin from turmeric (*Curcuma longa*), have also undergone clinical evaluation studies against viral diseases (Dhawan, 2012). *Embelia ribes*, also known as false black pepper, is used in Ayurveda to promote longevity and to treat diabetic ulcers, etc. An ethyl acetate fraction of fruits of *E. ribes* showed antiviral activity against the influenza virus. Its primary active compound, embelin, exhibited greatest activity when used at the early stages of infection (Hossan et al., 2018). Dried seeds of *Azadirachta indica* possesses many medicinal properties, such as anti-inflammatory, antiviral, antibacterial, anti-hyperglycaemic activities, etc. In a study conducted using Vero cells, a petroleum ether extract of *A. indica* oil (50 μg/ml) showed antiviral effects against poliovirus multiplication, whereas *Baccharis trinervis* exhibited antiviral activity against HSV-1 replication at concentrations of 50–200 μg/ml (Sai Ram et al., 2000). *Arisaema tortuosum* is widely found in India's Himalayas and Western Ghats and has been commonly used in traditional medicine to treat various ailments for many years. A chloroform-soluble fraction of leaves of *A. tortuosum* exhibited anti-HSV type 2 activity. The extract also showed antiviral activity against acyclovir-resistant HSV-2 and HSV-1. It was found that the flavones apigenin and luteolin are the two significant bioactives present in the extract responsible for this antiviral activity (Rittà et al., 2020). Some of the frequently studied medical plants have been shown to contain antiviral compounds, and their details are shown in Figure 3.1 and Table 3.1.

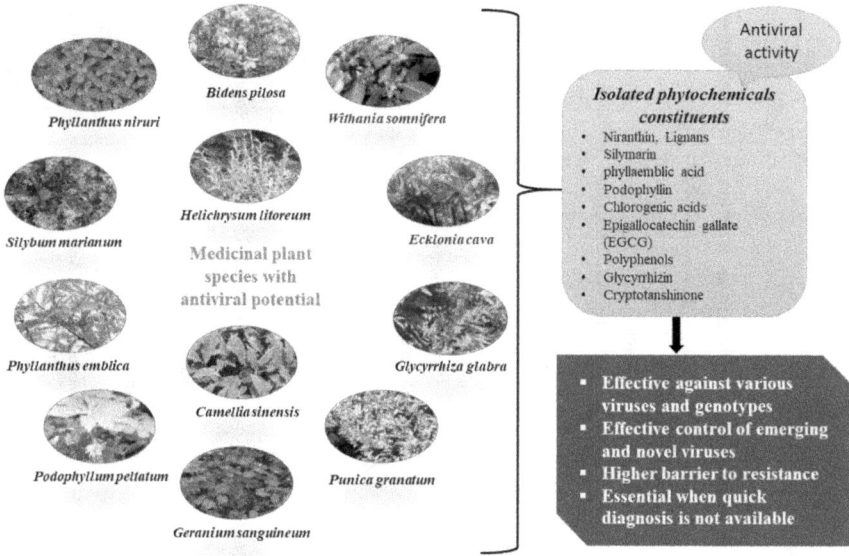

FIGURE 3.1   Plant-based antiviral compounds and their applications.

3.4   RECENT INSIGHTS ON ANTIVIRAL ACTIVITIES OF MEDICINAL PLANTS

3.4.1   MEDICINAL PLANTS FOR TREATMENT OF VIRAL HEPATITIS

The viral liver disease hepatitis is triggered by an inflamed liver and causes various infections, named hepatitis type A, B, C, D, and E. Although susceptibility to these viruses results in acute illness, types B, C, and D are uniquely correlated with a chronic condition. Conventional viral hepatitis medicines are based primarily on plants from the Euphorbiaceae family, particularly the genus *Phyllanthus*. Venkateswaran et al. (1987) showed that active components in the aqueous extract of *Phyllanthus niruri* inhibited replication of HBV and the woodchuck hepatitis virus (WHV). 3-Hydroxy caruilignan C (3-HCL-C), isolated from *Swietenia macrophylla* stems, exhibited potent anti-HCV activity by inhibiting HCV replication (Wu et al., 2012). *Embelia ribes* plant extracts enriched with quercetin inhibited non-structural protein 3 (NS3) which exhibits RNA helicase and serine protease activities, and heat shock proteins, thereby inhibiting HCV (Bachmetov et al., 2012). Wahyuni et al. (2013) conducted a study in Huh7.5 cells using nine strains of HCV (1a to 7a, 1b and 2b) with different genotypes. The ethanol extracts prepared from *Toona sureni* leaves, *Melicope latifolia* leaves, *Ficus fistulosa* leaves, and *Melanolepis multiglandulosa* stem prevented replication of all the nine genotypes of HCV. Niranthin extracted from *P. niruri* showed strong anti-HBV efficacy in both cell lines and animal models. Subsequently, niranthin demonstrated a defensive role against liver

TABLE 3.1

Ethnobotanical Data on Medicinal Plants Used Against Various Viral Diseases

Virus	Antiviral Plant Responsible	Antiviral Compound(s) Responsible	Plant Part(s)	Extract Type	Type of Test Model Studied	Mechanism of Action	References
HBV/HCV	*Phyllanthus niruri*	Niranthin, lignans	Whole plant	Aqueous	HepG2 cells	Inhibits replication of HBV DNA and expression of HBV antigen	Yong Li et al. (2017)
	Silybum marianum	Silymarin/silibinin	Seeds	Ethanol	HeLa cells	Serum ALT, AST reduction	Wagoner et al. (2010)
	Phyllanthus emblica	Phyllaemblic acid, phyllaemblic acids B and C, phyllaemblicin	Roots	70% ethanol	A549 cells	Inhibition of hepatitis C, HSV-1, and anti-CVB3	Lv et al. (2014)
HSV	*Podophyllum peltatum*	Podophyllin, deoxypodophyllotoxin	–	Ethanol	Lung fibroblast cells	Inhibition of HSV-1 and HSV-2 replication	Sudo et al. (1998)
	Bidens pilosa	Chlorogenic acid, feruloyl-caffeoylquinic acid	Seeds	Aqueous	Vero and RAW cells	Reduces the infectivity of HSV-1 strain, inhibits HSV-1 replication	Nakama et al. (2012)
	Helichrysum litoreum	6,11-Diacetyl-9,11-dihydroxydrimane	Leaves	Aqueous	Human lung fibroblasts	Reduction of HSV-1 viral replication	Guarino and Sciarrillo (2003)
Influenza virus	*Camellia sinensis*	EGCG, ECG, EGC	Leaves	Aqueous	MDCK cells	Inhibition of viral RNA synthesis, viral haemagglutinin and neuraminidase	Song et al. (2005)
	Geranium sanguineum	Polyphenols	Roots	Aqueous and alcohol	Mice	Inhibition of viral replication	Serkedjieva et al. (2008)
	Cistus incanus	Polyphenol-rich extract (CYSTUS052)	–	–	A549; MDCK cells	Reduction of influenza A viral replication	Ehrhardt et al. (2007)

(Continued)

TABLE 3.1 (CONTINUED)

Ethnobotanical Data on Medicinal Plants Used Against Various Viral Diseases

Virus	Antiviral Plant Responsible	Antiviral Compound(s) Responsible	Plant Part(s)	Extract Type	Type of Test Model Studied	Mechanism of Action	References
	Punica granatum	Ellagic acid, caffeic acid, luteolin and punicalagin	Fruit	-	MDCK cells	Inhibition of viral replication and viral entry	Haidari et al. (2009)
	Allium fistulosum	Fructans	-	-	Mice	Inhibition of viral replication	Lee et al., (2012)
	Sambucus nigra	-	Berry	Concentrated juice	Mice	Suppression of viral replication in the bronchoalveolar lavage fluids, and increased levels of the IFV-specific neutralizing antibody	Kinoshita et al. (2012)
	Shahakusan	Kampo medicine	Mori Cortex roots, Lycii Cortex roots, *Glycyrriza uralensis* roots, Oryzae Fructus caryopses	Aqueous	Mice	Immunomodulating activity through action of NK cells	Hokari et al. (2012)
	Rapanea melanophloeos and *Pittosporum viridiflorum*	-	-	Methanol, ethanol (100% and 30%), acetone, hot and cold water	MDCK cells	Modification of viral titre loads	Mehrbod et al. (2018)
	Geranium thunbergii	Kaempferitrin and geraniin	-	Ethanol	MDCK and A549 cells	Inhibition of neuraminidase	Choi et al. (2019)

(Continued)

TABLE 3.1 (CONTINUED)
Ethnobotanical Data on Medicinal Plants Used Against Various Viral Diseases

Virus	Antiviral Plant Responsible	Antiviral Compound(s) Responsible	Plant Part(s)	Extract Type	Type of Test Model Studied	Mechanism of Action	References
SARS-CoV	Glycyrrhiza glabra	Glycyrrhizin	Roots	Aqueous	Vero cells	Inhibition of SARS-associated virus replication	Cinatl et al. (2003)
	Withania somnifera	Withanoside V, somniferine	Roots	Aqueous	Molecular docking study	Binds to SARS virus	Shree et al. (2020)
	Ecklonia cava	Dieckol	Whole plant	Ethanol	SARS-CoV- 3CL (pro) cells	Inhibition of the SARS-CoV 3CL (pro) activity	Park et al. (2013)
	Salvia miltiorrhiza	Cryptotanshinone	Roots	Hexane	SARS-CoV PLpro	Dose- and time-dependent SARS-CoV inhibition in the slow- binding process of PLpro behaviour	Benarba and Pandiella (2020)

damage induced by HBV in ducklings (Liu et al., 2014). The ethanol fraction of *P. niruri*, enriched with ellagic acid, exerted cytotoxic effects against HepG2/C3A cells infected with HBV (Yong Li et al., 2017).

3.4.2 MEDICINAL PLANTS FOR TREATMENT OF HSV

HSV (both HSV-1 and HSV-2) are human pathogenic viruses that primarily affect adults. After latency has been developed, HSV can reactivate and cause repeated infections in some patients, whereas most people have few, if any, repeat episodes (Yoosook et al., 1989). Podophyllotoxin, a phytochemical extracted from the aqueous extract of *Podophyllum peltatum*, inhibited HSV-1 (Bedows and Hatfield, 1982). *Helichrysum litoreum* plant extracts (1.35 mg fresh weight/ml) exhibited antiviral activity against HSV-1 in human lung fibroblasts (Guarino and Sciarrillo, 2003). Lyu et al. (2005) performed a study to determine the anti-herpetic activities of flavonoids, using Vero cells infected with HSV-1 and HSV-2. Of the 18 flavonoids tested, epicatechin (EC), galangin, epicatechin gallate (ECG), and kaempferol showed potent antiviral activity against HSV-1. Aqueous and ethanolic extracts from *Pelargonium sidoides* demonstrated anti-HSV activity (Schnitzler et al., 2008). *Opuntia streptacantha* blocked virus multiplication and down-regulated extracellular viruses, such as HSV, equine herpes virus, pseudorabies virus, etc. *Bidens pilosa* extract showed potent virucidal activity against HSV-1 and HSV-2 (Marina et al., 2018).

3.4.3 MEDICINAL PLANTS FOR TREATING INFLUENZA VIRUS

Influenza viruses are universal and show marked annual morbidity and mortality worldwide (Cannell et al., 2008). Among the three types of influenza viruses, type A has caused significant health concerns to humans (Hudson, 2009). Song et al. (2005) demonstrated that aqueous extracts of *Camellia sinensis* (green tea) affected influenza A and B virus strains by inhibiting viral RNA synthesis, viral haemagglutinin and neuraminidase. Aqueous and alcoholic extracts of *Geranium sanguineum* aerial roots showed antiviral activities against influenza A virus, mainly by preventing virus multiplication (Serkedjieva et al., 2008). *Cistus incanus* extracts, rich in catechins, achieved its antiviral activity by reducing the replication of the influenza A virus (Ehrhardt et al., 2007). Haidari et al. (2009) showed that polyphenol-rich extracts of pomegranate exerted effects against the influenza virus by preventing virus replication and its entry into the host cell. Fructans isolated from a hot aqueous extract of the leafy part of *Allium fistulosum* inhibited virus replication in a mouse model and exhibited anti-influenza virus activity (Lee et al., 2012). Administration of concentrated elderberry juice (*Sambucus nigra*) to mice infected with influenza virus showed anti-influenza virus activity, with viral replication being suppressed (Kinoshita et al., 2012). Hokari et al. (2012) showed that Shahakusan, a Kampo (Japanese herbal) medicine, exhibited an anti-influenza virus effect in mice through NK cell action by altering immunomodulating activity. Five South African medicinal plants, extracted using methanol, ethanol (100% and 30%), acetone, hot and cold water, were screened for anti-influenza activity using Madin–Darby canine kidney

(MDCK) cells. Among the five plant species tested, *Rapanea melanophloeos* and *Pittosporum viridiflorum* showed strong anti-viral activity (Mehrbod et al., 2018). An ethanolic extract of the traditional Korean herbal preparation Geranii Herba, made from *Geranium* sp., showed higher anti-influenza activity in MDCK by inhibiting neuraminidase than was achieved with oseltamivir, the commercial synthetic anti-viral medication (Choi et al., 2019).

3.4.4   MEDICINAL PLANTS FOR TREATING SARS-CoV

The first coronavirus (SARS-CoV) outbreak was reported in 2002. MERS-CoV, first reported in 2012, has shown that coronaviruses can cross between hosts of different genera and appear as highly pathogenic viruses in humans (Lu et al., 2015). Recently, a very large number of cases of COVID-19 have been witnessed in many countries around the world since 2020. Hispidulin, a flavonoid found in *Salvia officinalis*, *Helichrysum bracteatum*, *Grindelia argentina*, *Crossostephium chinense*, and *Artemisia* spp., exhibits pharmacological activities, such as antioxidant, antifungal, anti-inflammatory, antimutagenic, and antiviral activites (Kavvadias et al., 2004). Studies in mice showed that hispudilin (50–150 mg/kg) prevented bromobenzene-induced liver damage and lipid oxidation, thereby acting against viral toxicity (Ferrándiz et al., 1994). Cirsimaritin is a bioflavonoid present in many medicinal plants, including *Cantuarea pseudosinaica*, *Micotea debilis*, *Salvia palaestina*, and *Scorparia centaurea* (Adeem Mahmood and Hamad Alkhathlan, 2020). An *in-silico* study evaluated the efficacy of phytochemicals against SARS-CoV-2 Mpro and ACE2, compared with hydroxychloroquine, showed that hispidulin, quercetin, and cirsimaritin exhibited greater inhibitory ability in terms of virus-binding affinity than did hydroxychloroquine (Shah et al., 2020). Jensenone is a monoterpenoid found in eucalyptus essential oil (Goodger et al., 2016). The potential of Jensenone as an inhibitor of SARS-CoV-2 Mpro was evaluated using an *in-silico* method, finding that Jensenone had a sizeable binding affinity with low binding energies (Sharma and Kaur, 2020). Glycyrrhizin, a triterpene saponin present in *Glycyrrhiza glabra*, could be a potential candidate for COVID-19 inhibition, based on its potential to bind to ACE2, thereby down-regulating levels of pro-inflammatory cytokines, preventing the accumulation of intracellular reactive oxygen species, inhibiting thrombin accumulation, and activating endogenous interferon (Luo et al., 2020).

3.5   SIGNIFICANCE OF ANTIVIRAL DRUGS FROM NATURAL SOURCES

The identification, supply, and use of effective medications are among the necessities for primary health care quality. Plants have long been an important source of drugs, be it in the context of conventional tissue extracts or as pure active constituents. For decades, the natural origin of medical substances, with many valuable medicines produced from plant sources, pioneered treatments against many important diseases

(Mushtaq et al., 2018). Consequently, it is appropriate for decision makers to include commonly available plants or plant extracts on the national list of medicinal products or to use them to substitute for those prescription preparations that need to be bought and imported. Around 12,000 secondary metabolites have been extracted from medicinal plants, but this amount is estimated to be only a small proportion (<10%) of the total phytochemicals, such as quinine, atropine, galantamine, vinblastine and vincristine, terpenoids, flavonoids, etc., which are a tremendous resource for human health researchers.

3.6   CLINICAL RATIONALE FOR ANTIVIRAL MEDICINAL PLANTS

There are many benefits to using natural medicines. Medicinal plants appear to be more successful for treating long-term health conditions which do not react adequately to conventional medication. Medicinal plants typically have adequate beneficial health effects and can be used more safely over time. For severe and abrupt infections, on the other hand, mainstream medicine usually prevails. New conventional treatments for treating disease and injuries are regarded as being far safer than natural or alternative therapies (Craig, 1999). Herbal medicine is now mostly regarded as an unsubstantiated, flawed topic. Whereas the past history of herbal medicine provides anecdotal evidence from many decades, centuries, or even millennia of use, the systematic research of herbal medicine is still in its adolescence. Although modern-day medical practitioners remain dismissive of herbal medicine, many conventional medicines used in practice today were originally extracted from plant resources.

3.7   CHALLENGES AND FUTURE PERSPECTIVES

Plant-based herbal antiviral drugs are released to the market without any compulsory protection or toxicological review of the impact of the medication. Many countries still lack reliable machinery for governing the activities and quality requirements of herbal medicines. Problems linked to regulatory status, protection, and effectiveness evaluation, quality management, and safety compliance abound, and incomplete or poor awareness of traditional, complementary or alternative medicines is prevalent in many countries (Zhou et al., 2013). The concept of dietary supplement is that of a food which is consumed which is meant to supplement the diet and includes a "dietary" ingredient, in which various vitamins, minerals, herbs, or other botanicals needed by the body can be used as a dietary supplement. No additional toxicity tests are usually needed under the Dietary Supplement Health and Education Act of 1994 (DSHEA) of the United States if the herb was on the market prior to 1994 (Dietary Supplements I FDA, 2020). The other significant problem in many countries is the reality that regulatory knowledge on herbal medicinal goods is often not exchanged amongst regulators and centres of safety testing or pharmacovigilance. No one can refute that the protection and efficacy assessment of herbal medicinal products, as well as the corresponding testing procedures, criteria, and methods, are far more complicated than those needed for conventional single-chemical pharmaceuticals (Dietary Supplement Fact Sheets, 2020).

There can be hundreds of natural constituents in a single herbal remedy or medicinal plant species, and a herbal medicinal substance blended from several herbal plant species can include many times the number present in a single species. It can be practically impossible to assess the effects, including safety, of individual active constituents, particularly if the herbal product consists of a mixture of two or more herbs. The consistency of the raw materials used in the manufacture of herbal medicinal products primarily determines the consistency of the safety and effectiveness of the preparation. The nature of the source or raw material depends not only on intrinsic (genetic) influences, but also on external factors, such as environmental conditions, farming and medicinal plant collecting practices, like selection of the correct plant and plant part, and cultivation conditions. This combination of several variables makes quality controls on the raw materials of herbal pharmaceutical goods impossible to carry out (Rodrigues and Barnes, 2013). A variety of causes are responsible for harmful effects resulting from the use of herbal medicinal products, including the use of incorrect plant species, adulteration of herbal products, undeclared medicinal products, poisoning, overdose, abuse of herbal medicinal products by health care practitioners or customers, and the use (and subsequent interaction) of herbal medicinal products with other medicinal products. There is a shortage of proper information on the significance of taxonomic botany and documentation in most herbal medicinal products manufacturers, which presents unique challenges in identifying and harvesting herbal plants (Farah et al., 2000; Bhardwaj et al., 2018).

3.8   CONCLUSION

The global disease burden caused by viral infection has encouraged researchers worldwide to develop novel and more effective antiviral drugs. Medicinal plants have provided ample scope for researchers to explore and establish viable alternative treatments for many emerging viral infections. In this chapter, the significance and treatment options of medicinal plants for managing various viral diseases have been discussed. Although the molecular mechanisms behind the antiviral effects of medicinal plants are often well documented, controlled human clinical trials are still warranted. Overall, this chapter should help current and future researchers to find, understand, and assess new molecules from the numerous antiviral medicinal plants available.

REFERENCES

Abad, M.J., P. Bermejo, S. Sanchez Palomino, X. Chiriboga, and L. Carrasco. 1999. "Antiviral activity of some South American medicinal plants." *Phytotherapy Research* 13 (2). John Wiley & Sons, Ltd: 142–46.

Adeem Mahmood, and Hamad Z. Alkhathlan. 2020. "Isolation, synthesis and pharmacological applications of Cirsimaritin – A short review." *Academia Journal of Medicinal Plants.* doi:10.15413/ajmp.2019.0159.

Akram, Muhammad, Imtiaz Mahmood Tahir, Syed Muhammad Ali Shah, Zahed Mahmood, Awais Altaf, Khalil Ahmad, Naveed Munir, Muhammad Daniyal, Suhaila Nasir, and Huma Mehboob. 2018. "Antiviral potential of medicinal plants against HIV,

HSV, Influenza, Hepatitis, and Coxsackievirus: A systematic review." *Phytotherapy Research*. John Wiley and Sons Ltd. doi:10.1002/ptr.6024.

Bachmetov, L., M. Gal-Tanamy, A. Shapira, M. Vorobeychik, T. Giterman-Galam, P. Sathiyamoorthy, A. Golan-Goldhirsh, I. Benhar, R. Tur-Kaspa, and R. Zemel. 2012. "Suppression of hepatitis C virus by the flavonoid Quercetin is mediated by inhibition of NS3 protease activity." *Journal of Viral Hepatitis* 19 (2). John Wiley & Sons, Ltd: e81–88. doi:10.1111/j.1365-2893.2011.01507.x.

Balasubramanian, G., M. Sarathi, S. R. Kumar, A.S. Sahul Hameed. 2007. "Screening the antiviral activity of Indian medicinal plants against white spot syndrome virus in shrimp". *Aquaculture*, 263 (1–4) (2007), pp. 15–19.

Bedows, E, and G.M. Hatfield. 1982. "An investigation of the antiviral activity of *Podophyllum peltatum*." *Journal of Natural Products* 45 (6). American Chemical Society: 725–29. doi:10.1021/np50024a015.

Benarba, Bachir and Atanasio Pandiella. 2020. "Medicinal plants as sources of active molecules against COVID-19." *Frontiers in Pharmacology*. Frontiers Media S.A. doi:10.3389/fphar.2020.01189.

Bhardwaj, Shubham, Rajeshwar Verma and Jyoti Gupta. 2018. "Challenges and future prospects of herbal medicine." *International Research in Medical and Health Science*, October. Academic and Scholar Publications. doi:10.36437/irmhs.2018.1.1.d.

Boukhatem, Mohamed Nadjib and William N. Setzer. 2020. "Aromatic herbs, medicinal plant-derived essential oils, and phytochemical extracts as potential therapies for coronaviruses: future perspectives." *Plants*. MDPI AG. doi:10.3390/PLANTS9060800.

Cannell, John J., Michael Zasloff, Cedric F. Garland, Robert Scragg, and Edward Giovannucci. 2008. "On the epidemiology of influenza." *Virology Journal*. BioMed Central. doi:10.1186/1743-422X-5-29.

Chantril, B.H., C.E. Coulthard, Oulthard, L. Dickinson, G.W. Inkley, W. Morris, and A.H. Pyle, 1952. "The action of plant extracts on a bacteriophage of *Pseudomonas pyocyanea* and on Influenza A virus." *Journal of General Microbiology* 6 (1–2). J Gen Microbiol: 74–84. doi:10.1099/00221287-6-1-2-74.

Chen, Jieliang. 2020. "Pathogenicity and transmissibility of 2019-NCoV—A quick overview and comparison with other emerging viruses." *Microbes and Infection* 22 (2). Elsevier Masson SAS: 69–71. doi:10.1016/j.micinf.2020.01.004.

Chisari, F.V., M. Isogawa, and S.F. Wieland. 2010. "Pathogenesis of Hepatitis B virus infection." *Pathologie Biologie*. NIH Public Access. doi:10.1016/j.patbio.2009.11.001.

Choi, Jang Gi, Young Soo Kim, Ji Hye Kim, and Hwan Suck Chung. 2019. "Antiviral activity of ethanol extract of geranii herba and its components against influenza viruses via neuraminidase inhibition." *Scientific Reports* 9 (1). Nature Publishing Group. doi:10.1038/s41598-019-48430-8.

Cinatl, J., B. Morgenstern, G. Bauer, P. Chandra, H. Rabenau, and H.W. Doerr. 2003. "Glycyrrhizin, an active component of Liquorice roots, and replication of SARS-associated Coronavirus." *Lancet* 361 (9374). Elsevier Limited: 2045–46. doi:10.1016/S0140-6736(03)13615-X.

Craig, Winston J. 1999. "Health-promoting properties of common herbs." In *American Journal of Clinical Nutrition*, 70 Supplement:491s–499s. American Society for Nutrition. doi:10.1093/ajcn/70.3.491s.

Dhawan, B.N. 2012. "Anti-viral activity of Indian plants." *Proceedings of the National Academy of Sciences India Section B - Biological Sciences*. Nature Publishing Group. doi:10.1007/s40011-011-0016-7.

"Dietary Supplement Fact Sheets." 2020. Accessed November 10. https://ods.od.nih.gov/factsheets/list-all/.

"Dietary Supplements I FDA." 2020. Accessed November 10. https://www.fda.gov/food/dietary-supplements.

Ehrhardt, Christina, Thorsten Wolff, Stephan Pleschka, Oliver Planz, Wiebke Beermann, Johannes G. Bode, Mirco Schmolke, and Stephan Ludwig. 2007. "Influenza A virus NS1 protein activates the PI3K/Akt pathway to mediate antiapoptotic signaling responses." *Journal of Virology* 81 (7). American Society for Microbiology: 3058–67. doi:10.1128/jvi.02082-06.

Farah, Mohamed H., Ralph Edwards, Marie Lindquist, Christine Leon, and Debbie Shaw. 2000. "International monitoring of adverse health effects associated with herbal medicines." *Pharmacoepidemiology and Drug Safety* 9 (2). Pharmacoepidemiol Drug Saf: 105–12. doi:10.1002/(SICI)1099-1557(200003/04)9:2<105::AID-PDS486>3.0. CO;2-2.

Faral-Tello, Paula, Santiago Mirazo, Carmelo Dutra, Andrés Pérez, Lucía Geis-Asteggiante, Sandra Frabasile, Elina Koncke, et al. 2012. "Cytotoxic, virucidal, and antiviral activity of South American plant and algae extracts." *The Scientific World Journal* 2012. doi:10.1100/2012/174837.

Ferrándiz, M.L., G. Bustos, M. Payá, R. Gunasegaran, and M.J. Alcaraz. 1994. "Hispidulin protection against hepatotoxicity induced by bromobenzene in mice." *Life Sciences* 55 (8). Pergamon: PL145–50. doi:10.1016/0024-3205(94)00490-0.

García-Sastre, Adolfo, Andrej Egorov, Demetrius Matassov, Sabine Brandt, David E. Levy, Joan E. Durbin, Peter Palese, and Thomas Muster. 1998. "Influenza A virus lacking the NS1 gene replicates in Interferon-deficient systems." *Virology* 252 (2). Academic Press Inc.: 324–30. doi:10.1006/viro.1998.9508.

Goodger, Jason Q.D., Samiddhi L. Seneratne, Dean Nicolle, and Ian E. Woodrow. 2016. "Foliar essential oil glands of Eucalyptus subgenus Eucalyptus (Myrtaceae) are a rich source of flavonoids and related non-volatile constituents." Edited by Björn Hamberger. *PLOS ONE* 11 (3). Public Library of Science: e0151432. doi:10.1371/journal.pone.0151432.

Guarino, C., and R. Sciarrillo. 2003. "Inhibition of Herpes Simplex Virus Type 1 by aqueous extracts from leaves of *Helichrysum litoreum* Guss." *Bollettino Chimico Farmaceutico* 142 (6): 242–43.

Haidari, Mehran, Muzammil Ali, Samuel Ward Casscells, and Mohammad Madjid. 2009. "Pomegranate (*Punica granatum*) purified polyphenol extract inhibits influenza virus and has a synergistic effect with oseltamivir." *Phytomedicine* 16 (12): 1127–36. doi:10.1016/j.phymed.2009.06.002.

Hamming, I., W. Timens, M. L.C. Bulthuis, A. T. Lely, G. J. Navis, and H. van Goor. 2004. "Tissue distribution of ACE2 protein, the functional receptor for SARS Coronavirus. A first step in understanding SARS pathogenesis." *Journal of Pathology* 203 (2): 631–37. doi:10.1002/path.1570.

Hokari, Rei, Takayuki Nagai, and Haruki Yamada. 2012. "In vivo anti-influenza virus activity of Japanese herbal (Kampo) medicine, 'Shahakusan,' and its possible mode of action." *Evidence-Based Complementary and Alternative Medicine* 2012. Hindawi Limited: 13. doi:10.1155/2012/794970.

Hossan, Md Shahadat, Ayesha Fatima, Mohammed Rahmatullah, Teng Jin Khoo, Veeranoot Nissapatorn, Anastasia V. Galochkina, Alexander V. Slita, et al. 2018. "Antiviral activity of *Embelia ribes Burm. F.* against Influenza Virus in vitro." *Archives of Virology* 163 (8). Springer-Verlag Wien: 2121–31. doi:10.1007/s00705-018-3842-6.

Hudson, James B. 2009. "The use of herbal extracts in the control of influenza." *Journal of Medicinal Plants Research* 3. Academic Journals. doi:10.5897/JMPR.9001242.

Jadhav, Priyanka, Natasha Kapoor, Becky Thomas, Hingorani Lal, and Nilima Kshirsagar. 2012. "Antiviral potential of selected Indian medicinal (Ayurvedic) plants against Herpes Simplex Virus 1 and 2." *North American Journal of Medical Sciences*. Wolters Kluwer -- Medknow Publications. doi:10.4103/1947-2714.104316.

Jassim, Sabah A.A., and M.A. Naji. 2003. "Novel antiviral agents: a medicinal plant perspective." *Journal of Applied Microbiology* 95 (3): 412–27. doi:10.1046/j.1365-2672.2003.02026.x.

Kalyani P. 2013. "Antiviral activity of some Indian medicinal herbs." *Indian Journal of Pharmacy Practice* 6 (2). doi:Nill.

Kavvadias, Dominique, Philipp Sand, Kuresh A. Youdim, M. Zeeshan Qaiser, Catherine Rice-Evans, Roland Baur, Erwin Sigel, Wolf Dieter Rausch, Peter Riederer, and Peter Schreier. 2004. "The flavone hispidulin, a benzodiazepine receptor ligand with positive allosteric properties, traverses the blood-brain barrier and exhibits anticonvulsive effects." *British Journal of Pharmacology* 142 (5). Wiley-Blackwell: 811–20. doi:10.1038/sj.bjp.0705828.

Kimura, Takashi, and Diane E. Griffin. 2003. "Extensive immune-mediated hippocampal damage in mice surviving infection with neuroadapted Sindbis virus." *Virology* 311 (1). Academic Press Inc.: 28–39. doi:10.1016/S0042-6822(03)00110-7.

Kinoshita, Emiko, Kyoko Hayashi, Hiroshi Katayama, Toshimitsu Hayashi, and Akio Obata. 2012. "Anti-influenza virus effects of elderberry juice and its fractions." *Bioscience, Biotechnology and Biochemistry* 76 (9): 1633–38. doi:10.1271/bbb.120112.

Lanford, Therapeutic silencing of microRNA-122 in primates with chronic hepatitis C virus infection Robert E., Elisabeth S. Hildebrandt-Eriksen, Andreas Petri, Robert Persson, Morten Lindow, Martin E. Munk, Sakari Kauppinen, and Henrik Rum. 2010. "Therapeutic silencing of MicroRNA-122 in primates with chronic Hepatitis C virus infection." *Science* 327 (5962). Science: 198–201. doi:10.1126/science.1178178.

Lee, Jung Bum, Sachi Miyake, Ryo Umetsu, Kyoko Hayashi, Takeshi Chijimatsu, and Toshimitsu Hayashi. 2012. "Anti-influenza A virus effects of fructan from Welsh onion (*Allium fistulosum* L.)." *Food Chemistry* 134 (4): 2164–68. doi:10.1016/j.foodchem.2012.04.016.

Li, Fu Shuang, and Jing Ke Weng. 2017. "Demystifying traditional herbal medicine with modern approaches." *Nature Plants*. Palgrave Macmillan Ltd. doi:10.1038/nplants.2017.109.

Li, Yaolan, Linda S.M. Ooi, Hua Wang, Paul P.H. But, and Vincent E.C. Ooi. 2004. "Antiviral activities of medicinal herbs traditionally used in Southern Mainland China." *Phytotherapy Research* 18 (9). Phytother Res: 718–22. doi:10.1002/ptr.1518.

Li, Yong, Xin Li, Jia Kun Wang, Yan Kuang, and Ming Xiu Qi. 2017. "Anti-Hepatitis B viral activity of *Phyllanthus niruri* L (Phyllanthaceae) in HepG2/C3A and SK-HEP-1 Cells." *Tropical Journal of Pharmaceutical Research* 16 (8). University of Benin: 1873–79. doi:10.4314/tjpr.v16i8.17.

Liu, Mingzhu, Qing Yu, Hehe Xiao, Yi Yi, Hao Cheng, Dedi Fazriansyah Putra, Yaming Huang, Qin Zhang, and Pengfei Li. 2020. "Antiviral activity of *Illicium verum* Hook. f. extracts against Grouper Iridovirus infection." *Journal of Fish Diseases* 43 (5). Blackwell Publishing Ltd: 531–40. doi:10.1111/jfd.13146.

Liu, Sheng, Wanxing Wei, Kaichuang Shi, Xun Cao, Min Zhou, and Zhiping Liu. 2014. "In vitro and in vivo anti-hepatitis B virus activities of the lignan Niranthin isolated from *Phyllanthus niruri* L." *Journal of Ethnopharmacology* 155 (2). Elsevier Ireland Ltd: 1061–67. doi:10.1016/j.jep.2014.05.064.

Lu, Guangwen, Qihui Wang, and George F. Gao. 2015. "Bat-to-Human: Spike features determining 'host Jump' of Coronaviruses SARS-CoV, MERS-CoV, and beyond." *Trends in Microbiology* 23 (8). Elsevier Ltd: 468–78. doi:10.1016/j.tim.2015.06.003.

Luo P, Liu D, and Li J. 2020. "Pharmacological perspective: glycyrrhizin may be an efficacious therapeutic agent for COVID-19." International Journal of Antimicrobial Agents 55(6):105995. doi:10.1016/j.ijantimicag.2020.105995

Lv, Jun Jiang, Ya Feng Wang, Jing Min Zhang, Shan Yu, Dong Wang, Hong Tao Zhu, Rong Rong Cheng, Chong Ren Yang, Min Xu, and Ying Jun Zhang. 2014. "Anti-Hepatitis B virus activities and absolute configurations of sesquiterpenoid glycosides from *Phyllanthus emblica*." *Organic and Biomolecular Chemistry* 12 (43). Royal Society of Chemistry: 8764–74. doi:10.1039/c4ob01196a.

Lyu, Su Yun, Jee Young Rhim, and Won Bong Park. 2005. "Antiherpetic activities of flavonoids against herpes simplex virus type 1 (HSV-1) and type 2 (HSV-2) in vitro." *Archives of Pharmacal Research* 28 (11). Pharmaceutical Society of Korea: 1293–1301. doi:10.1007/BF02978215.

Ma, Li, and Lei Yao. 2020. "Antiviral effects of plant-derived essential oils and their components: An updated review." *Molecules* 25 (11). NLM (Medline): 2627. doi:10.3390/molecules25112627.

Ma, Shuang Cheng, Jiang Du, Paul Pui Hay But, Xue Long Deng, Yong Wen Zhang, Vincent Eng Choon Ooi, Hong Xi Xu, Spencer Hon Sun Lee, and Song Fong Lee. 2002. "Antiviral Chinese medicinal herbs against Respiratory Syncytial Virus." *Journal of Ethnopharmacology* 79 (2). J Ethnopharmacol: 205–11. doi:10.1016/S0378-8741(01)00389-0.

Marina, A. Padilla, C. Simoni Isabela, Moreira H. Hoe Veronica, Judite B. Fernandes Maria, W. Arns Clarice, R. Brito Juliana, and Henrique G. Lago João. 2018. "In vitro antiviral activity of Brazilian Cerrado plant extracts against animal and human herpesviruses." *Journal of Medicinal Plants Research* 12 (10). Academic Journals: 106–15. doi:10.5897/jmpr2018.6567.

Maryam, Maqsood, Kian Keong TE, Fai Chu Wong, Tsun Thai CHAI, Gary K.K. Low, Seng Chiew Gan, and Hui yee Chee. 2020. "Antiviral activity of traditional Chinese medicinal plants *Dryopteris crassirhizoma* and *Morus alba* against dengue virus." *Journal of Integrative Agriculture* 19 (4). Chinese Academy of Agricultural Sciences: 1085–96. doi:10.1016/S2095-3119(19)62820-0.

McCutcheon, A.R., T.E. Roberts, E. Gibbons, S.M. Ellis, L.A. Babiuk, R.E.W. Hancock, and G.H.N. Towers. 1995. "Antiviral screening of British Columbian medicinal plants." *Journal of Ethnopharmacology* 49 (2): 101–10. doi:10.1016/0378-8741(95)90037-3.

Mehrbod, Parvaneh, Muna A. Abdalla, Emmanuel M. Njoya, Aroke S. Ahmed, Fatemeh Fotouhi, Behrokh Farahmand, Dorcas A. Gado, et al. 2018. "South African medicinal plant extracts active against influenza A virus." *BMC Complementary and Alternative Medicine* 18 (1). BioMed Central Ltd.: 1–10. doi:10.1186/s12906-018-2184-y.

McNab, Finlay W., Ricardo Rajsbaum, Jonathan P. Stoye, and Anne O'Garra. 2011. "Tripartite-Motif proteins and innate immune regulation." *Current Opinion in Immunology*. Curr Opin Immunol. doi:10.1016/j.coi.2010.10.021.

Mushtaq, Sadaf, Bilal Haider Abbasi, Bushra Uzair, and Rashda Abbasi. 2018. "Natural products as reservoirs of novel therapeutic agents." *EXCLI Journal*. Leibniz Research Centre for Working Environment and Human Factors. doi:10.17179/excli2018-1174.

Mutz, Pascal, Philippe Metz, Florian A. Lempp, Silke Bender, Bingqian Qu, Katrin Schöneweis, Stefan Seitz, et al. 2018. "HBV bypasses the innate immune response and does not protect HCV from antiviral activity of interferon." *Gastroenterology* 154 (6). W.B. Saunders: 1791–1804.e22. doi:10.1053/j.gastro.2018.01.044.

Nakama, Shinji, Kazumi Tamaki, Chie Ishikawa, Masayuki Tadano, and Naoki Mori. 2012. "Efficacy of *Bidens pilosa* extract against Herpes Simplex Virus infection in vitro and in vivo." *Evidence-Based Complementary and Alternative Medicine* 2012. doi:10.1155/2012/413453.

Nathanson, N. 2008. "Viral Pathogenesis." In *Encyclopedia of Virology*, 314–19. Elsevier Ltd. doi:10.1016/B978-012374410-4.00464-7.

Nebigil, Canan G., Christiane Moog, Stéphan Vagner, Nadia Benkirane-Jessel, Duncan R. Smith, and Laurent Désaubry. 2020. "Flavaglines as natural products targeting EIF4A and Prohibitins: From Traditional Chinese medicine to antiviral activity against Coronaviruses." *European Journal of Medicinal Chemistry* 203 (October). Elsevier Masson SAS. doi:10.1016/j.ejmech.2020.112653.

Park, Ji Young, Jang Hoon Kim, Jung Min Kwon, Hyung Jun Kwon, Hyung Jae Jeong, Young
   Min Kim, Doman Kim, Woo Song Lee, and Young Bae Ryu. 2013. "Dieckol, a SARS-CoV
   3CLpro inhibitor, isolated from the edible brown algae *Ecklonia cava*." *Bioorganic and
   Medicinal Chemistry* 21 (13). Bioorg Med Chem: 3730–37. doi:10.1016/j.bmc.2013.04.026.
Payne, Susan. 2017. "Introduction to Animal Viruses." In *Viruses*, 1–11. Elsevier. doi:10.1016/
   b978-0-12-803109-4.00001-5.
Porter, Randall S, and Robert F. Bode. 2017. "A review of the antiviral properties of black
   elder (*Sambucus Nigra* L.) products." *Phytotherapy Research* 31 (4). John Wiley and
   Sons Ltd: 533–54. doi:10.1002/ptr.5782.
Rittà, Massimo, Arianna Marengo, Andrea Civra, David Lembo, Cecilia Cagliero, Kamal
   Kant, Uma Ranjan Lal, Patrizia Rubiolo, Manik Ghosh, and Manuela Donalisio. 2020.
   "Antiviral activity of a *Arisaema tortuosum* leaf extract and some of its constituents
   against Herpes simplex virus type 2." *Planta Medica* 86 (4). Georg Thieme Verlag:
   267–75. doi:10.1055/a-1087-8303.
Rodrigues, Eliana, and Joanne Barnes. 2013. "Pharmacovigilance of herbal medicines: The
   potential contributions of ethnobotanical and ethnopharmacological studies." *Drug
   Safety* 36 (1). Drug Saf: 1–12. doi:10.1007/s40264-012-0005-7.
Rose, Patrick P., Sheri L. Hanna, Anna Spiridigliozzi, Nattha Wannissorn, Daniel P. Beiting,
   Susan R. Ross, Richard W. Hardy, Shelly A. Bambina, Mark T. Heise, and Sara Cherry.
   2011. "Natural resistance-associated macrophage protein is a cellular receptor for
   Sindbis virus in both insect and mammalian hosts." *Cell Host and Microbe* 10 (2). Cell
   Host Microbe: 97–104. doi:10.1016/j.chom.2011.06.009.
Rossmann, Michael G., Yongning He, and Richard J. Kuhn. 2002. "Picornavirus-
   receptor interactions." *Trends in Microbiology*. Trends Microbiol. doi:10.1016/
   S0966-842X(02)02383-1.
SaiRam M., G. Ilavazhagan, S.K. Sharma, S.A. Dhanraj, B. Suresh, M.M. Parida, A.M.
   Jana, K. Devendra, and W. Selvamurthy. 2000. "Anti-microbial activity of a new
   vaginal Contraceptive NIM-76 from neem oil (*Azadirachta indica*)." *Journal of
   Ethnopharmacology* 71 (3). J Ethnopharmacol. doi:10.1016/S0378-8741(99)00211-1.
Saklani, Arvind, and Samuel K. Kutty. 2008. "Plant-derived compounds in clinical trials."
   Drug Discovery Today. Drug Discov Today. doi:10.1016/j.drudis.2007.10.010.
Schnitzler, P., S. Schneider, F.C. Stintzing, R. Carle, and J. Reichling. 2008. "Efficacy of an
   aqueous *Pelargonium sidoides* extract against Herpesvirus." *Phytomedicine* 15 (12):
   1108–16. doi:10.1016/j.phymed.2008.06.009.
Serkedjieva, J., G. Gegova, and K. Mladenov. 2008. "Protective efficacy of an aerosol prepa-
   ration, obtained from *Geranium sanguineum* L., in experimental influenza infection."
   Pharmazie 63 (2): 160–63. doi:10.1691/ph.2008.7617.
Shah, Bhumi, Palmi Modi, and Sneha R. Sagar. 2020. "In silico studies on therapeutic
   agents for COVID-19: Drug repurposing approach." *Life Sciences* 252. doi:10.1016/j.
   lfs.2020.117652.
Sharifi-Rad, Javad, Marcello Iriti, William N. Setzer, Mehdi Sharifi-Rad, Amir Roointan,
   and Bahare Salehi. 2018. "Antiviral activity of *Veronica persica* Poir. on Herpes virus
   infection." *Cellular and Molecular Biology* 64 (8). Cellular and Molecular Biology
   Association: 11–17. doi:10.14715/cmb/2018.64.8.2.
Sharma, Arun Dev, and Inderjeet Kaur. 2020. "Molecular docking studies on Jensenone from
   Eucalyptus essential oil as a potential inhibitor of COVID 19 Coronavirus infection,"
   March. http://arxiv.org/abs/2004.00217.
Shree, Priya, Priyanka Mishra, Chandrabose Selvaraj, Sanjeev Kumar Singh, Radha Chaube,
   Neha Garg, and Yamini Bhusan Tripathi. 2020. "Targeting COVID-19 (SARS-CoV-2)
   Main protease through active phytochemicals of ayurvedic medicinal plants–*Withania*

somnifera (Ashwagandha), *Tinospora cordifolia* (Giloy) and *Ocimum sanctum* (Tulsi)–a Molecular docking study." *Journal of Biomolecular Structure and Dynamics*. Taylor and Francis Ltd. doi:10.1080/07391102.2020.1810778.

Song, Jae Min, Kwang Hee Lee, and Baik Lin Seong. 2005. "Antiviral effect of catechins in green tea on influenza virus." *Antiviral Research* 68 (2): 66–74. doi:10.1016/j. antiviral.2005.06.010.

Spear, Patricia G. 2004. "Herpes simplex virus: receptors and ligands for cell entry." *Cellular Microbiology*. Cell Microbiol. doi:10.1111/j.1462-5822.2004.00389.x.

Sudo, K., K. Konno, S. Shigeta, and T. Yokota. 1998. "Inhibitory effects of Podophyllotoxin derivatives on Herpes Simplex virus replication." *Antiviral Chemistry and Chemotherapy* 9 (3). International Medical Press Ltd: 263–67. doi:10.1177/095632029800900307.

Venkateswaran, P S, I Millman, and B S Blumberg. 1987. "Effects of an extract from *Phyllanthus niruri* on Hepatitis B and Woodchuck hepatitis viruses: In vitro and in vivo studies (Antiviral Agent/Marmota Monax/DNA Polymerase/Hepatitis B Surface Antigen/Woodchuck Hepatitis Surface Antigen)." Proceedings of the National Academy of Sciences Vol. 84.

Verma, H., P. Patil, R. Kolhapure, and V. Gopalkrishna. 2008. "Antiviral activity of the Indian medicinal plant extract, *Swertia chirata* against Herpes Simplex viruses: a study by in-vitro and molecular approach." *Indian Journal of Medical Microbiology* 26 (4). Medknow Publications and Media Pvt. Ltd: 322–26. doi:10.4103/0255-0857.43561.

Vicenzi, Elisa, Massimo Alfano, Silvia Ghezzi, and Guido Poli. 2007. "Immunopathogenesis of HIV infection." In *The Biology of Dendritic Cells and HIV Infection*, 245–95. Springer US. doi:10.1007/978-0-387-33785-2_7.

Vimalanathan, S., S. Ignacimuthu, and J.B. Hudson. 2009. "Medicinal plants of Tamil Nadu (Southern India) are a rich source of antiviral activities." *Pharmaceutical Biology* 47 (5). Taylor & Francis: 422–29. doi:10.1080/13880200902800196.

Virgin, Herbert W. 2014. "The Virome in mammalian physiology and disease." *Cell*. Cell Press. doi:10.1016/j.cell.2014.02.032.

Wagoner, Jessica, Amina Negash, Olivia J. Kane, Laura E. Martinez, Yaakov Nahmias, Nigel Bourne, David M. Owen, et al. 2010. "Multiple effects of Silymarin on the Hepatitis C virus lifecycle." *Hepatology* 51 (6). NIH Public Access: 1912–21. doi:10.1002/hep.23587.

Wahyuni, Tutik Sri, Lydia Tumewu, Adita Ayu Permanasari, Evhy Apriani, Myrna Adianti, Abdul Rahman, Aty Widyawaruyanti, et al. 2013. "Antiviral activities of Indonesian medicinal plants in the East Java region against Hepatitis C virus." *Virology Journal* 10 (1). BioMed Central Ltd.: 1–9. doi:10.1186/1743-422X-10-259.

Wasik, Brian R., Emmie de Wit, Vincent Munster, James O. Lloyd-Smith, Luis Martinez-Sobrido, and Colin R. Parrish. 2019. "Onward transmission of viruses: How do viruses emerge to cause epidemics after spillover?" *Philosophical Transactions of the Royal Society B: Biological Sciences* 374 (1782). Royal Society Publishing: 20190017. doi:10.1098/rstb.2019.0017.

Wu, S.F., C.K. Lin, Y.S. Chuang, F.R. Chang, C.K. Tseng, Y.C. Wu, and J.C. Lee. 2012. "Anti-hepatitis C virus activity of 3-hydroxy caruilignan C from swietenia macrophylla stems." *Journal of Viral Hepatitis* 19 (5): 364–70. doi:10.1111/j.1365-2893.2011.01558.x.

Yoosook, C., W. Chantratita, and P. Rimdusit. 1989. "Recovery frequencies of Herpes Simplex virus types 1 and 2 from symptomatic and asymptomatic genital Herpes cases and antiviral sensitivities of isolates." *Journal of the Medical Association of Thailand* 72 (10): 572–76. https://europepmc.org/article/med/2555430.

Zhou, Jue, Moustapha Ouedraogo, Fan Qu, and Pierre Duez. 2013. "Potential genotoxicity of traditional Chinese medicinal plants and phytochemicals: An overview." *Phytotherapy Research*. Phytother Res. doi:10.1002/ptr.4942.

4 Conventional Medicinal Plants
Boosting the Immune System in Humans

Antul Kumar, Anuj Choudhary, Harmanjot Kaur,
Asish Kumar Padhy, and Sahil Mehta

CONTENTS

4.1 INTRODUCTION

In humans, the immune system is a unique, complex network that helps to deal with various stresses, foreign particles, insults, and illnesses (Anywar et al. 2020). It regulates different pathways and interconnection processes involving microbial recognition, inflammation, microbial clearance, cell/tissue damage, and healing. This homoeostatic system entails the well-organized interplays of different classes of immune cells and their crosstalk with particular tissue microenvironments to sustain immune homoeostasis. The immune responses are rapid or slow, depending upon infection halting, infection rate, severity, and the memory of functions. In homoeostasis, immunity plays a pivotal role and can be categorized into two types: adaptive immunity or innate immunity (Singh et al. 2016). The acquired or adaptive immune system responses are relatively slow (and are coordinated by B cells and T cells) compared with the innate immunity system, (which includes basophils, dendritic cells, eosinophils, mast cells, macrophages, neutrophils, and invariant natural killer cells). Together, both immune systems help in regulating the activity of cells responsible for the elimination of pathogens and damaged cells, as well as tumour cells (Kumar et al. 2011; Uttpal et al. 2019).

Over the past few decades, paradigm shifts in the medical system have been reported, with changes in interest towards disease prevention. Interest has been boosted to a new level due to the recent catastrophic pandemic situation of COVID-19 (Khanal et al. 2020; Ahmad et al. 2021). In the traditional medicinal system, the disease ailment is based only on primary symptoms and not according to its evaluation or clinical diagnosis, in order to improve the overall quality of life and the maintenance of human health. Based on herbal formulations, various plant parts, ranging from roots, leaves, stems, berries, flowers, buds, twigs, barks, seeds to fruits and whole plants, are used in the treatment of diseases by naturally enhancing the human immune system as a result of supplying vitamins, flavonoids, carotenoids, alkaloids, or other secondary metabolites present in the herbal plant preparation (Archana et al. 2011; Thangadurai et al. 2018; Tuy et al. 2020).

Traditionally, inflammation is considered to be the first symptom and is characterized by pain, swelling, redness, heat, and other functional disturbances. During treatment, medicinal practitioners target such primary symptoms and prescribe herbal formulations (Cundell 2014). Conventional medical research expects that a single chemical compound confers low toxicity, high potency, and selectivity towards targeted cellular diseases. However, understanding the pathways of compounds involved in the immune response is difficult and needs more thorough research (Sultan et al. 2014; Sharma et al. 2017; Singh 2020). Overall, the present chapter highlights the potential of conventional medicinal plants, including members of the same family, major bioactive molecules, and their associated therapeutic role in a strong immune system in humans.

4.2   HISTORY OF MEDICINAL SYSTEMS

Folk or conventional medicine is based on the strategic utilization of basic ingredients of the traditional medicine system, i.e., herbal material and other herbal products that are enriched with bioactive phytochemicals. For example, aspirin was originally obtained from *Filipendula ulmaria* (as the herbal preparation Spiraea Ulmaria), which has been recommended for fever and pain swelling since being prescribed by Hippocrates as presented on Egyptian papyri. The medicinal practical system started in Iraq about 60,000 years ago and about 8,000 years ago in China. The medicinal practitioners used to gain knowledge through their parents/grandparents and recommended the specific herbal medicine formulations (or their products) without any hesitation to the various patients in local communities. Even after so many years of being in use, the conventional medicinal system still requires answers to a variety of questions related to the exact mechanism, functional response, and facts relying on the response of the immune systems, directly or indirectly (Thangadurai et al. 2018).

The concept of immunomodulation has been practiced by the Ayurvedicists for many decades (Sharma et al. 2017). The objective of Ayurvedic practices for immune systems is achieved *via* the implementation of Vajikarana and Rasayana therapy. Disease prevention is acceptable but how they regulate it is unclear and creates an enthusiasm for the endorsement of the traditional medicinal system. The conventional medicinal system is followed by many medicinal systems such as Ayurveda, Chinese, Siddha, Amachis, and Arabic herbal medicines, but the most widely accepted ones are the Ayurvedic and Chinese medicinal systems, which are described in the following sections.

4.2.1 Ayurvedic Medicinal System (AYMS)

The Charaka Samhita is considered to be a primary record that is fully devoted to practical and conceptual medicinal health care and longevity systems. AYMS believes that "every plant can be a medicinal plant" and has been deeply explained in the Indian culture. Medicinal practitioners have utilized these extensive collections of herbs, shrubs, climbers, lianas, etc. and have described their roles meticulously (Tripathi et al. 1999; Sharma et al. 2017). Reference to such plants was reported earliest in the publication known as Rig Veda in the Sanskrit literature. Another one is Bhava Prakasha (1550 Before the Common Era, BCE), which lists 470 Indian herbal medicines (IHMs), and is an important textbook on plants/herbs written by Bhava Mishra, which is held in great esteem by medicinal practitioners (Khodadadi et al. 2015; Anywar et al. 2020). Other important textbooks explaining IHMs are Sushruta Samhita (600 BCE), which describes 516 IHMs, Yajurveda (1000–600 BCE), that lists 87 IHMs, and Atharva Veda (4500–2500 BCE), which records 290 IHMs. Currently, 8,000 herbal remedies are confirmed in AYSM and are explained in Materia Medica of Ayurveda (Chulet and Pradhan 2010; Ven et al. 2010; Kumar et al. 2012; Anywar et al. 2020; Figure 4.1).

4.2.2 Traditional Chinese Medicinal (TCM) System

In the 18th century, a book known as Mian Yi Lei Fang or "Formulas for the Immunity from Plague" referred to a Chinese word for "immune" for the first time. For example, the variolation incubation against the smallpox method, in which the patient inhales the powdered vaccine *via* the nostrils with the aid of silver tubes, is of Chinese origin. However, the terminology from the Western world provided an

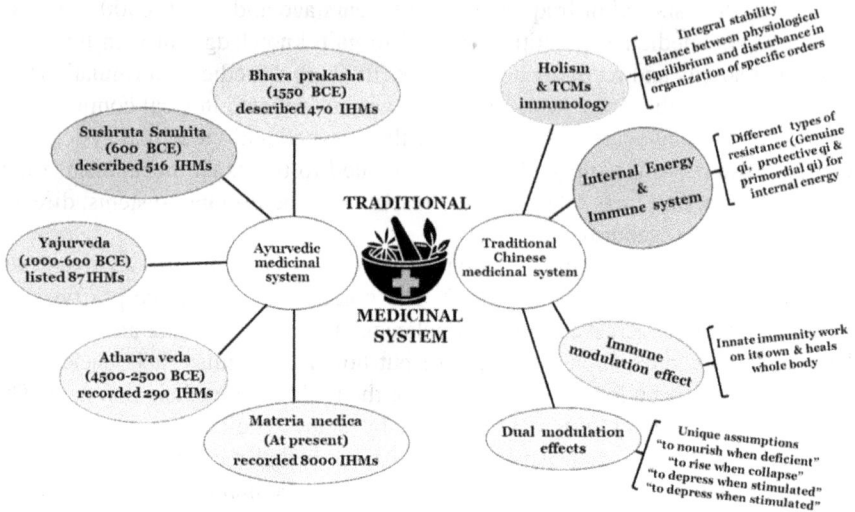

FIGURE 4.1 Contributions of different medicinal systems and their immunoprotective role.

explanation of immunology (Wang and Ren 2002). The TCM has various concepts, which are listed below:

- Holism and TCM immunology. The TCMs are based on holistic approaches and consider that the human body is composed of organic matter. The integral stability, balance between physiological equilibria, and disturbance in the organization of specific orders are the root cause of blockages of the the immune systems. According to Zheng Qi, healthy energy is the vital manifestation of immune functions (Wen et al. 2010).
- Internal energy and the immune system. Different types of resistance, such as genuine qi, protective qi, and primordial qi, are explained by TCMs for internal energy as the natural resistance mechanism of the body against disharmonized energy and diseases (Figure 4.1).
- Immune modulation effect and immune functionality. TCM's focus on energy flow is known as innate immunity, which works on its own, not to a specific system, but heals the whole body.

According to the yin yang theory, the equilibrium between yin and yang adjusts continuously and is most important to keep the body disease free. The approaches are mainly based on the possession and regulation of holism modulation that re-balance and remove extreme deficiencies. The TCM therapeutic immune system functions in dual states, including excessive hyper-functioning states and deficient or under-functioning states. The rehabilitation of the body occurs from an under-functional state to a Mohan normal state or from a hyper-functioning state to a normal state (Archana and Jatawa 2011; Venkatalakshmi et al. 2016).

This strategy manages to enhance our immune functions and to eliminate internal pathogenic factors with dual modulation effects. TCM has a unique assumption regarding immune functionality and regulatory properties in different actions; "to nourish when deficient", "to rise when collapsed", and "to depress when stimulated" (Cundell 2014; Tuy et al. 2020).

4.3   IMPORTANCE OF CONVENTIONAL MEDICINAL SYSTEMS

In modern-day disease management, immunomodulators of plant origin have been established to be the most potent tool, as they promote the non-specific activation of immune responses against pathogens. As a result, it became a scientific concept that has gained much attention in recent years (Thatte et al. 1997; Singh et al. 2016). The Ayurvedic principles (such as Ojas, Vyadhi-ksamatva, and Bala) and modern medicine concepts, including circadian rhythms, neuro-endocrine immune axis, seasonal variations, the influence of exercise, and different physiological states, are much closer to unfolding issues of immune systems (Chulet and Pradhan 2010; Doshi et al. 2013; Pan et al. 2014; Jantan et al. 2015; Utpal et al. 2019). The Vyadhi-ksamatva is regarded as immunity and is highly acceptable in Ayurveda, and also known as Vyadhibala. Charaka has also mentioned Bala as the component that eradicates the pathogens by killing them inside the body. The first action of Bala helps to inhibit, counteract, and overcome the disease-causing factors that cause degradation and cell death, such as anaemia, pulmonary tuberculosis, diabetes mellitus, premature senility, and malignant and other tumours. The second action of Bala relates to both humoral and cellular immunological factors that neutralize or destroy disease-causing agencies which attack the body. Furthermore, in clinical conditions, pathogen entry results in moderate or severe impairment of tissue, distribution in vessels, altered composition, and sometimes certain deficiencies. In addition, mental, physical, severe degenerative and wasting diseases, psychological diseases, starvation, and malnutrition also reduce immune functions (Sharma et al. 2007; Kulkarni et al. 2012).

The combination of four important medicinal plants are explained in Ayurveda, namely Tulsi (*Ocimum sanctum*), Amalaki (*Emblica officinalis*), Ashwagandha (*Withania somnifera*) and Guduchi (*Tinospora cordifolia*), mixed in equal proportions, is taken to elevate humoral and cellular components of the immune system (Reis et al. 2008; Rachh et al. 2014; Table 4.1). This preparation directly enhances the microbiocidal action of the neutrophil cells and increases the levels of globulin components in the circulatory system. Intake of the above medicinal plant preparation with the given composition results in increased levels of lymphocytes, which increase the memory of the T cells along with enhanced cell number and size of the macrophages (phagocytic cells) . The preparation is also helpful in improving our immune response and accelerating recovery when used as an adjunct to various immune-related disorders, such as multidrug-resistant tuberculosis, chronic wasting therapy, cancer, and other immunocompromized disorders (Chatterjee and Dass 1996; Tillu et al. 2020). The concept of Bala for innate immunity, acquired immunity, or immunological capabilities, playing a central role in disease and health, have to be appreciated and understood by Western immunologists. There is a wide range

TABLE 4.1

Comparative List of Conventional Medicinal Plants and Their Constituent Properties

S. No	Plant Species	Common Name	Family	Parts Used	Properties	Traditional Uses	Drug Derivatives	Commonly Used Drugs	References
1	*Atropa belladona*	Belladona	Solanaceae	Leaves and branches	• Pain reliever • Muscle relaxer • Anti-inflammatory • Treatment of menstrual problems	Treatment of headache, ulcers, typhoid, and scarlet fever	Atropine	Atroealth	Lanculov et al. (2004)
2	*Withania somnifera*	Ashwagandha	Solanaceae	Flower, root, bark, seeds, and leaves	• Antimicrobial • Anti-snake venom treatment • Antitumor • Anti-inflammatory	Treatment of asthma, diabetes, hypertension, stress, arthritic diseases, and cancer	Withanolides	Ashwagand harita	Gupta and Rana (2007)
3	*Andrographis paniculata*	Kalmegh	Acanthaceae	Leaf, roots, and aerial part	• Antimicrobial • Cytotoxicity • Antiprotozoan • Anti-inflammatory • Antioxidant • Immunostimulant • Antidiabetic • Anti-infective	Treatment of cancer, diabetes, high blood pressure, flatulence, ulcers, leprosy, skin diseases, colic, bronchitis, influenza, dysentery, dyspepsia, and malaria	Andrographolide	Jaborandi	Biswa et al. (2011)
4	*Andrographis paniculata*	Kalmegh	Acanthaceae	Leaves, roots, and whole plant	• Antimicrobial • Antiprotozoan • Anti-inflammatory • Anti-oxidant, • Immunostimulant, • Antidiabetic • Anti-infective	Treatment of cancer, high blood pressure, ulcer, leprosy, diabetes, bronchitis, dyspepsia skin diseases, flatulence, colic, influenza, dysentery, and malaria	Andrographolide	Fleximark	Biswa et al. (2011)

(Continued)

TABLE 4.1 (CONTINUED)
Comparative List of Conventional Medicinal Plants and Their Constituent Properties

S. No	Plant Species	Common Name	Family	Parts Used	Properties	Traditional Uses	Drug Derivatives	Commonly Used Drugs	References
5	*Berberis aristata*	Darhaid	Berberidaceae	Fruits, roots, leaves, stem, and bark	• Immunostimulant • Antidiabetic • Antimicrobial • Hepatoprotective • Antidepressant	Treatment of diarrhoea, jaundice, syphilis, chronic rheumatism, skin diseases, and urinary disorders	Berberine	Daruharida	Sharma et al. (2011)
6	*Nyctanthes arbos-tristis*	Parijat	Oleaceae	Leaves, flowers, seeds, stem, and bark	• Hepatoprotective • Antileishmaniasis • Antiviral • Antifungal • Antipyretic • Antihistaminic • Antimalarial • Antibacterial • Anti-inflammatory • Antioxidant activities	Reduce fever, enlargement of the spleen, malaria, blood dysentery, cough, and gastritis	Artemisinin and quinine	Harshingar	Rani et al. (2011)
7	*Ocimum sanctum*	Tulsi	Lamiaceae	Leaves, seeds, and root	• Analgesic • Anticancer • Antifertility • Antirheumatic • Antistress	Treatment of bronchitis, malaria, diarrhoea, dysentery, skin disease, arthritis, eye diseases, and insect bites	Monoterpenes and sesquiterpenes	Curill capsule	Vishwabhan et al. (2011)

(Continued)

TABLE 4.1 (CONTINUED)
Comparative List of Conventional Medicinal Plants and Their Constituent Properties

S. No	Plant Species	Common Name	Family	Parts Used	Properties	Traditional Uses	Drug Derivatives	Commonly Used Drugs	References
8	*Aegle marmelos*	Bael	Rutaceae	Leaves, bark, roots, fruits, and seeds	• Antidiarrhoeal • Antimicrobial • Antiviral • Radioprotective • Anticancer • Chemopreventive • Antipyretic • Ulcer healing	Treatment of asthma, jaundice, fever, and constipation	Dibutyl phthalate	WDPL Bilva	Atul et al. (2012)
9	*Acacia catechu*	Kattha	Fabaceae	Bark, fruits, and gum	• Antioxidant • Anti-inflammatory • Free radical scavenging • Tissue-protective effects	Reduce swelling of the nose, swelling of the colon (colitis), and throat, treat diarrhoea, dysentery, bleeding, osteoarthritis, and cancer.	Catechin, catechol, and catecholamine	Unibest	Verma (2012)
10	*Calotropis procera*	Aak	Apocynaceae	Root and root bark	• Antimicrobial • Anthelminthic • Anti-inflammatory • Analgesic • Antipyretic • Anticancer • Anti-angiogenic • Immunological • Antidiabetic • Gastroprotective,	Treatment of jaundice, diarrhoea, stomatic, sinus fistula, and skin disease	Cardiac glycosides	Calotropis 1000ch	Khairnar et al. (2012)

(Continued)

TABLE 4.1 (CONTINUED)
Comparative List of Conventional Medicinal Plants and Their Constituent Properties

S. No	Plant Species	Common Name	Family	Parts Used	Properties	Traditional Uses	Drug Derivatives	Commonly Used Drugs	References
11	Trachyspermum ammi	Ajwain	Apiaceae	Whole plant	• Stimulant • Antispasmodic • Carminative property	Acts as carminative, stimulant, antispasmodic, tonic, dyspepsia, and used to treat cholera	Glycosides, saponins, phenolic compounds	Ajwain oil	Jeet et al. (2012)
12	Trigonella foenum-graecum	Methi	Fabaceae	Seed	• Anticarcinogenic • Anti-diabetic • Antihelmintic • Anti-ulcer • Hypoglycaemic	Treatment of diarrhoea, dysentery, cough, liver, and spleen disorder	Trigonelline, iso-orientin, orientin, vitexin, and isovitexin	Indigo foenogreek tincture	Meghwal et al. (2012)
13	Commiphora wightii	Guggul	Burseraceae	Bark, leaves, and flowers	• Anti-inflammation • Anti-obesity • Antirheumatism • Gout treatment	Treatment of rheumatoid arthritis, neurological diseases, hypercholesterolaemia, leprosy, muscle and skin disorders, high blood pressure, and urine problems	Steroidal compounds	Gokshura	Ikram and Chahar (2013)
14	Eclipta alba	Vringraj	Asteraceae	Leaves, seed, and stem	• Antihepatotoxic • Antimicrobial • Antidiabetic • Anticancer • Analgesic • Anti-venom	Acts as liver tonic, to treat diabetes, eye health, and promote hair growth	Coumestan steroids	Bhringraj	Bhalerao (2013)

(Continued)

TABLE 4.1 (CONTINUED)
Comparative List of Conventional Medicinal Plants and Their Constituent Properties

S. No	Plant Species	Common Name	Family	Parts Used	Properties	Traditional Uses	Drug Derivatives	Commonly Used Drugs	References
15	*Datura metel*	Dhatura	Solanaceae	Leaves and flowers	• Analgesic • Antiviral • Anti-ulcer • Antistress • Antifungal • Anti-asthmatic	Treatment of Parkinson's disease, asthma, coughs, tuberculosis, and bronchitis	Withanolides and amides	Schwable Datura metel	Maheshwari et al. (2013)
16	*Aloe vera*	Gritkumari	Asphodelaceae	Leaf pulp	• Anti-inflammatory • Antiageing • Antitumour • Antibacterial • Antiseptic	Treatment for burns, skin irritations, cuts and insect bites, to relieve itching and skin swellings	Aloin	Clarina	Sahu et al. (2013)
17	*Abrus precatorius*	Gunja	Fabaceae	Roots, seeds, and leaves	• Antioxidative • Immunostimulant • Antimalarial • Anti-allergic • Anticataract	Treatment of tetanus, to cure fever, cough and cold, and to prevent rabies	Abrol, abrasine	Abrus precatorius	Bhatia et al. (2013)
18	*Azadirachta indica*	Neem	Meliaceae	Bark, leaves, and fruits	• Antibacterial • Antiviral • Antiparasitic • Anti-inflammatory • Anticarcinogenic • Antioxidant • Immune system upregulation • Anti-snake venom activity	Treatment of fungal infection, to reduce acne and nourish skin	Azadirachtin	Azadirachta indica tablets	Dubey et al. (2014)

(Continued)

TABLE 4.1 (CONTINUED)
Comparative List of Conventional Medicinal Plants and Their Constituent Properties

S. No	Plant Species	Common Name	Family	Parts Used	Properties	Traditional Uses	Drug Derivatives	Commonly Used Drugs	References
19	*Curcuma longa*	Haldi	Zingiberaceae	Rhizome	• Anti-inflammatory • Antioxidant • Antidiabetic • Click here to enter text. • Anti-asthmatic	Treat wounds infections, bruises, inflamed joints and sprains, treat various other illnesses	Curcuminoid	-	Nasri et al. (2014)
20	*Tinospora cordifolia*	Giloe	Menispermaceae	Roots, stem, and leaves	• Antiperiodic • Antispasmodic • Antimicrobial • Anti-osteoporotic • Anti-inflammatory • Anti-arthritic • Anti-allergic • Antidiabetic	Treatment of diabetes, high cholesterol, allergic rhinitis, upset stomach, gout, lymphoma and other cancers, rheumatoid arthritis, hepatitis, peptic ulcer disease, fever, gonorrhoea, and syphilis	Tinosporic acid, cordifoliosides	Himalaya Guduchi	Mittal (2014)
21	*Terminalia arjuna*	Arjuna	Combretaceae	Stem and bark	• Antioxidant • Hypotensive • Anti-atherogenic • Anti-inflammatory • Anticarcinogenic • Antimutagenic • Gastro-productive effect	Treatment of cardiovascular diseases (CVD), ulcers, diabetes, cough, excessive perspiration, asthma, tumour, inflammation, and skin disorders	Triterpenoids	Arjuna	Dwivedi and Chopra (2014)

(Continued)

TABLE 4.1 (CONTINUED)
Comparative List of Conventional Medicinal Plants and Their Constituent Properties

S. No	Plant Species	Common Name	Family	Parts Used	Properties	Traditional Uses	Drug Derivatives	Commonly Used Drugs	References
22	*Saraca asoca*	Ashoka	Fabaceae	Stem, bark, seeds, and leaves	• Anti-oestrogenic • Anti-inflammatory • Anti-implantation • Antioxidant • Antitumour • Anticancer	Treatment of neurological disorders, snake bites, fever, tumours, poisoning, diarrhoea, worm infestations, burning sensation, excessive menstrual bleeding, and abdominal swelling	Gallic acid	Ashoka powder	Singh et al. (2015)
23	*Abutilon indicum*	Kanghi	Malvaceae	Leaves, bark, and seeds	• Anti-inflammatory • Antiproliferative activity • Anti-arthritic activity • Analgesic and sedative property • Antioxidant • Antimicrobial activity • Hepatoprotective activity	Reduce toothache, tender gums, also used in treatment of ulcers	Palmitic acid, β-sitosterol, and stigmasteroid	Organic pure abutilon indicum powder	Raja and Kailasam (2015)
24	*Picrorhiza kurroa*	Kutaki	Plantaginaceae	Leaf, bark, root, and rhizhomes	• Immunostimulant • Antioxidant • Anti-inflammatory • Anti-allergic • Hepatoprotective • Choleretic • Anti-asthmatic • Anti-cancerous activity	Promote liver functioning, to treat dyspepsia, chronic diarrhoea, scorpion sting, and reduce fevers	Picrosides	Kutki	Qureshi et al. (2015)

(Continued)

TABLE 4.1 (CONTINUED)

Comparative List of Conventional Medicinal Plants and Their Constituent Properties

S. No	Plant Species	Common Name	Family	Parts Used	Properties	Traditional Uses	Drug Derivatives	Commonly Used Drugs	References
25	*Bryophyllum pinnatum*	Ghamari	Crassulaceae	Leaves	• Antimicrobial • Anticancer • Antihypertensive • Antidiabetic • Hepatoprotective • Anti-inflammatory	Treatment of earache, burns, abscesses, ulcer, insect bites, diarrhoea, and lithiasis	5- Methyl 4, 5, 7- trihydroxyl flavone 1 and 4-, 3, 5, 7 tetrahydroxy 5-methyl 5 1-propenamine anthocyanidins 2	SBL Bryophyllum calcynum	Nagaratna et al. (2015)
26	*Allium sativum*	Lasun	Amaryllidaceae	Bulb	• Hepatoprotective • Antioxidant • Anticarcinogenic • Antiprotozal • Diuretic	Treatment of fevers, dysentery, diabetes, rheumatism, intestinal worms, colic, flatulence, liver disorders, facial paralysis, tuberculosis, high blood pressure, and bronchitis	Allicin	Garlic oleoresin	Alam et al. (2016)
27	*Asparagus racemosus*	Satavari	Asparagaceae	Roots	• Anti-ulcer • Antioxidant • Antidiarrhoeal • Antidiabetic • Immunomodulatory	Treatment of dyspepsia, constipation, stomach spasms, stomach ulcers, cancer, diarrhoea, bronchitis, tuberculosis, dementia, and diabetes	Shatavarin	Spermon	Hasan et al. (2016)

(Continued)

TABLE 4.1 (CONTINUED)
Comparative List of Conventional Medicinal Plants and Their Constituent Properties

S. No	Plant Species	Common Name	Family	Parts Used	Properties	Traditional Uses	Drug Derivatives	Commonly Used Drugs	References
28	*Nardostachys jatamansi*	Jatamansi	Caprifoliaceae	Roots	• Antifungal • Antioxidant • Antidiabetic • Immunostimulant	Treatment of hysteria, syncope, epilepsy, and mental weakness	Sesquiterpene	Yuvika jatamansi	Sahu et al. (2016)
29	*Allium cepa*	Piyaz, onion	Amaryllidaceae	Bulb	• Anticholesterol • Anticancer • Antioxidant • Antibiotic • Antimicrobial • Antidiabetic	Help in scar removal, heal burns and wounds, reduce hair loss, treatment of diabetes, High cholesterol, blood pressure, asthma, whooping cough, sore throat, and bronchitis	SMCS (*S*-methyl cysteine sulfoxide)	SBL Allium Cepa Dilution 30 CH	Upadhyay et al. (2016)
30	*Cumanum cyminum*	Zira	Apiaceae	Seed	• Antimicrobial • Anti-inflammatory • Insecticidal • Antiplatelet • Diuretic	Treatment of stomach disorders, diuretic, carminative, stimulant	-	-	Al-Snafi (2016)
31	*Croton tiglium*	Jamalgota	Euphorbiaceae	Seeds	• Anti-tumour • Anti-inflammatory • Antioxidant • Antidermatophytic	Acts as purgative, stimulant, to treat bronchitis, asthma, paralysis, sciatica	Cardiac glycosides, phorbol esters, lectins, and cyanogenic glycoside	Croton tig 200	Sinsinwar et al. (2016)

(Continued)

TABLE 4.1 (CONTINUED)
Comparative List of Conventional Medicinal Plants and Their Constituent Properties

S. No	Plant Species	Common Name	Family	Parts Used	Properties	Traditional Uses	Drug Derivatives	Commonly Used Drugs	References
32	*Clitoria ternatea*	Aparjita	Fabaceae	Flower, roots, and seeds	• Immunostimulant • Antipyretic • Anti-inflammatory • Analgesic • Antimicrobial activity	Treatment of heart disease, depression, gonorrhoea, and other skin diseases	Finotin	-	Chauhan et al. (2017)
33	*Catharanthus roseus*	Sada bahar	Apocynaceae	Leaf, stem, root, and flower	• Antimalarial • Immunostimulant • Anticancer • Antihyperglycaemic • Analgesic	Help in relieving muscle pain, depression, diabetes, treatment of stomach ache, wasp stings, to heal wounds	Vinblastine, vincristine	Vincristine	Gupta et al. (2017)
34	*Bacopa monnieri*	Brahmi	Plantaginaceae	Twig, leaf, and flower	• Memory enhancing • Anti-inflammatory • Analgesic • Antipyretic • Sedative • Anti-epileptic agent	Acts as nervine tonic, diuretic, to treat asthma, epilepsy, insanity, and hoarseness	Baccosoids	Mentat	Rai et al. (2017)
35	*Zingiber officinale*	Adrak	Zingiberaceae	Rhizhome	• Antioxidant • Anticancer • Antipyretic • Anti-obesity • Gastroprotective • Analgesic • Antimigraine	To treat heart problems, stomach upset, diarrhoea, headache, and nausea	Gingerol	Organic ginger	Dhanik et al. (2017)

(Continued)

TABLE 4.1 (CONTINUED)

Comparative List of Conventional Medicinal Plants and Their Constituent Properties

S. No	Plant Species	Common Name	Family	Parts Used	Properties	Traditional Uses	Drug Derivatives	Commonly Used Drugs	References
36	*Cymbopogon martini*	Gandh	Poaceae	Leaves, rhizomes, roots	• Immunostimulant • Antimicrobial • Antifungal • Antiviral • Antihelmintic • Antioxidant	Treatment of scabies, asthma, rheumatism, arthritis, common cold, and reduce hair loss	Geraniol	Cymbopogon martini	Promila (2018)
37	*Hyoscyamus niger*	Parsikaya	Solanaceae	Roots, leaves, and seeds	• Immunostimulant • Anti-inflammatory • Analgesic • Antipyretic • Antiparkinsonism	Treatment during rheumatism, asthma, cough, nervous diseases, stomach pain, and toothache	Hyoscyamine	Hyoscyamine oral drops	Al-Snafi (2018)
38	*Terminalia chebula*	Harida	Combretaceae	Fruit	• Antibacterial • Antifungal • Antiviral • Antidiabetic • Antimutagenic • Antioxidant • Anti-ulcer • Wound healing	Treatment of dementia, constipation, and diabetes	Chebulagic acid, corilagin, mannitol, ascorbic acid	Haritaki capsules	Kolla and Kulkarni (2018)

(Continued)

TABLE 4.1 (CONTINUED)
Comparative List of Conventional Medicinal Plants and Their Constituent Properties

S. No	Plant Species	Common Name	Family	Parts Used	Properties	Traditional Uses	Drug Derivatives	Commonly Used Drugs	References
39	*Jatropha curcas*	Arandi	Euphorbiaceae	Leaves, fruit, seed, stem bark, branches, and roots	• Anti-inflammatory • Antioxidant • Antimicrobial • Antiviral • Anticancer • Antidiabetic • Anticoagulant • Hepatoprotective • Analgesic	Treatment of burn spot, chest inflammation, congestion, headache, hypertension, eczema, and galactogogue	Apigenin	Jatropha cur 30	Abobatta (2019)
40	*Cinnamomum zeylanicum*	Dalchini	Lauraceae	Bark and leaves	• Anti-bacterial • Anti-fungal • Antioxidant • Lowering cholesterol level	Treatment of nausea, vomiting, and diarrhoea.	Cinnamaldehyde	Ceylon cinnamon	Rawat et al. (2019)

of these herbal formulations and their derived drugs available in India, focusing on the nutritional dynamics that help to enhance the ability of the immune system to protect the body from infectious and communicable diseases and to act as a promoter of the treatment of the immunocompromized condition (Gan et al. 2003; Sharma et al. 2007; Archana et al. 2011; Derouiche 2020).

4.4 IMMUNITY-ENHANCING PLANT-DERIVED DRUGS

Plants synthesize a remarkably wide range of secondary metabolites. These secondary metabolites are mainly non-essential for the primary metabolism of plants, but play significant roles in defence by creating a strong immune response to pathogen infections, stress conditions, and environmental effects (Piasecka et al. 2015; Lokhande et al. 2019). The literature has tended to identify the active phytochemicals that are responsible for the therapeutic effects of most immunity-boosting plants, including Greco-Arab herbs (Venditti et al. 2016). They include flavonoids, tannins, terpenoids, steroids, and polysaccharides. Furthermore, the main immunity-enhancing drugs originated from plants are alkaloids, such as sophocarpine, chelerythrine, curcumin, peperine, sinomenine, quercitin, matrine, tetrandrine, berberine, capsaicin, colchicine, leonurine, gelselegine, pseudocoptisine, andrographolide, koumine, rhynchophylline, lycorine and genistein (Table 4.2). These chemicals can also be further categorized into other categories, such as:

- **Essential oil:** Tetramethylpyrazine and Z-ligustilide.
- **Flavonoids**: Dihydroxanthohumol, mallotophilippens C, D, E, licochalcone E, chalcone, butein, and xanthohumol.
- **Flavones:** Apigenin, baicalein, chrysin, oroxylin A, luteolin, nobiletin, and wogonin.
- **Flavonols**: Quercetin, rutin, and kaempferol.
- **Flavanols**: Epigallocatechin-3-gallate.
- **Isoflavones**: Daidzein, puerarin, and genistein.
- **Phloroglucinols:** Arzanol and myrtucommulone.
- **Quinones:** Emodin-8-O-β-D glucoside, shikonin, and thymoquinone.
- **Other Apocynins:** Piceatannol, resveratrol, and stilbenes.
- **Terpenoids:** Asiaticoside celastrol, demethylzelasteral, ginsan, oleanolic acid, echinocystic acid, triptolide, 11-keto-β-boswellic acid, 14-deoxyandrographolide,14-deoxy-11,12-didehydroandrographolide, and madecassoside (Table 4.2) (Cook and Samman 1996; Fernandez et al. 2001; Petronelli et al. 2009).

In all medicinal systems over the centuries, the treatment and prevention of disease, using plant-derived drugs, have been long-term processes but, using the immunity enhancer plants provides a better and more efficient way of achieving these goals than was previously possible in human history. Traditionally, these compounds were considered to be solely responsible for a strong immune system but validation by pre-clinical trials is needed (Kumar et al. 2011). As a result, much research

TABLE 4.2
Phytochemical Compounds, Derived from Medicinal Plants, as Immunity Boosters

S. No	Plant	Phytochemical Compounds	References
1.	Atropa belladona	Apoatropine, belladonine, scopolamine, tropine, 6β-hydroxyhyoscyamine, hyoscyamine and norhyoscyamine,	Lanculov et al. (2004)
2.	Withania somnifera	Anahygrine, anaferine, cysteine, chlorogenic acid, cuscohygrine, pseudotropine, withanine, tropanol, somniferiene, somniferinine, withanolides, withananine, scopoletin, iron and A-Y, β-sitosterol	Gupta and Rana (2007)
3.	Emblica officinalis	Ellagic acid, quercetin, gallic acid, 1-O galloyl-beta-D-glucose, chebulagic acid, 3,6-di-o-galloyl-D-glucose, 1,6- di-O-galloyl beta D-glucose, corilagin, chebulinic acid, isostrictiniin and 3-ethylgallic acid	Khan (2009)
4.	Piper longum	Asarinine, brachystamide-A, brachystine, brachystamide, fargesin, piperine, cinnamoyl-piperidine, iperonaline, piperlonguminine, piperlongumine, piperderidine, pipercide piperettine, pellitorine, 1-piperoyl piperidine, methyl pregumidiene, piperundecalidine refractomide A, longamide, dehydropipernonaline, tetrahydropiperine, terahydro piperlongumine, piperine, terahydropiperlongumine pulvuatiol, piperidine, trimethoxy piperlongumine and sesamin,	Zaveri et al. (2010)
5.	Centella asiatica	Asiaticoside, asiatic acid, α-pinene, brahmic acid, brahminoside, trans-β-farnesene, centellose, β-caryophyllene, bicycloelemene, brahmoside, bornyl acetate, campesterol, β-elemene, β-pinene, mesoinositol, myrcene, terpenic acetate, γ-terpinene, α-copaene, germacrene-D, sitosterol, glucose, saponin, and stigmasterol,	Singh et al. (2010)
6.	Berberis aristata	Aporphine, oxyberberine, palmatine, pseudopalmatine chloride, pseudoberberine chloride, aromoline, berberine, taxilamine, berbamine, oxyacanthine, proaporphine, protoberberine, 1-O-methyl pakistanine, pakistanine, and karachine,	Sharma et al. (2011)
7.	Nyctanthes arbos-tristis	Acetophenone, p-cymene, p-cymene, cineole, n-dodecanol, eugenol, (E)-β-damascone, methyl anthranilate, p-vinylquaiacol, camphor, nonanal 2-phenylethyl alcohol, α-pinene, nerol, limonene, α-terpineol, methyl salicylate, hexenyl acetate, 1,8-phenylacetaldehyde, hexenyl butanoate, hexenol, linalool, geraniol, m-cymen-8-ol, and (3Z)-hexenyl tiglate,	Rani et al. (2011)

(Continued)

TABLE 4.2 (CONTINUED)

Phytochemical Compounds, Derived from Medicinal Plants, as Immunity Boosters

S. No	Plant	Phytochemical Compounds	References
8.	*Ocimum sanctum*	Carvacrol, β caryophyllene, β-elemene, germacrene, ursolic acid, eugenol, linalool, oleanolic acid, and rosmarinic acid,	Vishwabhan et al. (2011)
9.	*Aristolochia indica*	Aristolochene, aristolactam IIa, Aristolindiquinone, aristolide, cephradione. methylaristolate, β-sitosterol-βD-glucoside aristolactam glycoside I, ishwarone, ishwarol, 2-hydroxy-1-methoxy-4H-dibenzo quinolone-4,5-(6H)- dione, stigmastenones II and III, and methylaristolate,	Dey and de (2011)
10.	*Andrographis paniculata*	Deoxyandrographolide, β–daucosterol, β-sitosterol, oleanolic acid, *trans*-cinnamic acid, neoandrographolide, isoandrographolide, 7-*O*-methylwogonin, 5-hydroxy-7,8,2′-trimethoxyflavone, 4-hydroxy-2- methoxycinnamaldehyde, 5-hydroxy-7,8,2′,5′-tetramethoxy flavone, 2′-methyl ether, 5-hydroxy7,8,2′,3′-tetramethoxyflavone, 5-hydroxy-7,8-dimethoxyflavone and 14-deoxy11,12-didehydroandrographide	Biswa et al. (2011)
11.	*Soymida febrifuga*	Deoxyandirobin-3-*O*-rutinoside, lupeol, methyl angolensate, sitosterol and quercetin-3-*O*-L-rhamnoside	Riazunnisa (2011)
12.	*Trachyspermum ammi*	Caryophyllene, β-pinene, cadinene, cadinol, *p*-cymene elemol, elemene, carvacrol, humulene, eudesmol, muurolene, γ-terpinene, muurolol, limonene, myrcene, limonene, and thymol	Jeet et al. (2012)
13.	*Trigonella foenum-graecum*	Coumarin, nicotinic acid, fenugreekine, scopoletin, phytic acid, trigonelline and saponins,	Meghwal et al. (2012)
14.	*Aegle marmelos*	Bicyclo heptane-2,3-diol, 2(4H)-benzofuranone, 2,3-dioxabicyclo oct-5-ene, cinnamic acid, 2-propenoic acid, phenol, 2,6-bis(1,1-dimethylethyl)-4-methyl-(BHT), 4-hydroxy-3-methyl-6-(1-methylethyl), 1-dodecanol, 2-cyclohexen-1-one, 2,3-dihydro-3,5-dihydroxy-6-methyl, 2-methyl-5-(1-methylethyl)-(1-phellandrene), myristic acid, 1,3-cyclohexadiene, 2,6,6-trimethyl (2,3-pinanediol), 5,6,7,7A-tetrah ydro-6-hydroxy-4,4,7a-trimethyl, 3-(4-hydroxy-3-methoxyphenyl)-, 3,7,11,15-tetramethyl-2-hexadecen-1-ol, 1-methyl-4-(1-methylethyl)-(limonene dioxide 1), methyl ester, marmelosin, 4H-pyran-4-one, psoralen, marmin, luvangetin, and tannins,	Atul et al. (2012)

(Continued)

TABLE 4.2 (CONTINUED)

Phytochemical Compounds, Derived from Medicinal Plants, as Immunity Boosters

S. No	Plant	Phytochemical Compounds	References
15.	*Calotropis procera*	Benzoyllineolone, benzoylisoloneolane, cardenolides, triterpenes, calotoxin, calotropaginin, calotropin, choline, glycoside-*O*-pyrocatechuric acid, alkaloids, triterpenoid, syriogenin, usechardin, uscharin, uzariganin, and phytosterols	Khairnar et al. (2012)
16.	*Commiphora wightii*	Steroids, amino acids, carbohydrates, aliphatic esters, diterpenoids, cholesterol and sesamin, E-guggulsterone, Z-guggulsterone, guggulsterol I, guggulsterol II, guggulsterol III	Ikram and Chahar (2013)
17.	*Eclipta alba*	Demethylwedelolactone, a-terthienylmethanol, stigmasterol, demethylwedelolactone-7-glucoside, and wedelolactone,	Bhalerao (2013)
18.	*Datura metel*	Adenosine, ilekudinoside C, pterodontriol B, scopolamine, dioscoroside D, thymidine, and disciferitriol	Maheshwari et al. (2013)
19.	*Abrus precatorious*	Abrine, abrusin, abrol, abraline, arabinose, abrasine, abruslactone, abrusoside A, abruslactone A, abrusoside B, abrusoside C, abrusoside D, Abrusin-2'-*O*-apioside, abricin, abrussic acid, anthocyanins, amyrin, abrusgenic-acid-methyl-ester, abrusgenic-acid, alanine, choline, choline, coumaroylgalloyl glucodelphinidin, cycloartenol, campesterol, D-mononethyl ether, delphinidin, *N*, *N*-dimethyl-tryptophan, kaikasaponin III, hederagenin, hemiphloin, hypaphorine, precatorine polysaccharide, precasine, precool, Protein P phosphorus, pectin, pentosans, precatorine, polygalacturonic acids, pinitol, glycyrrhizin, galactose, sophoradiol-2,2-*O*-acetate, sophoradiol, methyl ester, montanyl alcohol, serine, quinones, abruquinones, tryptophan, trigonelline, *N*-gallic-acid, *N*-dimethyl-tryptophan-metho-cation-m ethyl-ester, hypaphorine, ursolic acid, isoflavonoids, xylose, and valine.	Bhatia et al. (2013)
20.	*Aloe vera*	Sugars, amino acids, campesterol, choline, folic acid, vitamin B_{12}, cholesterol, β-sitosterol, 12 anthraquinones, lignin, saponins, salicylic acids, and lupeol	Sahu et al. (2013)
21.	*Azadirachta indica*	Ascorbic acid, quercetin, β-sitosterol, nimbiol, nimbin, nimbandiol, nimbanene, nimbolide, 7-desacetyl-7-benzoylazadiradirone, *N*-hexacosanol 6-desacetylnimbinene, flavonoids, polyphenolic compounds, 7-desacetyl-7-benzoylgedunin, amino acids, and 17-hydroxyazadiradione	Dubey et al. (2014)

(Continued)

TABLE 4.2 (CONTINUED)

Phytochemical Compounds, Derived from Medicinal Plants, as Immunity Boosters

S. No	Plant	Phytochemical Compounds	References
22.	*Curcuma longa*	α-turmerone, β-bisabolene, β-turmerone, curlone, *ar*-curcumene, 1,8-cineole β-caryophyllene, caryophyllene oxide, (*E*)-β-ocimene, (*Z*)-β-ocimene, α-santalene, β-sesquiphellandrene, (*E*)-γ-atlantone, α-zingiberene, β-selinene, β-sesquiphellandrene, santalenone, 1,8-cineole, α-phellandrene, *ar*-turmerone, (*Z*)-γ-atlantone, (*Z*)-β-farnesene, α-thujene, (*E*)-γ-atlantone, humulene oxide, β-myrcene, β-bisabolene, terpinolene, limonene, and zingiberene	Nasri et al. (2014)
23.	*Terminalia arjuna*	Arjungenin, arjunic acid, arjunone, arjunolone, arjunolic acid, arjun glycosides, luteolin, ellagic acid, oligomeric triterpenoid saponins, zinc, copper calcium and magnesium, gallic acid, phytosterols, flavonoids, proanthocyanidins and tannins,	Dwivedi and Chopra (2014)
24.	*Tinospora cordifolia*	Cordifolioside A, tinocordiside, formylannonain, *N*-methyl-2-pyrrolidone, hydroxymustakone, and syringine	Mittal (2014)
25.	*Saraca asoca*	Clerodane, catechin, duorene alkaloids, noroliveroline, 11'-deoxyprocyanidin B4, oliveroline-f3-*N*-oxide, epicatechin, procyanidin B-2, leucocyanidin, polyfothine and liriodenine,	Singh et al. (2015)
26.	*Picrorhiza kurroa*	Apocynin, kutki sterol kutkiol, D-mannitol and picrosides I and II	Qureshi et al. (2015)
27.	*Bryophyllum pinnatum*	α-D-Glucopyranoside, octadecanoic acid, benzaldehyde, *N*-hexadecanoic acid, 3,5-dihydroxy-6- methyl-2,3-dihydro-4H-pyran-4-one, and oleic acid	Nagaratna et al. (2015)
28.	*Abutilon indicum*	Aldehydes, amino acids, amyrin, capric acid, caprylic, eudesmic acid, flavonoids, ferulic acid, fatty acids, ketones, esters g–galactose, terpenes, caffeic acid, palmitic acid, 9, 10-methylene octadec-9-enoic (sterculic) acid, 13-epoxyoleic (vernolic) acid, 8, 9-methylene-heptadec-8-enoic (malvalic) acid, myristic, oleic, linoleic, palmitic, lauric, stearic acids, and sitosterol.	Raja and Kailasam (2015)
29.	*Allium sativum*	Ajoenes (*E*-ajoene, *Z*-ajoene), thiosulphinates (allicin), diallyl disulphide (DADS), diallyl trisulphide (DATS), vinyldithiins (2-vinyl-(4H)-1,3-dithiin, 3-vinyl-(4H)-1,2-dithiin)	Alam et al. (2016)
30.	*Croton tiglium*	Crotonic acid, crotonic resin, crotonoleic acid, crotonic acid, phorbol derivatives, and glyceryl crotonate,	Sinsinwar et al. (2016)

(Continued)

TABLE 4.2 (CONTINUED)

Phytochemical Compounds, Derived from Medicinal Plants, as Immunity Boosters

S. No	Plant	Phytochemical Compounds	References
31.	*Nardostachys jatamansi*	Alpha-patchoulene, angelicin, calarene, elemol, β-patchoulene, jatamansone, valeranal, nardostachone valeranone, β-sitosterol, jatamansinol, jatamansone, nardostachnol, hexacosane, patchouli alcohol, N- seychellene, N-hexaco-sanyl β-eudesemo, jatamansin, seychelane, and oroselol	Sahu et al. (2016)
32.	*Allium cepa*	Adenine riboside, allylsulfides, beta-sitosterol, 3-beta-glucopyranoside-6′-palmitate, cycloalliin, daucosterol, sitosterol, fructose, flavonoids, organosulphur compounds, sulphur, selenium, seleno compounds, S-alk(en)yl cysteine sulphoxides, N-trans-feruloyl tyramine, tryptophane, thiosulphinates, tianshic acid, quercetin, quercetin-3-glucoside, xylose, glucose, glucoside, galactose, and isorhamnetin-4-mannose	Upadhyay et al. (2016)
33.	*Asparagus racemosus*	Quercitin, racemosol, arsapogenin, asparagamine, kaempferol, flavonoids, racemoside A, B, C steroidal saponin, racemofuran, (α, α-diphenyl-β-picrylhydrazyl), hyperoside, sitosterol, 8-methoxy-5, 6, 4′-trihydroxyisoflavone, 4,6-dihydroxy benzaldehyde, 7-O-β-D-glucopyranoside, rutin, and saponins.	Hasan et al. (2016)
34.	*Zingiber officinale*	α-curcumene, β-bisabolene, α-farnesene, 6-dehydrogingerdione, gingerenone-A, β-sesquiphellandrene, quercetin, zingerone and zingiberene	Dhanik et al. (2017)
35.	*Clitoria ternatea*	Tannins, phlobatannin, carbohydrates, saponins, triterpenoids, phenols, flavonoids, flavonol glycosides, proteins, alkaloids, anthraquinones, anthocyanins, cardiac glycosides, stigmast-4-ene-3,6-dione, volatile oils and steroids	Chauhan et al. (2017)
36.	*Bacopa monnieri*	Bacosides A and B, betulinic acid, brahmine, nicotinine, stigmasterol, stigmastanol, triterpenoid saponins, D-mannitol, herpestine, saponins A, B, C, β-sitosterol, serine, glutamic acid, α-alanine, aspartic acid, and glycoside compounds	Rai et al. (2017)
37.	*Catharanthus roseus*	Ajmalicine, actineo plastidemeric, catharanthine, rosindin, raubasin, vindeline vineamine, vinceine, vincristine, vinblastine, vindesine, reserpine, and tabersonine	Gupta et al. (2017)
38.	*Hyoscyamus niger*	Atropine, choline, albumin, hyoscytricin, hyoscine, hyoscyamine, mucilage, and calcium oxalate	Al-Snafi (2018)

(Continued)

TABLE 4.2 (CONTINUED)
Phytochemical Compounds, Derived from Medicinal Plants, as Immunity Boosters

S. No	Plant	Phytochemical Compounds	References
39.	*Cymbopogon martini*	Camphene, carvone, *cis*-carveol, *trans*-carveol, durenol, delphone, limonene, *cis-p*-mentha-2,8-dien-1-ol, sabinol, and *trans-p*-mentha-2,8-dienol	Promila (2018)
40.	*Jatropha curcas*	α-cadinol, α-*epi*-cadinol, δ-cadinene, chrysanthenyl acetate, thymol, and pulegone,	Abobatta (2019)
41.	*Terminalia chebula*	Ascorbic acid, corilagin, chebulagic acid, chebulic acid, ellagic acid, ethyl gallate, gallic acid, tannic acid, and mannitol	Kolla and Kulkarni (2018)
42.	*Cinnamomum zeylanicum*	Caryophyllene oxide, (*E*)-cinnamyl acetate, and *trans*-α-bergamotene	Rawat et al. (2019)

still focuses on the single compounds as the key compounds that focus on a specific target associated with a particular disease (Thoppil et al. 2011; Swallah et al. 2020).

4.5 POTENTIAL OF LOCAL MEDICINAL PLANTS AS AN IMMUNITY ENHANCER

The immune system is the working house of the human body to maintain homoeostasis. The function and efficacy of the immune system are regulated by several endogenous and exogenous factors in order to achieve immunostimulation or immunosuppression. The agent which has the potential to modulate or normalize the pathophysiological processes is known as an immunomodulator (Jantan et al. 2015). Over the past several years, the immunomodulatory properties of numerous plant-derived compounds have been confirmed. The plant-based immunomodulators have a selective advantage over synthetic immunomodulators because of their minimal side effects and toxicity. There is a need for the discovery, identification, and isolation of specific immunomodulatory agents of plant origin with the potential to overcome the side effects of high-cost synthetic compounds. Thus, natural immunomodulators have great potential as substitutes for use in therapeutic procedures. The organic or synthetic biomolecules able to stimulate, suppress, or modulate the components of innate or adaptive immunity are known as immunomodulators, immune-augmenters, immunorestoratives, or biological response modifiers.

There are approximately 122 plant-derived chemicals which have been identified as therapeutic substances, which are used as commercially exploited drugs (Sorokina et al. 2020). For instance, willow tree bark is rich in the salicylic acid phytohormone, which is related to an active compound (acetyl salicylate) of aspirin. In the traditional medicinal system, the bark has been used as a painkiller and antipyretic substance from ancient times. The most frequent drugs prescribed by physicians are derived from plant sources, such as opium, quinine, digoxin, aspirin, etc. The immunomodulatory chemicals derived from plants are alkaloids, terpenoids, flavonoids, lactones, polysaccharides, and glycosidic products (Tiwari et al. 2018). The immunomodulators can be classified into immunostimulants, immunosuppressants, or immuno-adjuvants, examples of which have been listed in Table 4.2.

4.5.1 IMMUNOSTIMULANTS

The chemicals that induce or activate the components or mediators of the immune system are known as immunostimulants (Paul et al. 2020). Immunostimulants enhance the resistance against infection, allergy, cancer, and autoimmunity. Immunostimulants can be categorized into two categories, namely a) specific and b) non-specific immunostimulants. Specific immunostimulants can trigger the immune response, particularly with respect to antigenic type. Non-specific immunostimulants are not antigen-specific and are generally used for treatment of chronic infections, immune-deficiency diseases, and malignant or auto-immune diseases. The immunostimulants are recognized by the Toll-like receptors (TLR) to induce the TLR signalling for immune system initiation. Extracts of plants showing immunostimulant activity are *Allium sativum, Asparagus racemosus, Achyranthes aspera, Azadirachta indica, Aloe vera, Abutilon indicum, Andrographis paniculata, Aristolochia indica, Berberis aristata, Clitoria ternatea, Catharanthus roseus, Cymbopogon martini, Hyoscyamus niger, Nardostachys jatamansi, Picrorhiza kurroa, Cynodon dactylon, Curcuma longa, Embelia ribes, Ocimum sanctum, Sida cordifolia, Punica granatum, Piper longum, Nuctanthes arbor-tristis, Panax ginseng, Phyllanthus emblica, Saussurea costus, Withania somnifera,* and *Tinospora cordifolia* (Figure 4.2; Table 4.2).

4.5.2 Immunosuppressants

Immunosuppressants are the chemicals that inhibit the immune system and can be used to prevent pathological immune reactions after organ transplantation. These substances are used to treat infections related to immunopathology, auto-immune diseases, and hypersensitive reactions (Romanelli and Mascolo 2020). The activation of B and T lymphocytes, macrophages, and the imperfect apoptosis of immune effector cells play important roles in the pathogenesis of various disorders (Turner et al. 2016). Plants showing immunosuppressant activity include *Linum persicum, Salvia mirzayanii, Stachys obtusicrena, Andrographis paniculata, Bupleurum falcatum, Glycyrrhiza glabra, Dracocephalum kotschyi, Periploca sepium, Tripterygium wilfordii Echium amoenum, Salvia miltiorrhiza Argyrolobium roseum, Clerodendron trichotomum,* and *Campylotropis hirtella* (Figure 4.2).

4.5.3 Immuno-adjuvants

Immuno-adjuvants are the specific stimulators of the immune system which boost the efficacy of a vaccine and hence can be considered to be true modulators of the immune response. They can be exploited as immunoprotectives, immunodestructives, or selectors between the cellular and humoral helper (Th1 and Th2) cells (Banstola et al. 2020). The plants showing such activity include *Ziziphus jujube, Withania somnifera, Achyranthes bidentata, Astragalus membranaceus, Allium sativum, Calliandra pulcherrima, Hedera taurica, Aesculus hippocastanum, Bupleurum falcatum, Andrographis paniculata, Anemone raddeana, Echinacea purpurea, Grifola frondosa, Nigella sativa, Panax ginseng, Tinospora cordifolia, Platycodon grandiflorum, Astragalus membranaceus, Asparagus racemosus, Curcuma longa,* and *Hypericum perforatum* (Table 4.2; Figure 4.2) (Goldman 2001; Balunas 2005; Licciardi and Underwood 2011; Patel 2012; Banstola et al. 2020).

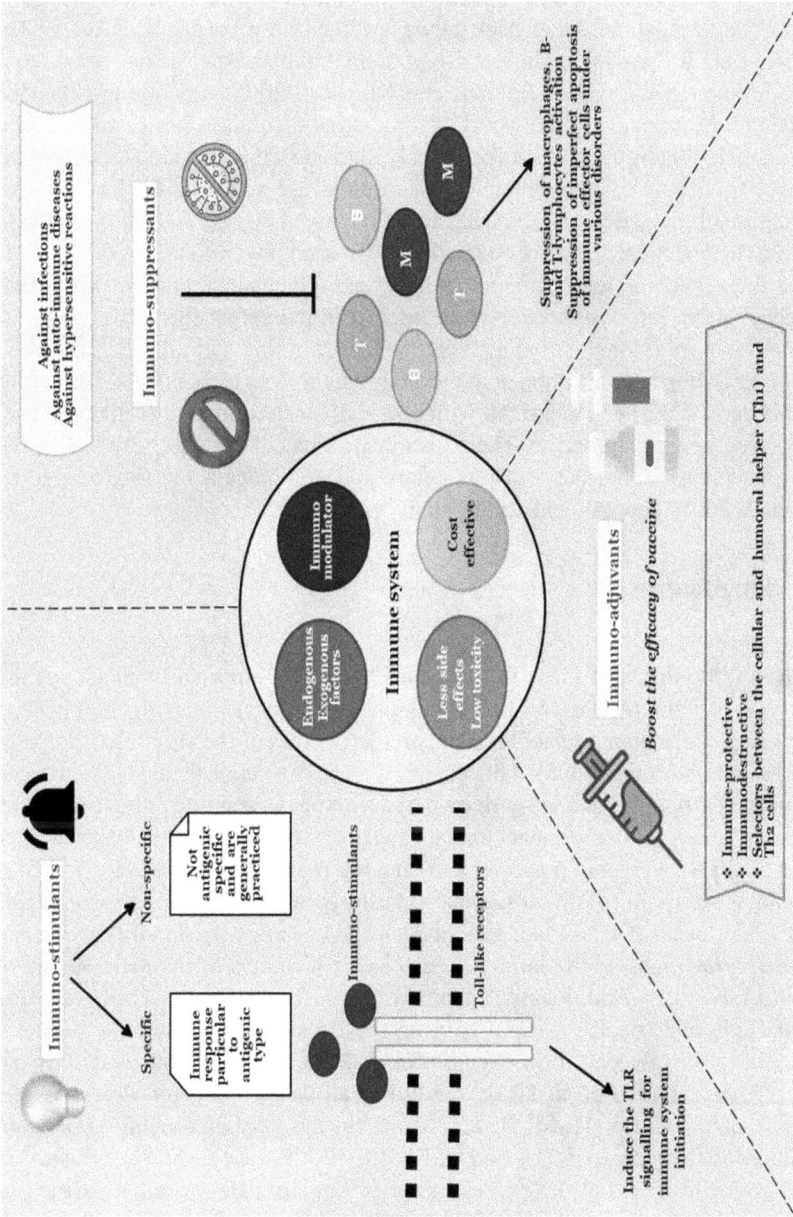

FIGURE 4.2 Different types of immunity-related chemicals and their role in disease treatment associated with weak immune systems.

4.6 PHYTOCHEMICAL EVIDENCE ASSOCIATED WITH TRADITIONAL MEDICINAL SYSTEMS

Plant-derived natural products have been used in medicine for more than 5,000 years, whereas Western medicines date back only a few hundred years ago (Goldman 2001; Atanasov et al. 2015). The medicinal use of > 85,000 plant species has been documented throughout the world (Balunas and Kinghorn 2005). According to WHO, more than 80% of people in the world rely on herbal medicines for treating several disorders, including immune disorders, mostly in the developing countries (Licciardi and Underwood 2011). Approximately 30% of the drugs approved by the Food and Drug Administration (FDA) of the USA are of botanical origin. Thus, it is crucial to determine the chemical structures of traditionally used phytomedicinal compounds to assess their potential for immunomodulatory activity against immune disorders.

Biochemists in the past developed an interest in extracting the active chemical molecules from traditional herbal medicines and examining them for their potential activities, and they began to notice additional roles for phytochemicals. Numerous phytochemicals have been identified with potential as an immunomodulator, a chemoprotective, or an adaptogenic. These chemicals include saponins, terpenoids, flavonoids, and polysaccharides, such as pectin and arabinogalactan (Sharma 2006; Rajput et al. 2007; Thoppil et al. 2011; Islam et al. 2020).

4.6.1 PHYTOCHEMISTRY

4.6.1.1 Flavonoids

More than 4,000 different kinds of flavonoids have been reported in plants and are known to contribute to leaf and flower colour. They are members of the phenolic group of secondary plant metabolites and are derivatives of the shikimic acid pathway (Cook and Samman 1996). This category of phytochemicals has gained much attention due to their antioxidant activity in scavenging oxygen free radicals and they have proven to be promising agents for anticancer therapy and anti-ageing properties (Bose et al. 2018). Apigenin poses tumour-suppressing activity by inhibiting TNF-α intra-cellular adhesion to inhibit tumour metastasis, while also suppressing angiogenesis (Patel et al. 2007). Plant genera such as *Artemisia*, *Achillea*, *Tanacetum*, and *Matricaria* belong to the family Asteraceae, which acts as the main source of apigenin (Table 4.1). Additionally, members of the Lamiaceae, such as *Sideritis* and *Teucrium*, and species of *Genista* from the Fabaceae also show the presence of apigenin in its aglycone form (Venditti et al. 2015, 2016a, 2016b, 2017; Ornano et al. 2016; Sharifi-Rad et al. 2018; Venditti et al. 2018). Apigenin decreases the expression of cytokines (IL-1α, IL-8, TNF-α) (in the case of *Cynodon dactylon*) and reduces the response of Th1 and Th17 cells (in the case of *Salvia officinalis*), as well as downregulating the expression of pro-inflammatory mediators such as inducible nitric oxide synthase (iNOS) and cyclooxygenase-2 (COX-2) (in *Portulaca oleracea*). Additionally, apigenin reduces the expression of the intracellular adhesion molecule (ICAM) and vascular cell adhesion molecule (VCAM) (in *Mentha longifolia*), resulting in lowered neutrophil chemotaxis (Nicholas et al. 2007; Kang et al. 2009). Similarly, quercetin decreases the expression of pro-inflammatory factors, such as cytokines, NF-κB, and iNOS. Luteolin (a type of flavone) adjusts the inflammatory environment of the brain by targeting brain chemistry. It inhibits the release of microbial IL-6 and mimics the activity of the brain-derived neurotrophilic factor. There is a decrease in the secretion of INF-γ, IL-6 inflammatory mediators and in the expression of COX-2 and ICAM-1 following exposure to a preparation of *Lonicera japonica* (Ziyan et al. 2007; Chen et al. 2014).

4.6.1.2 Terpenoids

Terpenoids are considered to be the largest family of natural phytochemicals, consisting of more than 30,000 compounds that vary and show specificity to particular plants (Dubey et al. 2003; Stephane and Jules 2020). Many herbal medicines include combinations of terpenoids and saponins (examples of triterpenes) that inhibit the faulty immune inflammation response during the development of neoplastic disease. Similarly, limonene, the monoterpene obtained from apricots, cherries, and citrus fruits, suppress NF-kB activation (Berchtold et al. 2005; Younis et al. 2020). Genopsida, obtained from *Gardenia jasminoides* fruits, can suppress the expression of iNOS and NF-kB expression, and is traditionally used in the treatment of headache, fever, inflammation, and hepatic disorders (Koo et al. 2004). Sesquiterpene lactones are potent medicinal phytochemicals and are used against inflammatory diseases and cancers (Salminen et al. 2008). The artemisinin isolated from the leaves of *Artemisia annua* (a traditional Chinese medicinal plant) is used as an effective antimalarial drug. Artemisinin and its derivatives show anticancer, antifungal, anti-angiogenesis, and immunosuppressive properties. It inhibits the NF-kB signalling system, with strong inhibition of inflammation (Cui and Su 2009). The elephantopin derivatives (isodeoxyelephantopin and deoxyelephantopin) isolated from *Elephantopus scaber* induce anti-inflammatory activities and anticancer activities *via* negatively targeting NF-kB activation (Huang et al. 2010; Su et al. 2011a). Similarly, paclitaxel, marketed under the brand name Taxol, is a polyoxygenated diterpenoid alkaloid originating from *Taxus brevifolia* (Pacific yew) bark, being used clinically as a drug against ovarian cancer and other cancers (Weaver 2014). Tanshinone IIA (a diterpenoid quinone), extracted from the roots of *Salvia miltiorrhiza*, is traditionally used against immunological disorders, osteoporosis, breast cancer, and cardiovascular diseases. It inhibits NF-kB signalling in the inflammation pathway (Gao et al. 2012). Carnosol and carnosic acid (abietane-type diterpenoids) are abundant in *Rosmarinus officinalis* and are frequently used traditionally as a result of their activity in inhibiting NF-kB signalling and inducing expression of the Nrf-2-activated HO-1 (Pan and Ho 2008; Yousef et al. 2020). Celastrol (a quinone methide pentacyclic triterpenoid) has shown anticancer and anti-inflammatory activities (Pinna et al. 2004). It suppresses NF-kB signalling in tumour growth and inflammation (Kim et al. 2009). Ursolic acid (a pentacyclic triterpene) is the main active ingredient in some traditional remedies used as an anticancer agent, with hepatoprotective activities, and for antihyperlipidaemia (Ikeda et al. 2008; Salminen et al. 2008). Ursolic acid inhibits the NF-kB activation that is involved in the inhibition of TPA-induced skin tumours and lipid polysaccharide (LPS)-induced pro-inflammatory mediators (Ikeda et al. 2008).

Betulinic acid (a lupane-type triterpenoid) and its derivatives show therapeutically potent activity against cancer, pathogen infections, and various kind of inflammations (Fulda 2009). Lupeol (a triterpenoid derivative) inhibits the Akt-dependent pathway, contributing to anti-inflammatory and anticancer activities (Fernandez et al. 2001; Salminen et al. 2008; Wang et al. 2020). The tetraterpenoid derivatives, such as lutein, lycopene, and β-carotene, modulate the redox-sensitive signalling pathways, including ROS signalling and NF-kB signalling pathways (Chew and Park 2004; Huang et al. 2007).

4.6.1.3   Organosulphur Compounds

The organosulphur compounds, derived from garlic and onion, have been shown to result in suppressed activities of cyclooxygenase and lipooxygenase (inflammatory enzymes) and decreased levels of inhibitory iNOS expression in the inflammatory macrophages (Dirsch et al. 1998; Ali et al. 2000; Ruhee et al. 2020). Garlic extract inhibits receptor NF-kB activity induced in response to receptor agonists, such as TNF-an and LPS, under anti-inflammatory responses (Keiss et al. 2003; Jo et al. 2020). Garlic extract can also modulate inflammatory responses through inhibition of TLR activation (Youn et al. 2008; Table 4.2; Figure 4.3).

4.6.2   Pharmacology

The use of plants as medicines for treating disease has been recorded since ancient times (Singh et al. 2016). In India, in particular, it has become an important system of health care, and approximately 70% of rural people in India use the traditional herbal medicinal system for treating disease. There are various medicinal systems mentioned in Vedas and other scriptures, dating from ancient times. Many conventional systems, such as Siddha, homoeopathy, naturopathy, Unani, Yoga, Ayurveda, Chinese, or Amachi medicines, have been well known and widely adopted for many years. Ayurveda is also known as the "science of longevity" because it helps to maintain a long, healthy life for any individual (Kumar et al. 2012).

In the conventional medicine system, there are easy and cheap treatment methods (derived from herbs and various plant parts) to treat many common diseases, such as cancer, food allergies, and another immune diseases, for which there are few modern treatments. The medicinal attributes of many plants are found in leaves, rhizomes, and roots, and can be used as a tonic, diuretic, blood purifier, and antiphlogistic. These are used as remedies for treating various diseases, like chronic eczema, chronic rheumatism, chronic nervous diseases, cholera amenorrhoea, chronic ulcers, etc. The powder of dried leaves of plants like *Catharanthus roseus, Clitoria ternatea,* etc., is used for the treatment of depression and for improving memory when the powder is consumed with milk. Similarly, the juice of the leaves of plants like *Ocimum sanctum* and *Tinospora cordifolia* are used as an alternative treatment of cases of jaundice, fever, or gonorrhoea. These plants are also helpful in improving the nervous system in children and for treating cutaneous diseases. There are more than 3,000 medicinal-value plant species in India that are used to prepare medicinal drugs, of which a number have been highlighted in Table 4.1.

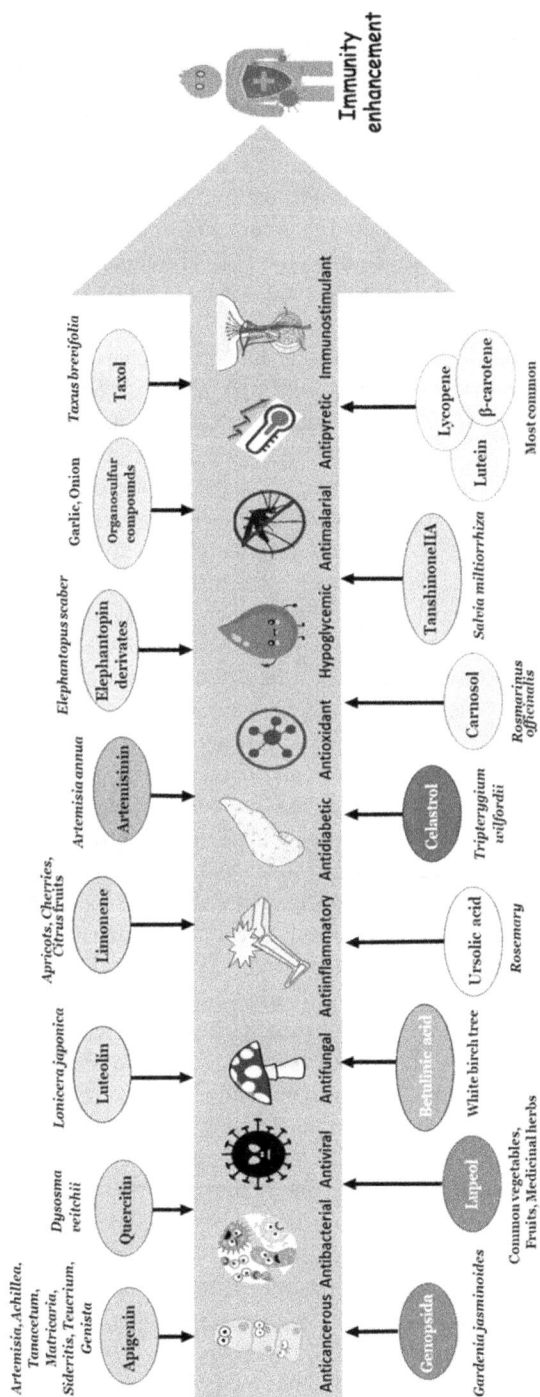

FIGURE 4.3 Phytochemical constituents obtained from various medicinal plant parts with special reference to immunity enhancement.

The effectiveness of medicinal plants varies from species to species and for the treatment of different conditions. For example, in the treatment of nervous disorders, the brain tonic, brahmi, is more effective than mandukparni. The brahmi plant is also used to reduce fatigue, and to treat asthma and depression. It energizes the central nervous system and improves the circulatory system, soothes and minimizes varicose veins, and helps to minimize scarring. Brahmi also proves useful in repairing skin and connective tissues in the body as well as smoothing out cellulite. In India, this plant has been used by Ayurvedic medicine for 3,000 years. The Ayurvedic treatise, the Charaka-samhta (100 AD) recommends Brahmi in formulations for a range of mental conditions, including treating anxiety and improving concentration.

Most of the valuable medicinal plants, like punarnava (*Boerhaavia diffusa*), gokhru (*Tribulus terrestris*), and ark (*Calotropis procera*), etc., grow in the wild, mainly because of the favorable climatic and edaphic conditions, as well as the reduced urbanization in these regions. Another important plant, ashwagandha (*Withania somnifera*) is widely used in the treatment of psoriasis, arthritis, and rheumatism. It is rich in valuable phytochemical constituents, like alkaloids (isopelletierine and anaferine), steroidal lactones (withanolides, withaferins), and saponins (sitoindosides VII and VIII). For treatment of arthritis, ginger (*Zingiber officinale*) is used because of its chemical constituent zingiberene, which is mainly responsible for reducing pain and inflammation by inhibiting the cyclooxygenase (COX) and lipoxygenase (LOX) pathways. Onion (*Allium cepa*) is also widely used to decrease the numbers of cancer cells, to effectively heal stomach ulcers, and inhibit the proliferation of cultured ovarian, breast, and colon cancer cells. This plant also reduces levels of cholesterol and blood pressure, and decreases symptoms associated with diabetes mellitus, inhibits platelet aggregation, and prevents inflammatory processes associated with asthma (Upadhyay et al. 2016). The fruit extract of the plant *Phyllanthus emblica* possesses antidiarrhoeal and spasmolytic activity, which is mediated possibly through the dual blockage of muscarinic receptors and Ca^{2+} channels, thus explaining its medicinal use in the treatment of diarrhoea. In addition, *P. emblica* has great potential to check cancer and tumour growth. In addition, extracts of sunflower (*Helianthus annuus*) seeds are used as a diuretic and to effectively cure coughs and lung infections. They are also used as an antiseptic, aphrodisiac, emollient, and as an anti-malarial. Leaves of neem (*Azadirachta indica*) are used in the treatment of numerous diseases, like eczema, ringworm, and acne, and they possess anti-inflammatory and antihyperglycaemic activities (Srivastava et al. 2020). Neem is used to treat chronic wounds, diabetes, and gangrene. It also helps to remove toxins from the body, quench free radicals, and to purify the blood (Dubey et al. 2014).

The high value of the conventional medicinal system, and its application in terms of derived drug phytochemistry, gained much attention in 2011 following a paper published by Dr. YY Tu in Nature Medicine. The discovery of artemisinin, from *Artemesia annua* plant, for the treatment of malaria resulted in the author winning the Lasker Award for medicinal research in 2011. The article explained the need for the re-recognition of the traditional medicinal system and its background to the identification of immunity boosters. In another report, published in Science Translation Medicine by YC Cheng and coworkers, highlighted the use of TCMs containing multiple formulations, including extracts of more than three or four plants, for the treatment of cancer instead of the use of a single chemical constituent. This report described experiments that provide strong evidence for identification of preparations with anti-inflammatory, anticancer, and molecular patterning activities based solely on metabolite profiling. The above reports, supported by clinical trials, attracted greater belief and interest from the medical community. In a case study, a methanolic extract of *Ocimum sanctum* samples (100 mg/kg body wt.) showed increased concentration of red blood cells (RBC) in sheep. The extract had a promotional effect on humoral-mediated immunity and expressed an immunomodulatory effect, enhancing the level of RBCs in sheep, and decreasing the amount of histamine released from the mast cells. The findings indicated the responses of both humoral- and cell-mediated immune responses to this herbal plant preparation. An alcoholic extract of *Achillea millefolium* (100 mg/kg, i.p.) exhibited a significant stimulatory effect on both cellular and humoral function in mice. The enhanced carbon clearance and neutrophile adhesion, and the decreased level of cyclophosphamide-induced neutropaenia reflects an immunomodulatory effect (Licciardi et al. 2011; Kumar et al. 2012) In mitogen-induced lymphocyte proliferation, the andrographolide compounds from *Andrographis paniculata* act as an inhibitor of TNF-an and a stimulator of both non-specific and antigen-specific types of immunostimulatory response in mice, exhibiting responses to a range of oncogenic and infectious agents. Treatment with an extract of *Gymnema sylvestre* showed immunomodulation *in vivo* and *in vitro*, with significant immunostimulatory activity, affecting the activities of neutrophils and phagocytes, as well as chemotaxis responses (Kumar et al. 2012; Table 4.3). The herbs used in conventional formulations or Rasayana seem to function by affecting the effector arm that regulates immunosuppressants, immunoadjuvants, and immunostimulant activities. Immunomodulation activities can be used to create a pathogen-free state inside the body of a diseased person.

Immunomodulation mechanisms are mainly regulated *via* the activities of various cellular functions, such as macrophage activation, increased antigen-specific immunoglobulin production, enhanced numbers of non-specific immunity mediators and natural killer cells, increased cellular immune function, increased non-specific cellular immune system effect, phagocytosis stimulation, immunostimulatory effect on peritoneal macrophages, lymphoid cells stimulation, reduction in chemotherapy-induced leukopaenia, and increased total white cell counts *via* circulating and interleukin-2 levels (Kumar et al. 2012).

It has become our main responsibility to highlight these valuable plant species, which would help herbal practitioners, conservationists, and environmentalists to narrow down their focus to such indigenous plant species, thereby ensuring protection of the medicinal flora. Many commercial products derived from herbal plants are sold in the markets these days (Table 4.3) and their demand, production, and consumption have been significantly boosted in the present COVID-19 situation.

TABLE 4.3
Commercially Available Products Derived from Traditional Medicinal Plants. Used as Immuno-protectants

S. No.	Plant Name	Market Products	References
1	*Withania somnifera* (ashwagandha)		Gupta and Rana (2007)
2	*Aloe barbadensis* (aloe vera)		Christaki and Panneri (2010)

(Continued)

TABLE 4.3 (CONTINUED)

Commercially Available Products Derived from Traditional Medicinal Plants. Used as Immuno-protectants

S. No.	Plant Name	Market Products	References
3	*Ocimum tenuiflorum* (tulsi)		Vishwabhan et al. (2011)
4	*Aegle marmelos* (bael)		Atul et al. (2012)

(Continued)

TABLE 4.3 (CONTINUED)
Commercially Available Products Derived from Traditional Medicinal Plants. Used as Immuno-protectants

S. No.	Plant Name	Market Products	References
5	*Azadirachta indica* (neem)		Dubey et al. (2014)
6	*Tinospora cordifolia* (giloy)		Mittal (2014)

(Continued)

TABLE 4.3 (CONTINUED)
Commercially Available Products Derived from Traditional Medicinal Plants. Used as Immuno-protectants

S. No.	Plant Name	Market Products	References
7	*Mentha arvensis* (mint)		Choudhary and Shah (2017)
8	*Olea europaea* (olive)		Sahin and Bilgin (2017)

(Continued)

TABLE 4.3 (CONTINUED)
Commercially Available Products Derived from Traditional Medicinal Plants. Used as Immuno-protectants

S. No.	Plant Name	Market Products	References
9	*Zingiber officinale* (ginger)		Bag (2018)
10	*Moringa oleifera* (moringa)		Sekhar and Arumugam (2019)

4.7   CONCLUSION

Herbalists widely recommend the use of specific traditional medicinal plants to enhance immunity and restrict the activities of cancer, HIV, and other conditions associated with pathogenic microbes. The reason for the importance of these medicinal-value plants is that they contain chemicals exhibiting important pharmacological properties. The repeated, conclusive findings on the various properties, including anti-inflammation, antioxidant, antitumour activities, serve as an effective way of boosting the immune system. Modern-day validations are based on the activities of secondary plant metabolites. As a result, the true specificity of the traditional medicinal system was questioned by Western medicine, which later confirmed it on the basis of bioactive plant extracts containing physiologically active phytochemicals. In a nutshell, the potent immunity-based anti-inflammation and anti-tumour activities can be harmful if not evaluated over a range of doses. By the same token, different herbal formulations are often recommended in conventional medicines for the treatment of specific diseases by targeting particular cellular and molecular pathways. The use of many plants in a single drug preparation in a conventional medicinal system lacks information on the primary drug, the adjuvant, and the delivery systems within the body. Therefore, it cannot be specific for particular targets and treats the problem indirectly. Firstly, the incomplete understanding of the chemical constituents and their mode of action needs clinical trialling, to identify the exact profile of immunomodulatory activities of various herbal formulations used in the conventional medicinal system. Secondly, the majority of herbal formulations and their extracts are typically considered to be less toxic than modern-day single-chemical pharmaceutical products. Thirdly, the drawback of the conventional medicinal system is hypersensitivity and allergies, such as skin allergies caused by the intake of products from chamomile and other members of the Asteraceae due to the high concentration of sesquiterpene lactones, although this response occurs in only a few patients. Fourthly, there is an issue with the misidentification of plants with similar phenologies, such as compendia by most of the herbalists which confuse the identity of *Parthenium integrifolium*. Fifthly, herbal formulations can effectively penetrate dermal regions and their immunomodulatory region as a drug delivery system. However, several compounds, such as ginsenosides and anolides, are able to enhance the inflammatory system during healing, infections, and to suppress chronic inflammation. The importance of ethnobotanists is underrated as much usage of the knowledge on medicinal plants comes from early cultures, which evaluated the potential role and effectiveness of herbal preparations based on information passed down from the ancestors. Most of these properties of medicinal herbs are positive, but why they are not completely accepted by the modern-day medicinal system is an unsolved question which needs resolution in the future. Properly conducted research and clinical trialling, carried out under strict guidelines, must be performed that will ultimately result in the acceptance of the value of medicinal herbs to Western medicine, in particular as well as in the appropriate recognition of ethnobotanists.

REFERENCES

Abobatta, W. 2019. *Jatropha curcas*: an overview. *Journal of Advances in Agriculture* 10: 1650–1656.

Ahmad, S., P. Chitkara, F.N. Khan, A. Kishan, V. Alok, A. Ramlal, and S. Mehta. 2021. Mobile technology solution for COVID-19: surveillance and prevention. In: *Computational Intelligence Methods in COVID-19: Surveillance, Prevention, Prediction and Diagnosis*. Ed. K. Raza. Springer, pp. 79–108.

Alam, M.K., M.O. Hoq, and M.S. Uddin. 2016. Medicinal plant *Allium sativum*: a Review. *Journal of Medicinal Plant Studies* 4: 72–79.

Ali, M., M. Thomson, and M. Afzal. 2000. Garlic and onions: their effect on eicosanoid metabolism and its clinical relevance. *Prostaglandins, Leukotrienes, and Essential Fatty Acids* 62: 55–73.

Al-snafi, A.E. 2016. The pharmacology activity of Cuminum cynimum: a review. *IOSR Journal of Pharmacy* 6: 46–65.

Al-Snafi, A.E. 2018. Therapeutic importance of *Hyoscyamus* species grown in Iraq (*Hyoscyamus albus, Hyoscyamus niger* and *Hyoscyamus reticulates*)-A review. *IOSR Journal of Pharmacy* 8: 18–32.

Anywar, G., E. Kakudidi, R. Byamukama, J. Mukonzo, A. Schubert, and H. Oryem-Origa. 2020. Medicinal plants used by traditional medicine practitioners to boost the immune system in people living with HIV/AIDS in Uganda. *European Journal of Integrative Medicine* 35: 101011.

Archana, S.J., P. Rajkumar, and T. Archana. 2011. Indian medicinal plants: a rich source of natural immuno-modulator. *International Journal of Pharmacology* 7: 198–205.

Atanasov, A.G., B. Waltenberger, E.M. Pferschy-Wenzig, T. Linder, C. Wawrosch, P. Uhrin, V. Temml, L. Wang, S. Schwaiger, E.H. Heiss, and J.M. Rollinger. 2015. Discovery and resupply of pharmacologically active plant-derived natural products: a review. *Biotechnology Advances* 33: 1582–1614.

Atul, N.P., V.D. Nilesh, A.R. Akkatai, and S.K. Kamlakar. 2012. A review on *Aegle marmelos*: a potential medicinal tree. *International Research Journal of Pharmacy* 3: 86–91.

Bag, B. 2018. Ginger processing in India (*Zingiber officinale*): a review. *International Journal of Current Microbiology and Applied Sciences* 7: 1639–1651.

Balunas, M.J. and A.D. Kinghorn. 2005. Drug discovery from medicinal plants. *Life Sciences* 78: 431–441.

Banstola, A., J.H. Jeong, and S. Yook. 2020. Immunoadjuvants for cancer immunotherapy: a review of recent developments. *Acta biomaterialia* 114: 16–30.

Berchtold, C.M., K.S. Chen, Miyamoto, S., and M.N. Gould. 2005. Perillyl alcohol inhibits a calcium-dependent constitutive nuclear factor-kappaB pathway. *Cancer Research* 65: 8558–8566.

Bhalerao, S. 2013. *Eclipta alba* (L.): an overview. *International Journal of Bioassays* 1443–1447.

Bhatia, M., N. Siddiqui, and S. Gupta. 2013. Abrus Precatorius (L.): an evaluation of traditional herb. Indo American Journal of Pharmaceutical Research 3: 3295–3315.

Biswa, D., P. Bharati, N. Kumar, and R. Dudhe. 2011. Pharmacological activity of *Andrographis paniculata*: a brief review. *Pharmacology Online* 2: 1–10.

Bose, S., D. Sarkar, A. Bose, and S.C. Mandal. 2018. Natural flavonoids and its pharmaceutical importance. *The Pharma Review* 61–75.

Chatterjee, S. and S.N. Das. 1996. Effect of herbal Immu-21 on murine peritoneal acrophages and splenic lymphocytes. *Ancient Science of Life* 15: 250253.

Chauhan, N., N. Singh, J. Gupta, K. Shah, P. Mishra, A. Tripathi, and N. Upmanyu. 2017. A review on *Clitoria ternatea* (Linn.): *Chemistry and Pharmacology* 1: 1–17.

Chen, D., A. Bi, X. Dong, Y. Jiang, B. Rui, and J. Liu. 2014. Luteolin exhibits anti-inflammatory effects by blocking the activity of heat shock protein 90 in macrophages. *Biochemical and Biophysical Research Communications* 443: 326–332.

Cheng, Y.C. and A. VanHook. 2010. Science translational medicine podcast: 18 August 2010. *Science Translational Medicine* 2(45): 45pc6.

Chew, B.P. and J.S. Park. 2004. Carotenoid action on the immune response. *The Journal of Nutrition* 134: 257S–261S.

Choudhary, H. and R. Shah. 2017. Marketing of Menthol Mint (*Mentha*) in Uttar Pradesh, India. *International Journal of Pure and Applied Bioscience* 5: 1323–1327.

Christaki, E. and P. Florou-Paneri. 2010. *Aloe vera*: a plant for many uses. *Journal of Food, Agriculture and Environment* 8: 245–249.

Chulet, R. and Pradhan, P. 2010. A review on rasayana. *Pharmacognosy Reviews* 3: 229e34.

Cook, N.C. and S. Samman. 1996. Flavonoids – chemistry, metabolism, cardioprotective effects and dietary sources. *The Journal of Nutritional Biochemistry* 7: 66–75

Cui, L. and X.Z. Su. 2009. Discovery, mechanisms of action and combination therapy of artemisinin. *Expert Review of Anti-Infective Therapy* 7: 999–1013.

Cundell, D.R. 2014. Herbal phytochemicals as immunomodulators. *Current Immunology Reviews* 10: 64–81.

Derouiche, S. 2020. Current review on herbal pharmaceutical improve immune responses against COVID-19 infection. *Research Journal of Pharmaceutical Dosage Forms and Technology* 12: 181–184.

Dey, A. and J. De 2011. *Aristolochia indica* L.: a review. *Asian Journal of Plant Sciences* 10: 108–116.

Dhanik, J., N. Arya, and V. Nand. 2017. A review on *Zingiber officinale*. *Journal of Pharmacognosy and Phytochemistry* 6: 174–184.

Dirsch, V.M., A.K. Kiemer, H. Wagner, and A.M. Vollmar. 1998. Effect of allicin and ajoene, two compounds of garlic, on inducible nitric oxide synthase. *Atherosclerosis* 139: 333–339.

Doshi, G.M., H.D. Une, and P.P. Shanbhag. 2013. Rasayans and non-rasayans herbs: future immunodrug - targets. *Pharmacognosy Reviews* 7: 92–96.

Dubey, S. and P. Kashyap. 2014. *Azadirachta indica*: a plant with versatile potential. *Journal of Pharmaceutical Sciences* 4: 39–46.

Dubey, V.S., R. Bhalla, and R. Luthra. 2003. An overview of the nonmevalonate pathway for terpenoid biosynthesis in plants. *Journal of Bioscience* 28: 637–646

Dwivedi, S. and D. Chopra. 2014. Revisiting *Terminalia arjuna*- an ancient cardiovascular drug. *Journal of Traditional and Complementary Medicine* 4: 224–231.

Fernandez, M.A., B. De Las Heras, M.D. Garcia, M.T. Saenz, and A. Villar. 2001. New insights into the mechanism of action of the anti-inflammatory triterpene lupeol. *The Journal of Pharmacy and Pharmacology* 53: 1533–1539.

Fulda, S. 2009. Betulinic acid: a natural product with anticancer activity. *Molecular Nutrition and Food Research* 53: 140–146.

Gan, L., S.H. Zhang, Q. Liu, and H.B. Xu. 2003. A polysaccharide-protein complex from *Lycium barbarum* upregulates cytokine expression in human peripheral blood mononuclear cells. *European Journal of Pharmacology* 471: 217e22.

Gao, S., Z. Liu, H. Li, P.J. Little, P. Liu, and S. Xu. 2012. Cardiovascular actions and therapeutic potential of tanshinone IIA. *Atherosclerosis* 220: 3–10.

Goldman, P. 2001. Herbal medicines today and the roots of modern pharmacology. *Annals of Internal Medicine* 135: 594–600.

Gupta, G. and A.C. Rana. 2007. *Withania somnifera* (Ashwagandha): a review. *Pharmacognosy Reviews* 1: 129–136.

Gupta, M., S. Kaushik, R. Tomar, and R. Mishra. 2017. An overview of *Catharanthus roseus* and medicinal properties of their metabolites against important diseases. *European Academic Research* 5: 1237–1247.

Hasan, N, N. Ahmad, S. Zohrameena, M. Khalid, and J. Akhtar. 2016. *Asparagus racemosus*: for medicinal uses & pharmacological actions. *International Journal of Advanced Research* 4: 259–267.

Huang, C.C., C.P. Lo, C.Y. Chiu, and L.F. Shyur. 2010. Deoxyelephantopin, a novel multifunctional agent, suppresses mammary tumour growth and lung metastasis and doubles survival time in mice. *British Journal of Pharmacology* 159: 856–871.

Huang, C.S., Y.E. Fan, C.Y. Lin, and M.L. Hu. 2007. Lycopene inhibits matrix metalloproteinase-9 expression and down-regulates the binding activity of nuclear factor-kappa B and stimulatory protein-1. *The Journal of Nutritional Biochemistry* 18: 449–456.

Ikeda, Y., A. Murakami, and H. Ohigashi. 2008. Ursolic acid: an anti- and proinflammatory triterpenoid. *Molecular Nutrition and Food Research* 52: 26–42.

Ikram, Q. and O.P. Chahar. 2013. Medicinal use of endangered plant *Commiphora wightii*. *Variorum Multi-Disciplinary e-Research Journal* 4: 1–5.

Islam, M.T., C. Sarkar, D.M. El-Kersh, S. Jamaddar, S.J. Uddin, J.A. Shilpi, and M.S. Mubarak. 2020. Natural products and their derivatives against coronavirus: a review of the non-clinical and pre-clinical data. *Phytotherapy Research* 34: 2471–2492.

Jantan, I., W. Ahmad, and S.N.A. Bukhari. 2015. Plant-derived immunomodulators: an insight on their preclinical evaluation and clinical trials. *Frontiers in Plant Science* 6: 655.

Jeet, K., N. Devi, N. Thakur, S. Tomar, L. Shalta, and R. Thakur. (2012). *Trachyspermum ammi*: A comprehensive review. *International Research Journal of Pharmacy* 3: 6.

Jo, E.S., N. Sp, D.Y. Kang, A. Rugamba, I.H. Kim, S.W. Bae, Q. Liu, K.J. Jang, and Y.M. Yang. 2020. Sulfur compounds inhibit high glucose-induced inflammation by regulating NF-κB signaling in human monocytes. *Molecules* 25: 2342.

Kang, H.-K., D. Ecklund, M. Liu, and S.K. Datta. 2009. Apigenin, a nonmutagenic dietary flavonoid, suppresses lupus by inhibiting autoantigen presentation for expansion of autoreactive Th1 and Th17 cells. *Arthritis Research Therapy* 11: R59.

Keiss, H.P., V.M. Dirsch, T. Hartung, T. Haffner, L. Trueman, J. Auger, R. Kahane, and A.M. Vollmar. 2003. Garlic (*Allium sativum* L.) modulates cytokine expression in lipopolysaccharide-activated human blood thereby inhibiting NF-kappaB activity. *The Journal of Nutrition* 133: 2171–2175.

Khairnar, A., S. Bhamare, and H. Bhamare. 2012. *Calotropis procera*: an ethnopharmacological update. *Advance Research in Pharmaceuticals and Biologicals* 2: 142–156.

Khan, K. 2009. Role of *Emblica officinalis* in medicine - a review. *Botany Research International* 2: 218–228.

Khanal, P., T. Duyu, Y.N. Dey, B.M. Patil, I. Pasha and M. Wanjari. 2020. Network pharmacology of AYUSH recommended immune-boosting medicinal plants against COVID-19. *Research Square* 1–12.

Khodadadi, S. 2015. Role of herbal medicine in boosting immune system. *Immunopathologia Persa* 1: e01.

Kim, D.H., E.K. Shin, Y.H. Kim, B.W. Lee, J.G. Jun, J.H. Park, and J.K. Kim. 2009. Suppression of inflammatory responses by celastrol, a quinone methide triterpenoid isolated from *Celastrus regelii*. *European Journal of Clinical Investigation* 39: 819–827.

Kolla J. and N. Kulkarni. 2018. *Terminalia chebula* Retz. – an important medicinal plant. *Herba Polonica* 63: 45–56.

Koo, H.J., Y.S. Song, H.J. Kim, Y.H. Lee, S.M. Hong, S.J. Kim, B.C. Kim, C. Jin, C.J. Lim, and E.H. Park. 2004. Antiinflammatory effects of genipin, an active principle of *Gardenia*. *European Journal of Pharmacology* 495: 201–208.

Kulkarni, R., K.J. Girish, and A. Kumar. 2012. Nootropic herbs (*Medhya Rasayana*) in Ayurveda: an update. *Pharmacognosy Reviews* 6: 147–153.

Kumar, D., A. Vikrant, K. Ranjeet, A.B. Zulfiqar, V.K. Gupta, and V. Kumar. 2012. A review of immunomodulators in the Indian traditional health care system. *Journal of Microbiology* 45: 165e184.

Kumar, S.V., P.K. Sharma, R. Dudhe, and N. Kumar. 2011. Immunomodulatory effects of some traditional medicinal plants. *Journal of Chemical and Pharmaceutical Research* 3: 675–84.

Kumar, D., V. Arya, R. Kaur, Z.A. Bhat, V.K. Gupta, and V. Kumar. 2012. A review of immunomodulators in the Indian traditional health care system. *Journal of Microbiology, Immunology and Infection* 45: 165–184.

Lanculov, I., I. Gergen, R. Palicica, M. Butnariu, D.G. Dumbravă, and L. Gabor. 2004. The determination of total alkaloids from *Atropa belladona* and *Lupinus* sp using various spectrophotometrical and gravimetrical methods. *Revista de Chimie* 55: 835–838.

Licciardi, P.V. and J.R. Underwood. 2011. Plant-derived medicines: a novel class of immunological adjuvants. *International Immunopharmacology* 11: 390–398.

Lokhande, P., A. Kharche, S.G. Wagh, D. Manithe, and S. Harke. 2019. Immune boosting super food supplement from natural resources. *Journal of Pharmacognosy and Phytochemistry* 8: 2108–2113.

Maheshwari, N.O., A. Khan, and B.A. Chopade. 2013. Rediscovering the medicinal properties of *Datura* sp.: a review. *Journal of Medicinal Plants Research* 7: 2885–2897.

Meghwal, M. and T.K. Goswami. 2012. A review on the functional properties, nutritional content, medicinal utilization and potential application of fenugreek. *Journal of Food Processing and Technology* 3: 1–10.

Mittal, J. 2014. *Tinospora cordifolia*: a multipurpose medicinal plant- a review. *Journal of Medicinal Plants Studies* 2: 32–47.

Nagaratna, A., and P. L. Hegde. 2015. A comprehensive review on Parnabeeja [Bryophyllum pinnatum (Lam.) Oken]. *Journal of Medicinal Plants Studies* 3(5): 166–71.

Nasri, H., N. Sahinfard, M. Rafieian, S. Rafieian, M. Shirzad, and M. Rafieian-Kopaei. 2014. Turmeric: a spice with multifunctional medicinal properties. *Journal of HerbMed Pharmacology* 3: 5–8.

Nicholas, C., S. Batra, M.A. Vargo, O.H. Voss, M.A. Gavrilin, and M.D. Wewers. 2007. Apigenin blocks lipopolysaccharide-induced lethality in vivo and proinflammatory cytokines expression by inactivating NF-κB through the suppression of p65 phosphorylation. *The Journal of Immunology* 179: 7121–7127.

Ornano, L., A. Venditti, Y. Donno, C. Sanna, M. Ballero, and A. Bianco. 2016. Phytochemical analysis of non-volatile fraction of *Artemisia caerulescens* subsp. *densiflora* (Viv.) (Asteraceae), an endemic species of La Maddalena Archipelago (Sardinia–Italy). *Natural Product Research* 30: 920–925.

Pan, S.Y., G. Litscher, S.H. Gao, S.F. Zhou, Z.L. Yu, H.Q. Chen, Z. Shuo-Feng, T. Min-Ke, S. Jian-Ning, and K. Kam-Ming. 2014. Historical perspective of traditional indigenous medical practices: the current renaissance and conservation of herbal resources. *Evidence-Based Complementary and Alternative Medicine* 2014.

Pan, M.H. and C.T. Ho. 2008. Chemopreventive effects of natural dietary compounds on cancer development. *Chemical Society Reviews* 37: 2558–2574.

Patel, D. and S. Gupta. 2007. Apigenin and cancer chemoprevention: progress, potential and future promise. *International Journal of Oncology* 30: 233–245.

Patel, K. 2012. A review on herbal immunoadjuvant. *International Journal of Pharmacy and Life Sciences* 3: 1568–1576.

Paul, S. and H.K.S. El Bethel Hmar. 2020. Strengthening immunity with immunostimulants: a. *Current Trends in Pharmaceutical Research* 7: 35–64.

Petronelli, A., G. Pannitteri, and U. Testa. 2009. Triterpenoids as new promising anticancer drugs. *Anticancer Drugs* 20: 880–892.

Piasecka, A., N. Jedrzejczak-Rey, and P. Bednarek. 2015. Secondary metabolites in plant innate immunity: conserved function of divergent chemicals. *New Phytologist* 206: 948–964.

Pinna, G.F., M. Fiorucci, J.M. Reimund, N. Taquet, Y. Arondel, and C.D. Muller. 2004. Celastrol inhibits pro-inflammatory cytokine secretion in Crohn's disease biopsies. *Biochemical and Biophysical Research Communications* 322: 778–786.

Promila, P. 2018. A review on the medicinal and aromatic plant- *Cymbopogon martinii* (Roxb.) Watson (Palmarosa) Promila. *International Journal of Chemical Studies* 6: 1311–1315.

Qureshi, H., Masood, M., Arshad, M., Qureshi, R., Sabir, S., Amjad, M., and Tahir, Z. 2015. *Picrorhiza kurroa*: an ethnopharmacologically important plant species of Himalayan region. *Pure and Applied Biology* 4: 407–417.

Rachh, P., Dhabaliya, F., Rachh, M., Lakhani, K., Kanani, A., and Limbani, D. 2014. Immunomodulatory medicinal plants: a review. *Pharmacognosy, Technology and Medicine* 1: 435–440.

Rai, K., N. Gupta, L. Dharamdasani, P. Nair, and P. Bodhankar. 2017. Bacopa monnieri: a wonder drug changing fortune of people. *International Journal of Applied Sciences and Biotechnology* 5(2): 127–132.

Raja, R. and K. Kailasam. 2015. Abutilon indicum L (Malvaceae)-medicinal potential review. *Pharmacognosy Journal* 7: 330–332.

Rajput, Z.I., H. Song-hua, and A.G. Arijo. 2007. Adjuvant effects of saponins on animal immune responses. *Journal of Zhejiang University Science B* 8: 153–161.

Rani, C., S. Chawla, M. Mangal, A. Mangal, S. Kajla, and A. Dhawan. 2011. *Nyctanthes arbor-tristis* Linn. (night jasmine): a sacred ornamental plant with immense medicinal potential. *Indian Journal of Traditional knowledge* 3: 427–435.

Rawat, I., N. Verma, and K. Joshi. 2019. Cinnamon (Cinnamomum zeylanicum). Jaya Publishing House, New Delhi.

Reis, L.S., N.M. Frazatti-Gallina, R.L. Paoli, A.A. Giuffrida, E. Oba, and P.E. Pardo 2008. Efficiency of *Matricaria chamomilla* CH12 and number of doses of rabies vaccine on the humoral immune response in cattle. *Journal of Veterinary Science* 9: 433e5.

Riazunnisa, K., U. Adilakshmamma, and C. Khadri. 2011. phytochemical analysis and in vitro antibacterial activity of *Soymida febrifuga* (Roxb.) Juss. and *Hemidesmus indicus* (L.). *Indian Journal of Applied Research* 3: 57–59.

Romanelli, A. and S. Mascolo. 2020. Immunosuppression drug-related and clinical manifestation of coronavirus disease 2019: a therapeutical hypothesis. *American Journal of Transplantation* 20: 2928–2932.

Ruhee, R.T., L.A. Roberts, S. Ma, and K. Suzuki. 2020. Organosulfur compounds: a review of their anti-inflammatory effects in human health. *Frontiers in Nutrition* 7: 64.

Şahin, S. and M. Bilgin. 2017. Olive tree (*Olea europaea* L.) leaf as a waste by-product of table olive and olive oil industry: a review. *Journal of the Science of Food and Agriculture* 98: 1271–1279.

Sahu, P.K., D.D. Giri, R. Singh, P. Pandey, S Gupta, A.K. Shrivastava, A. Kumar, and K.D. Pandey. 2013. Therapeutic and medicinal uses of *Aloe vera*: a review. *Pharmalogy and Pharmacy* 4: 599–610.

Sahu, R., H. Dhongade, A. Pandey, P. Sahu, V. Sahu, D. Patel and P. Kashyap. 2016. Medicinal properties of *Nardostachys jatamansi* (a review). *Oriental Journal of Chemistry* 32: 859–866.

Salminen, A., M. Lehtonen, T. Suuronen, K. Kaarniranta, and J. Huuskonen. 2008. Terpenoids: natural inhibitors of NF-kappaB signaling with antiinflammatory and anticancer potential. *Cellular and Molecular Life Sciences* 65: 2979–2999.

Sekhar, C. and V. Arumugam. 2019. Marketing of moringa. *Horticulture International Journal* 2: 212–21.

Sharifi-Rad, M., J. Nazaruk, L. Polito, M.F.B. Morais-Braga, J.E. Rocha, H.D.M. Coutinho, B. Salehi, G. Tabanelli, C. Montanari, M. Del Mar Contreras, Z. Yousaf, W.N. Setzer, D.R. Verma, M. Martorell, A. Sureda, and J. Sharifi-Rad. 2018. *Matricaria* genus as a source of antimicrobial agents: From farm to pharmacy and food applications. *Microbiology Research* 215: 76–88.

Sharma, D.K. 2006. Pharmacological properties of flavonoids including flavolignans – integration of petrocrops with drug development from plants. *Journal of Science Indian Research* 65: 477–484.

Sharma, H., H.M. Chandola, G. Singh, and G. Basisht. 2007. Utilization of Ayurveda in health care: an approach for prevention, health promotion, and treatment of disease. Part 1. Ayurveda, the science of life. *Journal of Alternative and Complementary* 13: 1011–1019.

Sharma, K., R. Bairwa, N. Chauhan, B. Shrivastava, and N. Saini. 2011. *Berberis aristata*: a review. *International Journal of Research in Ayurveda and Pharmacy* 2: 383–388.

Sharma, P., P. Kumar, R. Sharma, G. Gupta, and A. Chaudhary. 2017. Immunomodulators: role of medicinal plants in immune system. *National Journal of Physiology, Pharmacy and Pharmacology* 7: 552–556.

Singh, N., M.M. Tailang and S.C. Mehta. 2016. A review on herbal plants as immunomodulators. *International Journal of Pharmacy Science and Research* 7: 3602–3610.

Singh, S. 2020. Magical ayurvedic spices and herbs that can boost our immunity. *MOJ Food and Processing Technology* 8: 99–102.

Singh, S., A. Gautam, A. Sharma, and A. Batra. 2010. *Centella asiatica* (L): a plant with immense medicinal potential but threatened. *International Journal of Pharmaceutical Science Review and Research* 4: 9–17.

Singh, S., T.H. Krishna, S. Kamalraj, G. Kuriakose, V. Mathew, and C. Jayabaskaran. 2015. Phytomedicinal importance of *Saraca asoca* (Ashoka): an exciting past, an emerging present and a promising future. *Current Science* 109: 1760–1801.

Singh, N., M. Tailang, and S.C. Mehta. 2016. A review on herbal plants as immunomodulators. *International Journal of Pharmaceutical Sciences and Research* 7: 3602.

Sinsinwar, S., I. Paramasivam, and M. Muthuraman. 2016. An overview of the biological and chemical perspectives of *Croton tiglium*. *Der Pharmacia Lettre* 8: 324–328.

Sorokina, M. and C. Steinbeck. 2020. Review on natural products databases: where to find data in 2020. *Journal of Cheminformatics* 12: 1–51.

Srivastava, A.K., J.P. Chaurasia, R. Khan, C. Dhand, and S. Verma. 2020. Role of medicinal plants of traditional use in recuperating devastating COVID-19 situation. *Medicinal Aromatic Plants* 9: 2167

Stephane, F.F.Y. and B.K.J. Jules. 2020. Terpenoids as important bioactive constituents of essential oils. In: *Essential Oils-Bioactive Compounds. New Perspectives and Applications*. Eds. Fotsing, F., Y. Stephane, and B.K.J. Jules. IntechOpen, United Kingdom.

Su, M., H.Y. Chung, and Y. Li. 2011. Deoxyelephantopin from *Elephantopus scaber* L. induces cell-cycle arrest and apoptosis in the human nasopharyngeal cancer CNE cells. *Biochemical and Biophysical Research Communications* 411: 342–47.

Sultan, M.F., M.S. Buttxs, M. Mir, Q. Nasir, and H.A.R. Suleria. 2014. Immunity: plants as effective mediators. *Critical Reviews in Food Science and Nutrition* 54: 1298–1308.

Swallah, M.S., H. Sun, R. Affoh, H. Fu, and H. Yu. 2020. Antioxidant potential overviews of secondary metabolites (polyphenols) in fruits. *International Journal of Food Science* 2020: 1–8.

Thangadurai, K., R. Savitha, S. Rengasundari, K. Suresh, and V. Banumathi. 2018. International immunomodulatory action of traditional herbs for the management of acquired immunodeficiency syndrome: a review. *Journal of Herbal Medicine* 6: 10–14.

Thatte, U.M. and S.A. Dahanukar. 1997. Rasayana concept: clues from immunomodulatory therapy. In *Immunomodulation*. Narosa Publishing House, New Delhi, p. 41e148.

Thoppil, R.J. and A. Bishayee. 2011. Terpenoids as potential chemopreventive and therapeutic agents in liver cancer. *World Journal of Hepatology* 3: 228–249.

Tillu, G., S. Chaturvedi, A. Chopra, and B. Patwardhan. 2020. Public health approach of Ayurveda and Yoga for COVID-19 prophylaxis. *The Journal of Alternative and Complementary Medicine* 26: 360–364.

Tiwari, R., S.K. Latheef, I. Ahmed, H. Iqbal, M.H. Bule, K. Dhama, H.A. Samad, K. Karthik, M. Alagawany, M.E. El-Hack, and M.I. Yatoo. 2018. Herbal immunomodulators-A remedial panacea for designing and developing effective drugs and medicines: current scenario and future prospects. *Current Drug Metabolism* 19: 264–301.

Tripathi, J.S. and R.H. Singh. The concept and practice of immunomodulation in ayurveda and the role of Rasayanas as immunomodulators. *Ancient Science of Life* 19: 59.

Tu, Y. 2011. The discovery of artemisinin (qinghaosu) and gifts from Chinese medicine. *Nature Medicine* 17(10): 1217–1220.

Turner, J.E., G. Spielmann, A.J. Wadley, S. Aldred, R.J. Simpson, and J.P. Campbell. 2016. Exercise-induced B cell mobilisation: preliminary evidence for an influx of immature cells into the bloodstream. *Physiology and Behaviour* 164: 376–382.

Tuy, A.T., P. Jimin, H.O. Ji, S.P. Jung, L. Dahae, E.K. Chang, C. Han-Seok, C. Sang-Back Kim, G.S. Hwang, A.K. Bon, and K.S. Kang. 2020. Effect of herbal formulation on immune response enhancement in RAW 264.7 macrophages. *Biomolecules* 10: 424.

Uapadhyay, R.K. 2016. Nutraceutical, pharmaceutical and therapeutic uses of *Allium cepa*: a review. *International Journal of Green Pharmacy* 10: S46–S64.

Uttpal, A., N. Jacobo-Herrera, A. Ammar, and L. Naoufal. 2019. A comprehensive review on medicinal plants as antimicrobial therapeutics: potential avenues of biocompatible drug discovery. *Metabolites* 9: 258.

Ven, M.M.R., P.K. Ranjekar, C. Ramassamy and M. Deshpande. 2010. Scientific basis for the use of Indian ayurvedic medicinal plants. *Central Nervous System Agents in Medical Chemistry* 10: 238–246.

Venditti, A. 2017. Secondary metabolites from *Teucrium polium* L. collected in Southern Iran. *Arabian Journal of Medicinal and Aromatic Plants* 3: 108–123.

Venditti, A., C. Frezza, F. Sciubba, M. Serafini, A. Bianco, K. Cianfaglione and F. Maggi 2018. Volatile components, polar constituents and biological activity of tansy daisy (*Tanacetum macrophyllum* (Waldst. et Kit.) Schultz Bip). *Industrial Crops and Products* 118: 225–235.

Venditti, A., F. Maggi, S. Vittori, F. Papa, A.M. Serrilli, M. Di Cecco, G. Ciaschetti, M. Mandrone, F. Poli and A. Bianco. 2015. An antioxidant and α-glucosidase inhibitory activities of *Achillea tenorii*. *Pharmaceutical Biology* 53: 1505–1510.

Venkatalakshmi, P., V. Vadivel, and P. Brindha 2016. Role of phytochemicals as immunomodulatory agents. *International Journal of Green Pharmacy* 10: 1–17.

Verma, N. 2012. An overview on *Acacia catechu*. *International Journal of Research and Reviews in Pharmacy and Applied science* 2: 342–346.

Vishwabhan, S., V.K. Birendra, and S. Vishal. 2011. A review on ethnomedical uses of *Ocimum sanctum* (Tulsi). *International Research Journal of Pharmacy* 2: 1–3.

Wang, Z.G. and J. Ren. 2002. Current status and future direction of Chinese herbal medicine. *Trends in Pharmacology Science* 23: 347–348.

Wang, Z., Y. Han, S. Tian, J. Bao, Y. Wang, and J. Jiao. 2020. Lupeol Alleviates Cerebral Ischemia–Reperfusion Injury in Correlation with Modulation of PI3K/Akt Pathway. *Neuropsychiatric Disease and Treatment* 16: 1381–1390.

Weaver, B.A. 2014. How Taxol/paclitaxel kills cancer cells. *Molecular biology of the cell* 25: 2677–2681.

Wen, C.C., H.M. Chen, and N.S. Yang. 2010. Developing phytocompounds from medicinal plants as immunomodulators. *Advances in Botanical Research* 62: 197–272.

Youn, H.S., H.J. Lim, H.J. Lee, D. Hwang, M. Yang, R. Jeon, and J.H. Ryu. 2008. Garlic (*Allium sativum*) extract inhibits lipopolysaccharide-induced Toll-like receptor 4 dimerization. *Bioscience, Biotechnology, and Biochemistry* 72: 368–375.

Younis, N.S. 2020. D-Limonene mitigate myocardial injury in rats through MAPK/ERK/ NF-κB pathway inhibition. *The Korean journal of physiology and pharmacology* 24: 259.

Yousef, M., R.W. Crozier, N.J. Hicks, C.J. Watson, T. Boyd, E. Tsiani, and A.J. MacNeil 2020. Attenuation of allergen-mediated mast cell activation by rosemary extract (*Rosmarinus officinalis* L.). *Journal of Leukocyte Biology* 107: 843–857.

Zaveri, M., A. Khandhar, S. Patel, and A. Patel. 2010. Chemistry and pharmacology of Piper longum L. *International Journal of Pharmaceutical Sciences Review and Research* 5(1): 67–76.

Ziyan, L., Z. Yongmei, Z. Nan, T. Ning, and L. Baolin. 2007. Evaluation of the anti-inflammatory activity of luteolin in experimental animal models. *Planta Medica* 73: 221–226.

5 Medicinal Plants for Strong Immune System and Traditional Skin Therapy in South Africa
An Overview

Learnmore Kambizi and Callistus Bvenura

CONTENTS

5.1 INTRODUCTION

Without a doubt, skin care/therapy is one of the leading global markets and contributes significantly to economies today. The global value is estimated at 128.38 billion USD and is expected to rise to 189.3 billion USD by 2025 (Statista 2020a). The South African market, which was valued at 581.7 million USD in 2017, will have an estimated value of 839.2 million USD by the year 2023 (Statista 2020b). In fact, South Africa holds the largest share of the market in Africa. The major divisions of this market include anti-ageing, antipigmentation, antidehydration, and sun protection, with applications in beauty salons, medical institutions, and retail stores, among others. These figures are reflective of the role of the skin in the human body. The skin is indeed the human body's largest organ and acts as a gateway to the rest of the body. It is the body's first line of defence against pathogens and water loss,

DOI: 10.1201/9781003137955-5

regulating temperature and sensation, and providing insulation among its myriad functions. Nevertheless, the skin is also home to millions of complex communities of fungi, viruses, and bacteria, with most of the bacteria playing a beneficial role to the body and immune system. The communities of fungi, viruses, and bacteria are informed by a host of factors, which depend largely on environmental conditions and the ecology of the skin surface itself (Grice and Segre 2011). More specifically, Chen and Tsao (2013) reported that skin moisture content, temperature, skin physiology, including sebaceous gland density, and host genetics, as well as exogenous environmental factors are the major determinants of the composition of these communities. Furthermore, adaptive and cutaneous immune responses can moderate microbial communities, while they also inform the immune system (Grice and Segre 2011). An understanding of the skin microbiota would therefore open a window into the microbiota–skin interactions which lead to diseases and abnormalities, so that researchers can develop appropriate treatment approaches. Since the dawn of time, visible alterations of the skin surface have been recognized, with some being treated and others not.

Although medicinal plant use is as old as the story of civilisation, the specific modes of action involved in individual treatments have not always been fully understood (Grierson and Afolayan 1999). Mantle and Gok (2001) reported that almost one-third of known herbal medicines are used in the treatment of wounds and an assortment of skin disorders. The antioxidant and antimicrobial properties of the volatile compounds of these plants have proven effective in many herbal medicines used for dermatological purposes when topically applied to the skin (Quave et al. 2008). These compounds inhibit and/or eliminate pathogenic activities in the cells (Perumal Samy and Gopalakrishnakone 2010). The protective effects of antioxidants against cell damage caused by free radicals generated by metabolic processes have been widely reported (Adedapo et al. 2008), with antioxidants having a neutralizing effect on the free radicals. More recently, however, due to the recognized role of plant antioxidants in ameliorating skin damage from UV light, plants containing phytochemicals with antioxidant activity are receiving increased attention (Katiyar et al. 2001). Some of the compounds found in these plants also ameliorate the negative reactions caused by stings or insect bites by restricting diffusion of toxins, while they also reduce the effects of skin irritation and itching (Dawid-Pać 2013).

Statistics indicate that, currently, the largest antiretroviral (ARV) program globally is administered in South Africa. In fact, it is estimated that, in 2019, about 7.5 million people were infected with HIV and 70% (5,250,000) of these were on ARVs (UNAIDS 2020). However, the first-line ARVs, such as stavudine, lamivudine, and efavirenz, have been linked to both cutaneous and subcutaneous tissue disorders because of hypersensitivity reactions (Ranbaxy 2006; Adcock Ingram 2007). In addition to post-inflammatory hyperpigmentation and serious discomfort, some of the side effects of these ARVs include eczema, fungal dermatitis, itches, irritations, nail disorders, lesions and skin rashes, skin nodules, skin ulcers, herpes simplex pustular rush, and herpes zones (Pharmacare Limited 2003).

The global use of folkloric herbal medicines for ritual purposes and improvement of skin complexion and texture, as well as in the treatment of skin diseases, is prevalent, including in South Africa. The use of herbal medicines such as *Cassipourea flanaganii* in reducing blemishes, as well as pimples, and increasing complexion clarity and skin lightening have been widely reported in South Africa (Cocks and Dold 2000). Furthermore, annually, in various provinces/ regions in South Africa and according to traditions, young initiates (Abakhwethwa – Eastern Cape province; nghomeni – xiTsonga; bagadikana – siPedi) are circumcised, and the resultant wounds are treated and dressed using medicinal plants. The use of Western medicine and practices in traditional circumcision ceremonies is viewed as meaningless, unacceptable, and a taboo. South African traditional herbal medicinal knowledge has been handed down through generations and for centuries, making the country a rich source of this knowledge (Thirumalai et al. 2009). Herbalists, traditional healers, and spiritualists, including ordinary local people, exploit this knowledge in the treatment of various ailments. This knowledge is known to have been passed down through generations by oral tradition without the need for documentation (Perumal Samy and Ignacimuthu 2000). Therefore, fears that this knowledge might be lost because of the lack of documentation or if the current holders of the knowledge die without passing it on are not far fetched. In the worst cases, there are fears that the rural healthcare systems in South Africa could eventually fail.

Nevertheless, one of the most effective and reliable methods of bioprospecting for herbal medicines and their uses is through ethnobotanical surveys. These surveys have led to the incorporation of numerous herbal medicines into the mainstream healthcare systems. Interestingly, the use of herbal medicines, which are effective as well as affordable, is gaining attention in both urban and rural areas (Katewa et al. 2004). According to Grierson and Afolayan (1999), to protect traditional herbal knowledge from extinction, its documentation is essential. Although the ethnobotanical documentation may not provide an exhaustive list, these studies are essential not only in ensuring the continued existence of this important knowledge but also for biodiversity conservation and the sustainable utilization of scarce resources (Revathi and Parimelazhagan 2010).

Although several articles have documented some of these ethnobotanical surveys to reveal the plants of dermatological significance in South Africa, they have largely been regional, with a comprehensive national study being lacking. This chapter seeks, therefore, through an extensive literature survey, to reveal and document plants of dermatological significance in South Africa at a national level. To achieve this, Google Scholar, Europe PMC, PubMed, and Science Direct search engines were used. Phrases such as "plants used for the treatment of skin/wounds in the Eastern Cape/ Western Cape/ Northern Cape/ North West/ Gauteng/ Free State/ Limpopo/ Mpumalanga/ KwaZulu Natal", "plants of dermatological significance in South Africa", "herbal medicines for skin treatment in South Africa", "skin lightening in South Africa", "skin care in South Africa", "cosmetics in South Africa", and "herbal plants and the immune system", as well as "the skin, human immune system and herbal medicines", were used, among others. Although each search generated millions of hits at a time, these were further streamlined until, eventually, a total number of 26 articles published over a period of 21 years (1999–2020) were considered relevant and therefore used for purposes of the present study. Altogther, a total number of 57 articles are cited in the entire manuscript. Although these additional citations are relatively modern, some of the original ethnobotanical surveys cited in the present work date back fifty years.

5.2   CLASSIFICATION OF SKIN DISEASES

Diseases affecting the skin are so diverse and complex that there is a need to classify them. In fact, the Scottish Dermatological Society (2020) estimates that over 11,000 individual skin disease cases have been recorded, based on Thomas McCall Anderson's work, as shown in Table 5.1 (1887). The British Association of Dermatologists (Dermnet-NZ 2008) developed an index of twenty-five classification codes, whereas the American Academy of Dermatology (1999) developed sixteen classification codes. Furthermore, Dermnet-NZ (2008) considered (i) the site of involvement, (ii) the pathogenesis and (iii) the main structure affected as their main parameters for classification of skin diseases. The work to classify skin diseases is seemingly never ending. Tabassum and Hamdani (2014) reported nine common types of infections, including rashes, viral, bacterial, fungal, and parasitic infections, pigmentation disorders, tumours and cancers, and traumas, as well as other conditions that could not neatly be classified. These latter conditions include rosacea, spider and varicose veins, and wrinkles. But, more recently, due to advances in technology and the use of data mining and machine-learning techniques, some researchers have developed what are known as dermatological predictive classifications, which, in effect, classify skin diseases more accurately and effectively. For example, Verma et al. (2019) merged the Gradient Boosting Decision Tree, Random Forest, Decision Tree, Support Vector Machines, and the Classification and Regression Tree data mining techniques to develop an ensemble supervised learning model to predict skin diseases. These authors concluded that, although the individual data mining techniques worked in terms of skin disease prediction, the ensemble model was more accurate than the individual techniques.

Permanent skin diseases and conditions can be treated or managed using various means. Treatment can either be topical (application of creams to the affected body

TABLE 5.1
Major Classes of Skin Diseases

Organic	Functional
Inflammations	Affections of the skin
New formations and tumours	Affections of hair
Haemorrhages	Affections of the sebaceous glands
Diseases produced by uniform causes:	Affections of the sudoriparous glands
• Parasitic affections	
• Syphilitic affections	
• Strumous affections	
• Eruptive fevers	

part) or by oral ingestion of medication. Topical applications include antibacterials, anthralin, antifungal agents, benzoyl peroxide, coal tar, corticosteroids, retinoids, and salicylic acid (Tabassum and Hamdani 2014). Oral treatments include the use of antibiotics, antifungal agents, antiviral agents, immunosuppressants, and corticosteroids. More recently, some new oral therapies, known as biologics, have been developed to treat conditions such as psoriasis. Biologic drugs are produced from living organisms, such as microorganisms, animals and/or humans using biotechnology, or might themselves contain components of living organisms. Some common examples of biologics are Amevive, Enbrel, Stelara, Remicade and Humira. However, biologics are not exclusive to skin treatment but treat a host of other diseases and conditions that may not be related to the skin. On the other hand, temporary and/or cosmetic skin conditions can be treated by the application of medicated makeup, over-the-counter skin care products, good hygiene practices, and lifestyle adjustments, such as dietary changes. Medicinal plants, therefore, become the basis of development of the treatments.

5.3 LITERATURE SURVEY OF PLANTS OF DERMATOLOGICAL SIGNIFICANCE IN SOUTH AFRICA

Numerous South African studies have reported on the pharmacological aspects of some common plants used in skin therapy, while a handful of ethnobotanical surveys have been conducted under the same theme. The ethnobotanical surveys are notably provincial/ regional, with a lack of a comprehensive national study. We present here the first comprehensive list of plants of dermatological significance in South Africa (Table 5.2). The literature search revealed 431 species from 117 families that have been documented to date in South Africa as being used in skin therapy (Figure 5.1). In general, South Africa contains some 41,983 flowering plant species, of which well over 2,000 are of medicinal value or use (Street and Prinsloo, 2013; Raimondo 2015; SANBI 2020). Of the nine provinces, the Eastern Cape and KwaZulu Natal dominate this list, with the Gauteng and Northern Cape provinces being barely mentioned.

5.4 INDIGENOUS KNOWLEDGE OF SOUTH AFRICAN PLANTS FOR USE IN SKIN BEAUTY, THERAPY, AND THE IMMUNE SYSTEM

Although most plants reported in this survey are used for the treatment of skin diseases and conditions, about 8% are used for cosmetics. This is a significant proportion against the backdrop of the percentage of plants used for the treatment of wounds, making up 18% in the present study. Skin beauty plays an important role in current South African society, as it has for years. According to Davids et al. (2016), the perceived social benefits, including beauty, historical racism, and marketing strategies of multinational companies drive this industry's growth. The marketing strategies often involved local celebrities from whom most young people draw inspiration. In fact, despite the toxic systemic effects of skin lighteners, South Africa remains the

TABLE 5.2

South African Ethnomedicinal Plants of Dermatological and Immune Significance

Botanical Name	Family	Local Name	Part Used	Condition for Treatment	Mode of Administration	Ref
Acacia burkei Benth.	Fabaceae	Umkhaya wehlalahlathi (KZN)	Bark and leaves	Sores	Topical	10, 11
Acacia cinerea (L.) Spreng	Fabaceae	Murenzhe (L)	Twigs, fruits, bark	Ringworms, and wounds	Topical	16
Acacia erioloba Edgew.	Fabaceae	Kameeldoring (NC/WC)	Bark	Wounds	Topical	22, 26
Acacia karroo Hayne	Fabaceae	Umnga (EC)	Bark	Ringworm, clean, soften, and facial skin	Topical	5, 6, 9
Acalypha glabrata Thunb.	Euphorbiaceae	Umthombothi (EC)	Bark	Clean skin and rashes	Topical	5
Acmella caulirhiza Delile	Asteraceae	Tshishengeraphofu (L)	Leaves	Wounds and sores	Topical	16
Acokanthera oppositifolia (Lam.) Codd	Apocynaceae	Boesmansgif (WC/ NC)	Leaves	Accelerate hair growth, and snake bites	Topical	5, 6, 19, 22, 26
Acridocarpus natalitius A. Juss.	Malpighiaceae	Umabophe (EC)	Leaves	Skin allergies	Bathing	4
Acrotome inflata Benth.	Lamiaceae	Mogato (NW)	Rhizome	Albinism, burns, chickenpox, fleabites, sores, rash, and wounds	Topical	23
Adansonia digitata L.	Malvaceae	Ximuwu (L)	Fruit, bark	Toothache	Oral	14
Afroaster hispida (Thunb.) J.C. Manning & Goldblatt	Asteraceae	Phoa (FS)	Leaves	Sores, syphilitic sores, and wounds	Topical	24
Afzelia quanzensis Welw.	Fabaceae	Mdlavuza (KZN)	Bark	Eczema	Topical	19
Agapanthus africanus (L.) Hoffmanns	Amaryllidaceae	Isicakathi (EC)	Rhizome	Scabies, and boils	Bathing	5
Agapanthus campanulatus Leighton ssp. *campanulatus*	Amaryllidaceae	Leta-laphofu (FS); Bloulelie (WC/NC)	Leaves	Rash, and crust on infants' heads	Topical	24, 26

(Continued)

TABLE 5.2 (CONTINUED)
South African Ethnomedicinal Plants of Dermatological and Immune Significance

Botanical Name	Family	Local Name	Part Used	Condition for Treatment	Mode of Administration	Ref
Agathosma betulina (Berg.) Pillans	Rutaceae	Buchu (WC)	Leaves	Wounds, and bruises	Topical	20
Agave americana L.	Asparagaceae	Garamboom (NW); Lekhala (FS)	Leaves	Eczema	Topical	23, 24
Agave angustifolia Haw.	Asparagaceae	Xikwenga xa nhova (L)	Leaves	Sores	Topical	14
Agave sisalana Perrine.	Asparagaceae	Xikwenga (L)	Leaves	Black leg	Topical	14
Agrimonia eupatoria L.	Rosaceae	Inzinzinaba (EC)	Leaves	Burns	Topical	5
Albizia adianthifolia (Schumach.) W. Wight	Fabaceae	Umhlandlothi (EC); Umgadankawu/ igowane, umnalahanga/ umnebelele/ usolu (KZN)	Bark	Improves skin beauty, acne, eczema, and eye inflammation	Topical	9, 11
Albizia anthelmintica (A. Rich.) Brongn.	Fabaceae	Umnala (MP)	Stem	Lymphatic filariasis	Oral	25
Albizia harveyi E. Fourn.	Fabaceae	Molela (L)	Roots	Rash	Topical	16
Albizia versicolor Welw. ex Oliv.	Fabaceae	Umvangazi (KZN)	Bark	Sores	Topical	11
Albuca setosa Jacq.	Asparagaceae	Inqwebeba (EC); Wakgobaka-wa-seso (NW)	Leaves	Wounds, and Kaposi sarcoma	Topical	5, 23
Alepidea amatymbica Eckl. &Zeyh.	Apiaceae	Iqwili (EC)	Rhizome	Perfume skin	Topical	5, 9
Allium cepa L.	Amaryllidaceae	Onion	Bulb	Yaws	Topical	23
Aloe arborescens Mill.	Asphodelaceae	Ikalene (EC)	Leaves	Wounds, burns, acne, dreadlocks, skin moisturizer, and various skin ailments	Topical	6, 9, 13, 19, 22

(Continued)

TABLE 5.2 (CONTINUED)
South African Ethnomedicinal Plants of Dermatological and Immune Significance

Botanical Name	Family	Local Name	Part Used	Condition for Treatment	Mode of Administration	Ref
Aloe aristata Haw.	Asphodelaceae	Umathithibala (KZN)	Leaves	Dermatitis, wounds, burns, cuts and eczema, sunburn, insect stings, poison ivy skin irritations, abrasions, and numerous dermatological conditions	Topical	12, 13
Aloe barbadensis Mill.	Asphodelaceae	Mhangani/ Tshikopa (L)	Leaves	Ringworms, moisturize the skin, remove stretch marks, rash, burns, and wounds	Topical	16
Aloe ferox Mill.	Asphodelaceae	Umhlaba (EC), iNhlaba (KZN); Hlaba/ Lekhala La Quthing (FS)	Leaves, juice, Jel	Eczema, irritations, burns, wounds, insect bites, ringworm, boils pimples. Soften hair, foster hair growth, and prevent hair loss, and skin cleansing	Bathing	5, 6, 9, 12, 13, 24
Aloe greatheadii var. *davyana* (Schonland) Glen & D.S Hardy	Asphodelaceae	Kgopane	Leaf juice	Baruli ulcers, boils, chickenpox, eczema, and Steven Johnson syndrome	Topical	23
Aloe marlothii A. Berger	Asphodelaceae	Mhangane (L)	Leaves	Wounds	Topical	14, 17
Aloe turkanensis Christian	Asphodelaceae	Lekgala (NW)	Leaf juice	Eczema	Topical	23
Aloe vera (L.) Burm.f.	Asphodelaceae	Mhangani/ Tshikopa (L); Legkala (NW)	Leaves	Ringworms, moisturize the skin, remove stretch marks, rash, burns, and wounds	Topical	16, 23

(Continued)

TABLE 5.2 (CONTINUED)
South African Ethnomedicinal Plants of Dermatological and Immune Significance

Botanical Name	Family	Local Name	Part Used	Condition for Treatment	Mode of Administration	Ref
Aloe striatula Haw. var. striatula	Asphodelaceae	Serelei (FS)	Leaves	Burns, and wounds	Topical	24
Amaranthus caudatus L.	Amaranthaceae	Utyuthu (EC)	Leaves	Clean teeth	Bathing	5
Amaranthus hybridus L.	Amaranthaceae	Imbuya (EC)	Leaves	Clean facial skin	Bathing	5
Anagallis arvensis L.	Myrsinaceae	Umsobo (EC)	Leaves	Boils	Topical	5
Annona senegalensis Pers. ssp. senegalensis	Annonaceae	Umhlalajuba/ umphofu/ umthofa (KZN); Muembe (L)	Roots, twigs	Sores, and cleaning teeth	Topical, oral	11, 16
Aptenia cordifolia (L.f.) Schwant.	Mesembryanthemaceae	Ibohlololo (KZN/ MP)	Whole plant	Lymphatic filariasis	Topical	25
Aptosimum procumbens (Lehm.) Steud.	Scrophulariaceae	Brandbos	Leaves	Burns, and eczema	Topical	19
Aptosimum elongatum Engl.	Scrophulariaceae	Ditantanyane (NW)	Whole plant	Chicken pox, and yaws	Topical	23
Arctotis arctotoides (L.f.) O. Hoffm.	Asteraceae	Ubushwa (EC)	Leaves, juice,	Ringworm, insect bite, wound, pimples, and boils	Topical	5
Argyrolobium argenteum Eckl. & Zeyh.	Fabaceae	Umfanujacile (EC)	Leaves, juice,	Boils	Topical	5
Aristea ecklonii Baker	Iridaceae	Umhushuza (EC)	Whole plant	Shingles	Topical	22
Artemisia afra Jacq. ex Willd	Asteraceae	Umhlonyane (EC); Legana (NW)	Leaf decoctions	Acnes, boils, chicken pox, and rash	Bathing	6, 23
Arundinella nepalensis Trin.	Poaceae	Mahlakamane (FS)	Leaves	Wounds	Topical	24
Asclepias concolor (Decne.) Schltr.	Asclepiadaceae	Itshongwe (EC)		Pimples	Topical	5
Asclepias fruticosa L.	Asclepiadaceae	Igontsi (EC)	Leaves	Prevent hair loss	Topical	5

(Continued)

TABLE 5.2 (CONTINUED)
South African Ethnomedicinal Plants of Dermatological and Immune Significance

Botanical Name	Family	Local Name	Part Used	Condition for Treatment	Mode of Administration	Ref
Asparagus aethiopicus L.	Asparagaceae	Lelala-tau-le-leholo/leunyeli (L)	Roots	Skin protection against albinism	Topical	15
Asparagus africanus L.	Asparagaceae	Umathunga (EC)	Leaves	Eczema, and wounds	Topical	5, 6
Asparagus exuvialis Burch	Asparagaceae	Tlhkabotshwaro (NW)	Whole plant	Leprosy, impetigo, condylomata acuminata, and Madura foot	Topical	23
Asparagus nodulosus (Oberm) J.P. Lebrun & Stock	Asparagaceae	Radipolopolwane (NW)	Roots	Boils	Topical	23
Asparagus suaveolens Burch	Asparagaceae	Mothantanyane (NW)	Leaves	Leprosy, impetigo, and Madura foot	Topical	23
Athrixia phylicoides DC.	Asteraceae	Icholocholo (EC)	Leaves	Sores, and boils	Topical	6, 9, 22
Babiana hypogaea Burch.	Iridaceae	Thuge (NW)	Leaves	Burns	Topical	23
Barleria macrostegia Nees.	Acanthaceae	Magata (NW)	Rhizomes	Boils, burns chickenpox, and athlete's foot	Topical	23
Barleria obtusa Nees	Acanthaceae	Inzinziniba (EC); Thotshana tonya (NW)	Leaves	Burns	Topical	5, 23
Bauhinia bowkeri Harv.	Fabaceae	Umdlandlovu (EC)	Leaves and bark	Steaming, and bathing	Bathing	5
Bauhinia macranthera Benth. ex Hemsl	Fabaceae	–	Leaves	Wounds	Topical	22
Bauhinia thonningii Schum.	Fabaceae	Xidengana (L)	Fruit	Ringworms, sores, and skin irritation	Topical	16
Behnia reticulata (Thunb.) Didr.	Asparagaeae	Isilawu (EC)	Rhizome	Against hair loss	Bathing	5

(Continued)

TABLE 5.2 (CONTINUED)

South African Ethnomedicinal Plants of Dermatological and Immune Significance

Botanical Name	Family	Local Name	Part Used	Condition for Treatment	Mode of Administration	Ref
Berchemia discolor (Klotzsch) Hemsl.	Rhamnaceae	Ubalatsheni-omkhulu/ umadlozane/ umhlungulo/ uvuku (KZN)	Stem and twigs	Sores	Topical	10, 18
Berkheya setifera DC.	Asteraceae	Lelelemla-khomo/ ntsoantsane (FS); Mavumbuka (MP)	Whole plant	Herpes sores/ skin ulcers	Topical	24, 25
Bidens pilosa L.	Asteraceae	Uqaqadolo (KZN); Mushidzhi (L)	Leaves	Ringworms	Topical	10, 16
Boophone disticha (L.f.) Herb.	Amaryllidaceae	Gifbol (WC); Incwadi (KZN); kxutsana-yanaha/ motlatsisa (FS)	Bulb	Post-circumcision rites, wounds and draws out pus, boils, cuts, grazes, and abscesses	Topical	9, 12, 19, 22, 24
Bowiea volubilis Ex Hook.f. ssp. *volubilis*	Asparagaceae	Umagaqana (EC)	Bulb	Painkilling effect on skin	Topical	6, 9, 12
Brachylaena discolor DC.	Asteraceae	Isiduli (EC), Phahla (KZN)	Roots	Burns, wounds, and to clean facial skin	Topical	5, 11
Bridelia micrantha (Hochst.) Baill.	Euphorbiaceae	Umhlalimakwaba/ umshonge (KZN)	Leaves	Wounds, burns, and toothache	Topical	18, 22
Buddleja saligna Willd.	Scrophulariaceae	Igqange (EC)	Roots, leaves	Protect facial skin	Topical	5
Buddleja salviifolia (L.) Lam.	Scrophulariaceae	Bergsalie/ Kleinsalie (WC); Lelothwane (FS)	Leaves and stem	Sores	Topical	21, 24
Bulbine asphodeloides (L.) Spreng	Asphodelaceae	Uyakayakane/Intelezi (EC); Pekane (FS)	Leaves or leaf gel	Wounds, itches, burns, sunburns, rough skin, and insect bites	Topical	6, 9, 24
Bulbine abyssinica A. Rich	Asphodelaceae	Kgomo ya badisa (NW)	Leaves, roots	Chickenpox	Topical	23

(Continued)

TABLE 5.2 (CONTINUED)
South African Ethnomedicinal Plants of Dermatological and Immune Significance

Botanical Name	Family	Local Name	Part Used	Condition for Treatment	Mode of Administration	Ref
Bulbine capitata Poelln.	Asphodelaceae	Kgomo (NW)	Leaves	Chickenpox	Topical	23
Bulbine frutescens (L.) Willd.	Asphodelaceae	Itswelana (EC); Makgabinyane (NW)	Fresh leaf juice, slimy leaves	Cracked lips, wounds, and rash	Topical	6, 8, 9, 12, 13, 23, 24
Bulbine lagopus (Thunb.) N.E.Br.	Asphodelaceae	-	Leaves	Wounds, sores, and skin conditions	Topical	20
Bulbine latifolia (L.f.) Roem. et Schult.	Asphodelaceae	Ibhucu (EC)	Leaf sap	Wound, burns, eczema rashes, and itches	Topical	6
Bulbine natalensis Baker	Aspodelaceae	Ibhucu (KZN)	Leaves, bulbs, roots	Wounds, sores, burns, rashes, itches, ringworm, cracked lips and herpes, rheumatism, sunburn, itches, and mouth ulcers	Topical and oral	13
Buxus natalensis (Oliv.) Hutch.	Buxaceae	Isixhaza (EC)	Leaves	Ringworm, and boils	Topical	5
Cadaba aphylla (Thunb) Wild.	Capparaceae	Sekgalofatshe (male) (NW)	Whole plant	Sores, rashes, common warts, yaws	Topical	23
Cadaba aphylla (Thunb) Wild.	Capparaceae	Monnamontsho (female) (nW)	Leaves, roots	Chickenpox, Hermangioma, Kaposi sarcoma, and malignant melanoma	Topical	23
Calodendrum capense (L.f.) Thunb.	Rutaceae	Umemezi (EC)	Fruits	Soften hair, clean skin, clean teeth, and rashes	Topical	5, 6, 19
Calpurnia aurea (Ait.) Benth.	Fabaceae	Umbethe (EC)	Leaves, roots, Seeds	Accelerate hair growth, skin irritation, rashes, and boils	Topical	5

(Continued)

TABLE 5.2 (CONTINUED)
South African Ethnomedicinal Plants of Dermatological and Immune Significance

Botanical Name	Family	Local Name	Part Used	Condition for Treatment	Mode of Administration	Ref
Canthium inerme (L.f.) Kuntze	Rubiaceae	Isiphingo (EC); Isitobe (KZN)	Leaves	Ringworm, soften facial skin, pimples, Clean facial skin, and acne vulgaris	Bathing, topical	5, 10, 11
Capparis tomentosa Lam.	Capparaceae	Intsihlo (EC); Indoda-ebomvu (MP)	Roots, Powder	Sore throat, and wounds	Oral, topical	5, 25
Capsicum annuum L.	Solanaceae	Itshilisi (EC)	Fruits, Leaves	Sore throat	Oral	5
Carissa bispinosa (L.) Desf. Ex. Brenan	Apocynaceae	Isabetha (EC)	Fruits, juice	Soften facial skin	Topical	5
Carissa edulis (Forssk.) Vahl.	Apocynaceae	Mothokolo/ murungulu (L)	Leaves	Wounds	Topical	17
Carpobrotus dimidiatus (Haw.) L. Bolus	Mesembryanthemaceae	-	Leaf juice	Wounds, and burns	Topical	6, 20
Carpobrotus edulis L. Bolus	Aizoaceae	Unomatyumtyum (EC); sourfig/ suurvy (WC)	Leaves	Eczema, wounds, burns, and skin ulcers.	Topical	5, 6, 9, 19, 20
Cassiopourea flanaganii (Schinz) Alston	Rhizophoraceae	Umemeze (EC/WC)	Bark	Skin lightening, moisturizer, and pimples	Topical	2, 9, 19
Cassipourea flanaganii (Schinz). Alston	Rhizophoraceae	Umemezi (EC)	Bark, powder	Soften hair, and lighten skin	Topical	5, 6
Cassipourea flanaganii Alston.	Rhizophoraceae	Umemezi (EC)	Bark	Sunburn	Topical	3
Catha edulis (Vahl) Forssk. ex. Endl.	Celastraceae	Igqwakra (EC)	Leaves	Pimples	Topical	5
Catharanthus roseus (L.) G. Don	Apocynaceae	Lepolomo (L); Dabula (NW)	Fruits and leaves	Skin infections	Topical	17, 23
Centaurea benedicta (L.) L	Asteraceae	Ifinifini (EC)	Whole plant	Wounds	Topical	6, 9

(Continued)

TABLE 5.2 (CONTINUED)
South African Ethnomedicinal Plants of Dermatological and Immune Significance

Botanical Name	Family	Local Name	Part Used	Condition for Treatment	Mode of Administration	Ref
Centella asiatica (L.) Urban	Apiaceae	Imvumvu (EC); Setimamollo/pennywort (NW)	Whole plant	Wounds, insect bites, burns, genital warts, and skin itch	Topical	5, 6, 23
Cheilanthes viridis (Forssk.) Sw.	Pteridaceae	Unomlindana (EC)	Whole plant	Burns, wounds, and sores	Topical	6
Cheilanthes hastata (L.f.) Kunze	Pteridaceae	Isisefo (EC)	Leaves	Soften hair	Topical	5
Cheilanthes hirta Sw.	Pteridaceae		Leaves	Herpes sores/skin ulcers	Topical	24
Cheilanthes viridis (Forssk.) Sw.	Pteridaceae	Unomlindana (EC)	Fronds	Burns, wounds, and sores	Topical	7
Chenopodium ambrosioides Bert. ex Steud.	Amarathaceae	–	Leaves	Eczema, wounds, and skin infections	Topical	22
Chenopodium multifidum L	Amaranthaceae	Schalahalasamatlaka (NW)	Whole plant	Eczema, sores, and rash	Topical	23
Chironia baccifera L.	Gentianaceae	Aambeibossie (WC)	Leaves, stems	Acne, sores, and stiff muscles	Topical	20
Chlorophytum comosum (Thunb.) Jacques	Asparagaceae	Isicakathi (EC)	Tubers	Scabies	Topical	5
Chrysanthemum parthenium (L.) Pers.	Asteraceae	Ubushwa (EC)	Leaves	Wounds, and sores	Topical	3
Cinnamomum camphora L. Sieb.	Lauraceae	Urosalina (KZN)	Bark	Irritated skin, and perfume	Topical	19
Cissampelos capensis L.f.	Menispermaceae	Umayisake (EC; Dawidjies/ Dawidjieswortel/ Fynblaarklimop (WC)	Root, leaf	Wounds, sores, boils, and skin cancer	Topical	6, 21, 22

(Continued)

TABLE 5.2 (CONTINUED)
South African Ethnomedicinal Plants of Dermatological and Immune Significance

Botanical Name	Family	Local Name	Part Used	Condition for Treatment	Mode of Administration	Ref
Cissampelos torulosa E. Mey. Ex	Menispermaceae	Isitorhom (EC)	Roots	Toothache	Topical	6
Citrullus lanatus (Thunb.) Matsum. and Nakai	Cucurbitaceae	Umxoxozi (EC)	Flesh of fruits	Lotions, and sunburns	Topical	6
Citrus limon (L.) Burm.f.	Rutaceae	Lemon (EC); Tshikavhave (L)	Fruits, juice	Pimples, soften facial skin, wrinkles, and to clean facial skin	Bathing, topical	5, 16
Citrus reticulata Blanco.	Rutaceae	Swiri (L)	Fruit	Clean and soften skin	Topical	16
Clausena anisata (Willd.) Hook.f. ex Benth.	Rutaceae	Umfutho/Umtuto (EC)	Leaves, twigs, juice	Wounds, clean teeth	Topical	2, 5, 6
Clematis brachiata Thunb.	Ranunculaceae	Ityolo (EC)	Leaves, juice	Clean skin, perfume skin, and wrinkles	Bathing	5, 6
Clerodendrum glabrum E. Mey.	Lamiaceae	Umqwaqwanam (EC); Moswaapeba (FS)	Decoctions of leaves	Wounds	Topical	6, 24
Coddia rudis (E. Mey. ex Harv.) Verdc.	Rubiaceae	Intsinde (EC)	Twig, juice, fruit	Clean teeth; soften facial skin, and skin ulcer	Bathing, topical	5
Coleus kirkii (Baker) A.J. Paton	Lamiaceae	Umvuthuza/ uhlalawane (KZN)	Roots	Sores	Topical	10

(Continued)

TABLE 5.2 (CONTINUED)
South African Ethnomedicinal Plants of Dermatological and Immune Significance

Botanical Name	Family	Local Name	Part Used	Condition for Treatment	Mode of Administration	Ref
Combretum apiculatum Sond. ssp. *apiculatum*	Combretaceae	Tsholakhudu / Kgosi ya di thlare (NW)	Bark	Chickenpox, Kaposi sarcoma, flea bites, incision, molluscum contagiosum, malignant melanoma, rash, and sores	Topical	23
Combretum imberbe Wawra.	Combretaceae	Mondzo (L)	Bark	Sores	Topical	16
Commelina africana L.	Commelinaceae	Isicakathi (EC)	Roots	Scabies	Bathing	5
Commicarpus pentandrus (Burch) Heimerl	Nyctaginaceae	Moetapele (NW)	Whole plant	Burns, sores, warts, and wounds	Topical	23
Cotyledon orbiculata L.	Crassulaceae	Imphewula/kouterie/ plakkie (EC/ WC); Seredile (FS)	Leaves	Warts, corns, and sores	Topical	2, 6, 9, 19, 20, 22, 24
Crinum moorei Hook.F	Amaryllidaceae		Bulbs	Sores, and acne	Topical	6
Crossyne guttata (L.) D. Mull. -Doblies & U. Mull, -Doblies	Amaryllidaceae	Gifbol (WC)	Bulb	Post- circumcision rites, wounds and draws out pus	Topical	19
Croton sylvaticus Hochst.	Euphorbiaceae	Umfeze/Umagwaqane (EC)	Bark	Bleeding gums	Oral	6
Cryptocarya woodii Engl.	Lauraceae	Umnquma (EC)	Bark, infusion of powder	Eczema	Topical	5
Cucumis hirsutus Sond.	Cucurbitaceae		Leaves and roots	Inflammation	Topical	6
Cullen tomentosum (Thunb) J.W. Grimes	Fabaceae	Mojakubu (NW)	Whole plant	Rash, and sores	Topical	23

(Continued)

TABLE 5.2 (CONTINUED)
South African Ethnomedicinal Plants of Dermatological and Immune Significance

Botanical Name	Family	Local Name	Part Used	Condition for Treatment	Mode of Administration	Ref
Curtisia dentata C.A.Sm.	Curtisiaceae	Uzintlwa (EC)	Bark, infusion of powder	Eczema	Topical	5, 6, 9
Cussonia paniculata Eckl. Zeyh. ssp. *sinuata* (Reyneke & Kok) De Winter	Araliaceae		Leaves	Sores, and wounds	Topical	24
Cussonia spicata Thunb.	Araliaceae	Musenzhe (L)	Leaves	Ringworms	Topical	16
Cycnium racemosum Benth.	Orobanchaceae	Injanga (EC)	Leaves	Skin ulcers	Topical	5
Cymbopogon caesius (Hook. & Arn.) Stapf	Poaceae	Umqungu (EC)	Leaves	Skin itch	Topical	5
Cymbopogon dieterlenii Stapf. ex E. Phillips	Poaceae	Khotsoana (FS)	Whole plant	Wounds	Topical	24
Cymbopogon marginatus (Steud.) Stapf ex Burtt Davy	Poaceae	Umqungu (EC)	Leaves	Skin irritation	Bathing	5
Cynoglossum lanceolatum Forsk.	Boraginaceae		Roots	Wounds	Topical	24
Cyperus extilis Thunb.	Cyperaceae	Imizi (EC)	Leaves	Eczema	Topical	5
Cyrtanthus obliquus (L.f.) Aiton	Amaryllidaceae	Umathunga (EC)	Roots	Wounds	Topical	2
Dalbergia obovata E. Mey	Fabaceae	Umzungulu (EC); Udukuduku/ isibandhlube/ uphandlazi (KZN)	Stem	Sore mouths in infants		6, 11
Datura stramonium L.	Solanaceae	Umhlavuthwa (EC); Stinkblaar (WC)	Leaves	Boils, and wounds	Topical	5, 6, 9, 20, 24

(Continued)

TABLE 5.2 (CONTINUED)
South African Ethnomedicinal Plants of Dermatological and Immune Significance

Botanical Name	Family	Local Name	Part Used	Condition for Treatment	Mode of Administration	Ref
Dialium schlechteri Harms	Fabaceae	Umthiba (KZN)	Bark	Boils, burns, and wounds	Topical	11
Dianthus mooiensis F.N Williams ssp. *kirkii* (Burtt Davys) SS Hooper	Caryophyllaceae	Tlhokalatsela (NW)	Rhizome	Genital warts	Topical	23
Dianthus thunbergii (Thunb.) S.S. Hooper.	Caryophyllaceae	Ungcane (EC)	Leaves Infusion	Remove body odour	Bathing	5
Dicerocaryum zanguebarium (Lour.) Merr.	Pedaliaceae	Dinda (L)	Leaves	Shampoo	Bathing	14, 16
Dichrostachys cinerea (L.) Wight & Arn.	Fabaceae	Ugagane (KZN); Murenzhe (L)	Twigs, fruits, bark	Acne vulgaris, and wounds	Topical	10, 11, 16
Dicoma anomala Sond.	Asteraceae	Tlhonya (NW); Hloenya (FS)	Tuber	Wounds, skin ulcers, ringworm and head sores, albinism, boils, burns, flea bite, herpes zoster, condylomata acuminata, impetigo, Kaposi sarcoma, rash, and skin itching	Topical	22, 23, 24
Digitaria eriantha Steud.	Poaceae	Injica (EC)	Leaf decoction	Pimples	Topical	5
Dioscorea dregeana T. Durand & Schinz.	Dioscoreaceae	–	Tuber	Cuts and sores	Topical	22
Dioscorea elephantipes	Dioscoreaceae	Olifant foot (WC)	Bulb	Tired feet, athlete's foot, and blisters	Topical	19

(Continued)

TABLE 5.2 (CONTINUED)

South African Ethnomedicinal Plants of Dermatological and Immune Significance

Botanical Name	Family	Local Name	Part Used	Condition for Treatment	Mode of Administration	Ref
Dioscorea sylvatica (Kunth) Eckl.	Dioscoreaceae	Olifant foot (WC); Marakalla/ Leeto la tlou (FS)	Roots	Wounds	Topical	21, 25
Diospyros lycioides Desf.	Ebenaceae	Umbhongisa (EC); Muthala (L)	Bark and root	Inflammation, and wounds	Topical	6, 16
Diospyros mespiliformis Hochst.	Ebenaceae	Ntoma/ Musuma (L)	Bark, roots	Toothache	Oral	14, 16, 22
Diospyros natalensis (Harv.) Brenan	Ebenaceae	Xintomatomane (L)	Twigs	Clean teeth	Oral	16
Diospyros pubescens Pers.	Ebenaceae	Umbhongisa (EC)	Leaves	Strengthen nails	Topical	5
Dodonaea viscosa Jacq var. *angustifolia* (L.f) Benth.	Sapindaceae	-	Twigs, whole plant	Clean the teeth, and oral thrush	Oral	6, 22
Dombeya rotundifolia (Hochst.) Planch	Malvaceae	Tshiluvhari (L)	Leaves	Wash and dry hair	Bathing	16, 18
Drimia capensis (Burm.f.) Wijnands	Asparagaceae	Gifbol (WC)	Bulb	Post- circumcision rites, wounds, and draws out pus	Topical	19
Drimia altissima (LF) Ker Gawl.	Asparagaceae	Thobega (NW)	Leaves	Sores	Topical	23
Drimia delagoensis (Baker) Jessop	Asparagraceae	-	Bulb	Sores	Topical	10, 20
Drimia elata Jacq.	Asparagaceae	Red onion/ jeukoi/ roijukei (WC); Intelezi/ Mascaban (KZN)	Bulb	Opens pores, and swelling	Topical	19, 20

(Continued)

TABLE 5.2 (CONTINUED)
South African Ethnomedicinal Plants of Dermatological and Immune Significance

Botanical Name	Family	Local Name	Part Used	Condition for Treatment	Mode of Administration	Ref
Drimia sanguinea (Schinz) Jessop	Asparagaceae	Sekaname (NW)	Bark	Candidiasis, common warts, condylomata acuminata, genital warts, syphilis, and yaws	Topical	23
Dysphania ambrosioides (L.) Mosyakin & Clements	Amaranthaceae	Imboya (EC); Hlahlabadimo (NW)	Leaves, lotion	Skin itch, eczema, pimples, and clean skin	Bathing, topical	5, 23
Ekebergia capensis Sparrm.	Meliaceae	-	Bark	Boils, and acne	Topical	22
Elephantorrhiza elephantina (Burch.) Skeels.	Fabaceae	Intolwane (EC, KZN); Mositsane (FS/NW)	Roots and rhizomes	Acne, wounds, and burns	Topical	7, 9, 10, 11, 22, 24
Elephantorrhiza burchellii Benth (Burch). Skeels	Fabaceae	Mositsane (NW)	Roots	Chickenpox, condylomata acuminata, squamous carcinoma, malignant melanoma, infantile acropustulosis, Hermangioma, keratosis, Kaposi sarcoma, pearl penile papules, genital warts, madura foot, keratosis, and herpes simplex	Topical	23
Elytropappus rhinocerotis (L.f.) Less.	Asteraceae	Renosterbos (WC)	Leaves	Swollen hands and feet	Topical	19, 20
Embelia ruminata (E. Mey. ex A.Dc.) Mez	Myrsinaceae	-	Leaves	Wounds and leprosy	Topical	22

(Continued)

TABLE 5.2 (CONTINUED)
South African Ethnomedicinal Plants of Dermatological and Immune Significance

Botanical Name	Family	Local Name	Part Used	Condition for Treatment	Mode of Administration	Ref
Emex australis Steinh.	Polygonaceae	Inkunzane (EC)	Leaf decoction	Prevent hair loss	Topical	5
Eriocephalus africanus L.	Asteraceae	-	Essential oil	Skin care	Topical	16
Eriospermum lancifolium Jacq.	Asparagaceae	Babbejaanore (WC)	Bulb	Skin softening	Topical	19
Erythrina latissimi E. Mey.	Fabaceae	Umgqwabagqwaba/ umqonqazi (KZN)	Bark	Sores	Topical	18
Erythrina lysistemon Hutch.	Fabaceae	Umkuwane (EC); Umsinsi/ umsisi (KZN)	Bark powder	Wounds, skin irritation, abscesses, and sores	Topical	5, 6, 18, 22
Eucalyptus camaldulensis Dehnh.	Myrtaceae	-	Bark	Acne	Topical	22
Eucalyptus globulus Labill. Subsp. maidenii (F. Muell.) Kirkp.	Myrtaceae	Eucalyptus	Leaves	Wounds, muscle aches and pains, washing, and relaxation	Topical	19
Euclea divinorum Hiern	Ebenaceae	Nhlangula/ mutangule (L); Mokwere (NW)	Leaves	Skin irritation, ringworms, rash, pimples, chickenpox	Topical	16, 23
Euclea natalensis A.DC.	Ebenaceae	Umtshekesane (EC)	Root decoction, Wood	Sore throat and clean teeth	Oral	5
Eucomis autumnalis (Mill.) Chitt	Amaryllidaceae	Umathunga (EC); Mathubadifhala (NW)	Bulbs	Improve beauty and treat wounds	Topical	6, 9, 23
Eugenia capensis ssp. natalitia (Sond.) F. White	Myrtaceae	Tshitanzwatanzwane (L)	Roots	Sores	Topical	16
Eugenia natalitia Sond.	Myrtaceae	Tshitanzwatanzwane (L)	Roots	Sores	Topical	16

(Continued)

TABLE 5.2 (CONTINUED)
South African Ethnomedicinal Plants of Dermatological and Immune Significance

Botanical Name	Family	Local Name	Part Used	Condition for Treatment	Mode of Administration	Ref
Euphorbia bupleurifolia Jacq.	Euphorbiaceae	Intsema (EC)	Latex, leaves, twig	Pimples, wounds, rashes, and clean teeth	Bathing, topical	5
Euphorbia clavarioides Boiss var. *clavaroides*	Euphorbiaceae	Sehlehle/ Sehloko/ Thethebale (FS)	Stem	Acne, cancerous sores, cracked heels, herpes sores, leprosy, and skin rash in children	Topical	24, 25
Euphorbia hirta L.	Euphorbiaceae	Intsema (EC)	Roots	Wounds	Topical	2
Euphorbia inaequilatera Sond. var. *inaequilatera*	Euphorbiaceae	-	Rhizomes	Burns, sores, and rash	Topical	23
Euphorbia ingens	Euphorbiaceae	Umlonhlo (EC)	Stem	Skin rash post-inflammatory spots and promote healing without hyper pigmentation	Topical	9
Euphorbia mauritanica L. var. *mauritanica*	Euphorbiaceae	Milk thistle (WC)	Leaves	Warts	Topical	19
Euphorbia prostrata Aiton.	Asparagaceae	Letswetlane (NW)	Rhizomes	Candidiasis, syphilis, infantile cropustulosi, and chickenpox	Topical	23
Euphorbia serpen Kunths	Euphorbiaceae	Lwetsane (NW)	Leaves, roots	Athlete's foot and ringworm	Topical	23
Euphorbia tirucalli L.	Euphorbiaceae	Ingotsha (KZN)	Modified stem	Sores	Topical	10, 11
Euphorbia tuberosa L.	Euphorbiaceae	Milk root/ fennel (WC)	Root, whole plant	Warts	Topical	19
Ficus capensis Thunb.	Moraceae	Ikhiwane (EC)	Leaves	Pimples	Topical	3

(Continued)

TABLE 5.2 (CONTINUED)
South African Ethnomedicinal Plants of Dermatological and Immune Significance

Botanical Name	Family	Local Name	Part Used	Condition for Treatment	Mode of Administration	Ref
Ficus ingens (Miq.) Miq.	Moraceae	Mohlatsa/ motlhatsa/ tshikululu (L)	Bark	Sores	Topical	15
Ficus natalensis Hochst.	Moraceae	Umthombe (EC)	Leaf decoction	Clean skin	Bathing	5, 6, 22
Ficus sur Forssk.	Moraceae	Umkhiwane (KZN)	Bark	Sores	Topical	10, 22
Ficus sycomorus L.	Moraceae	Xirhomberhombe (L)	Leaves, bark, roots, sap	Dermatitis	Topical	14
Foeniculum vulgare Mill.	Apiaceae	-	Green dye from leaves	Fragrance component	Topical	6
Galenia africana L.	Aizoaceae	Kraalbos (WC)	Leaves	Skin ailments and toothache	Topical	19
Garcinia livingstonei T. Anderson.	Clusiaceae	Umphimbi/ ugobandlovu (KZN)	Bark	Burns	Topical	11
Gardenia volkensii K. Schum.	Rubiaceae	Tshiralala (L)	Flowers	Body odour	Bathing	16
Gasteria croucheri (Hook.f.) Baker	Asphodelaceae	Kannedot (WC); Intelezi (EC); Umathithibala (KZN)	Whole plant	Skin rash, warts, and ringworm.	Topical	19
Gasteria obliqua (Aiton) Duval	Asphodelaceae	Intelezi (EC)	Leaf decoction	Skin irritation, clean skin, eczema, and scabies	Bathing, topical	5
Gerbera piloselloides (L.) Cass	Asteraceae	Umsa (EC)	Root infusion	Post-inflammatory spots and pimples	Topical	6, 9
Gnidia anthylloides (L.f.) Gilg	Thymelaeaceae	Intozwane (EC)	Roots	Wounds and burns	Topical	6, 9
Gnidia capitata L.f.	Thymelaeaceae	Umsila (EC)	Roots	Wounds, rashes, fractures, snake bites, and sore throat		7, 9

(Continued)

TABLE 5.2 (CONTINUED)
South African Ethnomedicinal Plants of Dermatological and Immune Significance

Botanical Name	Family	Local Name	Part Used	Condition for Treatment	Mode of Administration	Ref
Gnidia gymnostachya (C.A. Mey) Gilg.	Thymelaeaceae	-	Leaves	Bruises and wounds	Topical	24
Gnidia kraussiana Meisn.	Thymelaeaceae	Iganna (EC)	Leaves	Protect facial skin, wounds, burns, boils, rashes, and sore throat	Topical, oral	5
Gompocarpus fruticosus (L) Aiton.f. ssp. *fruticosus*	Apocynaceae	Moetimolo (NW)	Whole plant	Burns, sores, and rash	Topical	23
Grewia occidentalis L.	Malvaceae	Umnqabaza (EC)	Bark	Wounds and shampoo	Topical and bathing	7, 18
Grewia caffra Meisn.	Tiliaceae	Iklolo/ ialanyathi/ iphata (KZN)	Bark	Wounds and shampoo	Topical and bathing	18
Grewia flava DC.	Malvaceae	Moretlwa (NW)	Roots	Pearl penile papules	Topical	23
Grewia flavescens Juss.	Malvaceae	Motsotsojane (NW)	Leaves	Candidiasis, common warts, and sores	Topical	23
Grewia occidentalis L.	Malvaceae	Umnqabaza (EC)	Bark	Wounds	Bathing	6
Greyia flanaganii Bolus	Francoaceae	Usinga/Lwamaxhegokazi (EC)	Leaves	Skin ailment	Topical	6
Gunnera perpensa L.	Gunneraceae	Iphuzi (EC); Qobo (FS)	Leaves	Insect bite	Topical	5, 9, 22, 24
Haemanthus albiflos Jacq.	Amaryllidaceae	Umathunga (EC)	Paste, leaf decoction	Skin ulcers, burns, and remove body odour	Bathing, topical	5
Halleria lucida L.	Stillbaceae	Inkobe (EC)	Leaf decoction	Scabies	Bathing	5, 6, 22
Haplocarpha scaposa Harv.	Asteraceae	Isicwe (EC)	Paste, leaves	Scabies and wounds	Bathing	5
Harpephyllum caffrum Bernh.	Anacardiaceae	Umgwenye (EC)	Bark decoction	Wounds, eczema, and pimples	Topical	5, 6, 9, 12, 22

(Continued)

TABLE 5.2 (CONTINUED)
South African Ethnomedicinal Plants of Dermatological and Immune Significance

Botanical Name	Family	Local Name	Part Used	Condition for Treatment	Mode of Administration	Ref
Haworthia limifolia Marloth.	Asphodelaceae	Isihlalakahle (KZN)	Leaves, stem, roots	Burns and sun burn	Topical	13
Hawthoria fasciata (Willd.) Haw.	Asphodelaceae	Kannedot (WC); Intelezi (EC)	Whole plant	Skin rash warts and ringworm	Topical	19
Helichrysum nudifolium (L.) Less.	Asteraceae	Indlebe (EC); Imphepho (NW)	Leaves, twig powder	Improve skin beauty and genital warts	Topical	6, 23
Helichrysum appendiculatum Less.	Asteraceae	Isicwe (EC)	Leaves	Circumcision wounds and sores	Topical	3, 21
Helichrysum leiopodium DC.	Asteraceae	Letapiso (EC)	Whole plant	Swollen feet	Bathing and Topical	3, 21
Helichrysum nudifolium	Asteraceae	Indlebe zebhokwe/Isicwe/Ichola chola (EC)	Leaves and twigs	Wound and improves skin beauty	Topical	9, 21
Helichrysum odoratissimum (L.) Sweet.	Asteraceae	Impepho (EC)	Infusions, lotion, leaves	Wounds, skin ulcers, scabies, protect facial skin, and perfumes of the skin	Topical	5, 6
Helichrysum paronychioides DC. Humbert	Asteraceae	Phate-ya-ngaka (NW)	Whole plant	Boils, candidiasis, eczema, Kaposi sarcoma, soils, rash, yaws, herpes zoster, ringworm, condylomata acuminata, eczema, and pearl penile papules	Topical	23
Helichrysum pedunculatum Hilliard & B.L. Burtt	Asteraceae	Isicwe (EC)	Leaves	Circumcision wounds	Topical	4

(Continued)

TABLE 5.2 (CONTINUED)
South African Ethnomedicinal Plants of Dermatological and Immune Significance

Botanical Name	Family	Local Name	Part Used	Condition for Treatment	Mode of Administration	Ref
Helichrysum petiolare Hilliard and B.L. Burtt	Asteraceae	Imphepho (EC)	Leaves	improve skin texture and beauty and to treat wounds	Topical	6, 9, 21
Helinus integrifolius (Lam.) Kuntze.	Rhamnaceae	Isilawu (EC); Mpupungwa/Mugumwa (L)	Leaves	Against hair loss	Topical	5, 16
Hermannia depressa N.E. Br	Malvaceae	Selejane (NW)	Whole plant	Sores	Topical	23
Hermania spp.	Malvaceae	8-days/ agdaegeeneesbos (WC)	Leaves	Ringworm, skin ailments, and sores	Topical	19
Hermannia coccocarpa K.Schum.	Malvaceae	–	Roots	Burns and wounds	Topical	24
Hermannia geniculata Eckl. &Zeyh.	Malvaceae	Impepho (EC)	Leaf paste	Boils	Topical	5
Heteromorpha arborescens (Spreng.) Cham. & Schltdl.	Apiaceae	Muthathavhanna (L)	Leaves	Skin burns	Topical	16
Hewittia malabarica L. (Suresh).	Convolvulaceae	Ihlanzandulo (KZN)	Leaves	Abscesses and boils	Topical	11
Hibiscus surattensis L.	Malvaceae	Indola ebomvu (KZN)	Roots	Burns and sores	Topical	11
Hilliardiella elaeagnoides (DC) Swelank & J.C. Manning	Asteraceae	Ntshikologa (NW)	Rhizomes	Scabies and eczema	Topical	23
Hydnora africana Thumb.	Hydnoraceae	Umavumbuka (EC)	Dried fruiting body	Acne and other skin blemishes	Topical	6
Hyperacanthus amoenus (Sims) Bridson.	Rubiaceae	Murombe (L)	Fruit	Pimples	Topical	16

(Continued)

TABLE 5.2 (CONTINUED)
South African Ethnomedicinal Plants of Dermatological and Immune Significance

Botanical Name	Family	Local Name	Part Used	Condition for Treatment	Mode of Administration	Ref
Hypericum aethiopicum Thunb.	Hypericaceae	Isimayisane/ Isimonyo/ Isivumelwane (KZN)	Leaves, stem, roots	Wounds and first-degree burns	Topical	13
Hypericum perforatum L.	Hypericaceae	-	Leaves	Wounds and first-degree burns	Topical	22
Hyphaene coriacea Gaertn.	Arecaceae	Ilala (EC)	Fruits, lotion, leaves, midrib	Soften hair and clean teeth	Bathing, topical	5
Hypoxis hemerocallidea Fisch. C.A. Mey. and Ave-Lall.	Hypoxidaceae	Inongwe (EC); Tshupoo ya poo (NW)	Corm	Pimples and improvement of beauty	Topical	6, 9, 23
Hypoxis argentea Harv. ex Baker	Hypoxidaceae	Inongwe (EC); Lotsane (FS)	Corm Infusion	Ringworm, eczema, pimples and to clean, and protect facial skin.	Topical	5, 24
Hypoxis hemerocallidea Fisch., C.A. Mey. & Ave-Lall.	Hypoxidaceae	Inkomfe/ inkomfe enkulu (KZN)	Corms	Boils, sores, and ringworm	Topical	10, 11
Hypoxis rigidula Baker var. *rigidula*	Hypoxidaceae	Moli-teane (FS)	Leaves	Wounds and rash	Topical	24
Ilex mitis (L.) Radlk.	Aquifoliaceae	Isidumo (EC); iphuphuma/ umdumo/ umdumowazo (KZN)	Leaf decoction	Rash and facial sores	Topical	5, 6, 18, 22
Indigofera arrecta Hochst. A. Rich	Fabaceae	Muswiswa (L)	Twigs and leaves	Cleaning and bathing	Orla and bathing	16
Ipomoea bolusiana Schinz.	Convolvulaceae	Mokutu (L)	Bulb	Foot ache	Topical	17

(Continued)

TABLE 5.2 (CONTINUED)
South African Ethnomedicinal Plants of Dermatological and Immune Significance

Botanical Name	Family	Local Name	Part Used	Condition for Treatment	Mode of Administration	Ref
Ipomoea oblongata E. Mey. ex Chiosy A.	Convolvulaceae	Morebe / Mokatelo (NW); Ubhoqo (MP); Mothokho (FS)	Rhizomes	Genital warts, leprosy, and scabies	Topical	23, 25
Ipomoea simplex Thunb.	Convolvulaceae	Igontsi (EC)	Corm, leaves	Hair loss, Clean skin, and protect facial skin	Topical	5
Jatropha brachyadenia Pax & K.Hoffm.	Euphorbiaceae	Xidemeja (L)	Leaves	Wounds	Topical	16
Jatropha curcas L.	Euphorbiaceae	Mupfure donga (L)	Stem, leaves, Roots	Skin moisturiser and wounds	Topical	16
Jatropha zeyheri Sond.	Euphorbiaceae	Modomeja/ Xidemeja (L); Seswagadi (NW)	Leaves	Wounds, acne vulgaris, albinism, boils, herpes zoster, genital warts, and yaws	Topical	14, 16, 23
Kedrotis nana var. *zeyheri*	Curcurbitaceae	Mpitike (NW)	Bulb	Eczema	Topical	23
Kigelia africana (Lam.) Benth.	Bignoniaceae	Umvunguta/ umfongothi (KZN); Umvongotsi (MP)	Bark	Ringworm	Topical	10, 11, 22, 25
Kniphofia laxifloria Kunth	Asphodelaceae	Inxonya (WC)	Root	Pimples	Topical	19
Kniphofia drepanophylla Baker.	Asphodelaceae	Ixonyi (EC)	Rhizomes	Ringworm, wounds, pimples, acne, and eczema	Topical	6, 9
Lannea discolor Engl.	Anacardiaceae		Bark	Boils and abscesses	Topical	22
Lannea schweinfurthii var. *stuhlmannii* (Engl.) Kokwaro	Anacardiaceae	Ndivata (L)	Leaves	Wounds	Topical	16
Lannea stuhlmannii Engl.	Anacardiaceae	Ndivata (L)	Leaves	Wounds	Topical	16
Lantana angolensis Moldenke	Verbenaceae	Selaole (NW)	Rhizome	Ringworm	Topical	23

(Continued)

TABLE 5.2 (CONTINUED)
South African Ethnomedicinal Plants of Dermatological and Immune Significance

Botanical Name	Family	Local Name	Part Used	Condition for Treatment	Mode of Administration	Ref
Lantana rugosa Thunb.	Verbenaceae	-	Leaves, stem, ripe fruits	Sores and cuts	Topical	22
Lasiosiphon kraussianus Hutch. & Dalz.	Thymelaeaceae	-	Whole plant	Wounds and bruises	Topical	24
Ledebouria revoluta (L.f.) Jessop	Hyacinthaceae	Icubudwana (KZN)	Bulb	Ringworm	Topical	10
Leonotis leonurus (L.) R.Br.	Lamiaceae	Umfincafincane/Umunyamunya (EC); Wild dagga (WC)	Leaves and stems	Itching, boils, eczema, and dandruff	Topical	6, 8, 9, 19
Leucosidea sericea Eckl. and Zeyh.	Rosaceae	Isidwadwa/Umyityi (EC); Mosino (FS)	Leaves	Acne	Topical	6, 24
Lippia javanica Burm.f. Spreng.	Verbenaceae	Inzinziniba (EC); Umsuzwane/ umswazi (KZN); Musudzungwane (L); Selaole / fever tea (NW)	Leaves	Boils, scabies, and wounds	Topical	5, 6, 9, 10, 11, 12, 16, 23
Lycium horridum Thunb.	Solanaceae	Motlhalawadikonyana (NW)	Whole plant	Kerotosis	Topical	23
Macaranga capensis (Baill.) Benth. ex Sim	Euphorbiaceae	Umpumelelo (EC)	Bark	Pimples, wounds eczema, and acne	Topical	6, 9
Malva neglecta Wallr.	Malvaceae	Tikamotse (NW)	Whole plant	Albinism, bullous dermatosis, herpes simplex, sores, and yaws	Topical	23
Malva parviflora L.	Malvaceae	Ijongilanga (EC)	Leaves	Pimples, insect bite, and wound boils	Topical	5, 6, 7, 22, 24
Melia azeadarach L.	Meliaceae	Mosara (L)	Leaves	Shingles	Bathing	17

(Continued)

TABLE 5.2 (CONTINUED)
South African Ethnomedicinal Plants of Dermatological and Immune Significance

Botanical Name	Family	Local Name	Part Used	Condition for Treatment	Mode of Administration	Ref
Melianthus comosus L.	Melianthaceae	Ubuhlungu bemamba (EC); Kruidjie roer my nie (WC)	Leaves	Wounds and Sores	Topical	6, 20, 22
Melianthus major L.	Melianthaceae	Ubuhlungubemamba/Ubutyayi (EC); kruidjie-roer-my-nie (WC)	Leaves	Wounds, sores and bruises	Topical	6, 8, 19, 21, 22
Mentha longifolia (L.)	Lamiaceae	Inixina/Inzinziniba (EC); Kruisement (WC)	Leaves	Wounds	Topical	6, 20, 22
Merwilla plumbea (Lindl.) Speta.	Asparagaceae	Ichitha/ Imbizenkulu/ Inguduza/ Ubulika (KZN)	Leaves, bulbs, roots	Boils, sores, wounds healing, sprains, and to remove scar tissue	Topical	13
Miscanthus capensis (Nees) Andersson.	Poaceae	Umpumelelo (EC)	Bark	Pimples, wounds eczema, and acne	Topical	6, 9
Momordica balsamina L.	Cucurbitaceae	Intshungu/ intshungwana yehlathi (KZN)	Leaves	Rash	Topical	11
Monadenium lugardiae N.E.Br.	Euphorbiaceae	Umhuwa (KZN)	Bark	Sunburn	Topical	19
Monsonia brevirostrata Knuth.	Geraniaceae	–	Leaves	Syphilitic sores	Topical	24
Musa acuminata Colla.	Musaceae	Muova (L.)	Flowers, leaves	Skin burns and wounds	Topical	16
Myrsine africana L.	Myrsinaceae	Moroko-pheleu/ semapo, sethakhisa/ thakisa (FS)	Leaves, fruits	Ringworm and skin diseases	Topical	24
Myrsine melanophloeos (L.) R. Br. Adamson	Primulaceae	Umaphipha (KZN)	Bark	Hair shampoo	Topical	19

(Continued)

TABLE 5.2 (CONTINUED)
South African Ethnomedicinal Plants of Dermatological and Immune Significance

Botanical Name	Family	Local Name	Part Used	Condition for Treatment	Mode of Administration	Ref
Nasturtium officinale W.T. Aiton	Brassicaceae	Umsobo (EC)	Whole plant	Antiseptic and blemishes	Topical	4
Nerium oleander L.	Apocynaceae	Five roses	Leaves	Toothache	Oral	17
Nicotiana tabacum L.	Solanaceae	Icuba (EC)	Paste	Wound	Topical	5
Obetia tenax Friis. Syn: *Urera tenax*	Urticaceae	Thanga (L)	Seeds	Skin moisturiser	Topical	16
Ochna serrulata (Hochst.) Walp.	Ochnaceae	Ilitye (EC)	Paste, leaves	Soften hair, strengthen nails, and to soften facial skin	Topical	5
Ocotea bullata	Lauraceae	Umnukani (KZN)	Bark	Pimples	Topical	12
Olea europaea L.	Oleaceae	Umquma (EC); Wild olive/ olienhout (WC); Modukguhlu (FS)	Leaf decoction	Remove body odour, sores, and skin ulcers	Bathing	5, 6, 21, 24
Ophioglossum vulgatum L.	Ophioglossaceae		Rhizomes	Boils	Topical	24
Opuntia aurantiaca Lindl.	Cactaceae	Itolofiya (EC)	Gel, Leaves	Soften hair, treat skin ulcers, and to protect facial skin	Topical	5
Opuntia ficus-indica (L.) Mill.	Cactaceae	Midhoro (L); Prickly pear (WC)	Leaves	Toothache	Oral	14, 17, 19, 22
Opuntia vulgaris Mill.	Cactaceae	Itolofiya (EC)	Stem	Wounds	Topical	2
Ozoroa engleri R. Fern. & A. Fern.	Anacardiaceae	Isifico/ Isifico (KZN)	Bark and leaves	Sores	Topical	10
Ozoroa engleri R. Fern. & A. Fern.	Anacardiaceae	-	Bark	Sores	Topical	11

(Continued)

TABLE 5.2 (CONTINUED)
South African Ethnomedicinal Plants of Dermatological and Immune Significance

Botanical Name	Family	Local Name	Part Used	Condition for Treatment	Mode of Administration	Ref
Ozoroa sphaerocarpa R. & A. Fern.	Anacardaceae	Isifice/ isifico (KZN)	Bark	Wounds	Topical	18
Parapodium costatum E. Mey	Apocynaceae	-	-	External tumours	Topical	24
Parinari capensis Harv. subsp. *capensis*	Chrysobalanaceae	-	Roots	Sores	Topical	11
Pavetta lanceolata Eckl.	Rubiaceae	Umhleza (EC)	Paste, leaves	Skin itch	Topical	5
Pelargonium lubridum (Andrews) Sweet	Geraniaceae	Thotamadi (NW)	Roots	Acne vulgaris, burns, eczema, pimples, and yaws	Topical	23
Pelargonium peltatum (L.) L.0Hér. ex	Geraniaceae	Ityolo (EC)	Tuber decoction	Clean the skin	Bathing	5, 20
Pelargonium sidoides DC.	Geraniaceae	Umsangela (EC)	Whole plant	Various skin disorders	Topical	6, 20
Pellaea calomelanos Link.	Adiantaceae	-	Leaves, rhizomes	Boils and abscesses	Topical	22
Peltophorum africanum Sond.	Fabaceae	Musese (L); Mosetlha (NW)	Bark, roots	Mouth sores, Kaposi sarcoma, and heat rash	Oral, topical	16, 17, 23
Pentanisia prunelloides (Klotzsch ex Xkl. and Zeyh.) Walp.	Rubiaceae	Icimamlilo/Irhubuxa (EC); Iscimamlilo (KZN)	Roots	Blisters, bruises, burns, cuts, insect, and stings/ bites	Topical	1, 6, 9, 19, 22, 24
Persea americana Mill.	Lauraceae	Avocado (EC); Afukhada (L)	Seed, leaves	Clean facial skin, protect facial skin, and wrinkles	Bathing, topical	5, 16
Phragmites australis (Cav.) Trin.ex Steud.	Poaceae	Ingcongolo (EC)	Paste of leaves	Protect facial skin	Topical	5

(Continued)

TABLE 5.2 (CONTINUED)
South African Ethnomedicinal Plants of Dermatological and Immune Significance

Botanical Name	Family	Local Name	Part Used	Condition for Treatment	Mode of Administration	Ref
Phragmites mauritianus Kunth.	Poaceae	Lutanga (L)	Thorns and whole plant	Moles and stretch marks	Topical	16
Phygelius capensis E. Mey.	Scrophulariaceae	Metsi-matsho (FS)	Leaves	Sores and skin ulcers	Topical	24
Phyllanthus maderaspatensis L.	Phyllanthaceae	Leestane (NW)	Leaves	Ringworm and eczema	Topical	23
Physalis angulata L.	Solanaceae	Itywabotywabo (EC)	Paste of leaves	Burns	Topical	5
Phytolacca americana L.	Phytolaccaceae	Umsobosobo (EC)	Paste of leaves	Boils	Topical	5
Phytolacca octandra L.	Phytolaccaceae	Amahashe ayatsala (EC)	Fruits	Wounds and sores	Topical	4
Piliostigma thonningii (Schum.) Milne- Redh	Fabaceae	Denga (L)	Fruit	Pimples and wounds	Topical	16
Pittosporum viridiflorum Sims.	Pittosporaceae	-	Roots, leaves	Boils	Topical	22
Plumbago auriculata Lam.	Plumbaginaceae	Umabophe (EC)	Roots /leaves	Warts, rashes, acne, and pimples	Topical	6, 9
Podocarpus latifolius (Thunb.) R.Br. ex Mirb.	Podocarpaceae	Umkhaba (EC)	Juice of leaves	Eczema	Topical	5
Polystichum pungens (Kaulf.) Presl.	Dryopteridaceae	Shield ferns (WC)	Leaves	Pain and inflammation	Topical	7, 26
Portulacaria afra Jacq.	Portulacaceae	Intelezi/ isidondwane/ isambilane/ indibili/ isicococo (KZN)	Leaves	Rash and chronic sores	Topical	11

(Continued)

TABLE 5.2 (CONTINUED)
South African Ethnomedicinal Plants of Dermatological and Immune Significance

Botanical Name	Family	Local Name	Part Used	Condition for Treatment	Mode of Administration	Ref
Pouzolzia mixta Solms	Urticaceae	Muthanzwa (L); Moreba (NW)	Roots	Wounds, abscess, boils, eczema, infantile acropustolosis, and pearl penile papules	Topical	16, 23
Protea repens (L.) L.	Proteaceae	Isadlungi (EC)	Whole plant	Inflammation	Topical	6
Protea simplex E. Phillips	Proteaceae	Isadlungi (EC)	Whole plant	Inflammation	Topical	6
Protorhus longifolia (Bernh.) Engl.	Anacardiaceae	Ikhubalo (EC)	Bark	Wounds, cuts, bruise, and graze ringworm, acne, and eczema	Topical	6
Pseudocrossidium crinitum (Schultz) R.H. Zander.	Pottiaceae	Ixolo lamatye (EC)	Infusion of leaves	Skin irritation	Topical	5
Pseudophyll anthusovalis (E. Mey. ex Sond.) Voronts. &Petra Hoffm.	Phyllanthaceae	Umbezo (EC)	Root decoction	Perfume skin	Topical	5
Psidium guajava L.	Myrtaceae	Gwabisi (KZN)	Leaves	Wounds	Topical	12
Psoralea pinnata L.	Fabaceae	Umhlonishwa (KZN)	Leaves	Shingles	Topical	10
Ptaeroxylon obliquum (Thunb.) Radlk.	Rutaceae	Umthathe (EC)	Bark Infusion	Remove body odour	Bathing	5
Pterocarpus angolensis DC.	Fabaceae	Indlandlovu/ umbilo/ umvangazi (KZN)	Bark	Sores	Topical	18
Pterocelastrus tricuspidatus (Lam.) Sond.	Celastraceae	Ibholo (EC)	Leaves, shrub Infusion	Sore throat and to protect facial skin	Topical	5
Ranunculus multifidus Forssk.	Ranunculaceae	Ishashakazane/ Isijojokazana/ Uxhaphozi (KZN),	Whole plant	Sores	Topical	10, 11

(Continued)

TABLE 5.2 (CONTINUED)
South African Ethnomedicinal Plants of Dermatological and Immune Significance

Botanical Name	Family	Local Name	Part Used	Condition for Treatment	Mode of Administration	Ref
Rapanea melanophloeos (L.) Mez.	Myrsinaceae	Umaphipha (EC); Ikhubalwane/ inhluthe (KZN)	Bark	Cosmetic paste to protect against evil, and wounds	Topical	6, 15, 18
Rauvolfia caffra Sond.	Apocynaceae	-	Bark	Measles, urticaria and other skin rashes	Topical	22, 23
Rawsonia lucida Harv. & Sond.	Achariaceae	Umlongo (EC)	Paste ofleaves	Ringworm	Topical	5
Rhamnus prinoides L'Her.	Rhamnaceae	Mofifi (FS)	Leaves	Sores	Topical	24
Rhus lucida L.	Anacardiaceae	Intlokoshane (EC)	Bark Infusion	Scabies	Topical	5
Ricinus communis L.	Euphorbiaceae	Umhlakuva (EC); Nhlampfurha/ mupfure (L); Olieblare/ kastorolie boom (WC); Mokhura (NW)	Roots and leaves	Wounds and sores	Topical	2, 16, 20, 23
Rothmannia capensis Thunb	Rubiaceae	Ibolo (EC)	Fruit juice	Wounds and burns	Topical	6, 22
Rubia horrid (Thunb.) Puff	Rubiaceae	Madi-a-phalane (NW)	Roots	Albinism	Topical	23
Rumex acetosella L.	Polygonaceae		Roots	Wounds and bruises	Topical	24
Rumex crispus L.	Polygonaceae	Ubuhlunga (EC)	Decoction of leaves	Treat hair loss	Topical	5
Rumex lanceolatus Thunb.	Rubiaceae	Dolonyana (EC)	Roots/leaves	Abscesses, boils, and bruises	Topical	7, 9, 24
Salacia rehmannii Schinz.	Celastraceae	Phathatsimima (L)	Roots	Sores	Topical	16
Salix mucronata Thunb.	Salicaceae	Mogokare (FS)	Leaves	Burn wounds	Topical	24
Salix babylonica L.	Salicaceae	Umngcunube (EC)	Bark	Wounds	Topical	2
Salvia africana-lutea L.	Lamiaceae	Red sage (WC)	Leaves	Sore legs	Topical	19, 21

(Continued)

TABLE 5.2 (CONTINUED)
South African Ethnomedicinal Plants of Dermatological and Immune Significance

Botanical Name	Family	Local Name	Part Used	Condition for Treatment	Mode of Administration	Ref
Salvia stenophylla Burch. ex Benth	Lamiaceae	–	Leaves	Wounds and sores	Topical	6
Sansevieria hyacinthoides (L.) Druce	Asparagaceae	Isikholokotho (EC); Mosekela tsebeng (NW)	Leaves	Swellings, burns, and wounds	Topical	6, 23
Sarcophyte sanguinea Sparrm. ssp. *sanguinea*	Balanophoraceae	Umavumbuka (EC)	Dried fruiting body	Acne and other skin blemishes	Topical	6, 25
Sarcostemma viminale L.	Apocynaceae	Umbelebele (EC)	Decoction of leaves	Skin itch	Topical	5
Scabiosa columbaria L.	Dipsacaceae	Makgha (EC); Tlhako- ea- pitsi/ selomi/ mamokhale/ moholungoane (FS)	Leaves, roots	Wounds, bruises, and cuts	Topical	6, 9, 24
Scadoxus multiflorus (Martyn) Raf.	Amaryllidaceae	Inkuphulwana (EC)	Bulb Infusion	Wounds and bruises	Topical	5
Scadoxus puniceus (L.) Friis and Nordal	Amaryllidaceae	Inkuphulwana (EC)	Bulbs and roots	Wound and skin ulcers	Topical	6, 22
Schinus molle L.	Anacardiaceae	Ipepile (EC): Pepper tree (WC)	Lotion of fruits	Eczema	Topical	5, 19
Schotia afra (L.) Thunb.	Fabaceae	Umquqoba (EC)	Bark decoction	Skin ulcers	Topical	5
Schotia brachypetala Sond.	Fabaceae	Ihluze/umgxamu/uvovovo (KZN)	Bark	Sores	Topical	10, 11, 12
Scilla natalensis Planch	Hyacinthaceae	–	Fresh bulbs	Boils and sores	Topical	6
Scilla nervosa (Burch.) Jessop	Asparagaceae	Inkwitelu (EC)	Bulb ointment	Wounds and ringworm	Topical	5

(Continued)

TABLE 5.2 (CONTINUED)
South African Ethnomedicinal Plants of Dermatological and Immune Significance

Botanical Name	Family	Local Name	Part Used	Condition for Treatment	Mode of Administration	Ref
Sclerocarya birrea (A. Rich) Hochst., ssp.*caffra*	Anacardiaceae	Umganu (KZN)	Bark and leaves	Sores	Topical	10, 11, 16, 23
Scutia myrtina (Burm.f.) Kurz	Rhamnaceae	Isiphingo (EC)	Paste Leaves	Ringworm	Topical	5
Searsia lancea (L.f.) F.A. Barkley	Anacardiaceae	Mushakaladzane (L); Mosinabele/ mosilabele (FS)	Leaves	Rash and pimples	Topical	16, 24
Selaginella caffrorum (Milde) Hieron	Selaginaceae		Leaves	Herps and ulcers	Topical	24
Senecio asperulus DC.	Asteraceae	Moferefere/ Letapisa (FS)	Whole plant	Herpes sores/skin ulcers, and mouth ulcers	Topical, oral	24
Senecio deltoideus Less.	Asteraceae	Ityolo (EC)	Leaf lotion	Scabies and burns	Topical	5
Senecio longiflorus (DC). Sch. Bip	Asteraceae	Mosiama (NW)	Whole plant	Athlete's foot, chicken pox, eczema, Kaposi sarcoma, molluscum contagiosum, rash syphilis, and yaws	Topical	23
Senecio serratuloides DC.	Asteraceae	Ichazampukane/ Insukumbili/ Umaphozisa/ Umkhuthelo (KZN)	Leaves	Sores and shingles	Topical	10, 11
Senecio speciosus Willd.	Asteraceae	Ustukumbini (EC)	Leaves, stem	Swellings, cuts, burns, and sores		7, 9
Senna italica Mill ssp. *arachoides* Burch Lock.	Fabaceae	Sebetebete (NW)	Whole plant	Chickenpox	Topical	23
Senna occidentalis (L.) Link	Fabaceae	Nembenembe/ Munembenembe (L)	Leaves	Skin burns and wounds	Topical	16

(Continued)

TABLE 5.2 (CONTINUED)
South African Ethnomedicinal Plants of Dermatological and Immune Significance

Botanical Name	Family	Local Name	Part Used	Condition for Treatment	Mode of Administration	Ref
Setaria acromelaena (Hochst.) T. Durand & Schinz	Poaceae	Xihovane (L)	Stem	Sores	Topical	16
Sida pseudocordifolia Hochr.	Malvaceae	Mutudo (L)	Whole plant	Ringworm	Topical	10, 16
Sideroxylon inerme C.A.Sm.	Sapotaceae	Unqwashu (EC)	Decoction of leaves	Remove body odour	Bathing	5, 6
Siphonochilus aethiopicus Schweif.	Zingiberaceae	Ingungulo/ isiphephetho (KZN); Serokolo (NW)	Leaves	Oral thrush and chickenpox	Oral, topical	6, 23
Solanum aculeastrum Dunal.	Solanaceae	Umthuma (EC); Gifapple (WC)	Decoction of fruit	Insect bite, strengthen nails, perfume skin, and skin ulcers	Topical	5, 19
Solanum aculeatissimum Jacq.	Solanaceae	-	Leaves	Wounds	Topical	24
Solanum catombelense Peyr	Solanaceae	Morolwana (NW)	Whole plant	Chickenpox, fleabites, Kaposi sarcoma, rash, and sores	Topical	23
Solanum incanum L. Ruiz and Pav.	Solanaceae	Umthuma (EC)	Leaves, roots, fruits	Wounds, furuncles, and ringworm, and scars	Topical	6, 9, 22
Solanum lichtensteinii Willd.	Solanaceae	Tolwane (NW)	Whole plant	Burns	Topical	23
Solanum nigrum L.	Solanaceae	Umsobosobo (EC); Morotho (FS)	Paste of leaves	Ringworm	Topical	5, 24
Solanum panduriforme E. Mey.	Solanaceae	Mututulwa (L)	Fruits	Warts	Topical	11, 14, 16
Solanum rigescens Jacq.	Solanaceae	Mtuma (KZN)	Fruits	Boils	Topical	10, 11
Solanum tuberosum L.	Solanaceae	Potato	Tubers	Rash	Topical	16

(Continued)

TABLE 5.2 (CONTINUED)
South African Ethnomedicinal Plants of Dermatological and Immune Significance

Botanical Name	Family	Local Name	Part Used	Condition for Treatment	Mode of Administration	Ref
Sonchus dregeanus DC.	Asteraceae	Leshoabe/ sentlokojane/ sethokojane (FS)	Leaves	Rash	Topical	24
Sorghum bicolour (L) Moench	Poaceae	Mabele (NW)	Grains	Chickenpox	Topical	23
Spirostachys africana Sond.	Euphorbiaceae	Umthombothi (EC)	Bark	Rashes on newborn babies, nappy rashes, wounds, birth wounds, and pimples	Topical	9
Stapelia gigantea N.E. Br	Apocynaceae	Menoanoga (NW)	Whole plant	Kaposi sarcoma and molluscum contagiosum		
Striga asiatica (L.) Kuntze	Orobanchaceae	Vhuri (L)	Whole plant	Wounds	Topical	16
Strychnos madagascariensis Poir.	Loganiaceae	Umgluguza/ umkwakwa (KZN)	Bark	Sores, burns, sores, and ringworm	Topical	10, 11
Strychnos spinosa Lam.	Loganiaceae	Ihlala (KZN); Muramba (L)	Fruit sap	Sores	Topical	10, 11, 16
Sutherlandia frutescens (L.) R.Br.	Fabaceae	Umnwele (EC); Cancer bush/ kankerbos (WC); Lerumolamadi (NW)	Leaves	Wounds and skin cancer	Topical	6, 9, 19, 23
Synadenium cupulare (Boiss.) L. C. Wheeler	Euphorbiaceae	Muswoswo (L)	Stem	Moles	Topical	16
Syzygium cordatum Hochst.ex C. Krauss	Myrtaceae	Umswi (EC); Umdoni (KZN)	Bark, leaves	Blisters, pimples, inflammations, acne, and eczema	Topical	6, 9, 10,11, 18
Tabernaemontana elegans Stapf.	Apocynaceae	Umkhahlwana/umkhadlu (KZN); Muhatu (L)	Bark and leaves	Sores and ringworms	Topical	10, 11, 16
Talinum portulacifolium (Forssk.) Asch. ex Schweinf.	Talinaceae	Umhlabelo (EC)	Paste of leaves	Skin itch	Topical	5

(Continued)

TABLE 5.2 (CONTINUED)
South African Ethnomedicinal Plants of Dermatological and Immune Significance

Botanical Name	Family	Local Name	Part Used	Condition for Treatment	Mode of Administration	Ref
Taraxacum officinale F.H. Wigg	Asteraceae	Ikhokhoyi (EC)	Decoction of leaves	Remove body odour	Bathing	5
Tarchonanthus camphoratus L.	Asteraceae	Mohatha Wadikonyana (NW)	Roots	Albinism	Topical	23
Tecomaria capensis (Thunb.) Spach.	Bignoniaceae	Umsilingi/Icakatha (EC)	Bark	Inflammation	Topical	6
Terminalia sericea Burch. ex DC.	Combretaceae	Nkonono (L)	Leaves	Burns	Topical	11, 16, 22
Tetradenia riparia (Hochst)	Lamiaceae	Iboza (EC)	Leaves	Mouth ulcers	Oral	6
Thesium strictum P.J. Bergius	Santalaceae	Umbiza (EC)	Paste of leaves	Boils, wounds	Topical	5
Trachyandra muricata (L.f.) Kunth	Asphodelaceae	Olifant foot (WC)	Rhizome	Tired feet, athlete's foot, and blisters	Topical	19
Tribulus terristris L.	Zygophylaceae	Tshetlho (NW); Inkunzane (EC)	Seeds, leaves	Chickenpox, eczema, infantile acropustulosis, hair loss, and scabies	Topical	5, 23
Trichilia dregeana Sond.	Meliaceae	Umkhuhlu (EC)	Seeds	Body ointment and hair oil	Topical	6
Trichilia emetica Vahl.	Meliaceae	Umkhuhlu (EC); Nkuhlu (L)	Leaves or fruits	Bruises and eczema	Topical	6, 9, 16, 22
Tulbaghia alliacea (L.f.) Thunb.	Amaryllidaceae	Itswele (EC)	Bulb	Boils, wounds, pimples, eczema, and herpes	Topical	6, 9
Tulbaghia violacea Harv.	Amaryllidaceae	Wildeknoffel/ wildeknoflok (WC); Utswelane (EC); Isihaqa/ incinsini (KZN)	Whole plant	Wounds	Topical	21, 23
Ursinia nana DC. ssp. *nana*	Asteraceae		Whole plant	Wounds	Topical	24

(Continued)

TABLE 5.2 (CONTINUED)
South African Ethnomedicinal Plants of Dermatological and Immune Significance

Botanical Name	Family	Local Name	Part Used	Condition for Treatment	Mode of Administration	Ref
Urtica urens L.	Urticaceae		Whole plant	Wounds	Topical	24
Vepris undulata (Thunb.) I. Verd.	Rutaceae	Ilatile lokuqhumisa (EC)	Decoction of leaves	Accelerate hair growth	Topical	5
Vernonia fastigiate Oliv. & Hiern	Asteraceae	Tanyi (L)	Leaves	Wound scars	Topical	16
Vernonia natalensis Sch.Bip. ex Walp	Valerianaceae	Umthi wezulu (EC)	Roots and leaves	Boils	Topical	6, 22
Viscum capense L.f.	Santalaceae	-	Whole plant	Warts	Topical	22
Viscum menyharthii Engl.& Schinz	Santalaceae	Lephakama (NW)	Stem	Kaposi sarcoma	Topical	23
Wahlenbergia banksiana A.DC.	Campanulaceae		Roots	Syphilitic sores	Topical	24
Waltheria indica L.	Malvaceae	-	Roots	Burns and wounds	Topical	11
Warburgia salutaris (Bertol. F.) Chiov.	Canellaceae	Manaka/ shibaha (L)	Bark	Various skin complaints	Topical	6, 15
Warburgia salutaris (G. Bertol.) Chiov.	Canellaceae	Isibhaha (KZN)	Bark	Mouth sores	Oral	12, 18, 22
Withania somnifera (L.) Dunal	Solanaceae	Ubuvimba/Ubushwa (EC, KZN); Geneesbos (WC); Bofepha (FS)	Leaves and berries	Cuts, wounds, abscesses, inflammation, and soap, douche	Topical	6, 9, 11, 19, 24
Ximenia americana L.	Olacaceae	Ntsenghele	Roots, leaves	Inflamed eyes	Bathing	14
Ximenia caffra Sond.	Olacaceae	Umthunduluka obomvu (KZN)	Twigs	Sores	Topical	11
Xysmalobium undulatum (L.) Aiton F.	Apocynaceae	Nwachaba/Ishongwane (EC)	Roots	Cuts and wounds	Topical	6

(Continued)

TABLE 5.2 (CONTINUED)
South African Ethnomedicinal Plants of Dermatological and Immune Significance

Botanical Name	Family	Local Name	Part Used	Condition for Treatment	Mode of Administration	Ref
Zantedeschia albomaculata (Hook.) Baill ssp. *albomaculata*	Araceae	Mohalalitoe (FS)	Leaves	Mouth ulcers	Oral	24
Zantedeschia aethiopica (L.) Spreng.	Araceae	Inyibiba (EC)	Leaves, rhizome	Wounds, burns, and sore throat	Topical	2, 6, 8, 13, 22
Zanthoxylum capense Harv.	Rutaceae	Isifutho (EC); Umnungamabele (KZN); Monokwane/ khunugumorupa (L); Knobwood (WC)	Leaves, roots, bark	Sores and toothache swollen feet	Topical	6, 11, 15, 19
Zanthoxylum davyi Waterm.	Rutaceae	Munungu (L)	Roots, Leaves, Stem	Wounds and teeth cleaning	Topical and oral	16
Zea mays L.	Poaceae	Umbona (EC); Mufhumbu ha mavhele (L)	Leaves, seeds	Wound, rash, and pimples	Topical	6, 16
Ziziphus mucronata Willd.	Rhamnaceae	Umphafa (EC); Umphafa/ umlahlankosi/ isilahla (KZN); Mokgalo/ mutshetshete/ mphasamhala/ mokgalô/ moonaona (L)	Leaves, roots, bark	Boils and swellings	Topical	6, 11, 15, 17, 22

Key: EC – Eastern Cape; FS – Free State; KZN – KwaZulu Natal; L – Limpopo; MP – Mpumalanga; NC – Northern Cape; NW – North West; WC – Western Cape 1. Maroyi (2019); 2. Buwa-Komoreng et al. (2019); 3. Bhat (2013); 4. Bhat (2014); 5. Afolayan et al. (2014); 6. Sagbo and Mbeng (2018); 7. Grierson and Afolayan (1999); 8. Weideman (2005); 9. Mahachi (2013); 10. de Wet et al. (2013); 11. Nciki et al. (2016); 12. Coopoosamy and Naidoo (2012); 13. Ghuman et al. (2016); 14. Shikwambana and Mahlo (2020); 15. Rasethe et al. (2019); 16. Setshego et al. (2020); 17. Mongalo and Makhafola (2018); 18. Grace et al. (2003); 19. Aston Philander (2011); 20. Thring and Weitz (2006); 21. Mintsa Mi Nzue (2009); 22. Mabona et al. (2013); 23. Asong et al. (2019); 24. Moteetee and Kose (2017); 25. Komoreng et al. (2019); 26. Lall and Kishore (2014).

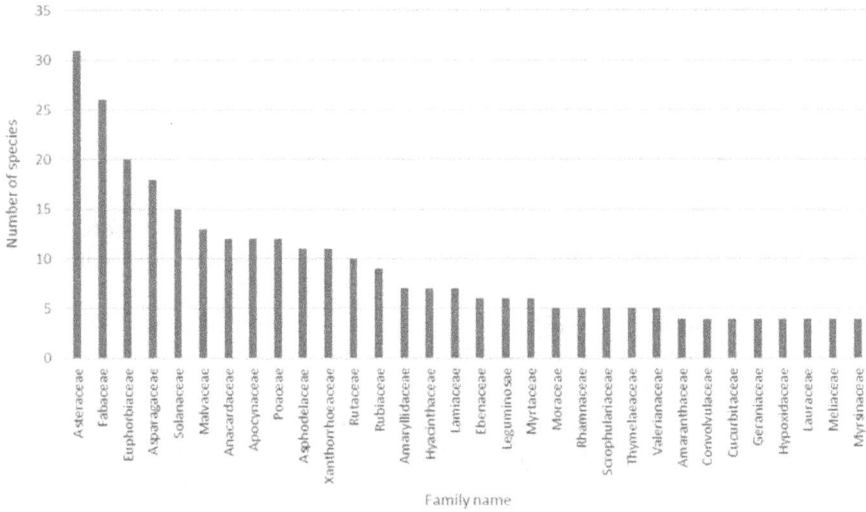

FIGURE 5.1 Some plant species of dermatological significance in South Africa.

world's largest documented consumer of these products (Davids et al., 2016). The use of chemicals, such as mercury and hydroquinone, are the major causes of these toxic effects. This led to the banning of hydroquinone in cosmetics in draft legislation in 1988 (Thomas, 2012). Nevertheless, history indicates the use of medicinal plants for skin lightening with little or no side effects. However, the use of herbs to boost the immune system achieves this goal by softening the skin and protecting the skin against ultraviolet (UV) radiation from the sun. Some compounds from these medicinal plants have been shown to inhibit UV-induced development of squamous cell carcinomas, or simply to guard against cutaneous damage caused by UV irradiation (Tabassum and Hamdani 2014). The study of Heo et al. (2001) was able to show that the ethanol extract of *Prunus persica* was able to inhibit UVB- or UVC-induced lipid peroxidation in skin fibroblast cells. Perhaps the revitalization of medicinal plant use in cosmetics could lead to other avenues, such as their domestication and eventual cultivation. These plants have little or no side effects, even after long-term use, in comparison with the harsh synthetic chemicals that often leave the skin without melanin and damaged beyond any prospects of repair. Most of the users of skin lightening products are poor and cannot afford the expensive treatment regimes. Some of the medicinal plants, such as lemons, avocados, potatoes, sorghum, and others reported in this work, are common foods which are highly nutritious and therefore play a dual role, as topical skincare applications and as a source of nutrition to boost the immune system. Orally administered medicines have, in times past, been reported to also possess nutritional benefits, so that, whereas the compounds target the pathogens, the nutritional composition of the medicine boosts the immune system, leading to a quicker recovery.

5.5 COMMON METHODS OF PREPARATION

The literature survey revealed that the medicinal plants identified as being effective in skincare strategies are used for wounds (18%), sores (11%), cosmetics (8%), burns (8%), allergies (8%), boils (6%) and eczema (5%), among other conditions, as shown in Figure 5.2. Other conditions that are treated by these medicinal plants and that appear in the literature search, as shown in Table 5.2, include leprosy, impetigo, condylomata acuminata, madura foot, painkilling effect on skin, sore throat, corns, drawing out pus, sore mouth, keratosis, pearl penile papules, and molluscum contagiosum.

Topical administration (84%) is the most common form of administering the medicinal plant preparation, followed by bathing (6%) and oral consumption (3%), as shown in Figure 5.3. The same plant preparation can be administered both topically and orally or in a bath and orally. However, *Albizia anthelmintica*, a plant mentioned in the treatment of lymphatic filariasis is also administered orally. Other orally administered plants are used either for cleaning teeth or for the treatment of gums, sore throat, oral thrush, and/or mouth ulcers. A total of six plant species are reportedly mixed with lotion/ glycerin to ensure that the product sticks to the skin. Several authors, including Lordani et al. (2018), reported on this mode of application of medicinal plant preparations.

5.6 SUSTAINABLE UTILIZATION AND CONSERVATION OF PLANTS FOR SKIN THERAPY

This current literature survey reveals that the leaves are the plant parts most used for herbal preparations, accounting for 47% of usage, while the bark (14%) and roots

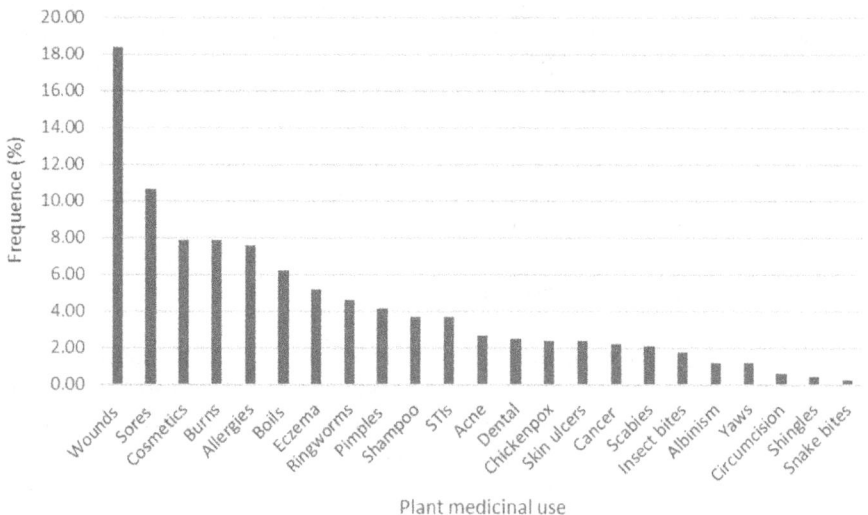

FIGURE 5.2 The medicinal uses of the plants.

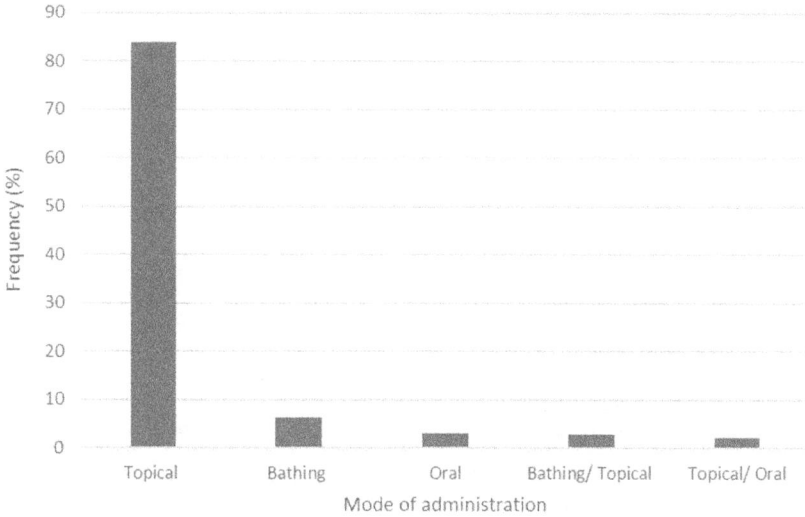

FIGURE 5.3 Mode of administration of medicinal plants.

(13%) also play a significant role (Figure 5.4), with other plant parts contributing less than 10% each. The use of the whole plant and roots is of significance. This is because these harvesting methods are destructive and therefore pay little attention to biodiversity conservation. In fact, the greatest proportion of documented plant species becoming extinct in the world has been reported in South Africa. A total of sixty-four plant species has not been seen in more than fifty years and their habitat has been destroyed, while thirty-nine species are extinct (Raimondo et al. 2013). As of 2020, SANBI (2020) lists South Africa's threatened flora in the order: Western Cape (63.8% species are threatened) > Northern Cape (13.9 %) > Eastern Cape (9.7%) > KwaZulu Natal (8.1%) > Mpumalanga (4.6%) > Limpopo (3.3%) > Gauteng (0.8%) > North West (0.7%) > Free State (0.2%). As of 2014, about 172 plant taxa had been listed as "protected" under the South African National Environmental Management: Biodiversity Act (NEMBA); Act No. 10 of 2004 (Raimondo 2015). However, the updated list (SANBI 2020) shows the proportion of protected taxa in each of South Africa's nine biomes as follows: Albany Thicket (11.9%), Desert (30.3%), Forest (40.8%), Fynbos (22.7%), Grassland (4.5%), Indian Ocean Coastal Belt (7.1%), Nama Karoo (1.6%), Savanna (13.4%), and Succulent Karoo (7.8%). Habitat loss, habitat degradation, invasive alien species, overharvesting of medicinal plants, demographic factors, pollution, climate change, and natural disasters are the major driving forces behind medicinal plant extinction in South Africa. Current SANBI (2020) statistics indicate that, between 1990 and 2018, about 5% of the taxa increased in threat status. Furthermore, about 40% of the increased threat to medicinal plants over the past twenty years has been caused by invasive species. Other threats, such as habitat invasion due to livestock overgrazing, urban development, and crop cultivation, has contributed 11, 20, and 33%, respectively.

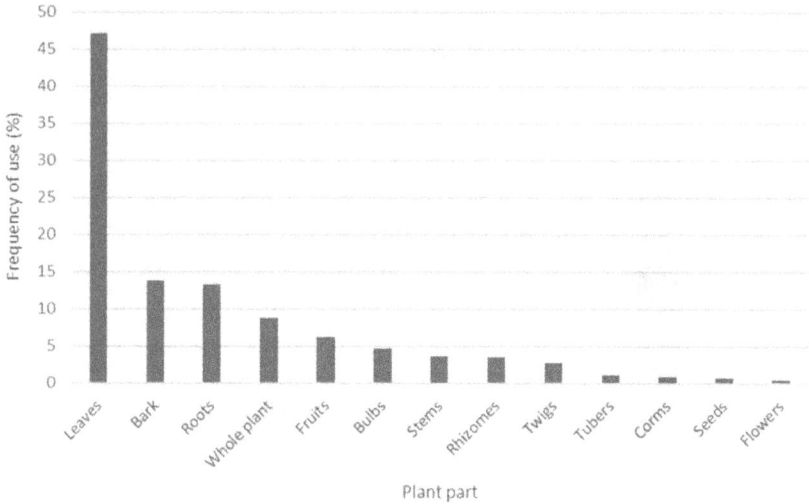

FIGURE 5.4 Plant parts used of plant species of dermatological significance in South Africa.

The need for protection of South Africa's biodiversity and for implementation of the various conservation strategies is clear. In fact, the draft policy on African Traditional Medicine Notice 906 of 2008 (South Africa 2008) is an attempt to protect not only biodiversity but also the African traditional herbal medicine knowledge. This legislation specifically makes it illegal to harvest plants from the wild without permission from the relevant authorities. To ensure protection of biodiversity due to habitat loss or degradation, *in-situ* and *ex-situ* conservation strategies have been put in place. South Africa currently has seventeen national parks, eight natural Transfrontier Conservation Areas, and numerous private parks, wild nurseries, and forest reserves. These *in-situ* conservation areas play a huge role in the protection of biodiversity, including that of medicinal plants. *Ex-situ* conservation strategies in place in South Africa include seventeen national botanic gardens and numerous seed banks. Research on the domestication of medicinal plants in South Africa has been on-going for more than ten years. This research aims to bring medicinal plants under cultivation to put less pressure on harvesting these resources from the wild. Although these strategies may not be able to replicate the exact growing conditions of plants in the wild, this a step in the right direction. Researchers now know that the polyphenolic compounds produced by plants in the wild change when these plants are cultivated either under controlled conditions or in environments other than their original habitats. Scientists therefore need to focus more on how to stimulate the production of specific bioactive compounds under controlled environments or in other habitats. More importantly, biodiversity protection rules and regulations put in place by the government need to be adhered to.

5.7   CONCLUSION

South Africa is richly endowed with numerous medicinal plants that are used in the treatment of various skin-related diseases and conditions. Most of the plants are used to treat wounds, although a sizeable proportion has immunological functions, for use, for example, in cosmetics. The preferred mode of administering medicinal plant preparations is topical, and the leaves are the most used plant parts. Although South Africa contains more than 400 species with dermatological uses, care needs to be taken to ensure that the legislation put in place by the government to protect these species is adhered to and administered. Habitat degradation and/or loss, overharvesting and natural disasters are some of the major threats to these plants' survival. There is therefore a need to constantly raise awareness of these important species by educating the public on the importance of protecting them. If these species are neglected and their knowledge is not passed on to future generations, their risk of extinction, which is already high, will increase further, and this will leave future generations with nothing.

REFERENCES

Adcock Ingram limited. 2007. Instruction paper. William Nicolrylaan 3011, Bryanston, Privaatsak X69, Bryanstan, 2021.

Adedapo, A.A., Jumoh, F.O., Koduro, S., Afolayan, A.J., and P. Masika. 2008. Antibacterial and antioxidant properties of the methanol extracts of the leaves and stems of Calpurnia aurea. *BMC Complementary and Alternative Medicine*, 8: 53.

Afolayan, A.J., Grierson, D.S., and W.O. Mbeng. 2014. Ethnobotanical survey of medicinal plants used in the management of skin disorders among the Xhosa communities of the Amathole District, Eastern Cape, South Africa. *Journal of Ethnopharmacology*, 153(1): 220–32.

American Academy of Dermatology. 1999. https://server.aad.org/DermLex/?#4945. [Accessed 8 October 2020].

Asong, J.A., Ndhlovu, P.T., Khosana, N.S., Aremua, A.O., and W. Otang-Mbeng. 2019. Medicinal plants used for skin-related diseases among the Batswanas in Ngaka Modiri Molema District Municipality, South Africa. *South African Journal of Botany*, 126: 11–20.

Aston Philander, L. 2011. An ethnobotany of Western Cape Rasta bush medicine. *Journal of Ethnopharmacology*, 138(2): 578–594.

Bhat, R.B. 2013. Plants of Xhosa people in the Transkei region of Eastern Cape (South Africa) with major pharmacological and therapeutic properties. *Journal of Medicinal Plants Research*, 7(20): 1474–1480.

Bhat, R.B. 2014. Medicinal plants and traditional practices of Xhosa people in the Transkei region of Eastern Cape, South Africa. *Indian Journal of Traditional Knowledge*, 13(2): 292–298.

Buwa-Komoreng, L.V., Mayekiso, B., Mhinana, Z., and A.L. Adeniran. 2019. An ethnobotanical and ethnomedicinal survey of traditionally used medicinal plants in Seymour, South Africa: An attempt toward digitization and preservation of ethnic knowledge. *Pharmacognosy Magazine*, 15: 115–123.

Chen, Y.E., and H. Tsao. 2013. The skin microbiome: current perspectives and future challenges. *Journal of the American Academy of Dermatology*, 69(1): 143–55.

Cock, M.L., and A.P. Dold. 2000. The medicinal plants traded in the Eastern Cape province. Unpublished report, Department of Water Affairs and Forestry, Pretoria.

Coopoosamy, R.M., and K.K. Naidoo. 2012. An ethnobotanical study of medicinal plants used by traditional healers in Durban, South Africa. *African Journal of Pharmacy and Pharmacology*, 6(11): 818–823.

Davids, L.M., van Wyk, J., Khumalo, N.P., and N.G. Jablonski. 2016. The phenomenon of skin lightening: Is it right to be light? *South African Journal of Science,* 112(11/12).

Dawid-Pać, R. 2013. Medicinal plants used in treatment of inflammatory skin diseases. *Postepy dermatologii i alergologii*, 30(3): 170–177.

De Wet H, Nciki S., and S.F. van Vuuren. 2013. Medicinal plants used for the treatment of various skin disorders by a rural community in northern Maputaland, South Africa. *Journal of Ethnobiology and Ethnomedicine*, 9: 51.

Dermnet-NZ. 2008. Principles of dermatological practice: an overview of dermatology. Available at: https://www.dermnetnz.org/cme/principles/an-overview-of-dermatology/. [Accessed 8 October 2020].

Ghuman, S., Ncube, B., Finnie, J.F., McGaw, L.J., Coopoosamy, R.M., and J. van Staden. 2016. Antimicrobial activity, phenolic content, and cytotoxicity of medicinal plant extracts used for treating dermatological diseases and wound healing in KwaZulu-Natal, South Africa. *Frontiers in Pharmacology*, 7: 320.

Grace, O.M., Prendergast, H.D.V., Jäger, A.K., and J. van Staden. 2003. Bark medicines used in traditional healthcare in KwaZulu-Natal, South Africa: an inventory. *South African Journal of Botany*, 69: 301–363.

Grice, E.A. and J.A., and J.A. Segre. 2011. The skin microbiome. *Nature Reviews Microbiology*, 9(4): 244–53. Erratum in: *Nature Reviews Microbiology*, 9(8): 626.

Grierson, D.S., and A.J. Afolayan. 1999. Antibacterial activity of some indigenous plants used for treatment of wounds in the Eastern Cape, South Africa. *Journal of Ethnopharmacology*, 66: 103–106.

Heo, M.Y., Kim, S.H., Yang, H.E., Lee, S.H., Jo, B.K., and H.P. Kim. 2001. Protection against ultraviolet B-and C-induced DNA damage and skin carcinogenesis by the flowers of Prunus persica extract. *Mutation Research*, 496: 47–59.

Katewa, S.S., Chaudhary, B.L., and J. Anita. 2004. Folk herbal medicine from tribal area of Rajastan, India. *Journal of Ethnopharmacology*, 92: 41–6.

Katiyar, S.K., Afaq, F., Perez, A., and H. Mukhtar. 2001. Green tea polyphenol (-)-epigallo-catechin3-gallate treatment of human skin inhibits ultra-violet radiation induced by oxidative stress. *Carcinogenesis*, 22(2): 287–294.

Komoreng, L., Thekisoe, O., Lehasa, S., Tiwani, T., Mzizi, N., Mokoena, N., Khambule, N., Ndebele, S., and N. Mdletshe. 2019. An ethnobotanical survey of traditional medicinal plants used against lymphatic filariasis in South Africa. *South African Journal of Botany*, 111: 12–16.

Lall, N., and N. Kishore. 2014. Are plants used for skin care in South Africa fully explored? *Journal of ethnopharmacology*, 153(1): 61–84.

Lordani, T.V.A., de Lara, C.E., Ferreira, F.B.P., de Souza Terron Monich, M., Mesquita da Silva, C., Felicetti Lordani, C.R., Giacomini Bueno, F., Vieira Teixeira, J.J., and M.V.C. Lonardoni. 2018. Therapeutic effects of medicinal plants on cutaneous wound healing in humans: a systematic review. *Mediators of inflammation*, 2018: 7354250.

Mabona, U., Viljoen, A., Shikanga, E., Marston, A., and S. van Vuuren. 2013. Antimicrobial activity of southern African medicinal plants with dermatological relevance: From an ethnopharmacological screening approach, to combination studies and the isolation of a bioactive compound. *Journal of Ethnopharmacology*, 148(1): 45–55.

Mahachi, J. 2013. Medicinal properties of some plants used for the treatment of skin disorders in the OR Tambo and Amathole municipalities of the Eastern Cape province, South Africa. Master of Science (MSc): Botany Dissertation, Walter Sisulu University. Available at: https://core.ac.uk/download/pdf/145036454.pdf. [Accessed 6 November 2020].

Mantle, D., and Gok, M.A. 2001. Adverse and beneficial effects of plant extracts on skin and skin disorders. *Adverse Drug Reactions and Toxicological Reviews*, 77: 89–103.

Maroyi, A. 2019. A review of botany, medicinal uses, and biological activities of Pentanisia prunelloides (Rubiaceae). *Asian Journal of Pharmaceutical and Clinical Research*, 12(8): 4–9.

Mintsa Mi Nzue, A.P. 2009. Use and conservation status of medicinal plants in the Cape Peninsula, Western Cape Province of South Africa. MSc Dissertation, University of Stellenbosch. Available at: https://core.ac.uk/download/pdf/37319949.pdf. [Accessed 5 November 2020].

Mongalo, N.I., and T.J. Makhafola. 2018. Ethnobotanical knowledge of the lay people of Blouberg area (Pedi tribe), Limpopo Province, South Africa. *Journal of Ethnobiology and Ethnomedicine*, 14: 46.

Moteetee, A., and Kose, L.S. 2017. A review of medicinal plants used by the Basotho for treatment of skin disorders: Their phytochemical, antimicrobial, and anti-inflammatory potential. *African Journal of Traditional, Complementary and Alternative Medicines*, 14(5): 121–137.

Nciki, N., Vuuren, S., van Eyk, A., and H. de Wet. 2016. Plants used to treat skin diseases in northern Maputaland, South Africa: antimicrobial activity and in vitro permeability studies. *Pharmaceutical Biology*, 54(11): 2420–2436.

Pharmcare limited. 2003. Building 12, Healthcare Park, Woodlands Drive, Woodmead, Sandton, 2148.

Quave, C.L., Plano, L.R.W., Pantuso, T., and C. Bradley. 2008. Effects of extracts from Italian medicinal plants on planktonic growth, biofilm and adherence of methicillin-resistant Staphylococcus aureus. *Journal of Ethnopharmacology*, 118(3): 418–28.

Raimondo, D. (ed.) 2015. South Africa's Strategy for Plant Conservation. South African National Biodiversity Institute and the Botanical Society of South Africa, Pretoria.

Raimondo, D.C., von Staden, L., and Donaldson, J.S. 2013. Lessons from the conservation assessment of the South African megaflora. *Annals of the Missouri Botanical Garden*, 99(2): 221–230.

Ranbaxy (SA) (PTY) LTD. 2006. Third Floor, Outspan House, 1006 Lenchen Avenue North, Centurion.

Rasethe, M.T., Semenya, S., and A. Maroyi. 2019. Medicinal Plants Traded in Informal Herbal Medicine Markets of the Limpopo Province, South Africa. Evidence-based Complementary and Alternative Medicine, eCAM, 2019.

Revathi, P., and T. Parimelazhagan. 2010. Traditional Knowledge on Plants Used by the Irula Tribe of Hasanur Hills, Erode District, Tamil Nadu, India. *Ethnobotanical Leaflets*, 14: 136–60.

Sagbo, I.J., and W.O. Mbeng. 2018. Plants used for cosmetics in the Eastern Cape Province of South Africa: a case study of skin care. *Pharmacognosy Reviews*, 12: 139–56.

Perumal Samy, R., and P. Gopalakrishnakone. 2010. Therapeutic potential of plants as anti-microbials for drug discovery. *Evidence-based Complementary and Alternative Medicine*, 7(3): 283–94.

Perumal Samy, R., and Ignacimuthu S. 2000. Antibacterial activity of some folklore medicinal plants used by tribals in Western Ghats of India. *Journal of Ethnopharmacology*, 69(1): 63–71.

SANBI. 2020. Statistics: Red List of South African Plants version 2020.1. Downloaded from Redlist.sanbi.org on 2020/11/12. Available at: http://redlist.sanbi.org/stats.php#Natio nal%20statistics. [Accessed 20 Nov 2020].

Scottish Dermatological Society. 2020. McCall Andersons Classification of Skin Diseases. Available at: https://www.sds.org.uk/history/mccall-andersons-classification-skin-di seases. [Accessed 8 October 2020].

Setshego, M.V., Aremu, A.O., Mooki, O., and W. Otang-Mbeng. 2020. Natural resources used as folk cosmeceuticals among rural communities in Vhembe district municipality, Limpopo province, South Africa. *BMC Complementary Medicine and Therapies*, 20: 81.

Shikwambana, N., and S.M. Mahlo. 2020. Mahlo A Survey of Antifungal Activity of Selected South African Plant Species Used for the Treatment of Skin Infections. *Natural Products Communications*, 15(5): 1–10.

South Africa, 2008. Notice: Draft policy on African traditional medicine for South Africa. Notice 906 of 2008 (49 pp.) Available at: https://tradmed.ukzn.ac.za/wp-content/ uploads/2018/05/Draft-Policy-on-African-Traditional-Healers.pdf, [Accessed 13 November 2020].

Statista. 2020a. Size of the global skin care market from 2012 to 2025 (in billion U.S. dollars). Available at: https://www.statista.com/statistics/254612/global-skin-care-market-size/. [Accessed 6 October 2020].

Statista. 2020b. Market value of the professional skin care market in South Africa from 2017 to 2023(in million U.S. dollars). Available at: https://www.statista.com/statistics/8638 32/skin-care-market-value-south-africa/. [Accessed 6 October 2020].

Street, R.A., and G. Prinsloo. 2013. Commercially important medicinal plants of South Africa: a review. *Journal of Chemistry*, Article ID 205048: 1–16.

Tabassum, N., and M. Hamdani. 2014. Plants used to treat skin diseases. *Pharmacognosy Reviews*, 8(15): 52–60.

Thirumalai, T., Kelumalail, B., Senthilkumar, E., and E. David. 2009. Ethnobotanical study of medicinal plants used by the local people in Vellore District, Tamilnadu, India. *Ethnobotanical Leaflets*, 13: 1302–11.

Thomas, L.M. 2012. Skin lighteners, black consumers and Jewish entrepreneurs in South Africa. *History Workshop Journal*, 73: 259–283.

Thring, T.S.A., and F.M. Weitz. 2006. Medicinal plant use in the Bredasdorp/Elim region of the Southern Overberg in the Western Cape Province of South Africa. *Journal of Ethnopharmacology*, 103: 261–275.

UNAIDS. 2020. HIV/AIDS estimates: Country factsheet- South Africa 2019. Available at: https://www.unaids.org/en/regionscountries/countries/southafrica. [Accessed 8/10/2020].

Verma, A.K., Pal, S., and S. Kumar. 2019. Classification of skin disease using ensemble data mining techniques. *Asian Pacific Journal of Cancer Prevention*, 20(6): 1887–1894.

Weideman, L. 2005. An investigation into the antibacterial activities of medicinal plants traditionally used in the Eastern Cape to treat secondary skin infections associated with burn wounds. Magister Technologiae Dissertation, Nelson Mandela Metropolitan University. Available at: https://core.ac.uk/download/pdf/145044672.pdf. [Accessed 5 November 2020].

6 Traditional African Medicinal Plants for a Strong Immune System

Anywar Godwin

CONTENTS

6.1 INTRODUCTION

Africa is disproportionately affected by diseases such as HIV/AIDS, which attack and destroy the immune system. More than 68% of the 38 million people globally affected by HIV/AIDS reside in sub-Saharan Africa (UNAIDS 2020). Furthermore, many of them do not have access to modern treatment facilities or medicines.

The immune system consists of a highly complex mechanism for defending the body against disease by identifying and killing pathogens or tumour cells (Gertsch et al. 2011; Wen et al. 2012; Wynn et al. 2013). It is composed of the innate and adaptive immune systems. The former is characterized by a non-specific response of cells *via* molecular interactions and the expression of inducible cytokines and chemokines, whereas the latter consists of specialized effector cells (T and B cells) which recognize antigens, that are processed and presented by macrophages and dendritic cells. This leads to the activation of cytotoxic T cells and generation of antibodies which are pivotal in eliminating or preventing pathogenic insults (Gertsch et al. 2011; Kuwabara et al. 2017).

Conventionally, disorders of he immune system are categorised as: (i) primary immune deficiencies, which occur when one is born with a weak immune system, such as severe combined immunodeficiency (SCID), (ii) acquired immune

DOI: 10.1201/9781003137955-6

deficiencies, which occur when one catches a disease that weakens the immune system, such as HIV/AIDS, (iii) overactive immune systems, which occur when one's immune system is too active, e.g., in allergic reactions, and (iv) autoimmune diseases, which occur when one's immune system attacks itself, e.g., type 1 diabetes and rheumatoid arthritis (Murphy and Weaver 2016). However, in African traditional medicine, diseases of the immune system are looked at from the perspective of immune deficiencies, particularly HIV/AIDS or cancer. This chapter focuses on the use of medicinal plants on immune disorders only in the category of acquired immune deficiencies.

Immunomodulators are biological or synthetic biomolecules which have the ability to regulate, suppress, or stimulate any components of the immune system (Puri et al. 1994; Jantan et al. 2015). They are also referred to as immunorestoratives, immunoaugmentors, or biological response modifiers (Jantan et al. 2015). Immunomodulators are categorized as immunostimulants, immunoadjuvants, or immunosuppressants. Immunostimulants activate or stimulate the immune system mediators, resulting in improved resistance against various infections and restoration of compromized immunity (Saxena et al. 2008; Kumar et al. 2011; Jantan et al. 2015; Raj and Gothandam 2015). Immunomodulators can be used to stimulate the immune system to reduce drug side effect (Prendergast and Jaffee 2007). Immunoadjuvants are specific immune stimulators which boost vaccine efficacy (Leroux-Roels 2010). Immunosuppressants inhibit the immune system and can be used to control pathological immune reactions (Chatterjee et al. 1988; Jantan et al. 2015). Overall, the present chapter explores the most recent scientific evidence supporting the employment of some widely used African medicinal plant species with proven immunomodulatory activity. Additionally, the phytochemistry, mode of action, and toxicity of these plant species are discussed in relation to traditional uses of these plant species.

6.2   IMMUNOMODULATORY AGENTS FROM PLANTS

Unfortunately, most immunostimulants and immunosuppressants in clinical use are cytotoxic (Leroux-Roels, 2010; Jantan et al. 2015). Many of the immunomodulating biological agents approved for use by the Food and Drug Authority in the USA have been reported to have a wide array of unintended, sometimes fatal side effects. For instance, rituximab use was associated with a higher incidence of serious infections, particularly in patients with profound CD4 lymphopaenia (Koo et al. 2010). On the contrary, natural products are known to have many advantages, such as nontoxicity, ease of preparation and application, and greater safety, and accessibility (Oršolić & Bašić 2003; Lotter-Stark et al. 2012; Mukherjee et al. 2014).

Several plant species have been regularly used in traditional medicine to treat immune system disorders (Fernandez et al. 2002; Sultan et al. 2014; Anywar et al. 2020a) and are a potential source of immunomodulating agents (Williams 2001). Different studies have shown novel and significant immunomodulatory activities from various plant species (Puri et al. 2000; Reis et al. 2008; Karunai Raj et al. 2012; Arthanari et al. 2013; Sultan et al. 2014; Mukherjee et al. 2015; Raj & Gothandam 2015;

Hasson et al. 2019; Olwenyi et al., 2021). This emphasizes the need to search for novel immunomodulatory agents from natural sources (Raj and Gothandam, 2015).

6.3 MECHANISMS OF ACTION OF IMMUNOMODULATORY AGENTS FROM PLANTS

A compromized immune system can lead to the development of several serious chronic diseases (Gertsch et al. 2011; Wen et al. 2012; Abbas et al. 2019) such as AIDS, the most widespread immunosuppressive disease globally (Gea-Banacloche 2006). In such cases, maintenance of the immune system by means of medication can be achieved, using herbal medicines. Herbal medicines which function as immunomodulators alter the activity of immune function through the dynamic regulation of informational molecules, such as cytokines (Spelman et al. 2006).

Cytokines are secreted proteins that regulate immune responses through growth, differentiation, and activation functions. They are involved in almost all aspects of immunity and inflammation. Different combinations of cytokines are produced in response to specific immune insults (Steinke and Borish 2006). The modulation of cytokine secretion may offer novel approaches in the treatment of a variety of diseases. The cytokines include interleukins (IL), such as IL-2, IL-4, IL-17 (Vitetta et al. 1985; Dembic 2015; Kuwabara et al. 2017), interferons (IFNs) such as IFN-γ (Tau and Rothman 1999; Kak et al. 2018) and TNF-α (Pfeffer 2003; Bradley 2008). Some of the better known and more widely used medicinal plant species in Africa for stimulating or modulating the immune system exert their immunomodulatory effects through various mechanisms, as illustrated in Table 6.1. Some of these mechanisms include the induction of various cytokines, such as IFN-α and -β (Beuscher et al. 1994; Ngure et al. 2014), triggering the alternative complement pathway, raising the number and distribution of white blood cells, stimulating phagocytosis, T-cell production, or lymphocytic activity (El-Ashmawy et al. 2015), inducing apoptosis, suppression of cell proliferation, inhibition of pro-inflammatory cytokine/chemokine production, and increasing anti-inflammatory cytokine production (Rieder et al. 2010).

6.4 MEDICINAL PLANTS USED IN AFRICAN TRADITIONAL MEDICINE FOR IMMUNOMODULATION

This review was carried out on the relevant articles, books, theses, dissertations, patents, and other English-only reports on ethnobotany, immunomodulatory profiles, pharmacological or biological activity, toxicity, or phytochemistry, of selected medicinal plant species in Africa used by herbalists in boosting or modulating the immune system. We searched databases, such as PubMed, Web of Science, Scopus, and Science Direct, and search engines, such as Google Scholar. **Table 6.1** shows nineteen medicinal plant species with proven immunomodulatory activity used in African traditional medicine for immune-related disorders. The table also shows their mode of action, the identity of their bioactive molecules, as well their toxicity *in vitro*.

TABLE 6.1
Medicinal Plant Species Used in African Traditional Medicine for Strong immunomodulation

Scientific name and Family	Traditional Uses Related to Immune Disorders	Immunomodulatory Activity and Mode of Action	Phytochemical Composition	Toxicity /cytotoxicity
1. *Aerva lanata* (L.) Juss. Amaranthaceae	Low/compromized immunity to HIV (Anywar et al. 2020a).	The ethanolic extract of the whole plant produced an increase in total WBC count, bone marrow cellularity, number of α-esterase-positive cells in BALB/c mice, proliferation of splenocytes, thymocytes and bone marrow cells (Nevin and Vijayammal, 2005; Siveen & Kuttan, 2011).	Phenolic compounds e.g. gallic acid, apigetrin, rutin, myricetin, saponins, flavonoids, tannins and phytosterols (Kumar et al. 2013)	The aqueous whole plant extract is relatively safe (LD_{50} = 22.62 g/kg bw) in albino mice (Omotoso et al. 2017). The aqueous stem extract was nontoxic to human erythrocytes (IC_{50}= 24.89 mg/ml) (Kumar et al. 2013). The ethanol extract is cytotoxic to Dalton's lymphoma ascites and Ehrlich ascites carcinoma cells at 500 μg/ ml. The extract was also cytotoxic to L929 and HeLa cells at higher concentrations (Siveen and Kuttan, 2011).

(*Continued*)

TABLE 6.1 (CONTINUED)
Medicinal Plant Species Used in African Traditional Medicine for Strong immunomodulation

Scientific name and Family	Traditional Uses Related to Immune Disorders	Immunomodulatory Activity and Mode of Action	Phytochemical Composition	Toxicity /cytotoxicity
2. *Aloe vera* (L.) Burm.f. Asphodolaceae	Low/compromized immunity to HIV (Anywar et al. 2020a)	The decolorized leaf extract of *A. vera* showed immunomodulatory activity by significantly increasing the activation of T lymphocytes, monocytes and expression of CD25 & CD69 glycoproteins of NK cells in PBMCs (Ingles et al. 2017). *A. vera* gel ameliorates cyclophosphamide-induced immunotoxicity in rats by activating Peyer's patch cells to produce cytokines (Im et al. 2014). Acemannan from *A. vera* reduced mortality in irradiated Swiss albino mice by inducing haematopoiesis and upregulation of cytokines e.g. TNF-α and IL-1 (Kumar and Tiku 2016).	Polysaccharides: glucomannan and acemannan; carboxypeptidase, saponins, sterols, amino acids, anthraquinone, enzymes, glycosides: aloin, aloe-emodin, barbaloin (Reynolds & Dweck, 1999; Reynolds, 2004; Augustino et al. 2011)	Acute and sub-acute tests on Wistar rats using the methanol extract (16 g/kg bw) did not show significant toxic effect (Saritha and Anilkumar, 2010). The aqueous leaf extract is toxic (LD_{50} = 120.65 g/lkg bw) in Swiss albino mice (Lagarto et al. 2001) and induces toxic hepatitis (Lee et al. 2014).
3. *Allium cepa* L. Amaryllidaceae	Tuberculosis (TB) (Nguta et al. 2015), low immunity in HIV (Anywar et al. 2020b)	Onion fructo-oligosaccharides from *A. cepa* significantly increased the proliferation of mouse splenocytes/ thymocytes, enhanced the production of NO, intracellular free radicals and phagocytic activity in Wistar rats (Kumar et al. 2015).	Quercetin, phenolics (Prakash et al. 2007).	The crude extract is cytotoxic against tumoral Lucena multidrug-resistant (MDR) human erythroleukaemic and K562 cell lines (Votto et al. 2010). Excessive

(Continued)

TABLE 6.1 (CONTINUED)
Medicinal Plant Species Used in African Traditional Medicine for Strong immunomodulation

Scientific name and Family	Traditional Uses Related to Immune Disorders	Immunomodulatory Activity and Mode of Action	Phytochemical Composition	Toxicity /cytotoxicity
4. *Allium sativum* L. Amaryllidaceae	Infections (Koch and Lawson, 1996), cough, low immunity (Anywar et al. 2020a)	Garlic organo-sulphur compounds cause various immune responses (Schafer and Kaschula, 2014). Incubation of PBMCs with alliin produced a significant increase in spontaneous IL-1b production (Salman et al. 1999).	Diallyl thio-sulphinate (allicin), allyl methyl thiosulphinate, methyl allyl thiosulphinate, ajoene, alliin, deoxyalliin, diallyl disulphide and diallyl trisulphide (Weber et al. 1992).	Generally safe (Borrelli et al 2007) but can cause gastrointestinal discomfort, nausea, bloating, headache, dizziness, profuse sweating when excessively consumed (Rose et al. 1990; Beck and Grunwald 1993; Borrelli et al. 2007).
5. *Carica papaya* L. Caricaceae	Cough, low immunity (Tugume et al. 2016), skin infections (Anywar et al. 2020a).	The aqueous extract of *C. papaya* (150 mg/kg) caused an increase in thrombocytes, delayed-type hypersensitivity response, and mediated the release of platelets in rats (Anjum et al. 2017). The extract caused a reduction in the production of IL-2 and IL-4, and an increase in IL-12p40, IL-12p70, IFN-γ and TNF-α in PBMC (Otsuki et al. 2010).	Polysaccharides, glycosides, saponins, flavonoids and phytosterols (Saeed et al. 2014), myricetin, caffeic acid, *trans*-ferulic acid and kaempferol (Anjum et al. 2017)	Sub-acute oral toxicity tests of the leaf extracts in Sprague Dawley rats at 14 times the levels used in traditional medicine in Malaysia is safe (Afzan et al. 2012; Ismail et al. 2014).
6. *Cannabis sativa* L. Cannabaceae	TB, low/compromized immunity in HIV (Anywar et al. 2020a; 2020b).	Cannabinoids modulate immune responses during inflammatory processes *via* (i) cell proliferation, (ii) inhibition of pro-inflammatory cytokine/chemokine production, (iii) increase in anti-inflammatory cytokines, (iv) induction of regulatory T cells (Rieder et al. 2010) and (v) epigenetic regulation involving histone modifications (Yang et al. 2014).	Phytocannabinoids, e.g., delta8-tetrahydrocannabinol, cannabigerol, cannabinol (Russo 2011).	Frequent and prolonged use produces both mental and physical impairment, mood disorders, exacerbation of psychotic disorders in vulnerable people, cannabis use disorders, withdrawal syndrome, neurocognitive impairments, cardiovascular, and respiratory diseases (Smith, 1968; Karila et al. 2014).

TABLE 6.1 (CONTINUED)
Medicinal Plant Species Used in African Traditional Medicine for Strong immunomodulation

Scientific name and Family	Traditional Uses Related to Immune Disorders	Immunomodulatory Activity and Mode of Action	Phytochemical Composition	Toxicity /cytotoxicity
7. *Centella asiatica* (L.) Urb. Apiaceae	Dermatitis (Ssegawa and Kasenene 2007), skin infections, low/ compromized immunity in HIV (Anywar et al. 2020a; 2020b)	*C. asiatica* produced non-specific cellular and humoral immune responses in PBMCs, significantly increased proliferation and production of IL-2 and TNF-α and showed higher responses to both primary and secondary antibodies against Bovine Serum Albumin antibodies in BALB/c mice (Punturee et al. 2005).	Asiaticoside, asiatic and madecassic acids (Kwon et al. 2014). Tannins, essential oils, phytosterols, mucilages, resins, flavonoids, alkaloids (hydrochotine), vallerine, fatty acids (linoleic, linoleic, oleic, palmitic, and stearic acids) (Srivastava and Vaidya 1999)	The acetone extract was non-toxic in Swiss mice (LD$_{50}$ < 4000mg/ kg bw) (Chauhan and Singh 2012) and the crude extracts were non-toxic to normal human lymphocytes (Babu et al. 1995).
8. *Curcuma longa* L. Zingiberaceae	Low/compromized immunity in HIV (Anywar et al. 2020a)	Alpha-turmerone and aromatic-turmerone showed stimulatory effects on human PBMC proliferation & cytokine production (Yue et al. 2010).	Curcuminoids, e.g., curcumin, demethoxycurcumin, bisdemethoxycurcumin and α-turmerone (Yue et al. 2010; Ankur et al. 2015), fisetin, quercetin, and myricetin (Lako et al. 2007), α- and β-turmerone, α–santalene, aromatic-curcumene, oleoresins (Singh et al. 2010).	Powder/ alcoholic extract is not toxic at 10 g/kg bw (LD$_{50}$ > 15 g/kg bw) in Swiss albino mice (Sittisomwong et al. 1990) or guinea pigs and monkeys (300 mg/kg – 2.5 g/kg, respectively) (Shankar et al. 1980). The essential oil is safe up to 0.5 g/kg bw in Wistar rats and is not mutagenic/genotoxic when orally administered (Liju et al. 2013).

(Continued)

TABLE 6.1 (CONTINUED)
Medicinal Plant Species Used in African Traditional Medicine for Strong immunomodulation

Scientific name and Family	Traditional Uses Related to Immune Disorders	Immunomodulatory Activity and Mode of Action	Phytochemical Composition	Toxicity /cytotoxicity
9. *Jatropha curcas* L. Euphorbiaceae	Low/compromized immunity in HIV (Anywar et al. 2020ba)	An 80% aqueous methanol extract & some of its compounds, e.g., biapigenin, apigenin, orientin and vitexin stimulated both humoral and cell-mediated seroresponse in one-day-old specific pathogen-free chicks (Abd-Alla et al. 2009).	Jatrophalactone, jatrophalone, jatrophadiketone (Liu et al. 2012), curcusone B (Devappa, et al. 2011), curcin (Luo et al. 2007), phorbol esters (Li et al. 2010), biflavone di-*C*-glucoside, apigenin 7-*O*-β-D- galactoside, orientin, vitexin, vicenin and apigenin (Abd-Alla et al. 2009).	Known to be toxic and causes nausea, vomiting, and abdominal cramps (Joubert et al. 1984; Mampane et al. 1987). The purified phorbol esters from the oil are highly toxic to Swiss Hauschka mice (LD_{50} = 27.34 mg/kg bw (Li et al. 2010).
10. *Mangifera indica* L. Anacardiaceae	Skin infections, low/compromized immunity in HIV (Anywar et al. 2020a; 2020b)	Has immunomodulatory properties (Núñez-Sellés 2005). An extract with 2.6 % mangiferin caused an increase in humoral antibody titre and delayed type- hypersensitivity in mice (Makare et al. 2001). Vimang, an extract from *M. indica* containing mangiferin, a glucosylxanthone, modulates the activation and functionality of macrophages, through partial inhibition of chemotactic migration, phagocytic activity, ROS & RNS production (García et al. 2002).	Protocatechic acid, catechin, mangiferin, alanine, glycine, γ–aminobutyric acid (Scartezzini and Speroni 2000), triterpenoids and flavonoids.	Leaf extracts are non-toxic in ICR mice in acute and long-term toxicity studies up to 18.4g/kg bw (Zhang et al. 2014) and are not genotoxic or clastogenic *in vivo* (Reddeman et al. 2019).

(Continued)

TABLE 6.1 (CONTINUED)
Medicinal Plant Species Used in African Traditional Medicine for Strong immunomodulation

Scientific name and Family	Traditional Uses Related to Immune Disorders	Immunomodulatory Activity and Mode of Action	Phytochemical Composition	Toxicity /cytotoxicity
11. *Moringa oleifera* Lam Moringaceae	Low/compromized immunity in HIV (Anywar et al. 2020b)	The methanolic leaf extract caused an increase in WBC, lymphocyte and neutrophil counts at 1000 mg/kg bw comparable to levamisole, the standard drug (Nfambi et al. 2015). The ethanolic extract stimulates IgG, IgM and IgA production in Sprague Dawley male ratsand neutralized haematoimmune toxic hazards (Abd-Elhakim et al. 2018). *M. oleifera* seed lectin protein induced the release of TNF-α, IL-2, IL-6, IL-10 and NO, and achieved activation of CD8+ T lymphocytes in PBMCs, promoting immunomodulation (Coriolano et al. 2018). A 50% ethanolic leaf extract caused a significant increase in WBC, neutrophils, thymus, and spleen weight in normal and cyclophosphamide-immunosuppressed mice (Anamika et al. 2010).	Alkaloids, polyphenols, flavonoids, anthraquinones, coumarins, tannins, triterpenes, sterols, and saponins (Dzotam et al. 2016).	Leaves are genotoxic at supra-supplementation levels of 3000 mg/kg bw but are safe at $\leq$ 1000 mg/kg bw in rats (Asare et al. 2012), in male Wistar albino mice (LD_{50} = 1585 mg/kg) (Awodele et al. 2012) and in Swiss albino mice (LD_{50} = 17.8 g/kg) (Kasolo et al. 2011).

(Continued)

TABLE 6.1 (CONTINUED)
Medicinal Plant Species Used in African Traditional Medicine for Strong immunomodulation

Scientific name and Family	Traditional Uses Related to Immune Disorders	Immunomodulatory Activity and Mode of Action	Phytochemical Composition	Toxicity /cytotoxicity
12. *Pelargonium sidoides* DC. Geraniaceae	Respiratory tract infections, e.g., TB (Brendler and van Wyk, 2008)	EPs® 7630, an aqueous-ethanolic formulation of *P. sidoides* extracts, induced TNF and IF in activated bone marrow-derived macrophages (Kolodziej et al. 2003). Has significant immunomodulatory properties (Kolodziej and Kiderlen 2007)	Coumarins, simple phenolics, gallic acid and proanthocyanidins (Kolodziej and Kayser 1998).	No evident toxic effect in mice (Theisen and Muller 2012)
13. *Persea americana* Mill. Lauraceae	HIV/AIDS infections (Nyamukuru et al. 2017), TB (Anywar et al. 2020a).	An arabinogalactan-protein-rich fraction showed inhibitory effects on the complement system (Yamassaki et al. 2018).	Quercetin, rutin, luteolin, apigenin (Owolabi et al. 2010).	Seed (LD$_{50}$ > 10 g/kg) and leaf extracts (LD$_{50}$ > 10 g/kg) were not toxic in rats (Adeyemi et al. 2002; Ozoluaet al. 2009).
14. *Psidium guajava* L. Myrtaceae	Low/compromized immunity in HIV (Anywar et al. 2020b)	A fraction of guava seed polysaccharide (GSPS), GSF3, has potent immunomodulatory effects in female BALB/c mice against LPS-stimulated inflammation in macrophages *via* decreasing IL-6/IL-10 secretion ratio (Lin and Lin 2020)	Meroterpenoids (Qin et al. 2017).	The aqueous leaf extracts were not-toxic to rats/mice (LD$_{50}$ > 5 g/kg, p.o.) **at** 100 times the recommended dose for treatment of diarrhoea (Jaiarj et al. 1999).

(Continued)

TABLE 6.1 (CONTINUED)
Medicinal Plant Species Used in African Traditional Medicine for Strong immunomodulation

Scientific name and Family	Traditional Uses Related to Immune Disorders	Immunomodulatory Activity and Mode of Action	Phytochemical Composition	Toxicity /cytotoxicity
15. *Punica granatum* L. Lythraceae	Inflammation, infections (Cowan 1999; Braga et al. 2005), low/ compromized immunity in HIV (Anywar et al. 2020a)	The fruit rind powder stimulates cell-mediated and humoral components of the immune system in rabbits by provoking an increase in antibody titre to typhoid-H antigen and enhanced the inhibition of leucocyte migration (Gracious et al. 2001). A polysaccharide (PSP001) from *P. granatum* showed a stimulatory effect on the growth of isolated normal lymphocytes and haemagglutinating antibodies in Wistar male rats (Sin et al. 2019).	Phenolics (Rout & Banerjee 2007), gallotannins, ellagitannins, ellagic acid, and anthocyanins (Madrigal-Carballo et al. 2009).	The fruit extract was not toxic to the chick embryo model or at doses < 0.1 mg/g in either male or female OF-1 mice (LD_{50} = 731 mg/kg) i.p (Vidal et al. 2003).
16. *Sutherlandia frutescens* (L.) R.Br. Fabaceae	Cancers, infections, and inflammatory conditions insouthern Africa (Lei et al. 2016).	The crude aqueous extract or polysaccharide- enriched fraction of *S. frutescens* increased macrophage production of ROS and NO. *S. frutescens* activated NF-κB signalling in murine macrophages, resulting in an increased production of TNF-α (Lei et al. 2016).	Triterpenoids, saponins, flavonoids, c-aminobutyric acid, pinitol and L-canavanine (van Wyk & Albrecht, 2008).	Potentially toxic because of L-canavanine (Rosenthal 1977). However, no toxicity or side effects were observed at the maximal dose of 81 mg/kg in vervet monkeys (Fernandes et al. 2004).

(Continued)

TABLE 6.1 (CONTINUED)
Medicinal Plant Species Used in African Traditional Medicine for Strong immunomodulation

Scientific name and Family	Traditional Uses Related to Immune Disorders	Immunomodulatory Activity and Mode of Action	Phytochemical Composition	Toxicity /cytotoxicity
17. *Tamarindus indica* L. Fabaceae	Low/compromized immunity in HIV (Godwin Anywar et al. 2020b)	Galactoxyloglucan (PST001), isolated from seed kernel stimulates the immune system (Manu et al. 2016). Another polysaccharide exhibited immunomodulatory activity by enhancing phagocytic activity, inhibition of leukocyte migration, and cell proliferation (Sreelekha et al. 1993). The seed kernel extract increased total WBC, CD4+ T-cell population, and bone marrow cellularity (Manu et al. 2013; 2016).	Phenolics, proanthocyanidins, arabinose, triterpenes, apigenin, luteolin (Bhadoriya et al. 2012).	Generally safe with no signs of toxicity up to 2000 mg/kg/p.o (Martinello et al. 2006; Agnihotri & Singh, 2013; Martinello et al. 2017)
18. *Warburgia ugandensis* Sprague Canellaceae	TB and HIV/AIDS, low immunity (Nyamukuru et al. 2017; Anywar et al. 2020a; 2020b), cancer (Schultz et al. 2020).	Stimulated moderate production of IFN-γ and low levels of IL-4 in BALB/c mice (Ngure et al. 2014)	Ugandensolide, ugandensidial, muzigadial, polygodial, warburganal, cinnamolide, mukaadial, muzigadiolide (Kioy et al. 1990; Wube et al. 2005).	Extracts are safe to use (LD$_{50}$ > 5000 mg/kg bw) in BALB/c mice (Karani et al. 2013). Different extracts of *W. ugandensis* were non-cytotoxic to human keratinocyte cells (IC$_{50}$ > 512 μg/ml) (Schultz et al. 2020). Anywar et al. 2021 found the the DMSO (CC$_{50}$ = 1.5 μg/ml) and the ethanol (CC$_{50}$ = 7.6 μg/ml) root extracts were highly cytotoxic to U87CD4CXCR4 cells.

(Continued)

TABLE 6.1 (CONTINUED)
Medicinal Plant Species Used in African Traditional Medicine for Strong immunomodulation

Scientific name and Family	Traditional Uses Related to Immune Disorders	Immunomodulatory Activity and Mode of Action	Phytochemical Composition	Toxicity /cytotoxicity
Azadirachta indica A. *Juss.* Meliaceae	HIV/AIDS opportunistic ailments (Anywar et al. 2020a)	Neem extract leaf has immunoactivating activity in BALB/c-mice. It caused spleen and thymus enlargement (Beuth et al., 2006). The ethanol-aqueous extract of *A. indica* contains down-regulates chronic HIV associated CD4+ T cell activation/ exhaustion (Olweny et al., 2021).	triterpenes, flavonoids and saponins, limonoids, tannins, alkaloids, sterols and gallic acid catechins and nimbins (Cesa et al., 2019; Schumacher et al., 2011; van der Nat et al., 1991).	An aqueous extracts of *A. indica* leaves was not toxic in mice (LD_{50} < 2500 mg/kg) (Dorababu et al., 2006). Another study showed the LD_{50} values of neem oil to be 31.95 g/kg (Deng et al., 2013). The queous wood ash extract posses damaging effects on sperms and testicular tissues in male albino mice (Auta and Hassan, 2016). Different biochemical parameters of toxicity indicated that the aqueous stem bark has some oral toxicity at the doses of 50, 100, 200 and 300 mg/kg body weight in mice (Auta and Hassan, 2016).

Key: PBMCs = Peripheral Blood Mononuclear Cells; bw= body weight, NO = nitric oxide, WBC = White Blood Cells, i.p = Intraperitoneal, ROS = reactive oxygen species, RNS= Reactive Nitrogen Species

All the medicinal plant species recorded are either traditionally used to treat an immunity-related disorder, such as immunodeficiency, especially HIV/AIDS, or to treat symptoms associated with low immunity and cancer. All the plant species are also widely used across the continent and have been scientifically researched to confirm their immunomodulatory properties and modes of action. However, despite several other medicinal plant species being recorded as immune boosters in African traditional medicine, they have not been subjected to any scientific investigations to verify these claims (Nalumansi et al. 2016; Anywar et al. 2020b, 2020c). Unfortunately, even when some plant species have been scientifically shown to possess immunomodulatory properties, such as *Tamarindus indica,* they have generally not been fully exploited and are often underlitilised (Tugume et al. 2020).

6.5 COMMERCIAL FORMULATIONS OF AFRICAN MEDICINAL PLANTS FOR STRENGTHENING IMMUNITY

Different herbal formulations of African medicinal plants have been tested for improving immunity and approved by regulatory authorities in some countries. Such products are now commercially available in different countries. Two prominent examples from South Africa are a traditional energy tonic formulation and *uMakhonya®*.

A traditional South African energy tonic formulation of equal measures of six different medicinal plants (*Eriosema salignum* E. Mey., *Tragia meyeriana* Müll.Arg., *Gladiolus sericeovillosus* Hook.f., *Rapanea melanophloeos* (L.) Mez, *Grewia occidentalis* var. *occidentalis* L., and *Zanthoxylum capense* (Thunb.) Harv.) produced immunomodulatory effects on isolated immune cells and modulated the immune response of rat models infected with *Staphylococcus aureus*. It further stimulated secretion of cytokines and increased sIL-2R levels at doses of 10–100 µg/ml. It also caused an increase in Nuclear Factor Kappa Beta (*NF-κβ*) transcription in lipopolysaccharide-stimulated THP-1 cells with minimal cytotoxicity in mitogen- and peptidoglycan-stimulated PBMCs, with no significant toxicity at doses of up to 2000 mg/ml/kg of body weight (Ngcobo et al. 2017).

Another herbal immune booster from South Africa called *uMakhonya®*, containing *Artemisia afra* Jacq., menthol, guava (*P. guajava*), the seaweed *Chondrus crispus*, and *Uncaria tomentosa* induced a significant increase in secretion of chemokines in unstimulated THP-1 cells when compared with untreated or cyclosporine-treated cells at lower doses. The lowest dose of *uMakhonya®* increased transcriptional activity of the NF-κβ gene in both unstimulated and lipopolysaccharide-stimulated THP-1 cells. This may explain the increase in chemokines secretion observed. However, *uMakhonya®* significantly induces dose-dependent cytotoxicity with high-dose cytotoxicity to monocytes (half maximal inhibitory concentration, IC_{50} = 100.08 and 107.68 µg/ml for normal and LPS- stimulated THP-1 cells, respectively((Ngcobo et al. 2016).

6.6 CONCLUSION

Medicinal plant species with proven immunomodulating properties have great potential in treating cancer patients or people with low or compromized immune systems, without having to resort to expensive and sometimes toxic conventional medicines. Such medicinal plants have the potential to be developed into modern drugs or improved herbal medicine products, as has been demonstrated with individual medicinal plant species, such as *P. sidoides,* in polyherbal formulations, especially in poor African nations.

REFERENCES

Abbas, A.K., Lichtman, A.H., & Pillai, S. (2019). *Basic Immunology E-Book: Functions and Disorders of the Immune System.* Elsevier Health Sciences.

Abd-Alla, H.I., Moharram, F.A., Gaara, A.H., & El-Safty, M.M. (2009). Phytoconstituents of *Jatropha curcas* L. leaves and their immunomodulatory activity on humoral and cell-mediated immune response in chicks. *Zeitschrift Für Naturforschung C, 64*(7–8), 495–501.

Abd-Elhakim, Y.M., El Bohi, K.M., Hassan, S.K., El Sayed, S., & Abd-Elmotal, S.M. (2018). Palliative effects of Moringa olifera ethanolic extract on hemato-immunologic impacts of melamine in rats. *Food and Chemical Toxicology, 114*, 1–10. https://doi.org/10.1016/j.fct.2018.02.020

Adeyemi, O.O., Okpo, S.O., & Ogunti, O.O. (2002). Analgesic and anti-inflammatory effects of the aqueous extract of leaves of *Persea americana* mill (Lauraceae). *Fitoterapia, 73*(5), 375–380.

Afzan, A., Abdullah, N.R., Halim, S.Z., Rashid, B.A., Semail, R.H.R., Abdullah, N., ... Ismail, Z. (2012). Repeated dose 28-days oral toxicity study of *Carica papaya* L. leaf extract in Sprague Dawley rats. *Molecules, 17*(4), 4326–4342.

Agnihotri, A., & Singh, V. (2013). Effect of *Tamarindus indica* Linn. and *Cassia fistula* Linn. stem bark extracts on oxidative stress and diabetic conditions. *Acta Pol Pharm, 70*(6), 1011–1019.

Anjum, V., Arora, P., Ansari, S.H., Najmi, A.K., & Ahmad, S. (2017). Antithrombocytopenic and immunomodulatory potential of metabolically characterized aqueous extract of Carica papaya leaves. *Pharmaceutical Biology, 55*(1), 2043–2056. https://doi.org/10.1080/13880209.2017.1346690

Anywar, Godwin, Kakudidi, E., Byamukama, R., Mukonzo, J., Schubert, A., & Oryem-Origa, H. (2020a). Medicinal plants used by traditional medicine practitioners to boost the immune system in people living with HIV/AIDS in Uganda. *European Journal of Integrative Medicine, 35*, 101011. https://doi.org/10.1016/j.eujim.2019.101011

Anywar, G., Kakudidi, E., Byamukama, R., Mukonzo, J., Schubert, A., & Oryem-Origa, H. (2020b). Indigenous traditional knowledge of medicinal plants used by herbalists in treating opportunistic infections among people living with HIV/AIDS in Uganda. *Journal of Ethnopharmacology, 246*, 112205. https://doi.org/https://doi.org/10.1016/j.jep.2019.112205

Anywar, G., Kakudidi, E., Byamukama, R., Mukonzo, J., Schubert, A., & Oryem-Origa, H. (2020c). Data on medicinal plants used by herbalists for boosting immunity in people living with HIV/AIDS in Uganda. *Data in Brief*, 105097. https://doi.org/https://doi.org/10.1016/j.dib.2019.105097

Anywar, G., Kakudidi,KK., Byamukama, R., Mukonzo, JK., Schubert, A., Oryem-Origa, H., & Jassoy, C. (2021). A review of the toxicity and phytochemistry of medicinal plant species used by herbalists in treating people living with HIV/AIDS in Uganda. *Frontiers in Pharmacology, 12*, 435. http://doi.org/10.3389/fphar.2021.615147

Arthanari, S., Vanitha, J., Krishnaswami, V., Renukadevi, P., Deivasigamani, K., & De Clercq, E. (2013). *In vitro* antiviral and cytotoxic screening of methanolic extract of *Cassia auriculata* flowers in HeLa, Vero, CRFK and HEL cell lines. *Drug Invention Today, 5*(1), 28–31. https://doi.org/http://dx.doi.org/10.1016/j.dit.2013.03.001

Asare, G.A., Gyan, B., Bugyei, K., Adjei, S., Mahama, R., Addo, P., ... Nyarko, A. (2012). Toxicity potentials of the nutraceutical Moringa oleifera at supra-supplementation levels. *Journal of Ethnopharmacology, 139*(1), 265–272.

Augustino, S., Hall, J.B., Makonda, F.B.S., & Ishengoma, R.C. (2011). Medicinal resources of the Miombo woodlands of Urumwa, Tanzania: plants and its uses. *Journal of Medicinal Plants Research, 5*(27), 6352–6372.

Auta, T., & Hassan, A.T. (2016). Reproductive toxicity of aqueous wood-ash extract of Azadirachta indica (neem) on male albino mice. *Asian Pacific Journal of Reproduction, 5*, 111–115. https://doi.org/10.1016/j.apjr.2016.01.005.

Awodele, O., Oreagba, I.A., Odoma, S., da Silva, J.A.T., & Osunkalu, V.O. (2012). Toxicological evaluation of the aqueous leaf extract of *Moringa oleifera* Lam.(Moringaceae). *Journal of Ethnopharmacology, 139*(2), 330–336.

Babu, T.D., Kuttan, G., & Padikkala, J. (1995). Cytotoxic and anti-tumour properties of certain taxa of Umbelliferae with special reference to *Centella asiatica* (L.) Urban. *Journal of Ethnopharmacology, 48*(1), 53–57. https://doi.org/https://doi.org/10.1016/0378-8741(95)01284-K

Beck, E., & Grunwald, J. (1993). Allium sativum in der stufentherapie der hyperlipidamie: studie mit 1997 patienten belegt wirksamkeit und vertraglichkeit. *Medizinische Welt, 44*(8), 516–520.

Beuscher, N., Bodinet, C., Neumann-Haefelin, D., Marston, A., & Hostettmann, K. (1994). Antiviral activity of African medicinal plants. Journal of Ethnopharmacology, *42*(2), 101–109.

Beuth, J., Schneider, H., & Ko, H.L. (2006). Enhancement of immune responses to neem leaf extract (*Azadirachta indica*) correlates with antineoplastic activity in BALB/c-mice. *In Vivo, 20*, 247–251.

Bhadoriya, S.S., Mishra, V., Raut, S., Ganeshpurkar, A., & Jain, S.K. (2012). Anti-inflammatory and antinociceptive activities of a hydroethanolic extract of *Tamarindus indica* Leaves. Scientia pharmaceutica, *80*(3), 685–700. https://doi.org/10.3797/scipharm.1110-09

Borrelli, F., Capasso, R., & Izzo, A.A. (2007). Garlic (*Allium sativum* L.): adverse effects and drug interactions in humans. *Molecular Nutrition & Food Research, 51*(11), 1386–1397. https://doi.org/10.1002/mnfr.200700072

Bradley, J.R. (2008). TNF-mediated inflammatory disease. *The Journal of Pathology, 214*(2), 149–160. https://doi.org/10.1002/path.2287

Braga, L.C., Shupp, J.W., Cummings, C., Jett, M., Takahashi, J.A., Carmo, L.S., ... Nascimento, A.M. (2005). Pomegranate extract inhibits *Staphylococcus aureus* growth and subsequent enterotoxin production. *Journal of Ethnopharmacology, 96*(1–2), 335–339. https://doi.org/10.1016/j.jep.2004.08.034

Brendler, T., & van Wyk, B.-E. (2008). A historical, scientific and commercial perspective on the medicinal use of *Pelargonium sidoides* (Geraniaceae). *Journal of Ethnopharmacology, 119*(3), 420–433. https://doi.org/https://doi.org/10.1016/j.jep.2008.07.037

Cesa, S., Sisto, F., Zengin, G., Scaccabarozzi, D., Kokolakis, A.K., Scaltrito, M.M., Grande, R., Locatelli, M., Cacciagrano, F., & Angiolella, L. (2019). Phytochemical analyses and pharmacological screening of Neem oil. *South African ournal of Botany, 120*, 331–337.

Chatterjee, R.K., Fatma, N., Jain, R.K., Gupta, C.M., & Anand, N. (1988). Litomosoides carinii in rodents: immunomodulation in potentiating action of diethylcarbamazine. *The Japanese Journal of Experimental Medicine, 58*(6), 243–248.

Chauhan, P.K., & Singh, V. (2012). Acute and Subacute Toxicity study of the Acetone Leaf extract of *Centella asiatica* in Experimental Animal Models. *Asian Pacific Journal of Tropical Biomedicine, 2*(2, Supplement), S511–S513. https://doi.org/https://doi.org/10.1016/S2221-1691(12)60263-9

Coriolano, M.C., de Santana Brito, J., de Siqueira Patriota, L.L., de Araujo Soares, A.K., de Lorena, V., Paiva, P.M.G., … de Melo, C.M.L. (2018). Immunomodulatory effects of the water-soluble lectin from *Moringa oleifera* seeds (WSMoL) on human peripheral blood mononuclear cells (PBMC). *Protein and Peptide Letters*, *25*(3), 295–301.

Cowan, M.M. (1999). Plant products as antimicrobial agents. Clinical Microbiology Reviews, *12*(4), 564–582.

Dembic, Z. (2015). *The Cytokines of the Immune System: The Role of Cytokines in Disease Related to Immune Response*. Academic Press.

Deng, Y., Cao, M., Shi, D., Yin, Z., Jia, R., Xu, J., Wang, C., Lv, C., Liang, X., He, C., Yang, Z., & Zhao, J. (2013). Toxicological evaluation of neem (*Azadirachta indica*) oil: Acute and subacute toxicity. *Environmental Toxicology and Pharmacology*, *35*, 240–246. https://doi.org/10.1016/j.etap.2012.12.015.

Devappa, R.K., Makkar, H.P.S., & Becker, K. (2011). Jatropha diterpenes: a review. *Journal of the American Oil Chemists' Society*, *88*(3), 301–322. https://doi.org/doi:10.1007/s11746-010-1720-9

Dorababu, M., Joshi, M.C., Bhawani, G., Kumar, M.M., Chaturvedi, A., & Goel, R.K. (2006). Effect of aqueous extract of neem (*Azadirachta indica*) leaves on offensive and diffensive gastric mucosal factors in rats. *Indian Journal of Physiology and Pharmacology*, *50*, 241–249.

Dzotam, J.K., Touani, F.K., & Kuete, V. (2016). Antibacterial and antibiotic-modifying activities of three food plants (*Xanthosoma mafaffa* Lam., *Moringa oleifera* (L.) Schott and *Passiflora edulis* Sims) against multidrug-resistant (MDR) Gram-negative bacteria. BMC complementary and Alternative Medicine, *16*. https://doi.org/10.1186/s12906-016-0990-7

El-Ashmawy, N.E., El-Zamarany, E.A., Salem, M.L., El-Bahrawy, H.A., & Al-Ashmawy, G.M. (2015). In vitro and in vivo studies of the immunomodulatory effect of Echinacea purpurea on dendritic cells. *Journal of Genetic Engineering and Biotechnology*, *13*(2), 185–192. https://doi.org/http://dx.doi.org/10.1016/j.jgeb.2015.05.002

Fernandes, A.C., Cromarty, A.D., Albrecht, C., & van Rensburg, C.E. (2004). The antioxidant potential of *Sutherlandia frutescens*. *Journal of Ethnopharmacology*, *95*. https://doi.org/10.1016/j.jep.2004.05.024

Fernandez, T., Cerda Zolezzi, P., Risco, E., Martino, V., Lopez, P., Clavin, M., … Alvarez, E. (2002). Immunomodulating properties of Argentine plants with ethnomedicinal use. *Phytomedicine*, *9*(6), 546–552. https://doi.org/10.1078/09447110260573182

García, D., Delgado, R., Ubeira, F.M., & Leiro, J. (2002). Modulation of rat macrophage function by the *Mangifera indica* L. extracts Vimang and mangiferin. *International Immunopharmacology*, *2*(6), 797–806. https://doi.org/https://doi.org/10.1016/S1567-5769(02)00018-8

Gea-Banacloche, J.C. (2006). Immunomodulation. In *Principles of Molecular Medicine* (pp. 893–904). Springer.

Gertsch, J., Viveros-Paredes, J.M., & Taylor, P. (2011). Plant immunostimulants—Scientific paradigm or myth? *Journal of Ethnopharmacology*, *136*(3), 385–391. https://doi.org/http://dx.doi.org/10.1016/j.jep.2010.06.044

Gracious Ross, R., Selvasubramanian, S., & Jayasundar, S. (2001). Immunomodulatory activity of *Punica granatum* in rabbits—a preliminary study. *Journal of Ethnopharmacology*, *78*(1), 85–87. https://doi.org/https://doi.org/10.1016/S0378-8741(01)00287-2

Gupta, Anamika, Gautam, M.K., Singh, R.K., Kumar, M.V., Rao, C.V., Goel, R.K., & Anupurba, S. (2010). *Immunomodulatory effect of Moringa oleifera Lam. extract on cyclophosphamide induced toxicity in mice.*

Gupta, Ankur, Mahajan, S., & Sharma, R. (2015). Evaluation of antimicrobial activity of Curcuma longa rhizome extract against *Staphylococcus aureus*. *Biotechnology Reports*, *6*, 51–55. https://doi.org/https://doi.org/10.1016/j.btre.2015.02.001

Hasson, S.S., Al Manthari, A.A., Idris, M.A., Al-Busaidi, J.Z., Al-Balushi, M.S., & Aleemallah, G.M. (2019). Immunomodulatory potential of combining some traditional medicinal plants in vivo. *Ann Microbiol Immunol. 2*(1), 1014.

Im, S.A., Kim, K.H., Kim, H.S., Lee, K.H., Shin, E., Do, S.G., … Lee, C.K. (2014). Processed *Aloe vera* gel ameliorates cyclophosphamide-induced immunotoxicity. International Journal of Molecular Sciences, *15*(11), 19342–19354. https://doi.org/10.3390/ijms1511 19342

Ingles, C., Benson, K.F., Jensen, G.S., Smillie, T., & Tornadu, I.G. (2017). Antioxidant and immune-modulatory effects of *Aloe vera* decolorized leaf juice vs. inner leaf juice. *The FASEB Journal, 31*(S1), lb400–lb400. https://doi.org/10.1096/fasebj.31.1_supplement. lb400

Ismail, Z., Halim, S.Z., Abdullah, N.R., Afzan, A., Rashid, A., Amini, B., & Jantan, I. (2014). Safety evaluation of oral toxicity of *Carica papaya* Linn. leaves: a subchronic toxicity study in sprague dawley rats. *Evidence-Based Complementary and Alternative Medicine, 2014.*

Jaiarj, P., Khoohaswan, P., Wongkrajang, Y., Peungvicha, P., Suriyawong, P., Saraya, M.L.S., & Ruangsomboon, O. (1999). Anticough and antimicrobial activities of *Psidium guajava* Linn. leaf extract. *Journal of Ethnopharmacology, 67*(2), 203–212.

Jantan, I., Ahmad, W., & Bukhari, S.N.A. (2015). Plant-derived immunomodulators: an insight on their preclinical evaluation and clinical trials. *Frontiers in Plant Science, 6.* https://doi.org/10.3389/fpls.2015.00655

Joubert, P.H., Brown, J.M., Hay, I.T., & Sebata, P.D. (1984). Acute poisoning with *Jatropha curcas* (purging nut tree) in children. *South African Medical Journal= Suid-Afrikaanse Tydskrif Vir Geneeskunde, 65*(18), 729–730.

Kak, G., Raza, M., & Tiwari, B.K. (2018). Interferon-gamma (IFN-γ): exploring its implications in infectious diseases. *Biomolecular Concepts, 9*(1), 64–79.

Karani, L.W., Tolo, F.M., Karanja, S.M., & Khayeka–Wandabwa, C. (2013). Safety of Prunus africana and Warburgia ugandensis in asthma treatment. *South African Journal of Botany, 88*, 183–190. https://doi.org/https://doi.org/10.1016/j.sajb.2013.07.007

Karila, L., Roux, P., Rolland, B., Benyamina, A., Reynaud, M., Aubin, H.-J., & Lancon, C. (2014). Acute and long-term effects of cannabis use: a review. *Current Pharmaceutical Design, 20*(25), 4112–4118.

Karunai Raj, M., Balachandran, C., Duraipandiyan, V., Agastian, P., & Ignacimuthu, S. (2012). Antimicrobial activity of Ulopterol isolated from *Toddalia asiatica* (L.) Lam.: a traditional medicinal plant. *Journal of Ethnopharmacology, 140*(1), 161–165. https://doi.org/http://dx.doi.org/10.1016/j.jep.2012.01.005

Kasolo, J.N., Bimenya, G.S., Ojok, L., & Ogwal-Okeng, J.W. (2011). Phytochemicals and acute toxicity of *Moringa oleifera* roots in mice. *Journal of Pharmacognosy and Phytotherapy, 3*(3), 38–42.

Kioy, D., Gray, A.I., & Waterman, P.G. (1990). A comparative study of the stem-bark drimane sesquiterpenes and leaf volatile oils of *Warburgia ugandensis and W. Stuhlmannii. Phytochemistry, 29*(11), 3535–3538. https://doi.org/https://doi.org/10.1016/0031-9422 (90)85270-P

Koch, H.P., & Lawson, L.D. (1996). *Garlic: The Science and Therapeutic Application of Allium sativum L. and Related Species.* Lippincott Williams & Wilkins.

Kolodziej, H, & Kayser, O. (1998). *Pelargonium sidoides* DC. Zeitschrift Fur Phytotherapie, *19*, 141–151.

Kolodziej, Herbert, Kayser, O., Radtke, O.A., Kiderlen, A.F., & Koch, E. (2003). Pharmacological profile of extracts of *Pelargonium sidoides* and their constituents. *Phytomedicine, 10* Supplement 4, 18–24. https://doi.org/https://doi.org/10.1078/1433-187X-00307

Kolodziej, Herbert, & Kiderlen, A.F. (2007). In vitro evaluation of antibacterial and immuno-modulatory activities of Pelargonium reniforme, *Pelargonium sidoides* and the related herbal drug preparation EPs® 7630. *Phytomedicine, 14,* 18–26.

Koo, S., Marty, F.M., & Baden, L.R. (2010). Infectious complications associated with immunomodulating biologic agents. *Infectious Disease Clinics of North America, 24*(2), 285–306. https://doi.org/http://dx.doi.org/10.1016/j.idc.2010.01.006

Kumar, G., Karthik, L., & Rao, K.V.B. (2013). Phytochemical composition and *in vitro* antioxidant activity of aqueous extract of *Aerva lanata* (L.) Juss. ex Schult. Stem (Amaranthaceae). *Asian Pacific Journal of Tropical Medicine, 6*(3), 180–187. https://doi.org/https://doi.org/10.1016/S1995-7645(13)60020-6

Kumar, S., & Tiku, A.B. (2016). Immunomodulatory potential of acemannan (polysaccharide from Aloe vera) against radiation induced mortality in Swiss albino mice. *Food and Agricultural Immunology, 27*(1), 72–86. https://doi.org/10.1080/09540105.2015.1079594

Kumar, S.V., Kumar, S.P., Rupesh, D., & Nitin, K. (2011). Immunomodulatory effects of some traditional medicinal plants. *J Chem Pharm Res, 3*(1), 675–684.

Kumar, V.P., Prashanth, K.V.H., & Venkatesh, Y.P. (2015). Structural analyses and immunomodulatory properties of fructo-oligosaccharides from onion (*Allium cepa*). *Carbohydrate Polymers, 117,* 115–122. https://doi.org/https://doi.org/10.1016/j.carbpol.2014.09.039

Kuwabara, T., Ishikawa, F., Kondo, M., & Kakiuchi, T. (2017). The Role of IL-17 and Related Cytokines in Inflammatory Autoimmune Diseases. *Mediators of Inflammation, 2017,* 3908061. https://doi.org/10.1155/2017/3908061

Kwon, K.J., Bae, S., Kim, K., An, I.S., Ahn, K.J., An, S., & Cha, H.J. (2014). Asiaticoside, a component of *Centella asiatica*, inhibits melanogenesis in B16F10 mouse melanoma. *Molecular Medicine Reports, 10*(1), 503–507.

Lagarto Parra, A., Silva Yhebra, R., Guerra Sardiñas, I., & Iglesias Buela, L. (2001). Comparative study of the assay of *Artemia salina* L. and the estimate of the medium lethal dose (LD50 value) in mice, to determine oral acute toxicity of plant extracts. *Phytomedicine, 8*(5), 395–400. https://doi.org/https://doi.org/10.1078/0944-7113-00044

Lako, J., Trenerry, V.C., Wahlqvist, M., Wattanapenpaiboon, N., Sotheeswaran, S., & Premier, R. (2007). Phytochemical flavonols, carotenoids and the antioxidant properties of a wide selection of Fijian fruit, vegetables and other readily available foods. *Food Chemistry, 101*(4), 1727–1741. https://doi.org/https://doi.org/10.1016/j.foodchem.2006.01.031

Lee, J., Lee, M.S., & Nam, K.W. (2014). Acute toxic hepatitis caused by an aloe vera preparation in a young patient: a case report with a literature review. *The Korean Journal of Gastroenterology, 64*(1), 54–58.

Lei, W., Browning Jr., J.D., Eichen, P.A., Folk, W.R., Sun, G.Y., Lubahn, D.B., & Fritsche, K.L. (2016). An Investigation into the Immunomodulatory Activities of Sutherlandia frutescens in Healthy Mice. *PLOS ONE, 11*(8), e0160994. Retrieved from https://doi.org/10.1371/journal.pone.0160994

Leroux-Roels, G. (2010). Unmet needs in modern vaccinology: Adjuvants to improve the immune response. *Vaccine, 28* Supplement 3, Supple, C25–C36. https://doi.org/http://dx.doi.org/10.1016/j.vaccine.2010.07.021

Li, C.-Y., Devappa, R.K., Liu, J.-X., Lv, J.-M., Makkar, H.P.S., & Becker, K. (2010). Toxicity of *Jatropha curcas* phorbol esters in mice. *Food and Chemical Toxicology, 48*(2), 620–625.

Liju, V.B., Jeena, K., & Kuttan, R. (2013). Acute and subchronic toxicity as well as mutagenic evaluation of essential oil from turmeric (*Curcuma longa* L). *Food and Chemical Toxicology, 53,* 52–61.

Lin, H.-C., & Lin, J.-Y. (2020). Characterization of guava (*Psidium guajava* Linn) seed poly-saccharides with an immunomodulatory activity. *International Journal of Biological Macromolecules*, *154*, 511–520. https://doi.org/https://doi.org/10.1016/j.ijbiomac.2020.03.137

Liu, J.-Q., Yang, Y.-F., Wang, C.-F., Li, Y., & Qiu, M.-H. (2012). Three new diterpenes from *Jatropha curcas*. *Tetrahedron*, *68*(4), 972–976. https://doi.org/https://doi.org/10.1016/j.tet.2011.12.006

Lotter-Stark, H.C.T., Rybicki, E.P., & Chikwamba, R.K. (2012). Plant made anti-HIV micro-bicides—A field of opportunity. *Biotechnology Advances*, *30*(6), 1614–1626. https://doi.org/http://dx.doi.org/10.1016/j.biotechadv.2012.06.002

Luo, M.J., Liu, W.X., Yang, X.Y., Xu, Y., Yan, F., Huang, P., & Chen, F. (2007). Cloning, expression, and antitumor activity of recombinant protein of curcin. *Russian Journal of Plant Physiology*, *54*(2), 202–206. https://doi.org/10.1134/s1021443707020070

Madrigal-Carballo, S., Rodriguez, G., Krueger, C.G., Dreher, M., & Reed, J.D. (2009). Pomegranate (Punica granatum) supplements: Authenticity, antioxidant and polyphenol composition. *Journal of Functional Foods*, *1*(3), 324–329. https://doi.org/https://doi.org/10.1016/j.jff.2009.02.005

Makare, N., Bodhankar, S., & Rangari, V. (2001). Immunomodulatory activity of alcoholic extract of Mangifera indica L. in mice. *Journal of Ethnopharmacology*, *78*(2), 133–137. https://doi.org/https://doi.org/10.1016/S0378-8741(01)00326-9

Mampane, K.J., Joubert, P.H., & Hay, I.T. (1987). *Jatropha curcas*: use as a traditional Tswana medicine and its role as a cause of acute poisoning. *Phytotherapy Research*, *1*(1), 50–51.

Manu, Joseph, M., Aravind, S.R., Varghese, S., Mini, S., & Sreelekha, T.T. (2013). PST-Gold nanoparticle as an effective anticancer agent with immunomodulatory properties. *Colloids and Surfaces. B, Biointerfaces*, *104*, 32–39. https://doi.org/10.1016/j.colsurfb.2012.11.046

Manu, J.M., Aravind R., S., Varghese, S., Mini, S., & Sreelekha T., T. (2012). Evaluation of antioxidant, antitumor and immunomodulatory properties of polysaccharide iso-lated from fruit rind of Punica granatum. Molecular Medicine Reports, 5(2), 489–496. https://doi.org/10.3892/mmr.2011.638

Manu, J.M., Aswathy, G., Manojkumar, T.K., & Sreelekha, T.T. (2016). Galactoxyloglucan-doxorubicin nanoparticles exerts superior cytotoxic effects on cancer cells-A mecha-nistic and in silico approach. *International Journal of Biological Macromolecules*, *92*, 20–29. https://doi.org/10.1016/j.ijbiomac.2016.06.093

Martinello, F., Kannen, V., Franco, J.J., Gasparotto, B., Sakita, J.Y., Sugohara, A., ... Uyemura, S.A. (2017). Chemopreventive effects of a *Tamarindus indica* fruit extract against colon carcinogenesis depends on the dietary cholesterol levels in hamsters. Food and Chemical Toxicology, *107*(Pt A), 261–269. https://doi.org/10.1016/j.fct.2017.07.005

Martinello, F., Soares, S.M., Franco, J.J., Santos, A.C. dos, Sugohara, A., Garcia, S.B., ... Uyemura, S.A. (2006). Hypolipemic and antioxidant activities from *Tamarindus indica* L. pulp fruit extract in hypercholesterolemic hamsters. *Food and Chemical Toxicology*, *44*(6), 810–818.

Mukherjee, K., Biswas, R., Chaudhary, S.K., & Mukherjee, P.K. (2015). Chapter 18 - Botanicals as Medicinal Food and Their Effects against Obesity. In P.K. Mukherjee (Ed.), *Evidence-Based Validation of Herbal Medicine* (pp. 373–403). https://doi.org/https://doi.org/10.1016/B978-0-12-800874-4.00018-0

Mukherjee, P.K., Nema, N.K., Bhadra, S., Mukherjee, D., Braga, F.C., & Matsabisa, M.G. (2014). *Immunomodulatory leads from medicinal plants.*

Murphy, K., & Weaver, C. (2016). *Janeway's Immunobiology.* Garland science.

Nalumansi, P., Kamatenesi-Mugisha, M., & Anywar, G. (2016). Medicinal Plants Used in Paediatric Health Care in Namungalwe Sub County, Iganga District, Uganda, 3(2). https://doi.org/10.20286/nova-jmbs-030234

Nevin, K.G., & Vijayammal, P.L. (2005). Pharmacological and Immunomodulatory Effects of Aerva lanata. in Daltons Lymphoma Ascites–Bearing Mice. Pharmaceutical Biology, 43(7), 640–646. https://doi.org/10.1080/13880200500303858

Nfambi, J., Bbosa, G.S., Sembajwe, L.F., Gakunga, J., & Kasolo, J.N. (2015). Immunomodulatory activity of methanolic leaf extract of Moringa oleifera in Wistar albino rats. Journal of Basic and Clinical Physiology and Pharmacology, 26(6), 603–611. https://doi.org/10.1515/jbcpp-2014-0104

Ngcobo, M, Gqaleni, N., Ndlovu, V., Serumula, M., & Sibiya, N. (2016). Immunomodulatory effects of Umakhonya®: a South African commercial traditional immune booster. South African Journal of Botany, 102, 26–32. https://doi.org/https://doi.org/10.1016/j.sajb.2015.07.014

Ngcobo, Mlungisi, Gqaleni, N., Naidoo, V., & Cele, P. (2017). The immune effects of an african traditional energy tonic in in vitro and in vivo models. Evidence-Based Complementary and Alternative Medicine : ECAM, 2017, 6310967. https://doi.org/10.1155/2017/6310967

Ngure, P., Ng'ang'a, Z., Kimutai, A., Kepha, S., Mong'are, S., Ingonga, J., & Tonui, W. (2014). Immunostimulatory responses to crude extracts of Warburgia ugandensis (Sprague) subsp ugandensis (Canellaceae) by BALB/c mice infected with Leishmania major. The Pan African Medical Journal, 17 Suppl 1, 15. https://doi.org/10.11694/pamj.supp.2014.17.1.3638

Nguta, J.M., Appiah-Opong, R., Nyarko, A.K., Yeboah-Manu, D., & Addo, P.G.A. (2015). Medicinal plants used to treat TB in Ghana. International Journal of Mycobacteriology, 4(2), 116–123. https://doi.org/https://doi.org/10.1016/j.ijmyco.2015.02.003

Núñez-Sellés, A.J. (2005). Antioxidant therapy: myth or reality? Journal of the Brazilian Chemical Society, 16, 699–710. Retrieved from http://www.scielo.br/scielo.php?script=sci_arttext&pid=S0103-50532005000500004&nrm=iso

Nyamukuru, A., Tabuti, J.R.S., Lamorde, M., Kato, B., Sekagya, Y., & Aduma, P.R. (2017). Medicinal plants and traditional treatment practices used in the management of HIV/AIDS clients in Mpigi District, Uganda. Journal of Herbal Medicine, 7, 51–58. https://doi.org/https://doi.org/10.1016/j.hermed.2016.10.001

Olwenyi, O.A., Asingura, B., Naluyima, P., Anywar, G.U., Nalunga, J., Nakabuye, M., Semwogerere, M., Bagaya, B., Cham, F., Tindikahwa, A., Kiweewa, F., Lichter, E.Z., Podany, A.T., Fletcher, C.V., Byrareddy, S.N., & Kibuuka, H. (2021). In-vitro immunomodulatory activity of Azadirachta indica A. Juss. Ethanol: Water mixture against HIV associated chronic CD4+ T-cell activation/exhaustion. BMC Complementary Medicine and Therapies, 21(1), 114. https://doi.org/10.1186/s12906-021-03288-0

Omotoso, K.S., Aigbe, F.R., Salako, O.A., Chijioke, M.C., & Adeyemi, O.O. (2017). Toxicological evaluation of the aqueous whole plant extract of Aerva lanata (l.) Juss. ex Schult (Amaranthaceae). Journal of Ethnopharmacology, 208, 174–184. https://doi.org/https://doi.org/10.1016/j.jep.2017.06.032

Oršolić, N., & Bašić, I. (2003). Immunomodulation by water-soluble derivative of propolis: a factor of antitumor reactivity. Journal of Ethnopharmacology, 84(2–3), 265–273. https://doi.org/http://dx.doi.org/10.1016/S0378-8741(02)00329-X

Otsuki, N., Dang, N.H., Kumagai, E., Kondo, A., Iwata, S., & Morimoto, C. (2010). Aqueous extract of Carica papaya leaves exhibits anti-tumor activity and immunomodulatory effects. Journal of Ethnopharmacology, 127(3), 760–767. https://doi.org/https://doi.org/10.1016/j.jep.2009.11.024

Owolabi, M.A., Coker, H.A.B., & Jaja, S.I. (2010). Bioactivity of the phytoconstituents of the leaves of *Persea americana*. *Journal of Medicinal Plants Research, 4*(12), 1130–1135.

Ozolua, R.I., Anaka, O.N., Okpo, S.O., & Idogun, S.E. (2009). Acute and sub-acute toxicological assessment of the aqueous seed extract of *Persea americana* Mill (Lauraceae) in rats. African Journal of Traditional, Complementary and Alternative Medicines, 6.

Pfeffer, K. (2003). Biological functions of tumor necrosis factor cytokines and their receptors. *Cytokine & Growth Factor Reviews, 14*(3), 185–191. https://doi.org/https://doi.org/10.1016/S1359-6101(03)00022-4

Prakash, D., Singh, B.N., & Upadhyay, G. (2007). Antioxidant and free radical scavenging activities of phenols from onion (*Allium cepa*). *Food Chemistry, 102*(4), 1389–1393. https://doi.org/https://doi.org/10.1016/j.foodchem.2006.06.063

Prendergast, G.C., & Jaffee, E.M. (2007). Cancer immunologists and cancer biologists: why we didn't talk then but need to now. Cancer Research, 67(8), 3500–3504. https://doi.org/10.1158/0008-5472.can-06-4626

Punturee, K., Wild, C.P., Kasinrerk, W., & Vinitketkumnuen, U. (2005). Immunomodulatory activities of *Centella asiatica* and *Rhinacanthus nasutus* extracts. Asian Pacific Journal of Cancer Prevention, 6(3), 396–400.

Puri, A, Saxena, R., Saxena, R.P., Saxena, K.C., Srivastava, V., & Tandon, J.S. (1994). Immunostimulant activity of Nyctanthes arbor-tristis L. *Journal of Ethnopharmacology, 42*(1), 31–37. https://doi.org/10.1016/0378-8741(94)90020-5

Puri, A, Sahai, R., Singh, K.L., Saxena, R.P., Tandon, J.S., & Saxena, K.C. (2000). Immunostimulant activity of dry fruits and plant materials used in Indian traditional medical system for mothers after child birth and invalids. *Journal of Ethnopharmacology, 71*(1–2), 89–92. https://doi.org/http://dx.doi.org/10.1016/S0378-8741(99)00181-6

Qin, X.-J.J., Yu, Q., Yan, H., Khan, A., Feng, M.-Y.Y., Li, P.-P.P., … Liu, H.-Y.Y. (2017). Meroterpenoids with Antitumor Activities from Guava (*Psidium guajava*). *Journal of Agricultural and Food Chemistry, 65*(24), 4993–4999. https://doi.org/10.1021/acs.jafc.7b01762

Raj, S., & Gothandam, K.M. (2015). Immunomodulatory activity of methanolic extract of *Amorphophallus commutatus* var. *wayanadensis* under normal and cyclophosphamide induced immunosuppressive conditions in mice models. Food and Chemical Toxicology, 81, 151–159. https://doi.org/10.1016/j.fct.2015.04.026

Reddeman, R.A., Glávits, R., Endres, J.R., Clewell, A.E., Hirka, G., Vértesi, A., … Szakonyiné, I.P. (2019). A Toxicological Evaluation of Mango Leaf Extract (Mangifera indica) Containing 60% Mangiferin. *Journal of Toxicology, 2019*.

Reis, S.R.I.N., Valente, L.M.M., Sampaio, A.L., Siani, A.C., Gandini, M., Azeredo, E.L., … Kubelka, C.F. (2008). Immunomodulating and antiviral activities of *Uncaria tomentosa* on human monocytes infected with Dengue Virus-2. *International Immunopharmacology, 8*(3), 468–476. https://doi.org/http://dx.doi.org/10.1016/j.intimp.2007.11.010

Reynolds, T, & Dweck, A.C. (1999). Aloe vera leaf gel: a review update. *Journal of Ethnopharmacology, 68*(1–3), 3–37.

Reynolds, T. (2004). *Aloes: The Genus Aloe*. CRC press.

Rieder, S.A., Chauhan, A., Singh, U., Nagarkatti, M., & Nagarkatti, P. (2010). Cannabinoid-induced apoptosis in immune cells as a pathway to immunosuppression. *Immunobiology, 215*(8), 598–605. https://doi.org/https://doi.org/10.1016/j.imbio.2009.04.001

Rose, K.D., Croissant, P.D., Parliament, C.F., & Levin, M.B. (1990). Spontaneous spinal epidural hematoma with associated platelet dysfunction from excessive garlic ingestion: a case report. *Neurosurgery, 26*(5), 880–882.

Rosenthal, G.A. (1977). The biological effects and mode of action of L-canavanine, a structural analogue of L-arginine. *The Quarterly Review of Biology*, *52*(2), 155–178. https://doi.org/10.1086/409853

Rout, S., & Banerjee, R. (2007). Free radical scavenging, anti-glycation and tyrosinase inhibition properties of a polysaccharide fraction isolated from the rind from Punica granatum. *Bioresource Technology*, *98*(16), 3159–3163. https://doi.org/https://doi.org/10.1016/j.biortech.2006.10.011

Russo, E.B. (2011). Taming THC: potential cannabis synergy and phytocannabinoid-terpenoid entourage effects. *Br J Pharmacol*, *163*(7), 1344–1364. https://doi.org/10.1111/j.1476-5381.2011.01238.x

Saeed, F., Arshad, M.U., Pasha, I., Naz, R., Batool, R., Khan, A.A., … Shafique, B. (2014). Nutritional and phyto-therapeutic potential of papaya (*Carica Papaya* Linn.): an overview. *International Journal of Food Properties*, *17*(7), 1637–1653. https://doi.org/10.1080/10942912.2012.709210

Salman, H., Bergman, M., Bessler, H., Punsky, I., & Djaldetti, M. (1999). Effect of a garlic derivative (alliin) on peripheral blood cell immune responses. *International Journal of Immunopharmacology*, *21*(9), 589–597. https://doi.org/https://doi.org/10.1016/S0192-0561(99)00038-7

Saritha, V., & Anilakumar, K.R. (2010). Toxicological evaluation of methanol extract of Aloe vera in rats. *International Journal of Pharmacy & Biomedical Research*, *1*, 142–149.

Saxena, A., Dixit, S., Aggarwal, S., Seenu, V., Prashad, R., Bhushan, S.M., … Srivastava, A. (2008). An ayurvedic herbal compound to reduce toxicity to cancer chemotherapy: a randomized controlled trial. *Indian Journal of Medical and Paediatric Oncology*, *29*(2), 11.

Scartezzini, P., & Speroni, E. (2000). Review on some plants of Indian traditional medicine with antioxidant activity. *Journal of Ethnopharmacology*, *71*(1–2), 23–43.

Schafer, G., & Kaschula, C.H. (2014). The immunomodulation and anti-inflammatory effects of garlic organosulfur compounds in cancer chemoprevention. Anti-Cancer Agents in Medicinal Chemistry, *14*(2), 233–240.

Schultz, F., Anywar, G., Tang, H., Chassagne, F., Lyles, J.T., Garbe, L.-A., & Quave, C.L. (2020). Targeting ESKAPE pathogens with anti-infective medicinal plants from the Greater Mpigi region in Uganda. *Scientific Reports*, *10*(1), 11935. https://doi.org/10.1038/s41598-020-67572-8

Schultz, F., Anywar, G., Wack, B., Quave, C.L., & Garbe, L.-A. (2020). Ethnobotanical study of selected medicinal plants traditionally used in the rural Greater Mpigi region of Uganda. *Journal of Ethnopharmacology*, 112742. https://doi.org/https://doi.org/10.1016/j.jep.2020.112742

Schumacher, M., Cerella, C., Reuter, S., Dicato, M., & Diederich, M. (2011). Anti-inflammatory, pro-apoptotic, and anti-proliferative effects of a methanolic neem (*Azadirachta indica*) leaf extract are mediated via modulation of the nuclear factor-κB pathway. *Genes & Nutrition*, *6*, 149–160.

Shankar, T.N.B., Shantha, N.V., Ramesh, H.P., Murthy, I.A.S., & Murthy, V.S. (1980). Toxicity studies on turmeric (*Curcuma longa*): acute toxicity studies in rats, guineapigs and monkeys. *Indian Journal of Experimental Biology*, *18*(1), 73–75.

Sin Mayor, A. del C., Díaz Gálvez, M., Sebazco Perna, C., & Jiménez Martínez, M. del C. (2019). Evaluation of the immunomodulatory activity of dry powder of *Punica granatum* Linn in an experimental model of immunosuppression. *Revista Cubana de Medicina Militar*, *48*(2), 177–186. https://doi.org/http://dx.doi.org/10.1016/j.jep.2014.12.025

Singh, G., Kapoor, I.P.S., Singh, P., de Heluani, C.S., de Lampasona, M.P., & Catalan, C.A.N. (2010). Comparative study of chemical composition and antioxidant activity of fresh and dry rhizomes of turmeric (*Curcuma longa* Linn.). *Food and Chemical Toxicology*, *48*(4), 1026–1031. https://doi.org/https://doi.org/10.1016/j.fct.2010.01.015

Sittisomwong, N., Leelasangaluk, V., Chivapat, S., Wangmad, A., Ragsaman, P., & Chuntarachaya, C. (1990). Acute and subchronic toxicity of turmeric. *Bull Dept Med Sci*, *32*(8), 101–111.

Siveen, K.S., & Kuttan, G. (2011). Immunomodulatory and antitumor activity of Aerva lanata ethanolic extract. *Immunopharmacology and Immunotoxicology*, *33*(3), 423–432. https://doi.org/10.3109/08923973.2010.526614

Smith, D.E. (1968). Acute and chronic toxicity of marijuana. *Journal of Psychedelic Drugs*, *2*(1), 37–48.

Spelman, K., Burns, J.J., Nichols, D., Winters, N., Ottersberg, S., & Tenborg, M. (2006). Modulation of cytokine expression by traditional medicines: a review of herbal immunomodulators. *Alternative Medicine Review*, *11*(2), 128.

Sreelekha, T.T., Vijayakumar, T., Ankanthil, R., Vijayan, K.K., & Nair, M.K. (1993). Immunomodulatory effects of a polysaccharide from *Tamarindus indica*. *Anticancer Drugs*, *4*(2), 209–212.

Srivastava, I.K., & Vaidya, A.B. (1999). A mechanism for the synergistic antimalarial action of atovaquone and proguanil. *Antimicrob Agents Chemother*, *43*.

Ssegawa, P., & Kasenene, J.M. (2007). Medicinal plant diversity and uses in the Sango bay area, Southern Uganda. *Journal of Ethnopharmacology*, *113*(3), 521–540. https://doi.org/http://dx.doi.org/10.1016/j.jep.2007.07.014

Steinke, J.W., & Borish, L. (2006). 3. Cytokines and chemokines. *Journal of Allergy and Clinical Immunology*, *117*(2) Supplement Mini-Primer, S441–S445. https://doi.org/10.1016/j.jaci.2005.07.001

Sultan, M.T., Butt, M.S., Qayyum, M.M., & Suleria, H.A. (2014). Immunity: plants as effective mediators. *Critical Reviews in Food Science and Nutrition*, *54*(10), 1298–1308. https://doi.org/10.1080/10408398.2011.633249

Tau, G., & Rothman, P. (1999). Biologic functions of the IFN-γ receptors. *Allergy*, *54*(12), 1233.

Theisen, L.L., & Muller, C.P. (2012). EPs® 7630 (Umckaloabo®), an extract from Pelargonium sidoides roots, exerts anti-influenza virus activity in vitro and in vivo. *Antiviral Research*, *94*(2), 147–156. https://doi.org/https://doi.org/10.1016/j.antiviral.2012.03.006

Tugume, P., Anywar, G., Ojelel, S., & K., K.E. (2020). *Science of Spices and Culinary Herbs Latest Laboratory, Pre-clinical, and Clinical Studies (Volume 2)* (S.Y. Eds: Atta-ur-Rahma, M. Iqbal Choudhary, Ed.). https://doi.org/10.2174/97898114441493120020003

Tugume, Patience, Kakudidi, E.K., Buyinza, M., Namaalwa, J., Kamatenesi, M., Mucunguzi, P., & Kalema, J. (2016). Ethnobotanical survey of medicinal plant species used by communities around Mabira Central Forest Reserve, Uganda. *Journal of Ethnobiology and Ethnomedicine*, *12*(1), 1–28. https://doi.org/10.1186/s13002-015-0077-4

UNAIDS. (2020). Global HIV & AIDS statistics — 2020 fact sheet. Retrieved from https://www.unaids.org/en/resources/fact-sheet

van der Nat, J.M., van der Sluis, W.G., de Silva, K.T.D., & Labadie, R.P., 1991. Ethnopharmacognostical survey of Azadirachta indica A. Juss (Meliaceae). *Journal of Ethnopharmacology*, *35*, 1–24. http://doi.org/10.1016/0378-8741(91)90131-V

van Wyk, B.-E., & Albrecht, C. (2008). A review of the taxonomy, ethnobotany, chemistry and pharmacology of *Sutherlandia frutescens* (Fabaceae). *Journal of Ethnopharmacology*, *119*(3), 620–629. https://doi.org/https://doi.org/10.1016/j.jep.2008.08.003

Vidal, A., Fallarero, A., Peña, B.R., Medina, M.E., Gra, B., Rivera, F., … Vuorela, P.M. (2003). Studies on the toxicity of *Punica granatum* L.(Punicaceae) whole fruit extracts. *Journal of Ethnopharmacology*, *89*(2–3), 295–300.

Vitetta, E.S., Ohara, J., Myers, C.D., Layton, J.E., Krammer, P.H., & Paul, W.E. (1985). Serological, biochemical, and functional identity of B cell-stimulatory factor 1 and B cell differentiation factor for IgG1. *The Journal of Experimental Medicine*, *162*(5), 1726–1731.

Votto, A.P.S., Domingues, B.S., de Souza, M.M., da Silva Júnior, F.M.R., Caldas, S.S., Filgueira, D., ... Furlong, E.B. (2010). Toxicity mechanisms of onion (*Allium cepa*) extracts and compounds in multidrug resistant erythroleukemic cell line. *Biological Research*, *43*(4), 429–437.

Weber, N.D., Andersen, D.O., North, J.A., Murray, B.K., Lawson, L.D., & Hughes, B.G. (1992). In vitro virucidal effects of *Allium sativum* (garlic) extract and compounds. *Planta Med*, *58*(5), 417–423. https://doi.org/10.1055/s-2006-961504

Wen, C.-C., Chen, H.-M., & Yang, N.-S. (2012). Chapter 6 - Developing Phytocompounds from Medicinal Plants as Immunomodulators. In S. Lie-Fen & S.Y.L. Allan (Eds.), *Advances in Botanical Research, Volume 62* (pp. 197–272). https://doi.org/http://dx.do i.org/10.1016/B978-0-12-394591-4.00004-0

Williams, J.E. (2001). Review of antiviral and immunomodulating properties of plants of the Peruvian rainforest with a particular emphasis on Una de Gato and Sangre de Grado. Alternative Medicine Review, *6*(6), 567–579.

Wube, A.A., Bucar, F., Gibbons, S., & Asres, K. (2005). Sesquiterpenes from *Warburgia ugandensis* and their antimycobacterial activity. *Phytochemistry*, *66*(19), 2309–2315. https://doi.org/10.1016/j.phytochem.2005.07.018

Wynn, T.A., Chawla, A., & Pollard, J.W. (2013). Macrophage biology in development, homeostasis and disease. *Nature*, *496*(7446), 445–455.

Yamassaki, F.T., Campestrini, L.H., Zawadzki-Baggio, S.F., & Maurer, J.B.B. (2018). Chemical characterization and complement modulating activities of an arabinogalactan-protein-rich fraction from an aqueous extract of avocado leaves. International Journal of Biological Macromolecules, *120*(Pt A), 513–521. https://doi.org/10.1016/j.ijbi omac.2018.08.072

Yang, X., Hegde, V.L., Rao, R., Zhang, J., Nagarkatti, P.S., & Nagarkatti, M. (2014). Histone modifications are associated with Delta9-tetrahydrocannabinol-mediated alterations in antigen-specific T cell responses. *J Biol Chem*, *289*(27), 18707–18718. https://doi.org/ 10.1074/jbc.M113.545210

Yue, G.G.L., Chan, B.C.L., Hon, P.-M., Lee, M.Y.H., Fung, K.-P., Leung, P.-C., & Lau, C.B.S. (2010). Evaluation of in vitro anti-proliferative and immunomodulatory activities of compounds isolated from Curcuma longa. *Food and Chemical Toxicology*, *48*(8), 2011–2020. https://doi.org/https://doi.org/10.1016/j.fct.2010.04.039

Zhang, Y., Li, J., Wu, Z., Liu, E., Shi, P., Han, L., ... Wang, T. (2014). Acute and long-term toxicity of mango leaves extract in mice and rats. *Evidence-Based Complementary and Alternative Medicine*, *2014*.

7 Traditional Brazilian Medicinal Plants for a Strong Immune System

José Crisólogo de Sales Silva,
Solma Lúcia Souto Maior de Araújo Baltar,
and Maria Lusia de Morais Belo Bezerra

CONTENTS

7.1 INTRODUCTION

On the South American continent, Brazil is the largest country, with regard to both its population size and its geographic dimensions. Brazil is not only a large country, but, because of its diverse topographic conditions and habitats, it also has a diverse flora, which are of medicinal interest and are strongly associated with human and animal immunity in general.

Public knowledge of the extreme and unique plant diversity, as well as the rich traditions of their use by the native, and later settler, populations in Brazil is relatively scarce in relation to its value. The aim of the present chapter is to serve as a modest introduction to this wonderful natural resource, with a special focus on medicinal plants and the immune system. In this sense, Brazil is presented as the richest country in terms of flora, with 40,989 species, of which 18,932 are endemic, according to Mathé and Silva (2018).

We can highlight that all plants contain bioactive chemicals which can be useful for conventional and/or traditional medicine. Even plants called weeds in the diverse biomes of Brazil can have an important function, and can be valued according to their specific contribution to the development of the ecosystems present there.

DOI: 10.1201/9781003137955-7

An herbaceous plant in a pasture can be invasive, whereas, in another context, it can heal an animal or a human being. On the other hand, it can be toxic at high dosages, whereas, in lower dosages, it can function, say, as a vermifuge or as a booster of immunity.

The Brazilian nation, having indigenous roots in people who valued and healed diseases and other conditions through their knowledge of the many useful species from the local flora, has, in its health system, many plants authorized for use in traditional medicine. In the Atenção Básica à Saúde (Primary Health Care) system, some native species have been recognized for treatment of certain conditions as the first step of emergency care. Local populans use teas and infusions of specific medicinal plants, for example, for the treatment of inflammatory symptoms.

This chapter provides a quick overview of the Brazilian medicinal flora and of those species that have an important phytotherapeutic property to treat particular conditions, as a source of drugs and useful substances for treating people, with particular reference to the maintenance of immunological health.

7.2   BRAZILIAN MEDICINAL FLORA: NATIVE AND EXOTIC

Endemic Brazilian plants, that compose much of its flora, have medicinal tendencies or are suppliers of substances of value in medicine. The fact that there are no scientific references to the medicinal function of a particular plant does not mean that it cannot be used with these objectives in the future. In principle, all plants from the Brazilian flora could have active components that are essential for the development of either medicines or nutrition, which, consequently, could strengthen human immunity; even toxic plants could have a function in parasite control. Most plants that compose the Brazilian medicinal flora are species endemic to South America, particularly from the biomes of the Atlantic Forest, the cerrado, and the caatinga, with some being from the Pantanal tropical wetlands or the Amazon tropical rainforests. Some plants can carry out important immunological functions through their active principles, acting in a partial or indirect way, combating diseases, particularly those related to the urban environment. Some of these species are listed in Table 7.1, with their scientific and popular names and the conditions which they are used to treat.

In this sense, plants with the ability to stimulate the immunoregulatory action of the liver and pancreas present themselves as natural, cheap alternatives, that, in safe dosages, contribute to the preventive balance of the health of many organs. However, for this to happen, it is necessary to return to the traditions of using plant teas and infusions to promote natural health. These immunity regulators need to be present daily in the diet of both the urban and rural people, in the form of refreshing drinks, without preservatives or industrialized products, so that they can regulate, slowly and in keeping with the body's timing, any dysfunctions provoked by the consumption of fibre-free food, by excessive work, sleepless nights, and the fast-paced routine which is part of the modern day. Daily breaks can be accompanied by teas and infusions that reduce inflammation of the cardiovascular, hepatic, pancreatic, and urinary systems, as healthy organs and bowels are rarely affected by infections and diseases. As

TABLE 7.1

Native and Exotic Brazilian Plants With Medicinal Potential to Strengthen the Immune System (adapted from Americano 2015)

Scientific Name	Popular Name in Brazil	Principal Use
Aloe vera arborensis Miller	Babosa	Immunological, vitamin A, B and C tonic
Annona muricata L.	Graviola	Antibiotic, anticancer, hypotensive, hypoglycaemic
Annona sylvatica A. St. Hill.	Araticum-do-campo	Immunogenic, antihypertensive
Baccaris dracunculifolia DC	Alecrim silvestre	General tonic, digestive
Baccharis trimera (Less) DC	Carqueja	Immunity control, cardiovascular, and glycaemic
Bidens pilosa L.	Picão	Antibiotic, hypoglycaemic, hypotensive
Chiococa racemose Jacq.	Cainana, Cainca	Anti-inflammatory and antibiotic
Cochlospermum insigne St. Hill.	Algodão-do-campo	Anti-inflammatory and antibiotic
Copaifera officinalis L.	Copaiba	Anti-inflammatory, immunogenic
Dipteryx alata Vog.	Baru	Antitumour, anti-inflammatory
Hancornia speciosa Muell.	Mangabeira	Hormonal control, protective effect on the liver and pancreas
Lychnophora ericoides Mart.	Arnica campestre	Anti-inflammatory, general tonic
Macrosiphonia velama St. Hill.	Velame	Antibiotic, tonic, immunoregulator
Maytenus ilicifolia Martius ex Reiss	Espinheira santa	Antibiogenic, liver tonic
Myracrodruon urundeuva Allem.	Aroeirinha-do-campo	Anti-inflammatory, anti-diarrhoeal
Ocimum gratissimum Fr. All.	Alfavaca	General tonic, antimicrobial
Persea americana Will.	Abacateira	Antioxidant, cholesterol control
Rosmarinus officinalis L.	Alecrim	Hepatotonic, digestive
Stryphnodendron adstringens (Mart.) Coville	Barbatimão	Anti-inflammatory, antibiogenic
Vernonia condensata Baker	Alumã	Protective of the liver

a reflection of the power of the native and exotic plants of the Brazilian flora plants, Table 7.1 lists some species that have medicinal properties that can strengthen the immune system.

7.2.1 ETHNOBOTANIC ASPECTS OF BRAZILIAN MEDICINAL PLANTS

Ethnobotany involves the study of human societies, with its main characteristic being the direct contact with traditional populations through knowledge of the interaction between people and local plants from a community, and their mores, uses, and peculiarities, searching for information that can be beneficial with regard to the use of the medicinal plants (Rodrigues and Andrade 2014; Tomazi et al. 2014). This relationship involves ecological, evolutionary, genetic, and cultural interactions, and contributes to our understanding of the many plant species with medicinal properties (Alves and Povh 2013).

In the communities, local knowledge about the use of medicinal plants is transmitted from generation to generation, through contact between older and younger members, socialization within the family group, or between individuals from the same generation (Amorozo 1996; Lozada et al. 2006). However, the conservation of this local knowledge represents a medicinal alternative for families, particularly for those with low purchasing power, since herbal medicine is cheaper and more accessible than pharmaceutical medicines (Silva and Proença 2008).

In this context, Brazil stands out as the country with the greatest diversity of biological species in the world, and its importance for ethnobotanical research is related to its botanical and cultural diversity, represented by indigenous peoples, quilombola communities of artisanal fishermen, family farmers, sertanejos and riverside dwellers, that, through their human and environmental relationships (Albuquerque et al. 2011), discover the potential of local plants for the development of new drugs, and develop information on the different ways of the handling and use of plant preparations (Feijo et al. 2013; Ribeiro et al. 2014; Vasquez et al. 2014).

Research shows that most of the medicinal species known and studied today were identified with the help of ethnobotanical surveys. The contribution of these studies highlights the practices of medicinal plant use, explaining the traditional medicinal systems of the local populations (Albuquerque et al. 2010; Oliveira and Menini Neto 2012; Ribeiro et al. 2014). However, some medicinal plants require special care in their administration, and this care is directly related to their medicinal and toxicological characteristics, and to the way the natural remedy is prepared and applied (Rehman et al. 2017).

According to the Brazilian Institute of Geography and Statistic (IBGE, in Portuguese), Brazil is formed of six natural regions, known as biomes (the Amazon, caatinga, cerrado, Atlantic forest, pampa, and wetland). These biomes harbor different types of vegetation, each with their own characteristics, and this biodiversity has allowed separate ethnobotanical studies to be carried out in different Brazilian regions (Albuquerque and Andrade 2002; Pasa et al. 2005; Miranda and Hanazaki 2008); among the many categories of use of these plants, the work with medicinal plants dominates (Oliveira et al. 2009). The approach to this topic allows the research to be planned from a pre-existing empirical knowledge, confirmed many times by regular medicinal use of these plants, which should then be tested on a scientific basis (Amorozo 1996).

7.3 MEDICINAL PLANTS WITHIN THE SCOPE OF THE BRAZILIAN HEALTH SYSTEM

Brazilian's Health System, SUS in Portuguese, is one of the world's largest and most complex systems of public health. It was created in 1998 by the Brazilian Federal Constitution to address the constitutional article that classifies health as a people's right and a state duty, regulated by the law n°. 8.080/1990 (Brasil 2000).

From the creation of the Brazilian Federal Constitution, all of the Brazilian populations were guaranteed the right to universal free healthcare, financed by the Union resources, the states, the Federal District, and the counties, according to article 195 of the Constitution, that establishes five basic principles: the universality (article 196), integrality (article 198–II), equity (article 196–'universal and egalitarian access'), decentralization (article 198–I), and social participation (article 198–III).

SUS care is performed in health centres and unities, in public hospitals, including the university hospitals, and the laboratories and blood banks in the service of the health, epidemiological, and environmental departments, other than academic and scientific research foundations and institutes. With the goal of offering a wider service to the population, SUS has been opening opportunities for treatments with alternative medicine, such as aromatherapy, meditation, and yoga, and expanding the accessibility to patients of medicines based on medicinal plants and herbal medicines (http://bvsms.saude.gov.br).

For the Ministry of Health, the benefits of natural treatments are recognized throughout the country for their relevance in preventing diseases, promoting health, and aiding recuperation from illness. To this end, the federal government published, in 2006, the National Policy of Integrative and Complementary Practices (PNPIC, in Portuguese), and, two years later, approved the National Program of Medicinal Plants and Phytotherapies, that details the guidelines of the policy in the form of concrete actions. The goal of this regulation is to guarantee safe access to medicinal plants and phytotherapy for the population, to assure the rational use of these resources, to promote the sustainable use of the biodiversity, and to develop the chain of production and the national industry.

To the National Health Surveillance Agency (Anvisa, in Portuguese), a medicinal plant is every plant or part of a plant that contains substances or classes of substance responsible for therapeutic action (Brasil 2009), and phytotherapy is the result of the transformation of the properties of a medicinal herb into a medicine.

Medicinal plants and phytotherapy are important for treatment of numerous conditions (infection, inflammation, pain, and control of blood pressure, among others). The regulation of the medicinal herbal products is done by Anvisa and by the County and State Health Surveillance agencies; therefore, all industrialized phytotherapies are regulated by Anvisa before being made available on the market. Nowadays, SUS lists 71 medicinal plants and phytotherapies that are disseminated by the National Program of Medicinal Plants and Phytotherapies from the Health Ministry.

SUS phytotherapies are approved by Anvisa, and are considered safe and effective for the population. This list has the goal of guiding studies and research that can subsidize the preparation of phytotherapies available to the population to be used safely and effectively for the treatment of a certain condition (http://bvsms.saude.gov.br).

7.4 IMMUNOMODULATORY PROPERTIES OF MEDICINAL PLANTS

From what has been described here, it is undeniable that the Brazilian flora contains a wide range of species with considerable medicinal potential, capable of generating innovative products, and which has benefitted many people throughout the national territory. Popular wisdom on the therapeutic effects of many Brazilian plants, especially those associated with the immune system, has been confirmed by numerous scientific studies (Zandonai et al. 2010; Seyfried et al. 2016; Ribeiro Neto et al. 2020).

The ability that the human body has to respond, in a protective way, against many biotic attacks, especially by bacteria, viruses, fungi, and parasitic infections (protozoa, helminths, and ectoparasites), is essential for its maintenance (Coelho-Castelo et al. 2009; Chen et al. 2018). The functional complexity of the immune system involves molecules, cells, and organs, integrating two types of immunity, the innate, and the acquired or adaptive, that act simultaneously during the control of an infection.

The innate response constitutes the first defensive line in a tissue, with the involvement of physical, chemical, and biological barriers, as well as the effects of local cells and molecules. In this way, the inflammatory response, phagocytosis (by dendritic cells, neutrophils, and macrophages), and the liberation of mediators (complement system molecules, cytokines, and chemokines) are mechanisms of innate immunity. In addition to acting as an alert for the immune system, innate immunity allows a quick response against the pathogen, until the activation of the adaptive immune response can happen (Nunes-Pinheiro et al. 2003; Coelho-Castelo et al. 2009; Cruvinel et al. 2010).

In turn, the adaptive immunity response involves humoral and cellular immune actions. The first is characterized by the production and secretion of antibodies by B lymphocytes. The antibodies facilitate phagocytosis and activate cytotoxicity mechanisms mediated by the complement system, neutrophils, macrophages, and natural killer cell (NK). The cellular immune action, on the other hand, is mediated by various types of T lymphocytes (Nunes-Pinheiro et al. 2003; Cruvinel et al. 2010).

In popular herbal medicine, numerous phytochemicals stand out, such as peptides, polysaccharides, lectins, terpenoids, saponins, oils, alkaloids, flavonoids, and others, with properties that act on the immune system (Nunes-Pinheiro et al. 2003; Seyfried et al. 2016). The immunomodulatory activity of primary and secondary metabolites from extracts of medicinal plants has been confirmed by research from Brazil and around the world (Zandonai et al. 2010; Seyfried et al. 2016; Wangchuk et al. 2018; Andrade et al. 2020). In this modulation process, the substances act as immunoregulatory, immunostimulatory, and/ or immunosuppressive factors, heightening or lowering the immune response (Amirghofran et al. 2009; Zandonai et al. 2010).

Pereskia aculeata Miller is a scrambling plant from the Cactaceae family, common in the Atlantic forest, and popularly known in Brazil as Ora-pro-nobis. Its leaves, apart from being used in cooking, are used to help in the reduction of signals and inflammatory symptoms, and in wound healing (Pinto and Scio 2014; Ribeiro Neto et al. 2020). The immunomodulatory effect of this plant's leaves has been demonstrated by Andrade and collaborators (Andrade et al. 2020), and is related to its capacity to stimulate the proliferation of human peripheral blood mononuclear cells.

Plantago major L., known as tanchagem in Brazil, is an herb native to Europe, but naturalized in the south of Brazil. In addition to immunostimulatory biological properties, the *P. major* extract exhibits healing, analgesic, antioxidant, anti-ulcerogenic, antibiotic, and anti-inflammatory activities (Samuelsen 2000; Lorenzi and Matos 2002). Studies show that polysaccharides extracted from the African locust bean (*Parkia biglobosa*), the cashew nut (*Anacardium occidentale*), and from noni (*Morinda citrifolia*) show promising immunomodulatory properties, regulating mainly the activity of macrophages and the release of effector cell mediators (Hirazumi and Furuzawa 1999; Zou et al. 2014; Yamassaki et al. 2015). Table 7.2

TABLE 7.2
Immunomodulatory Activities of Herbaceous, Shrub, and Tree Plants of Native and Exotic Brazilian Flora

Type of Plant/ Popular Name in Brazil	Scientific Name	Immunomodulatory Activity	References
Herbs			
Salsa-de-praia, pé-de-cabra	*Ipomea pés-caprae* (L.) R. Br.	Increased proliferation of T lymphocytes	Zandonai et al. (2010)
Unha de gato	*Uncaria tomentosa* (Willd.) DC	Immunostimulatory activity in macrophages, T and B lymphocytes with induction of cytokine production	Lenzi et al. (2013); Domingues et al. (2011)
Marcela	*Achyrocline satureioides* (Lam.) DC.	Operates in the complement system	Puhlmann et al. (1992)
Tanchagem	*Plantago major* L.	Immunostimulant. Complement system activator	Samuelsen (2000); Michaelsen et al. (2000)
Shrubs			
Ora-pro-nobis	*Pereskia aculeata* Miller	Proliferation of human peripheral blood mononuclear cells	Andrade et al. (2020)
Amoreira-rosa	*Rubus imperialis* Cham. & Schltdl.	T lymphocyte inhibition	Zandonai et al. (2010)
Malva branca	*Althaea officinalis* L.	Effect on the complement system	Al-Snafi (2013)
Erva-preá, Erva-de-são-Simeão	*Vernonia scorpioides* (Lam.) Pers.	Reduces T lymphocyte proliferation	Zandonai et al. (2010)
Trees			
Guanandi or jacareúba	*Callophyllum brasiliensis* Cambess.	Induces T lymphocyte proliferation	Zandonai et al. (2010)
Noni	*Morinda citrifolia* L.	Production of cytokines by macrophages. Stimulates the release of chemical mediators	Hirazumi and Furuzawa (1999); Mufidah et al. (2013)
Miguel-pintado, Cambuatá-branco	*Matayba elaeagnoides* Radlk.	Stimulates T lymphocyte proliferation	Zandonai et al. (2010)
Cajueiro	*Anacardium occidentale* L.	Regulation of macrophage activity	Yamassaki et al. (2015)
Coração-de-bugre, cafezinho-do- mato	*Maytenus robusta* Reissek.	T lymphocyte inhibition	Zandonai et al. (2010)

(Continued)

TABLE 7.2 (CONTINUED)
Immunomodulatory Activities of Herbaceous, Shrub, and Tree Plants of Native and Exotic Brazilian Flora

Type of Plant/ Popular Name in Brazil	Scientific Name	Immunomodulatory Activity	References
Visgueiro	*Parkia biglobosa* (Jacq.) R.Br. ex G. Don	Complement system effect, macrophage activation	Zou et al. (2014)
Aroeira	*Myracroduon urundeuva* Allem.	Modulates macrophage activation	Carvalho et al. (2017)
Babosa	*Aloe arborescens* Mill.	Induces the production of various cytokines and the tumour necrosis factor	Nazeam et al. (2020)
Carqueja	*Baccharis trimera* (Less.) DC.	Inhibitory effect on T lymphocyte proliferation	Paul et al. (2009)

lists various herbaceous, shrub, and tree species, native and exotic, in the Brazilian flora that contain substances with immunomodulatory properties. Countless plant species have been indicated and used in traditional medicine and have had their medicinal properties confirmed, but many are still unknown, especially with reference to those with immunomodulatory activity. Conducting medicinal plant research focused on immunomodulatory activity is essential, though challenging, since it involves high costs, considering that such research requires both *in vivo* and *in vitro* experiments. To achieve developments in this scientific field, greater investment is needed, whether from governmental or other funding agencies.

7.5 CONCLUSION

Medicinal Brazilian flora is a source of powerful therapeutic chemicals capable of acting on the molecular and cellular mechanisms of organic defence, either stimulating or inhibiting the immune system. Biologically active compounds can be obtained from fruit plants, ornamental plants, and species of no current economic importance, which are used daily for medical purposes by the local populations distributed throughout the national territory. In view of the great botanical diversity in this country, studies on the immunomodulatory properties of Brazilian plant extracts are still preliminary, representing a research niche that urgently needs to be expanded and increasingly explored.

REFERENCES

Albuquerque, U.P., Lucena, R.F.P., Alencar, N.L. 2010. Métodos e técnicas para coleta de dados etnobiológicos. *In* Albuquerque UP de org., Lucena, R.F.P., Cunha, L.V.F.C. Métodos e técnicas na pesquisa etnobiológica e etnoecológica. Núcleo Publicações em Ecologia e Etnobotânica Aplicada (NUPEEA). 39–64. Recife-PE, Brazil.

Albuquerque, U.P., Soldati, G.T., Sieber, S.S., Ramos, M.A., Sá, J.C., Souza, L.C. 2011. The use of plants in the medical system of the Fulni-ô people (NE Brazil): a perspective on age and gender. *Journal of Ethnopharmacology*, 133(2): 866–873.

Albuquerque, U.P. and Andrade, L.H.C. 2002. Conhecimento botânico tradicional e conservação em uma área de caatinga no Estado de Pernambuco, Nordeste do Brasil. *Acta Botanica Brasilica* 16(3): 273–285.

Al-Snafi, A.E. 2013. The pharmaceutical importance of Althaea officinalis and Althaea rosea: A review. *International Journal of PharmTech Research*, 5(3): 1387–1385.

Alves, G.S.P. and Povh, J.A. Estudo etnobotânico de plantas medicinais na comunidade de Santa Rita, *Revista Biotemas*, 26(3), 232–242. Ituiutaba, MG. 2013. ISSN 2175-7925.

Americano, T. 2015. Fitoterapia brasileira: uma abordagem energética. Cidade Grafica ed., Brazil.

Amirghofran, Z., Bahmani, M., Azadmehr, A., Javidnia, K., and Miri, R. 2009. Immunomodulatory activities of various medicinal plant extracts: effects on human lymphocytes apoptosis. *Immunological investigations*, 38(2): 181–192.

Amorozo, M.C.M. 1996. A abordagem Etnobotânica na Pesquisa de Plantas Medicinais. 47–67. In: Di-Stasi, L.C. Plantas Medicinais: Arte e Ciência: um guia de estudo interdisciplinar. São Paulo, Editora da Universidade Estadual Paulista.

Andrade, T.C., de Freitas, P.H.S., Ribeiro, J.M., de Faria Pinto, P., de Souza-Fagundes, E.M., Scio, E., and Ribeiro, A. 2020. Avaliação da atividade antioxidante e imunomoduladora dos metabólitos primários de Pereskia aculeata Miller. *Journal of Biology & Pharmacy and Agricultural Management*, 17(2): 358–376.

Brasil. Constituição 1988. 2000. Constituição da República Federativa do Brasil. 16. ed. Organização de Alexandre de Moraes. São Paulo: Atlas. p. 58.

Brasil. Agência Saúde. MS elabora Relação de Plantas Medicinais de Interesse ao SUS. 2009. Available in: http://bvsms.saude.gov.br/bvs/sus/pdf/marco/ms_relacao_plantas_medic inais_sus_0603.pdf

Carvalho, C.E.S., Sobrinho-Junior, E.P.C., Brito, L.M., Nicolau, L.A.D., Carvalho, T.P., Moura, A.K.S., ... and Carvalho, F.A.A. 2017. Anti-Leishmania activity of essential oil of Myracrodruon urundeuva (Engl.) Fr. All.: Composition, cytotoxity and possible mechanisms of action. *Experimental Parasitology*, 175, 59–67.

Chen, X., Liu, S., Goraya, M.U., Maarouf, M., Huang, S., and Chen, J.L. 2018. Host immune response to influenza A virus infection. *Frontiers in Immunology*, 9: 320.

Coelho-Castelo, A.A., Trombone, A.P., Rocha, C.D. and Lorenzi, J.C. 2009. Resposta imune a doenças infecciosas. *Medicina (Ribeirao Preto. Online)*, 42(2): 127–142.

Cruvinel, W.D.M., Mesquita Júnior, D., Araújo, J.A.P., Catelan, T.T.T., Souza, A.W.S.D., Silva, N.P.D. and Andrade, L.E.C. 2010. Sistema imunitário: Parte I. Fundamentos da imunidade inata com ênfase nos mecanismos moleculares e celulares da resposta inflamatória. *Revista Brasileira de Reumatologia*, 50(4): 434–447.

Domingues, A., Sartori, A., Valente, L.M.M., Golim, M.A., Siani, A.C. and Viero, R.M. 2011. *Uncaria tomentosa* Aqueous ethanol Extract Triggers an Immunomodulation toward a Th2 Cytokine Profile. *Phytotherapy Research*, 25(8), 1229–1235.

Feijo, E.V.R.S., Pereira, A.S., Souza, L.R., Silva, L.A.M. and Costa, L.C.B. 2013. Levantamento preliminar sobre plantas medicinais utilizadas no bairro Salobrinho no município de Ilhéus, Bahia. *Revista Brasileira de Plantas Medicinais*, v. 15(4): 595–604.

Hirazumi, A., and Furusawa, E. 1999. An immunomodulatory polysaccharide-rich substance from the fruit juice of Morinda citrifolia (noni) with antitumour activity. *Phytotherapy Research*, 13(5): 380–387. http://bvsms.saude.gov.br/bvs/sus/pdf/marco/ms_relacao_ plantas_medicinais_sus_0603.pdf https://antigo.saude.gov.br/sistema-unico-de-saude (accessed 10 Nov, 2020).

Lenzi, R.M., Campestrini, L.H., Okumura, L.M., Bertol, G., Kaiser, S., Ortega, G.G., ... and Maurer, J.B.B. 2013. Effects of aqueous fractions of Uncaria tomentosa (Willd.) DC on macrophage modulatory activities. *Food Research International*, 53(2): 767–779.

Lorenzi, H. and Matos, F.J.A. 2002. Plantas medicinais no Brasil: nativas e exóticas. Nova Odessa-SP: Instituto Plantarum. Brazil.

Lozada, M.; Ladio, A. and Weigandt, M. 2006. Cultural transmission of ethnobotanical knowledge in a rural community of northwestern Patagonia, Argentina. *Economic Botany* 60: 374–385.

Mathé, A. and Silva, J.C.S. 2018. Introduction to Medicinal and Aromatic Plants in Brazil. 47–69. U.P. Albuquerque et al. (eds.), *Medicinal and Aromatic Plants of South America, Medicinal and Aromatic Plants of the World 5*. Springer Nature B.V. https://doi.org/10.1007/978-94-024-1552-0_3

Michaelsen, T.E., Gilje, A., Samuelsen, A.B., Høgåsen, K. and Paulsen, B.S. 2000. Interaction between human complement and a pectin type polysaccharide fraction, PMII, from the leaves of *Plantago major* L. *Scandinavian Journal of Immunology*, 52(5): 483–490.

Miranda, T.M. and Hanazaki, N. 2008. Conhecimento e uso de recursos vegetais de restinga por comunidades das ilhas do Cardoso (SP) e de Santa Catarina (SC), Brasil. *Acta Botanica Brasilica* 22: 203–215.

Mufidah, Z., Rifa'i, M. and Rahayu, S. 2013. Immunomodulators activity of noni (Morinda citrifolia L.) fruit extract in mice infected with Staphylococcus aureus. *Jurnal Veteriner*, 14(4): 501–510.

Nazeam, J.A., El-Hefnawy, H.M. and Singab, A.N.B. 2020. Structural Elucidation of Immunomodulators, Acetylated Heteroglycan and Galactosamine, Isolated from Aloe arborescens Leaves. *Journal of Medicinal Food*, 23 (8): 895–901.

Nunes-Pinheiro, Diana Célia Sousa et al. Atividade imunomoduladora das plantas medicinais: perspectivas em medicina veterinária. *Ciência Animal*, 13(1):23–32, 2003.

Oliveira, E.R. and Minini Neto, L. 2012. Levantamento etnobotânico de plantas medicinais utilizadas pelos moradores do povoado de manejo, Lima Duarte – MG. *Revista Brasileira de Plantas Medicinais*, 14(2): 311–320.

Oliveira, F.C., Albuquerque, U.P., Fonseca-Kruel, V.S. and Hanazaki, N. 2009. Avanços nas pesquisas etnobotânicas no Brasil. *Acta Botanica Brasilica* 23(2): 590–605.

Pasa, M.C.; Soares, J.J. and Guarim Neto, G. 2005. Ethnobotany study in community of Conceição-Açu (on the upper basin of the River Aricá Açu, MT, Brazil). *Acta Botanica Brasilica* 19(2): 195–207.

Paul, E.L., Lunardelli, A., Caberlon, E., de Oliveira, C.B., Santos, R.C.V., Biolchi, V., ... and de Oliveira, J.R. 2009. Anti-inflammatory and immunomodulatory effects of Baccharis trimera aqueous extract on induced pleurisy in rats and lymphoproliferation in vitro. *Inflammation*, 32(6): 419.

Pinto, N.D.C.C. and Scio, E. 2014. The biological activities and chemical composition of Pereskia species (Cactaceae)—A review. *Plant Foods for Human Nutrition*, 69(3): 189–195.

Puhlmann, J., Knaus, U., Tubaro, L., Schaefer, W. and Wagner, H. 1992. Immunologically active metallic ion-containing polysaccharides of Achyrocline satureioides. *Phytochemistry*, 31(8): 2617–2621.

Rehman, S.; Latief, R.; Bhat, K.A.; Khuroo, M.A.; Shawl, A.S. and Chandra, S. 2017. Comparative analysis of the aroma chemicals of Melissa offinalis using hydrodistillation and HS-SPME techniques. *Arabian Journal of Chemistry*, 10: 2485–2490.

Ribeiro Neto, J.A., Tarôco, B.R.P., dos Santos, H.B., Thomé, R.G., Wolfram, E. and Ribeiro, R.I.M.D.A. 2020. Using the plants of Brazilian Cerrado for wound healing: From traditional use to scientific approach. *Journal of Ethnopharmacology*, 260(112547): 1–18.

Ribeiro, D.A., Macedo, D.G., Saraiva, M.E., Oliveira, S.F., Souza, M.M.A. and Menezes, I.R.A. 2014. Potencial terapêutico e uso de plantas medicinais em uma área de Caatinga no estado do Ceará, Nordeste do Brasil. *Revista Brasileira de Plantas Medicinais*, 16(4): 912–930.

Rodrigues, A.P. and Andrade, L.H.C. 2014. Levantamento etnobotânico das plantas medicinais utilizadas pela comunidade de Inhamã, Pernambuco, Nordeste do Brasil. *Revista Brasileira de Plantas Medicinais*, 16(3): 721–730.

Samuelsen, A.B. 2000. The traditional uses, chemical constituents and biological activities of Plantago major L. A review. *Journal of Ethnopharmacology*, 71(1–2): 1–21.

Seyfried, M., Soldera-Silva, A., Bovo, F., Stevan-Hancke, F.R., Maurer, J.B.B. and Zawadzki-Baggio, S.F. 2016. Pectinas de plantas medicinais: características estruturais e atividades imunomoduladoras. *Revista Brasileira de Plantas Medicinais*, 18(1): 201–214.

Silva, C.S.P. and Proença, C.E.B. 2008. Uso e disponibilidade de recursos medicinais no município de Ouro Verde de Goiás, GO, Brasil. *Acta Botanica Brasilica*, 22(2): 481–492.

Tomazi, L.B.; Aguiar, P.A.; Citadini-Zanette, V. and Rossato, A.E. 2014. Estudo etnobotânico das árvores medicinais do Parque Ecológico Municipal José Milanese, Criciúma, Santa Catarina, Brasil. *Revista Brasileira de Plantas Medicinais*, 16(2) Supplement 1: 450–461.

Vasquez, S. P. F., Mendoça, M. S., and Noda, S. N. 2014. Etnobotânica de plantas medicinais em comunidades ribeirinhas do Município de Manacapuru, Amazonas, Brasil. *Acta Amazonica*, 44(4): 457–472.

Wangchuk, P., Apte, S.H., Smout, M.J., Groves, P.L., Loukas, A. and Doolan, D.L. 2018. Defined small molecules produced by Himalayan medicinal plants display immunomodulatory properties. *International Journal of Molecular Sciences*, 19(11): 3490.

Yamassaki, F.T., Lenzi, R.M., Campestrini, L.H., Bovo, F., Seyfried, M., Soldera-Silva, A., ... and Maurer, J.B.B. 2015. Effect of the native polysaccharide of cashew-nut tree gum exudate on murine peritoneal macrophage modulatory activities. *Carbohydrate polymers*, 125: 241–248.

Zandonai, R.H., Coelho, F., Ferreira, J., Mendes, A.K.B., Biavatti, M.W., Niero, R., ... and Bueno, E.C. 2010. Evaluation of the proliferative activity of methanol extracts from six medicinal plants in murine spleen cells. *Brazilian Journal of Pharmaceutical Sciences*, 46(2): 323–333.

Zou, Y.F., Zhang, B.Z., Inngjerdingen, K.T., Barsett, H., Diallo, D., Michaelsen, T.E., ... and Paulsen, B.S. 2014. Polysaccharides with immunomodulating properties from the bark of Parkia biglobosa. *Carbohydrate polymers*, 101, 457–463.

Traditional
Himalayan Plants
*Nature's Gift for Maintaining
a Strong Immune System*

*Antul Kumar, Anuj Choudhary, Harmanjot Kaur,
Atul Arya, Baljinder Singh, and Sahil Mehta*

CONTENTS

8.1   INTRODUCTION

In the past fifty years, climate change has become the most recognized challenge to Sustainable Development Goal 15 (or Global Goal 15) that relates to the halting of biodiversity loss. It not only affects plant distribution, global temperature, and ice cover, but also pushes the vulnerable species towards extinction (Mehta et al. 2019;

DOI: 10.1201/9781003137955-8   **211**

Sharma et al. 2020; Bharti et al. 2021). The Himalayas ('Third Pole of the Earth'), harboring around 600 BT (billion tons) of ice glaciers, seems to have been affected by unpredictable changes in temperature since the 20th century, where the global warming trend began at 0.16°C (Viste and Sorteberg 2015). Later on, the temperature increase rate doubled by the start of the 21st century leading to further melting of glaciers. This has been highlighted by reports presented by many agencies and international organizations. For example, China, India, Bhutan, Nepal, and Pakistan account for the most glacier losses, occurring at a pace that has been accelerating since the year 1975. Significant increases in surface temperature have been reported from each of the past six decades and currently there is an annual mean temperature increase of 0.2°–0.3°C across the Hindu Kush Himalayan (HKH) Region (Mohamed et al. 2017; Islam et al. 2018). The Tibetan Plateau and the Himalayas have experienced a temperature increase of 0.5°C/decade, termed the EDW (elevation-dependent warming). The resulting increase in the glacial melt (especially of the HKH) has also resulted in increased (by nearly 17.4%) river flows for ten major Himalayan-region-dependent rivers, namely the Tarim, Amu Darya, Indus, Brahmaputra, Irrawaddy, Yangtze, Yellow, Mekong, Salween, and Ganges. Together, these rivers contribute more than 50% of the total utilizable water. The changes in the glacier melting pace and water levels, coupled with varying rainfall, climate, and soil degradation, have resulted in the Himalayan region rapidly losing its precious flora and fauna (Ridley et al. 2013; Hui et al. 2018; Dimri and Allen 2020).

One of the most frightening recent observations is the influence of ice melting, inadequate water supply, dry summers, and intense climatic conditions on the flowering of many medicinal plants in the Himalayan regions. All these factors together affect the plant's morphology, phenology, reproduction, and ability to complete their life cycle. Furthermore, these factors indirectly impact tree lines, ecosystem compositions, tribal livelihoods, and faunal diversity (Durcan et al. 2016; Bitew et al. 2019). In this regard, conserving the medicinal plants of the Himalayan regions under the changing climate is of utmost priority. The reason lies in the fact that many medicinal plants, including *Fritillaria roylei*, *Lilium polyphyllum*, *Habenaria edgeworthii*, *Habenaria intermedia*, *Malaxis muscifera*, *Malaxis acuminata*, *Polygonatum verticillatum*, and *Polygonatum cirrhifolium* (together termed Astavarga), have been used in Ayurveda for many centuries. Astavarga is important in treating seminal weakness, abnormal thirst, and fever, in healing fractures, reducing elevated body fat, and improving diabetic conditions. Plants listed in Astavarga are described as having rich antioxidant properties and can restore a range of health issues (Dhyani et al. 2010). Due to their potent medicinal properties, Astavarga plants are used in various forms, such as powder (churana), butter (clarified butter), extracted oils (taila), and other herbal formulation in the conventional herbal medical system (CMS), such as chyavanprasha, a well-known, immunostimulatory, and health-promoting agent. Taking together, these species are regarded as valuable 'Rasayana', with considerable health-improving and rejuvenating properties that together strengthen the immune system, including the capacity for cell regeneration.

Over the past two decades, many exploration-cum-documentation surveys have been conducted on tribal and conventional knowledge of Himalayan medicinal plants (Samal and Dhyani 2006; Kala and Sajwan 2007; Singh et al. 2018; Kumar et al. 2020). Findings indicate that the western Himalayas (including India, Pakistan, Nepal, and Bhutan) hold a prime position in harbouring high concentrations of medicinal plant species, as compared with the global distribution of such plants. This knowledge has been conserved and passed on to the next generation by the tribal communities as a result of the area's inaccessibility to tourism, its harsh environmental conditions, difficult survival conditions, and comparatively low rate of development (Kala et al. 2006; Rai 2017).

8.2   BACKGROUND

The tradition of treating diseases with preparations of plants growing at high altitude is not a new concept. The use of Himalayan medicinal plants was already documented early in the Vedic period in the Charaka Samhita (300 BC), Sushruta Samhita (1300 BC), Atharvaveda (2000 BC), and other Brahminic treatises (Figure 8.1.). Over the years, the tribal communities relied on traditional practitioners who developed medicinal plant preparations of various compositions to treat a number of diseases, like diabetes, renal disorders, hepatic ulcers, sexual debility, and neurological disorders that suppress immune function. The Himalayas are often known as the "Rooftop of the World" and contain a very high biodiversity of medicinal plants, and they are considered to be repositories of unique medicinal plants (Hemant and Aitken 2003; Yadav et al. 2017). Due to the remoteness of the area and the lack of conventional medical resources and facilities, the local communities are treated by traditional medicinal healers, known as Amachis or vaids, who are experts in herbal formulations based on local plants. According to a Chinese proverb:

'If you are thirsty and digging a well is like you start boosting your immune system when you are ill'.

Archaeological findings on folk medicines which are still in use, such as *Papaver somniferum*, date back more than 8,000 years. Concomitantly, the documentation on traditional plants obtained from the Himalayas is also found in the Atharvaveda, Rigveda, and Ayurveda. Hippocrates (c.460–c.370 BC) explained the role of a willow tree in curing fever, cold, and energy flow *via* an elevated immune system. Even before the 19th century, these plants were the major agents used by communities to treat sick people, and still, their importance is immense. Several plant-derived drugs, such as colchicine (an immunomodulator, preventing the development of a 'cytokine storm'), ephedrine (an immunostimulant), and quinine (an antimalarial drug), which were used in herbal preparations by tribal communities, are currently being manufactured by pharmaceutical companies commercially. Various other conventional healing therapies based on Himalayan plants, like *Rauwolfia serpentina* (to treat hypertension), *Mucuna pruriens* (Parkinson's disease), *Artemisia annua* (an antimalarial), *Holarrhena* sp. (amoebiasis), and *Commiphora* (an hypolipidaemic) are currently being used too. Furthermore, some renowned bioactive compounds present in Himalayan medicinal plants are also used in folk medicine practices, including

Ayurveda (6000 BC)

Panch bhutas (five elements: air, sky, water, fire and earth), of which the body is composed

Panch bhutas (five elements: air, sky, water, fire and earth), of which the body is composed

Dhatus (related to structural components of body) refers to vital body organ or parts : Rash (body fluid), Rakta (blood), Mansa (muscular tissue), Asthi (bone tissue), Majja (nerve tissue and bone marrow) and Sukra (generative tissue including sperm and ova)

Malas deals with production and excretion of waste products by different organs and body

Rasayana is an important therapy in Ayurveda (preparations are inducers of enzymes and hormones)

Acorus calamus, Asparagus racemosus, Centella asiatica, Commiphora wightii, Emblica officinalis, Ocimum sanctum, Piper longum, Semecarpus anacardium, Sida cordyfolla, Tinospora cordyfolia and Withania somnifera

Atharvaveda (2000BC)

The last of the four great bodies of knowledge-known as Vedas, which forms the backbone of Indian civilization, contains 114 hymns related to formulations for the treatment of different diseases. From the knowledge gathered and nurtured over centuries two major schools and eight specializations got evolved

Sushruta Samhita (1300BC)

Sushrutaa Samhita remained preserved for many centuries exclusively in the Sanskrit language. In the eight century AD, Sushrutaa Samhita was translated into Arabic as "Kitab Shah −Hindi" and "Kitab − I − Susurud." The first European translation of Sushrutaa Samhita was published by Hessler in the early 19th century; the complete English literature was done by Kaviraj Kunja Lal Bhishagratna in the three volumes in 1907 at Calcutta

Charaka Samhita (300BC)

Describes the work of ancient medical practitioners such as Acharya Atreya and Acharya Agnivesh of 800 BC and contains the Principle of Ayurveda. It remained the standard textbook of Ayurveda for almost for 2000 years.

Unani system of medicine (11th century)

Introduced in India by Arab and Persians prescribes daily diet quantity to patient and also depends on whole drug therapy in which the active principle of drug is not isolated

Siddha medical system (10-15th century)

Any ailment in human body is thought as a result of imbalance of three humors – bile (pitta), wind (vayu) and phlegm (kaph).

Tibetan medical system

Trans-Himalayan region, especially in Tibet, Ladakh and Lahaul/Spiti Plant forms major ingredient in Tibetan medicine

Modern medicine (or Allopathy) (in 1842 by C.F.S. Hahnemann)

Indian Medicine Central Council Act, 1970

Registered practitioners of Ayurveda, Siddha, and Unani called as Vaidyas, Siddhas and Hakeems, respectively, who prepare medicines on their own to distribute among their patients and not selling such drugs in the market are exempted from the purview of good manufacturing practices

Kuth (Repeal) Act 2002

Repealing Kuth Act is being projected as a way to encourage local people for cultivation of medicinal plants on their own land

Drugs & Cosmetics Act, 1940

Prescribes the specifications with respect to the good manufacturing practices for manufacturing Ayurvedic, Siddha and Unani medicines in India

The Biological Diversity Act, 2002

Framed many rules for sustainable utilization of medicinal plants and to mitigate the chances of bio-piracy

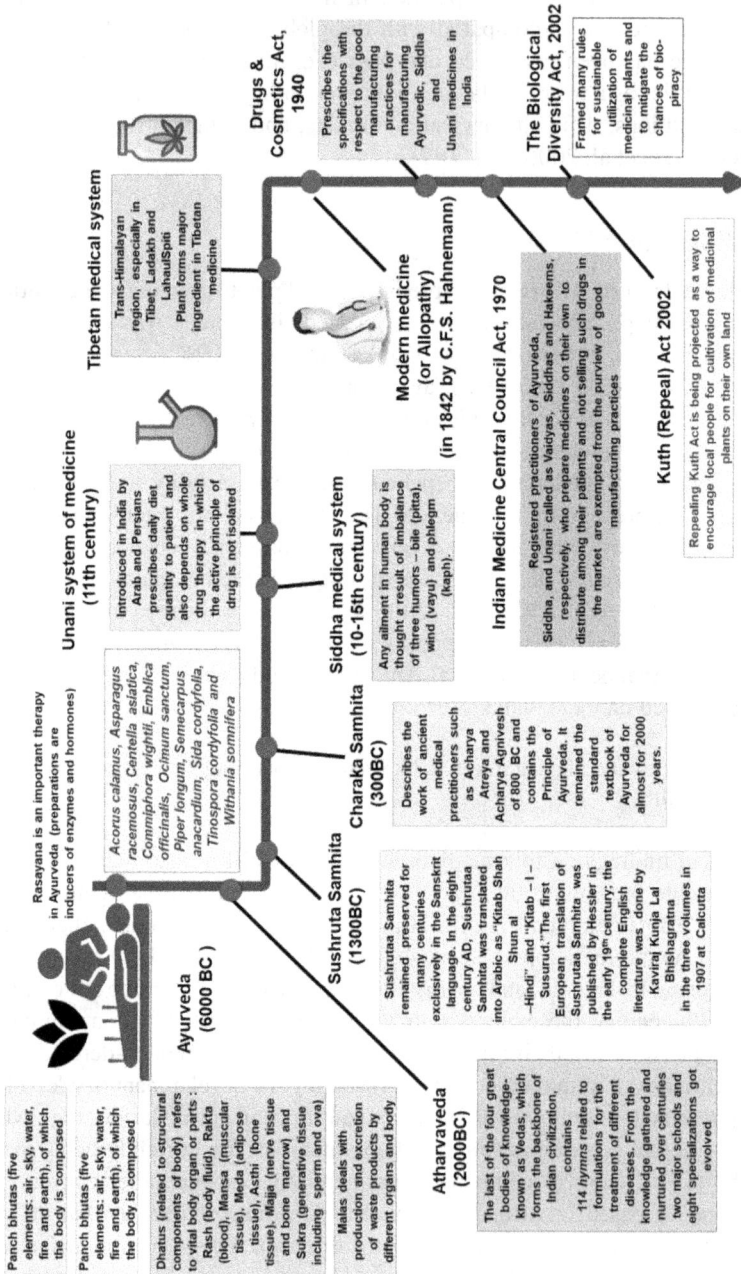

FIGURE 8.1 Historical milestones in immunity-boosting during research-cum-exploration mining of Himalayan plants.

guggulsterones (an hypolipidaemic), curcumin (an anti-inflammatory), asclepias (for mental retention), psoralens (for vitiligo), asarone (against hallucinations and for mental stability), picrosides (as a cardiotonic), withanolides (anticancer agents) and dirubin (an anti-tumour agent and to treat other immunomodulatory disorders). According to charaka system of medicine, exogenous diseases, or Agantuja Vyadhi and Rasayana chikitsa, are explained in Ayurveda in terms of diseases related to the immune system (Dhyani et al. 2010; Rana and Samant 2011; Sharma et al. 2017). At the medical level, modulation of cytokine activity is seen to be primarily targeted in both *in-vivo* and *in-vitro* studies that were conducted to assess the effect of herbal formulations on the immune system. These cytokines are glycoproteins or extracellular soluble proteins in the form of chemokines, interferons, and interleukins (ILs), which play a central role in both acquired and innate types of immune response (Joshi et al. 2010; Sharma et al. 2010). Furthermore, immunomodulation mediated by Himalayan medicinal plants was also observed to be associated with polysaccharides in the preparation, which caused a release of cytokines from IDCs (intestinal dendritic cells), reduced the levels of IL-6, IL-10, IL-1, IL-12, IL-8, IL-6, MCP-1 (monocyte chemoattractant protein-1), and lipopeptides. There was also an increase in levels of CD3-CD4-CD8-triple-negative thymocytes and natural killer (NK) cells, as well as in the activity of B lymphocytes, helper, and killer T cells (Ernst 2003; Namtak et al. 2018).

8.3 TRADITIONAL HIMALAYAN MEDICINAL PLANTS

More than 130 chemical compounds derived from medicinal plants have been recognized as valuable therapeutic agents and a number are established as well-known drugs in conventional medicine. For example, salicylic acid, extracted from the bark of the willow tree, is an important ingredient of skin ointments, pain killers, and as an antipyretic substance, marketed as aspirin. The bark has been used as an important herbal preparation for treating fever and pain by local communities since ancient times. Many drugs like opium, quinine, digoxin, etc. are frequently used by both herbal medicinal practitioners and conventional physicians for treating the same diseases.

Extracts of a number of medicinal plants have been used for studies on tumour necrotic factors, interleukins 1, IL-6, and interferons (Spelman et al. 2006; Wu et al. 2007; Dhyani et al. 2010; Chaurasia and Singh 2010; Kumar et al. 2019; Janifer et al. 2020), and are listed in Table 8.1: *Aconitum heterophyllum, Tinospora cordifolia, Atropa acuminata, Acalypha wilkesiana, Rheum australe, Fritillaria cirrhosa, Picrorhiza kurroa, Withania somnifera, Dactylorhiza hatagirea, Podophyllum hexandrum, Acanthopanax gracilistylus, Swertia chirayita, Allium sativum, Saussurea gossypiphora, Pleurospermum brunonis, Harpagophytum procumbens, Dioscorea deltoidea, Nardostachys grandiflora, Echinacea purpurea, Saussurea royleii, Uncaria tomentosa, Saussurea obvallata, Ananus comosus, Cissampelos sympodialis, Valeriana hardwickii, Silybum marianum, Polygala tenuifolia, Codonopsis ovata, Polygonatum cirrhifolium, Curcuma longa, Poria cocos, Jurinea dolomiaea, Smilax glabra, Panax ginseng, Grifola frondosa,* and *Coriolus versicolor*

TABLE 8.1

Comparison of Medicinal Plants, Based on Characters Like Pharmacological Properties, Folk Uses, and Herbal Formulations Used During Treatment of Various Health Issues

Botanical Name	Vernacular Name	Family	Part Used	Medicinal System	Part Administered	Uses/properties	References
Corydalis govaniana Wall.	Bhutjatta	Fumariaceae	Juice/ Roots	Tibetan	Root extract	Antiperiodic, diuretic, alterative antisyphilitic properties, to treat dermal allergies, and infections	Mukhopadhyay et al. (2004)
Inula orientalis Lam.	Poshkar/ Puskarmool (H) Manu (L)	Asteraceae	Roots	Ayurveda	Root extract	Anti-inflammatory, antiseptic, expectorant, and diuretic properties	Wani et al. (2006)
Achillea millefolium L.	Chuang/ biranjasif/ yarrow/ millefoeil	Asteraceae	Leaves/ flowers	Ayurveda	Crushed herb formulation (flowers and leaves)	To treat cardiovascular diseases, epilepsy, hysteria, antipyretic, to treat rheumatism, sleeping syndromes, tooth-ache, and bleeding piles	Benedek et al. (2008)
Rubia cordifolia L.	Manjith (H), Indian Maddar (E), Btsod (L)	Rubiaceae	Stems and roots	Ayurveda	Leaf extract	To treat urino-genital problems, stomach ache, chest complaints, menstrual disorders, ulcers, leukoderma, and blood-related diseases	Patil et al. (2009)

(Continued)

TABLE 8.1 (CONTINUED)

Comparison of Medicinal Plants, Based on Characters Like Pharmacological Properties, Folk Uses, and Herbal Formulations Used During Treatment of Various Health Issues

Botanical Name	Vernacular Name	Family	Part Used	Medicinal System	Part Administered	Uses/properties	References
Xanthium strumarium L.	Banokra	Asteraceae	Leaves, roots, fruits, and seeds	Chinese Medicine	Plant extract	To treat urinary diseases, diaphoretic properties, antimalarial, and leucorrhoea	Kamboj et al. (2010)
Piper longum L.	Pippali	Piperaceae	Fruits	Ayurveda	Plant extract	Immunomodulatory, antidiarrhoeal, antimicrobial, and antitumour activity	Khandhar et al. (2010)
Arctium lappa L.	Burdock/bankuth /jari	Asteraceae	Leaves, fruits, flowers, and roots	Tibetan	Root extract, crushed seeds	To treat cutaneous eruptions, rheumatism, eczema skin allergies, psoriasis inflammations, cystitis, gout, urinary infections, toothaches, and to maintain blood sugar levels	Chan et al. (2011)
Piper kadsura L.	Pippali	Piperaceae	Stem	Tibetan	Plant extract	Anti-irritant, analgesic, anti-asthmatic properties, and to treat bronchitis	Kim et al. (2011)

(Continued)

TABLE 8.1 (CONTINUED)

Comparison of Medicinal Plants, Based on Characters Like Pharmacological Properties, Folk Uses, and Herbal Formulations Used During Treatment of Various Health Issues

Botanical Name	Vernacular Name	Family	Part Used	Medicinal System	Part Administered	Uses/properties	References
Fritillaria cirrhosa D.Don	Hadjod	Liliaceae	Bulbs	Tibetan	Bulb paste	To treat respiratory syndromes, tuberculosis, asthma, fractured bones, joints, and bronchitis	Konchar et al. (2011)
Withania somnifera (L.) Dunal	Ashgandh/ ashwagandha	Solanaceae	Leaves, stem, flower, root, seeds, bark	Ayurveda	Dried root powder (mixed in milk)	Diuretic, hypnotic, sedative, abortifacient, immunostimulant, restorative, aphrodisiac, narcotic properties; to treat dropsy, weakness, rheumatism, coughs, and constipation	Verma et al. (2011)
Ferula jaeskiana L.	Jangli Heeng/ chuklam (L)	Apiaceae	Stem/roots	Ayurveda	Plant extract	To treat septic wounds, diabetes, antipyretic, rheumatism, and tooth problems	Mahendra et al. (2012)
Dactylorhiza hatagirea (D.Don) Soó	Hathpanja/ salampanja	Orchidaceae	Root/flowers	Unani/Ayurveda and Chinese medicine	Tubers	To treat chronic diarrhoea, dysentery, nerve debility, nerve stimulation, seminal debility, weakness in women after delivery, and other sexual problems	Pant et al. (2012)

(Continued)

TABLE 8.1 (CONTINUED)

Comparison of Medicinal Plants, Based on Characters Like Pharmacological Properties, Folk Uses, and Herbal Formulations Used During Treatment of Various Health Issues

Botanical Name	Vernacular Name	Family	Part Used	Medicinal System	Part Administered	Uses/properties	References
Anaphalis contorta (D.Don) Hook. f.	Rui-ghas	Asteraceae	Leaves, roots, flowers, and seeds	Ayurveda and Chinese medicine	Flower extract	Anti-bacterial properties, to treat burns, sores, ulcers, swellings, and rheumatic joints	Joshi (2013)
Scutellaria angulosa Benth.	Skullcap	Lamiaceae	Stem, flower	Tibetan	Plant extract	Febrifuge, nervine, antispasmodic, stomachic, laxative properties, microbiome modulation, and stimulation of immunoreactivity	Joshee et al. (2013)
Aloe vera (L.) Burm. F.	Aloe vera	Aloaceae	Leaves	Ayurvedic/homoeopathic	Aloe vera gel is used both, topically (treatment of wounds, minor burns, and skin irritation. Plant extract	Used to treat ulcers, arthritis, abdominal tumours, and burns	Sahu et al. (2013)
Jurinea dolomiaea Boiss.	Dhoop	Asteraceae	Roots/leaves	Tibetan	Plant extract	Antipyretic, to treat rheumatism, joint pains, colic, and gout	Asma et al. (2014)

(Continued)

TABLE 8.1 (CONTINUED)

Comparison of Medicinal Plants, Based on Characters Like Pharmacological Properties, Folk Uses, and Herbal Formulations Used During Treatment of Various Health Issues

Botanical Name	Vernacular Name	Family	Part Used	Medicinal System	Part Administered	Uses/properties	References
Fragaria vesca L.	Wild strawberry	Rosaceae	Roots/fruits	Ayurveda	Root extract	Antibacterial, angioprotective, to improve blood circulation, and treat urinary problems	Dhole et al. (2014)
Arnebia benthamii (Wall. ex G. Don)	Ratanjot	Boraginaceae	Roots, flowers	Ayurveda / Chinese medicine	Extract of plant aerial parts	Antiseptic, antibiotic, and anti-microbial properties	Ganie et al. (2014)
Arisaema tortuosum (Wall.) Schott	Samp ki kumb/ kidajadi	Araceae	Roots, seeds	Chinese medicine	Seeds, tubers	Antidote, neurotoxic injuries, and to maintain blood flow	Nile et al. (2015)
Thymus serpyllum L.	Banjwain	Lamiaceae	Stem, roots	Ayurveda	Dried root powder (mixed in tea)	Antispasmodic, anthelmintic, antiseptic, expectorant, carminative, cell regeneration, stimulant properties, to treat colds, coughs, fever, and stomach-ache	Jaric et al. (2015)

(Continued)

TABLE 8.1 (CONTINUED)

Comparison of Medicinal Plants, Based on Characters Like Pharmacological Properties, Folk Uses, and Herbal Formulations Used During Treatment of Various Health Issues

Botanical Name	Vernacular Name	Family	Part Used	Medicinal System	Part Administered	Uses/properties	References
Malaxis muscifera (Lindl.) Kuntze	Rishbhak	Orchidaceae	Leaves, flowers, fruits	Ayurveda	Plant extract	Antipyretic, to treat, dysentery, fever, burning, haematemesis, seminal weakness, dipsia, and emaciation	Kant (2015)
Lilium polyphyllum D. Don	Ksirakakoli	Liliaceae	Leaves, stem	Ayurveda	Plant extract	Anti-inflammatory, antipyretic, galactogogue, expectorant, aphrodisiac, diuretic, seminal weakness, haematemesis, to treat intermittent fever, and rheumatism	Sourabh (2015)
Prunella vulgaris L.	Ustakha-ddus	Labiatae	Leaves, flowers, roots	Chinese medicine	Plant juice (mixed with rose oil)	To treat haemorrhages, spasmodic, bleeding piles, fevers, cough stimulant; antiseptic, anti-rheumatic, carminative, diarrhoea, headache tonic, astringent, and expectorant property	Bai et al. (2016)

(Continued)

TABLE 8.1 (CONTINUED)

Comparison of Medicinal Plants, Based on Characters Like Pharmacological Properties, Folk Uses, and Herbal Formulations Used During Treatment of Various Health Issues

Botanical Name	Vernacular Name	Family	Part Used	Medicinal System	Part Administered	Uses/properties	References
Meconopsis aculeata Royle	Blue poppy	Papaveraceae	Roots/flower	Tibetan	Plant extract	To treat inflammation, fractures, and pain	Ganaie et al. (2016)
Roscoea capitata Sm.	Kakoli	Zingiberaceae	Tuber/rhizome	Ayurveda	Plant extract	Diabetes, diarrhoea, malaria, and antioxidants	Rawat et al. (2016)
Geranium wallichianum D.Don ex Sweet	Ratanjot	Geraniaceae	Rootstock	Chinese medicine	Plant extract	Mouth ulceration, joint pain, dysentery, diarrhoea, passive toothache, colic, jaundice, haemorrhage, kidney disorder, and eye troubles	Shaheen et al. (2017)
Swertia chirata L.	Chirayita	Gentianaceae	Leaves, fruit	Ayurveda	Plant extract	To treat anaemia, antipyretic, liver disorders, and respiratory disorders	Aleem et al. (2018)
Rosa webbiana Wall. ex Royle	Wild rose (E) / Siah (L)	Rosaceae	Seed/fruit	Chinese medicine	Plant extract	To treat antidote, jaundice, viral fever, hepatitis, and liver inflammation	Ayati et al. (2018)

(Continued)

TABLE 8.1 (CONTINUED)

Comparison of Medicinal Plants, Based on Characters Like Pharmacological Properties, Folk Uses, and Herbal Formulations Used During Treatment of Various Health Issues

Botanical Name	Vernacular Name	Family	Part Used	Medicinal System	Part Administered	Uses/properties	References
Origanum vulgare L.	Sathra/Sathra/ Banajwain, Baslughas/Wild oregano / marjoram	Lamiaceae	Leaves	Chinese medicine	Leaves, root paste	Diaphoretic, carminative, diuretic, emmenagogue properties; to treat diarrhoea, whooping cough, tuberculosis, bronchitis, spasmodic earache, and conjunctivitis	Bahmani et al. (2018)
Rhodiola imbricata Edgew.	Rose root or stonecrop (E)/ Shrolo (L)	Crassulaceae	Leaves/roots	Amchi	Plant extract	Anti-inflammatory properties, to treat lung problems, colds, coughs, to restore memory, and to maintain blood cell number during altitude sickness	Bhardwaj et al. (2018)
Carum carvi L.	Konyot/ban jeera	Apiaceae	Seeds	Chinese medicine	Seeds (mixed with butter)	Febrifuge, digestive problems, eye syndromes, and to prevent cardiac arrest	Goyal et al. (2018)

(Continued)

TABLE 8.1 (CONTINUED)

Comparison of Medicinal Plants, Based on Characters Like Pharmacological Properties, Folk Uses, and Herbal Formulations Used During Treatment of Various Health Issues

Botanical Name	Vernacular Name	Family	Part Used	Medicinal System	Part Administered	Uses/properties	References
Bistorta affinis L.	Banmundu/ sarbguni	Polygonaceae	Flowers/roots	Ayurveda/unani	Plant extract	To treat coughs, cold, tonsillitis, fever, diarrhoea, abdominal, and back pain	Paul et al. (2018)
Bergenia ciliata (Haw.) Sternb.	Pashanbhed/ patharchatta/ takli	Saxifragaceae	Leaves, rhizomes	Chinese medicine	Root extract (mixed with milk or curd), rhizome paste	To treat piles, as a laxative, heart diseases, spleen enlargement, diarrhoea, respiratory diseases, diuretic affections, renal stones and diabetes	Singh et al. (2018)
Plantago major L.	Isabgol	Plantaginaceae	Roots, leaves, flowers	Homoeopathy	Seeds	Dermatological inflammation, earache, toothache, and gastric allergies	Najafian et al. (2018)

(Continued)

TABLE 8.1 (CONTINUED)

Comparison of Medicinal Plants, Based on Characters Like Pharmacological Properties, Folk Uses, and Herbal Formulations Used During Treatment of Various Health Issues

Botanical Name	Vernacular Name	Family	Part Used	Medicinal System	Part Administered	Uses/properties	References
Rheum australe L.	Chuchi, chukri, leechu	Polygonaceae	Roots/flowers	Unani, Tibetan, homoeopathy	Dilute extract	Astringent, laxative properties; to treat muscular injury, Stomach pains, constipation, mumps dysentery, headache inflammation, blood purification, rheumatic earache and swelling of throat	Pandith et al. (2018)
Zanthoxylum armatum DC.	Tirmira/timru	Rutaceae	Leaves, bark, root	Ayurveda/Chinese Medicine	Leaf extract, bark	Dyspepsia, abdominal pains, dysentery, diarrhoea, asthma, antiplaque, diaphoretic, spasmolytic, hepatoprotective, anti-inflammatory, skin diseases, anthelmintic, and antispasmodic properties	Paul et al. (2018)
Hedychium spicatum Sm.	Kapur-Kachri	Zingiberaceae	Rhizomes	Tibetan	Rhizome extract	Dyspepsia, carminative, and spasmodic disorders	Utami et al. (2018)

(Continued)

TABLE 8.1 (CONTINUED)

Comparison of Medicinal Plants, Based on Characters Like Pharmacological Properties, Folk Uses, and Herbal Formulations Used During Treatment of Various Health Issues

Botanical Name	Vernacular Name	Family	Part Used	Medicinal System	Part Administered	Uses/properties	References
Tinospora cordifolia (Willd.) Miers	Giloe, gurcha, guluchi, amrita, gilo	Menispermaceae	Stem, leaves, roots	Ayurveda	Root extract	Gastrointestinal, anti-ulcer activity, chronic cough treatment, diabetes, rheumatoid arthritis, cardiac disorder, diuretic, stomachic, antidote, neuro-pharmacological activities, anaemia, stimulates bile secretion, gout, respiratory tract infections, antidote, anti-inflammatory activity, maintain cholesterol content, anti-asthmatic, antileprotic, anti-hyperglycaemic, hepatoprotective activity, and anticancer activity	Kumar et al. (2019)

(Continued)

TABLE 8.1 (CONTINUED)

Comparison of Medicinal Plants, Based on Characters Like Pharmacological Properties, Folk Uses, and Herbal Formulations Used During Treatment of Various Health Issues

Botanical Name	Vernacular Name	Family	Part Used	Medicinal System	Part Administered	Uses/properties	References
Echinops niveus Wall. ex Wall.	Untkandara	Asteraceae	Fruits/roots	Ayurveda	Root bark (mixed with honey)	Ophthalmia, indigestion, urinary, neural, respiratory and mild antibiotic properties, to treat asthma, cough, and chest infections	Bitew et al. (2019)
Artemesia dracunculus L.	Burtse/kundia/ Shersing	Asteraceae	Leaves/roots	Ayurveda/Chinese Medicine	Root extract	To treat urinary diseases, toothache, sexual problems, respiratory problems (especially lung infections), and menstrual problems	Fildan et al. (2019)
Dracocephalum heterophyllum Benth.	Zinkzer	Laminaceae	Leaves/ flowers	Ayurveda/Tibetan	Plant extract	To treat cold, headache, cough, and fever	Raj et al. (2009)
Ficus benghalensis L.	Banyan	Moraceae	Aerial roots	Ayurveda	Bark extract	Treatment of gonorrhoea, vomiting, and diabetes	Tripathi et al. 2019
Sinopodophyllum hexandrum (Royle) T.S. Ying	Bankakri	Berberidaceae	Roots, Rhizomes	Ayurveda	Dried root powder, fruits	Anticancer, gastric ulcers, hepatic problems, and tissue regeneration properties	Kumar et al. (2020)

(Continued)

TABLE 8.1 (CONTINUED)

Comparison of Medicinal Plants, Based on Characters Like Pharmacological Properties, Folk Uses, and Herbal Formulations Used During Treatment of Various Health Issues

Botanical Name	Vernacular Name	Family	Part Used	Medicinal System	Part Administered	Uses/properties	References
Hippophaë rhamnoides L.	Sea buckthorn, Tsermang	Elagnaceae	Leaves, berries, pulp, and seed residue	Ayurveda/Chinese edicine	Berries	Inflammatory, lung disorders, blood purifier, peptic ulcer, antiseptic, antimicrobial activities, improves digestion, nutrient deficiencies, and blood circulation	Kumar et al. (2020)
Polygonatum verticillatum (L.) All.	Mahameda, salammisri	Asparagaceae	Rhizomes	Ayurveda/Chinese medicine	Rhizomes	Used for urino-genital disorders, nerve tonic, general weakness, spermatorrhoea, haemorrhoids, leucorrhoea, anaemia, gastric problems, wounds, rheumatism, aphrodisiac, kidney problems (stones), and fever	Kumar et al. (2020)

These reports validate the therapeutic success of traditional medicinal theories in treatment of a range of autoimmune illnesses and cytokine-associated syndromes or diseases. The treatment based on conventional medicinal plants, including immuno-modulation, is effective due to the presence of different phytochemical compounds in a single dose of the preparation given to the patient. So, researchers are working on the isolation of single compounds that target particular diseases, using phytotherapy. Herbal practitioners use herbal compositions; single compounds may not work, and this has always been a point of criticism for conventional medicinal systems (Kala et al. 2006; Sharma et al. 2010; Rai 2017). The hypothesis underlying multi-component remedies proposes that dilute mixtures of more than four or five traditional medicinal plants representing the 'crude drug', consisting of many chemical constituents, show therapeutic and pharmacological effect as a result of synergistic activity. Equally, this complex combination of compounds is reflected in the effect of many compounds, regulating signalling cascades, cytokine receptors, and protein regulation. Studies on the dilution of biologically active chemical compounds suggest that subclinical concentrations of oral interferon-α can provide a wide range of useful benefits (Sharma et al. 2010). The strategy of using multiple immuno-modulatory compounds in a single dose regulates the activity of various cytokines. Currently, this knowledge is restricted to phytochemicals used by people in tribal regions in treatments based on multi-component plant extracts. Recently, due to the onset of the global COVID-19 pandemic, there has been increased attention being paid towards employing such immunomodulatory plants to boost the immune system (Ernst 2003; Rastogi et al. 2020).

8.4 ROLES OF HIMALAYAN MEDICINAL FLORA IN DISEASE TREATMENT

Plant extracts of various Himalayan herbal formulations have been regularly evaluated for their role as chemoprotective and immunomodulation agents (Mohan et al. 2019). The compounds in these plants modify and induce anti-tumour effects by enhancing the activities of the host immune response against the tumour. These plants show direct antiproliferative roles on cyst-like cells and also increase the ability of the host cells to resist or counteract toxic damage that may be crucial to the damage caused by the tumour cells (Janifer et al. 2020).

Immunomodulatory therapy could offer an efficient and effective approach over conventional chemotherapy for numerous conditions resulting from poor immune responsiveness or where targetted immunosuppression has to be initiated to treat the condition, as in auto-immune disorders, inflammatory diseases, or following bone marrow or organ transplantation. Numerous medicinal plants from temperate and sub-temperate zones have been claimed to exhibit immunostimulatory activities, supporting the evidence of local herbal medicinal practitioners. These well-known medicinal plants include *Achillea wilhelmsii*, *Caesalpinia bonducella*, *Astragalus membranaceus*, *Jatropha curcas*, *Picrorhiza scrophulariiflora*, *Bergenia ciliata*, *Tinospora cordifolia*, *Plantago asiatica*, *Panax ginseng*, *Sophora subprostrata*, *Mangifera indica*, *Morus alba*, and *Withania somnifera* (Singh et al. 2018; Kumar et al. 2020; Niraj and Varsha 2020). Several of these plants are described below:

8.4.1 ASTRAGALUS MEMBRANACEUS

In the Chinese medicine system, the roots are well known as a spleen tonic and for treating different wasting or deficiency conditions. Using an extract of *A. membranaceus, in-vitro* experiments showed lower levels of interleukin-6, one of the best-known signalling compounds involved in inflammatory disorders. The decline in content of interleukin-6 validates the long-held rationale of their role in wasting and deficiency disorders. Moreover, increased concentrations of C-reactive proteins and interleukin-6 are associated with significant increases in cardiovascular disorders (Hong et al. 2018; Riaz et al. 2019). The tribal communities use these plants in the treatment of oedema and respiratory syndromes, which could be associated with cardiovascular disorders due to poor immune response. Thus, a predictable mechanism of reduced interleukin-6 content in cardiovascular disorders underlines the effective role of *A. membranaceus* as an immunomodulatory agent (Rios 2010; Sharma et al. 2017; Niraj and Varsha 2020).

8.4.2 ALLIUM SATIVUM

Allium sativum, or garlic, is one of the most commonly used cooking ingredients as well as one of the most widely used medicinal plants available in the temperate, sub-temperate, and tropical areas of Asia. Garlic is effective at regulating the functions of multiple cytokines. Studies on the addition of garlic extract to *in-vitro* cell cultures showed a lowering in the concentration of interleukin-6 and lower antioxidant activity, lower cholesterol level, and lower acetylcholinesterase (ACE)-inhibition activity, which are associated with improved cardiovascular activity (Sharma et al. 2017). However, in another model, the use of *A. sativum* extract caused a decrease in the concentration of the pro-inflammatory cytokine-like interleukin-1 that is involved in the elimination of pancreatic β cells. Garlic extract also induced changes in alloxan-based diabetes and activity towards hypoglycaemia, which may cause inhibition of IL-2. It also reduced the activities of interleukin-1, IL-8, and TNF but increased the production of IL-10 (an antiproinflammatory cytokine). Moreover, interleukin-10 also plays a role in immunopathological (inflammatory bowel and microbial infection) and immunomodulatory disorders (Alzheimer's disease), both of which support the finding that *A. sativum* acts as a cytokine stimulatory agent (Villinger 2003; Spelman et al. 2006; Rastogi et al. 2020).

8.4.3 TYLOPHORA ASTHMATICA

This medicinal plant is traditionally used for treating respiratory disorders, such as asthma, chest infections, allergies, and other immune-related disorders. In the Ayurveda medicinal system, *T. asthmatica* is known as anthrapachaka and is used to boost circulation in terms of internal energy flow. *T. asthmatica* shows a biphasic effect in *in-vitro* studies; it increases the interleukin-2 level when used at a lower dosage, but a decline in interleukin-2 level is observed on application of high dosages of *T. asthmatica* extract (Nair et al. 2004; Chlubnova et al. 2011; Jantan et al. 2015;

Abbas et al. 2016). This paradoxical effect of the plant suggests that researchers need to maintain an optimum concentration during drug formulation (Sotto et al. 2020). However, the high dosage may lead to activation of the mechanism that upregulates cytokine activity. The *T. asthmatica* dosage recommended by herbal practitioners is still questionable, given the contradictory effects of other plant compounds in a single dose (Ganguly et al. 2001; Gilbert and Alves 2003; Villinger 2003; Nazar et al. 2020).

8.4.4 *WITHANIA SOMNIFERA*

W. somnifera (ashwagandha) has held a prime position in terms of health benefits from ancient times and its use is well documented in Ayurveda, Chinese, Siddha, Unani, and almost all medicinal systems, as well as being a well-known immunity booster plant. *W. somnifera* also shows biphasic dosage-response effects, and influences TNF expression in a concentration-dependent manner, thus restoring chemotactic activity (Cundell et al. 2014; Chandran et al. 2017; Kalra and Kaushik 2017). An *in-vitro* investigation showed the suppression of TNF and IL-1 activity against murine macrophages, using the carcinogenic ochratoxin A (OTA). The immunosuppressive action of ochratoxin A, elevating TNF expression, confirms the chemotactic role of W. *somnifera* (Singh et al. 2016). The above findings confirm the immunological properties of an extract of W. *somnifera,* which is exploited as an immunomodulatory agent in folk medicinal systems (Davis and Kuttan 1999; Niraj and Varsha 2020).

8.4.5 *PANAX GINSENG*

Ginseng plant parts are one of the most common ingredients of many local Chinese herb formulations used by the Tibetan herbal practitioners, the Amchis, and are also well represented in the soya-rigpa medicinal systems of Ladakh. The ginsenosides are active constituents and are believed to have a diverse role in addressing health issues. *P. ginseng* is prescribed to treat inflammation and is thus predicted to exert possible functionality in terms of immunomodulatory activities. In clinical studies, the ginseng extract inhibits the stimulation of cytokine-like TNF-α levels and decreases the expression and secretion expression of C-X-C motif chemokine ligand 10 (CXCL-10) (Sun et al. 2018). In another study, seven out of nine ginsenosides (Rh1, Rf, Rg1, Rb1, Rb2, Rd, Rg3, Rc, and Re) caused stimulation of the cytokine-like TNF-α and decreased the production and secretion of CXCL-10. Such suppression of CXCL-10 can directly be inter-linked with the inactivation of several oncogenes and could ultimately activate immune responses (Singh et al. 2016; Sotto et al. 2020).

8.4.6 *TINOSPORA CORDIFOLIA*

Historically, guduchi (or giloy) is considered to be the first medicinal plant that appeared in the Vedic period during samundra manthna, as explained in bhagavata-purana (the oldest Hindu scripture), so is referred to as amrita booti. *T. cordifolia* is used in many traditional healing therapies, conferring chemoprotectivity and treating immunological disorders (Aranha et al. 2012). The diverse range of functionalities of *T. cordifolia* is well known and helps to treat hyperglycaemia, alopecia, diabetes, hirsutism, hyperuricaemia, hyperkalaemia, renal dysfunction, hypercholesterolaemia, hypertension, elevated low-density lipoprotein (LDL) cholesterol, hyperlipidaemia, gum hyperplasia, nephrotoxicity, pulmonary toxicity, hepatic fibrosis, lymphoma nephrotoxicity, neurotoxicity, and to lower the risk of infection. Studies confirmed that macrophage activation and lymphoproliferative activities occurred in response to giloy preparations in the various herbal formulations, supporting the concept of an immunoprotective agent (Kumar et al. 2019; Sotto et al. 2020; Figure 8.2).

8.4.7 *BOERHAAVIA DIFFUSA*

Punarnavine is a commercial drug obtained from *B. diffusa* and is considered to play a valuable role in immunity enhancement. Several folk communities ingest leaves of this plant in the form of a herbal formulation as well as in the raw form. In sheep, treatment with the punarnavine extract causes increases in the circulation of antibodies, red blood cell (RBC) count, and numbers of plaque-forming cells (PFC) in spleen tissue. It also results in an increased number of bone marrow cells and thymocytes, as well as increased splenocyte proliferation under both *in-vitro* and *in-vivo* conditions. Punarnavine significantly reduces the concentrations of various proinflammatory cytokines like interleukin-6, IL-1β, and TNF-α in mice. The above findings suggest an immunomodulatory function of *B. diffusa* extracts (Rios 2010; Sharma et al. 2017; Thangadurai et al. 2018; Sotto et al. 2020).

8.4.8 *PICRORHIZA SCROPHULARIIFLORA*

Species of the genus *Picrorhiza* are mainly found in high-altitude regions and are utilized by tribal people of the Himalayan regions. The scrocaffeside A present in the *P. scrophulariiflora* extract induces immunostimulatory functions under laboratory conditions. The compound scrocaffeside A increased splenocyte proliferation and their effect on lipopolysaccharides (LPS) and ConA (concanavalin A), along with increased activity of NK (natural killer) cells, mature T cells, and peritoneal macrophage cells. The concentration of interferons and interleukins (IL12, IL-2, IL-4) responded *via* splenocytes to the extract containing scrocaffeside A, identifying a functional role for scrocaffeside A in stimulating the immune system (Spelman et al. 2006; Aranha et al. 2012; Singh et al. 2016; Smit 2020).

8.4.9 *ACTINIDIA ERIANTHA*

This plant species has been used for treating several serious diseases, such as cancer, as described in the traditional Chinese medicine system. The roots of *A. eriantha* are rich in polysaccharides, that suppress tumour activity in mice, indicating their

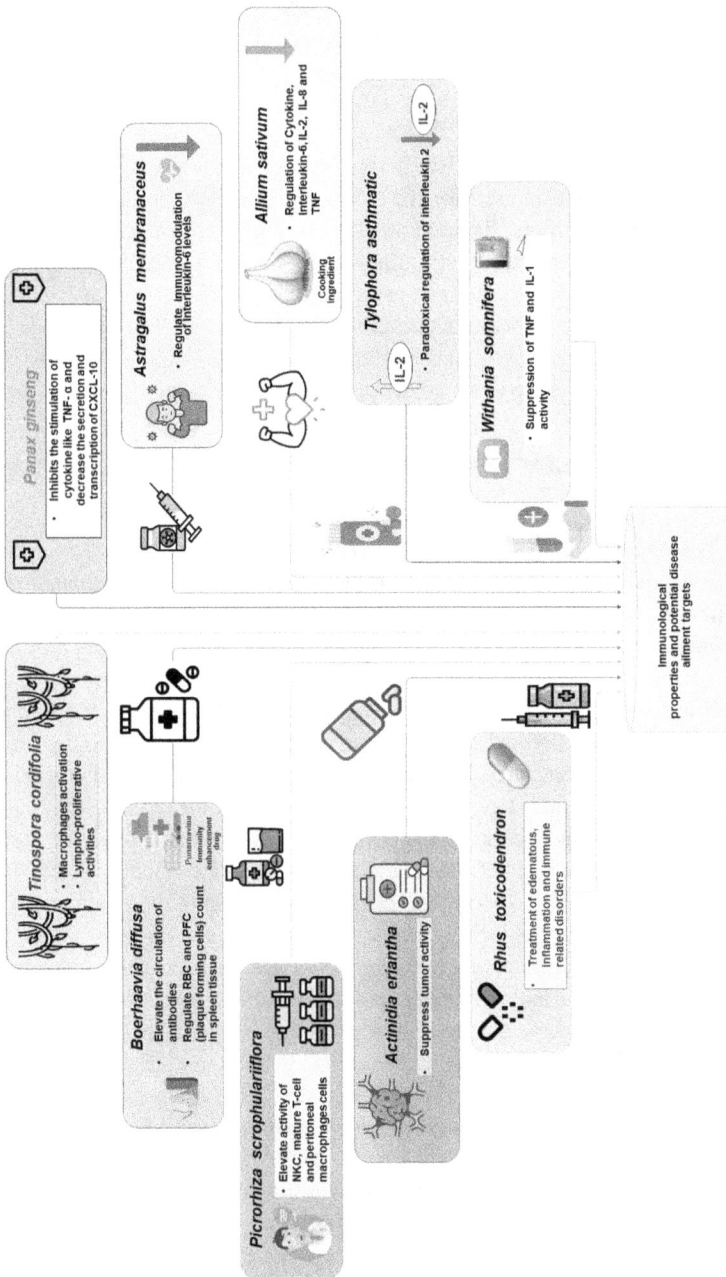

FIGURE 8.2 Immunological properties and potential disease treatment targets of Himalayan medicinal plants.

positive role in the immunostimulatory mechanism. In mice, the extract shows anti-tumour activity *via* improving immune response and is rich in uronic acid, several monosaccharides, and polysaccharides, which exhibit immunostimulatory activities (Thangadurai et al. 2018; Hasson et al. 2019; Sotto et al. 2020).

8.4.10 *RHUS TOXICODENDRON*

This plant is present in the Rhus Tox herbal formulation used by homoeopathic medicine practitioners and is used for the treatment of oedematous, inflammatory, and immune-related disorders. Treatment of mice with various concentrations of the derived compounds resulted in stimulation of both cellular and humoral types of immune response. Similar findings were also reported in humans, showing enhanced phagocytosis and chemotactic activities, confirming *R. toxicodendron* to be an important plant in conventional medicinal systems (Singh et al. 2000; Rios 2010; Hasson et al. 2019; Sotto et al. 2020).

8.5 ETHANOPHARMACOLOGY

Himalayan medicinal plants, such as *Inula racemosa, Rosa macrophylla, Mentha longifolia, Nepeta podostachys, Peganum harmala, Origanum vulgare, Utrica hyperborea, Gallium pauciflorum, Heracleum pinnatum, Rosa webbiana, Hippophaë rhamnoides, Dracocephalum heterophyllum, Tanacetum gracile, Artemesia dracunculus, Achillea millefolium, Bidens pilosa, Carum carvi, Ferula jaeskiana, Rubia cordifolia, Rhodiola imbricata,* and *Rhodiola heterodenta*, are endemic to high-altitude regions and are well utilized by folk medicinal practitioners, such as Amachis and Ladhakis (Wangchuk et al. 2018; Sotto et al. 2020). These plants are rich in flavonoids, tannins, alkaloids, steroids, saponins, terpenoids, cardiac glycosides, and other phytochemical compounds. These compounds have demonstrated promising results in the treatment of microbial infections, wounds, deficiencies, syndromes, and immune-related disorders. The herbal formulations of high-altitude plants contain phenolic compounds like flavanones, flavones, isoflavones, flavonols, and chalcones that help in the treatment of several diseases; these preparations include roots of *Ferula jaeskiana* (to treat rheumatism), *Heracleum pinnatum* (inflammation), and *Hippophaë rhaminoides* (to achieve immunostimulation). Therapeutic and ethnobotanical studies report the claims by traditional healers of the potential of these preparations to treat diseases like diabetes, cancer, and immune-related syndromes. Saponins in root extracts show anti-diabetic properties, whereas root extracts show other medicinal effects, as with *Dracocephalum heterophyllum* and *Inula racemosa* (to treat coughs, cold, and fever) and *Peganum harmala* (to treat cardiac arrhythmia and cardiac arrest). Tannins and flavonoids show astringent properties (leaves of *Achillea millefolium*), antifungal, and antimicrobial properties, and are used to treat toothache, menstrual problems (*Artemisia dracunculus*), gum problems (resin and stem gum of *Ferula jaeskiana*), and circulatory system problems, and to increase blood cell concentrations (*Rubia cordifolia*) (Surya et al. 2017). Some other pharmacological activities reported are antimicrobial effects, and protection from mutagenesis, carcinogenesis and ageing (*Rhus parviflora*), as well as anti-inflammatory effects, maintenance of blood glucose level, and treatment of hypertension (*Inula racemosa*). Polysaccharides show immunomodulatory properties, activating macrophages, dendritic cells, NK cells, B cells, T cells, and inflammatory pathways, and regulating cytokine gene expression (Joshi et al. 2016; Rastogi et al. 2020).

8.6   RECENT ADVANCES IN IMMUNOMODULATORY RESEARCH

Recently, the interest in immunity booster plants has gradually increased, and sales of such herbal plant-based medicines have increased, with annual growth of 20% in the Indian market, as well as increases in the international herbal market *via* indigenous and ethnopharmacological expansion. With enhanced conventional herbal therapies based on Himalayan plants, the documents confirming their efficacy require the verification of modern-day phytochemical extraction. The tribal therapies, based on diet, drug, and treatment, have been questioned, due to scarce research, poor document evaluation, and limited *in-vivo* studies. Several Himalayan plants which have recently been overexploited for immunomodulatory drug extraction include *Rubus ellipticus* for its abortifacient activity and its action as an anti-implantation agent, whereas the caterpillar fungus, *Ophiocordyceps sinensis*, is used to enhance memory, as a haemostatic, anticancer, anti-asthamatic, antioxidant, mycolytic, or antitumour agent, as well as stimulating the immune response (Janifer et al. 2020). Another plant species, *Plantago major*, is used in herbal medicine for its antibacterial, oestrogenic, anti-inflammatory, antitumour, and antiviral activities, and its functions as a wound healer, diuretic, as an agent to achieve renal stone disintegration, and to treat hypotension,. *Tinospora cordifolia* is used to inhibit COX-2, IL-6, IL-1 β, and TNF-α, increase the level of NF-κB in the blood, increase TNF-α/ DNA binding, cell-cycle arrest, and to treat Parkinsonism. The immunomodulatory drug derived from *T. cordifolia* enhances the number of T cells (Spelman et al. 2006; Chaurasia and Singh 2010; Haque et al. 2017; Kumar et al. 2019). *Boerhaavia diffusa* is a well-known immunomodulatory plant that inhibits cell proliferation, while the root extract inhibits the production of tumour necrosis factors, shows cytotoxicity towards natural killer cells, and interleukins (Janifer et al. 2020). *Centella asiatica* increases the concentration of antibodies, phagocytosis cells, and white blood cells (Kumar et al. 2020). A rhizome extract of *Rhodiola imbricata* causes stimulation of TNF-α and IL-6, and inhibits expression of the NF-κB transcription factor, demonstrating the immunosupportive properties of *R. imbricata* (Niraj et al. 2020). *Boswellia serrata*, a Chinese herb, is used to treat inflammatory arthritis and to inhibit the cellular toxicity of various cytokines, like IFN-γ, TH2, IL-2, IL-4, and IL-10. The inhibition is based solely on the anticancer properties that help to suppress carcinogenic cells *via* influence on the immune system (Sotto et al. 2020). Ginsenosides obtained from the ginseng plant *Panax ginseng* regulate the gene expression involved in cell growth, coagulation, cell adherence, and vascular contractions, and stimulates signalling by TNF-α (Sun et al. 2018; Riaz et al. 2019). In *Astragalus membranaceus,* the polysaccharides in the extract increase the nitrous oxide concentration in macrophage cells to increase phagocytic activity *via* activating transcription factors like NF-κB. Furthermore, the extract enhances the activity of NK cells, complement defence systems in peripheral lymphocytes, and upregulated B lymphocyte proliferation (Zheng et al. 2020). *Andrographia paniculata* shows antinociceptive, anticancer, antiplatelet-aggregation, anti-inflammatory, and antihyperglycaemic pharmacological activities and is also used for treating encephalomyelitis immune diseases, suppressing LPS-induced expression, and inhibiting levels of IL-6, TNF, and IL-1. To date, labdane diterpenes, polysaccharides, and fatty acids are mainly responsible for the immunomodulation properties from *A. paniculata*, where labdane diterpenes and polysaccharides are immunosuppressors, and fatty acids show immunostimulatory and immunosuppressive activities (Hong et al. 2018; Riaz et al. 2019). Much research of higher quality is needed to support the concepts and validity of the use of these plants in the fields of immunology and pharmaceutical sciences (Islam et al. 2017; Thangadurai et al. 2018; Sotto et al. 2020).

8.7   HIMALAYAN MEDICINAL PLANTS AND THEIR DECLINE

The survival of humans depends upon their capability to defend themselves against foreign particles or organisms, external factors, and toxic or allergenic compounds *via* a strong immune system. Once the infectious agent penetrates the host after suppressing its defence barriers, only the immune system can protect the body from severe damage. Without doubt, the native medicinal plants have a great ability to heal diseases exogenously as well as endogenously. The various plant parts, such as roots, shoots, leaves, and fruits, are used to increase the concentrations of specialized cell types associated with boosting the immune system and hence cope with disease and energy loss (Abbas et al. 2016). The fragile melting glacier in the Himalayas has resulted in the decline of many wild species, evolving into subspecies that remained stationary. The combination of habitat isolation, elevation gradient, and climate compression often increase endemism at a single topographical level. Among species, the endemic plants of some regions in the Himalayas face barriers to migrating further up the mountains to avoid the increasing temperatures, and become extinct (Ayati et al. 2018). Plant genera, such as *Meconopsis*, *Aconitum*, *Pedicularis*, and *Pleurospermum*, and many more, face the situation of 'climb or die': either they trek towards higher altitudes or die out at their native growing level (Khuroo et al. 2020). The species extinction rate in high-altitude regions is high, with two drug plants disappearing from their native habitat globally.

Climate change, overgrazing, and the unsustainable overexploitation of medicinal plants are major threats concerning the ecology of these high-altitude regions. As the global market for herbal plants expands, the population pressure on native herbal farming becomes more intense. The increase in farming of vegetables and exotic varieties also affects the farming of local wild medicinal plants.

8.8   CONCLUSION

At present, the global warming trends are visible in Himalayan regions in terms of the loss of species habitat, species shifts, and increasing dominance of sub-temperate species, habitat fragmentation, and endemism at high altitudes. These warming changes threaten not only the local ecology but also the survival of tribal communities that depend on local resources for their livelihood. Across the globe, but especially in the Asian Himalayas, communities living at high altitude, and which depend primarily on local flora for their disease treatment systems, are facing many problems. These plant resources are used effectively and sustainably by local communities and are an integral part of their life cycle. The use of medicinal plants also depends upon reachable sources, livelihood strategies, customs, and spiritual mythologies. Immunostimulation using Himalayan medicinal plants can achieve valuable treatment sources for chemotherapy of several diseases involving poor immune responses or immune-related disorders. In modern times, the pharmacological analysis of traditional immunomodulatory plants are playing an important role in the inhibition of several inflammatory factors, such as interleukins, tumour necrotic factors, cyclooxygenase, lipoxygenase, prostaglandins, and leukotrienes. These plants hold promise for the development of new drugs capable of relieving, reducing, or suppressing inflammation as well as pain. Still, many high-altitude plants are unavailable for research due to their endemicity to tribal regions, and these can have properties that antagonize the effects of interleukins and cytokines by improving the immune system. Conventional herbal formulations are very effective and act in multiple ways to target different ligands associated with various cellular receptors. However, the hidden fact of potency and effectiveness of the herbal formulation is that many chemical constituents are involved in treatment, rather than a single, active compound. Advances in biotechnologies and genetics can help to decipher the concept of ethnomedicine in terms of differential gene expression involved in an immune response. Polysaccharides show immunomodulatory properties, by activating macrophages, dendritic cells, natural killer cells, B cells, T cells, and inflammatory pathways, and by regulating cytokine-related gene expression. In the future, proper research with strict guidelines needs to be carried out that will ultimately result in conserving every Himalayan medicinal plant as well as generating a curated compendium of Himalayan medicinal herb knowledge, combining local medicinal knowledge with modern, pharmacological, and genetic knowledge, to include their bioactives, medicinal uses, and growing areas.

REFERENCES

Abbas, A.K., A.H.H. Lichtman, and P. Shiv. 2016. *Basic Immunology: Functions and Disorders of the Immune System.* 5th ed. Philadelphia, PA: Saunders. Ed. Elsevier Science. 239–243.

Aleem, A., and H. Kabir. 2018. Review on *Swertia chirata* as traditional uses to its phytochemistry and pharmacological activity. *Journal of Drug Delivery and Therapeutics* 8: 73–78.

Aranha, I., F. Clement, and Y.P. Venkatesh. 2012. Immunostimulatory properties of the major protein from the stem of the Ayurvedic medicinal herb, Guduchi (*Tinospora cordifolia*). *Journal of Ethnopharmacology* 31: 366–372.

Asma, B., A. I. Nawchoo, Z. Kaloo, P. Shabir, and A. Ali. 2014. Efficient propagation of an endangered medicinal plant *Jurinea dolomiaea* Boiss in the North Western Himalaya using rhizome cuttings under ex situ conditions. *Journal of Plant Breeding and Crop Science* 6: 114–118.

Ayati, Z., M.S. Amiri, M. Ramezani, E. Delshad, A. Sahebkar, and S.E. Emami. 2018. Phytochemistry, traditional uses and pharmacological profile of rose hip: a review. *Current Pharmaceutical Design* 24: 4101–4124.

Bahmani, M., M. Khaksarian, K.M. Rafieian, and N Abbasi. 2018. Overview of the therapeutic effects of *Origanum vulgare* and *hypericum perforatum* based on iran's ethnopharmacological documents. *Journal of clinical and diagnostic research* 12: 1–4.

Bai, Y., X. Bohou, Wenjian, Y. Zhou, J. Xie, H. Li, D. Liao, L. Lin, and C. Li. 2016. Phytochemistry and pharmacological activities of the genus *Prunella*. *Food Chemistry* 204: 483–496.

Benedek, B., K. Rothwangl-Wiltschnigg, E. Rozema, N. Gjoncaj, G. Reznicek, J. Jurenitsch, B. Kopp, and S. Glasl. 2008. Yarrow (*Achillea millefolium* L.): pharmaceutical quality of commercial samples. *Die Pharmazie* 63: 23–26.

Bhardwaj, P., G. Bhardwaj, R. Raghuvanshi, M.K. Thakur, and O. Chaurasia. 2018. *Rhodiola*: an overview of phytochemistry and pharmacological applications. In: *New Age Herbals*. Eds. Singh B., Peter K. Springer, Singapore, pp. 71–113.

Bharti, J., S. Mehta, S. Ahmad, B. Singh, A.K. Padhy, N. Srivastava, and V. Pandey. 2021. Mitogen-activated protein kinase, Plants and Heat stress. In: *Resilient Environment and Plant Potential*. Ed. A. Husen. Springer, Switzerland. ISBN-978-3-030-65911-0.

Bitew, H., and A. Hymete. 2019. The Genus *Echinops*: phytochemistry and biological activities: a review. *Frontiers in Pharmacology* 10: 1234.

Chan, Y.S., L.N. Cheng, J.H. Wu, E. Chan, Y.W. Kwan, S.M. Lee, G.P. Leung, P.H. Yu, and S.W. Chan. 2011. A review of the pharmacological effects of *Arctium lappa* (burdock). *Inflammopharmacology* 19: 245–254.

Chandran, U., and B. Patwardhan. 2017. Network ethnopharmacological evaluation of the immunomodulatory activity of *Withania somnifera*. *Journal of Ethnopharmacology* 197: 250–256.

Chaurasia, S., and B. Singh. 2010. *(India) Screening Phytochemical Constituents of 21 Medicinal Plants of Trans-Himalayan Region Medicinal Plants of the Himalayas: Advances and Insights*. UK: Global Science Books. 90–93.

Chlubnova, I., B. Sylla, C. Nugier-Chauvin, R. Daniellou, L. Legentil, B. Kralová, and V. Ferrières. 2011. Natural glycans and glycoconjugates as immunomodulating agents. *Natural Product Reports* 28: 937–952.

Cundell, R.D. 2014. Herbal Phytochemicals as Immunomodulators. *Current Immunology Reviews* 10: 64–81.

Davis, L., and G. Kuttan. 1999. Effect of *Withania somnifera* on cytokine production in normal and cyclophosphamide treated mice. *Immunotoxicology* 21: 695–703.

Dhole, A., S.K. Mohite, and C. Magdum. 2014. Pharmacognostical evalution of *Fragaria vesca* linn leaf. *International Journal of Phytopharmacy* 4: 1–4.

Dhyani, A., B.P. Nautiyal, and M.C. Nautiyal. 2010. Importance of Astavarga plants in traditional systems of medicine in Garhwal, Indian Himalaya. *International Journal of Biodiversity Science* 6: 13–19.

Dimri, A.P., and S. Allen. 2020. Himalayan climate interaction. *Frontiers in Environmental Science* 8: 96.

Durcan, L., and M. Petri. 2016. Immunomodulators in SLE: clinical evidence and immunologic actions. *Journal of Autoimmunology* 74: 73–84.

Ernst, E. 2003. Herbal medicines put into context. *BMJ* 327: 881–882.

Fildan, A., I. Pet, D. Stoin, G. Bujanca, A. Lukinich-Gruia, C. Jianu, A. Jianu, D. Radulescu, and D. Tofolean. 2019. *Artemisia dracunculus* essential oil chemical composition and antioxidant properties. *Revista de Chimie* 70: 59–62.

Ganaie, H., D. Ahmad, Z. Kaloo, B. Ganai, and S. Singh. 2016. Phytochemical screening of *Meconopsis aculeate* Royle an important medicinal plant of Kashmir himalaya: a perspective. *Research Journal of Phytochemistry* 10: 1–9.

Ganguly, T., L.P. Badheka, and K.B. Sainis. 2001. Immunomodulatory effect of *Tylophora indica* on Con A induced lymphoproliferation. *Phytomedicine* 8: 431–437.

Ganie, S., T. Dar, R. Hamid, O. Zargar, S. Abeer, A. Masood, S. Amin, and M. Zargar. 2014. In vitro antioxidant and cytotoxic activities of *Arnebia benthamii* (Wall ex. G. Don): a critically endangered medicinal plant of Kashmir valley. *Oxidative Medicine and Cellular Longevity* 2014: 792574.

Gilbert, B., and L.F. Alves. 2003. Synergy in plant medicines. *Current Medicinal Chemistry* 10: 13–20.

Goyal, M., V. Gupta, N. Singh, and M. Sharma. 2018. *Carum carvi*-an updated review. *Indian Journal of Pharmaceutical and Biological Research* 6: 14–24.

Haque, M.A., I. Jantan, and S.N. Abbas Bukhari. 2017. *Tinospora* species: an overview of their modulating effects on the immune system. *Journal of Ethnopharmacology* 207: 67–85.

Hasson, S.S., A.A. Al Manthari, M.A. Idri, J.Z. Al-Busaidi, M.S. Al-Balushi, and G.M. Aleemallah. 2019. Immunomodulatory potential of combining some traditional medicinal plants in vivo. *Annals in Microbiology and Immunology* 2: 1–8.

Hemant, K.B., and A. Stephen. 2003. The Himalayas of India: a treasury of medicinal plants under siege. *Biodiversity* 4: 3–13.

Hong, H., J. Kim, T. Lim, Y. Song, C. Cho, and M. Jang. 2018. Mixing ratio optimization for functional complex extracts of *Rhodiola crenulata*, *Panax quinquefolius*, and *Astragalus membranaceus* using mixture design and verification of immune functional efficacy in animal models. *Journal of Functional Foods* 40: 447–454.

Hui, D.S., N. Lee, P.K. Chan, and J.H. Beigel. 2018. The role of adjuvant immunomodulatory agents for treatment of severe influenza. *Antiviral Research* 150: 202–216.

Islam, M.T., E.S. Ali, S.J. Uddin, M.A. Islam, S. Shaw, I.N. Khan, S.S.S. Saravi, S. Ahmad, S. Rehman, V.K. Gupta, and M.A. Găman. 2018. Andrographolide, a diterpene lactone from *Andrographis paniculata* and its therapeutic promises in cancer. *Cancer Letters* 420: 129–145.

Islam, M.T., E.S. Ali, S.J. Uddin, M.A. Islam, S. Shaw, I.N. Khan, S.S.S. Saravi, S. Ahmad, S. Rehman, V.K. Gupta, and M.A. Găman. 2017. Labdane diterpenoids as potential anti-inflammatory agents. *Pharmacology Research* 124: 43–63.

Janifer, R., B. Basant, M. Pal, J.A. Murugan, T.D. Silva, K. Saurav, O.P. Chaurasia, S.B. Singh. 2020. Screening phytochemical constituents of medicinal plants of Trans-Himalayan Region. In: *Medicinal Plants of the Himalayas: Advances and Insights*. Ed. A.M. Husaini. Global Science Books, pp. 88–90.

Jantan, I., W. Ahmad, and S.N.A. Bukhari. 2015. Plant-derived immunomodulators: An insight on their preclinical evaluation and clinical trials. *Frontiers in Plant Science* 25: 655.

Jarić, S., M. Mitrović, and P. Pavlović, 2015. Review of ethnobotanical, phytochemical, and pharmacological study of *Thymus serpyllum* L. *Evidence-based Complementary and Alternative Medicine:eCAM* 101978.

Joshee, N., A. Tascan, F. Medina-Bolivar, R. Parajuli, D. Shannon, and J. Adelberg. 2013. Scutellaria: biotechnology, phytochemistry and its potential as a commercial medicinal crop. 10.1007/978-3-642-29974-2_3.

Joshi R.K., P. Satyal, and W.N. Setzer. 2016. Himalayan aromatic medicinal plants: a review of their ethanopharmacology, volatile phytochemistry, and biological activities. *Medicines* 6: 1–55.

Joshi, M., M. Kumar, W. Rainer, and Bussmann. 2010. *Ethnomedicinal Uses of Plant Resources of the Haigad Watershed in Kumaun Himalaya, India Medicinal Plants of the Himalayas: Advances and Insights*. Global Science Books, UK, 43–46.

Joshi, R.K. 2013. Essential oil of flowers of anaphalis contorta, an aromatic and medicinal plant from India. *Natural Product Communications* 8: 225–226.

Kala, C.P., P.P. Dhyani, and B.S. Sajwan. 2006. Developing the medicinal plants sector in northern India: challenges and opportunities. *Journal of Ethnobiology and Ethnomedicine* 2: 1–15.

Kalra, R., and N. Kaushik. 2017. *Withania somnifera* (Linn.) Dunal: a review of chemical and pharmacological diversity. *Phytochemistry Reviews* 16: 953–987.

Kamboj, A., Saluja, and K. Ajay. 2010. Phytopharmacological review of *Xanthium strumarium* L. (Cocklebur). *International Journal of Green Pharmacy* 4: 129–139.

Kant, R. 2015. Survival threats and conservation of *Malaxis muscifera* (Lindl.) Kuntze, a threatened medicinal orchid at Fagu, Himachal Pradesh. 1.

Khandhar, A., S. Patel, A. Patel, M. Zaveri, and S. Lecturer. 2010. Chemistry and pharmacology of Piper Longum L. *International Journal of Pharmaceutical Sciences Review and Research* 5: 67–76.

Khuroo, A., and G.H. Dar. 2020. Biodiversity of the Himalaya: Jammu and Kashmir State. Doi: 10.1007/978-981-32-9174-4.

Kim, K.H., J. Choi, S. Choi, S.K. Ha, S. Kim, H.L. Park, K. Lee. 2011. The chemical constituents of *Piper kadsura* and their cytotoxic and anti-neuroinflammtaory activities. *Journal of Enzyme Inhibition and Medicinal Chemistry* 26: 254–60.

Konchar, K., X.L. Li, Y.P. Yang, and E. Emshwiller. 2011. Phytochemical variation in *Fritillaria cirrhosa* D. Don (ChuanBei Mu) in relation to plant reproductive stage and timing of harvest. *Economic Botany* 65: 283–294.

Kumar A., A. Choudhary, and H. Kaur. 2020. Diversity of wild medicinal flora in Lahaul valley of Himachal Pradesh. *International Journal of Current Microbiology and Applied Sciences* 9: 48–62.

Kumar, A., A. Paul, G. Singh, and A. Choudhary. 2019. Review on pharmacological profile of medicinal vine: *Tinospora cordifolia. Current Journal of Applied Science and Technology* 35: 1–11.

Kumar A., A. Choudhary, and H. Kaur. 2020. *Podophyllum hexandrum*: the treasure of trans Himalayas. *International Journal of Ecology and Environmental Sciences* 2:191–196.

Mahendra, P., and S. Bisht. 2012. *Ferula asafoetida*: traditional uses and pharmacological activity. *Pharmacogn Reviews* 6: 141–146.

Mehta, S., D. James, and M.K. Reddy. 2019. Omics technologies for abiotic stress tolerance in plants: current status and prospects. In *Recent Approaches in Omics for Plant Resilience to Climate Change* (pp. 1–34). Springer, Cham.

Mohamed, S.I.A., I. Jantan, and M.A. Haque. 2017. Naturally occurring immunomodulators with antitumor activity: an insight on their mechanisms of action. *International Journal of Immunopharmacology* 50: 291–304.

Mohan, R., B. Garige, S. Rao, N. Boggula, A. Chettupalli, V. Kumar, V. Rao, and Bakshi. 2019. Indian medicinal plants used as immunomodulatory agents: a review. *International Journal of Green Pharmacy (IJGP)* 13: 312–318.

Mukhopadhyay, S., S. Banerjee, C. Atal, L.J. Lin, and G. Cordell. 2004. Alkaloids of *Corydalis govaniana* (Berberidaceae). *Journal of Natural Products* 50: 270–272.

Nair, P.K.R., S. Rodriguez, R. Ramachandran, A. Alamo, S.J. Melnick, E. Escalon, P.I. Garcia, J Wnuk, and S.F. Ramachandran. 2004. Immune stimulating properties of a novel polysaccharide from the medicinal plant *Tinospora cordifolia. International Journal of Immunopharmacology* 4: 1645–1659.

Najafian, Y., S.S. Hamedi, M.K. Farshchi, and Z. Feyzabadi. 2018. *Plantago major* in traditional persian medicine and modern phytotherapy: a narrative review. *Electron Physician* 10: 6390–6399.

Namtak, S., and R.C. Sharma. 2018. Medicinal plant resources in Skuru watershed of Karakoram wildlife sanctuary and their uses in traditional medicines system of Ladakh, India. *International Journal of Complementary and Alternative Medicine* 11: 294–302.

Nazar, S., M.A. Hussain, A. Khan, G. Muhammad, and S.N.A. Bukhari. 2020. Alkaloid-rich plant *Tylophora indica*: current trends in isolation strategies, chemical profiling and medicinal applications. *Arabian Journal of Chemistry* 13: 6348–6365.

Nile, S.H., and S.W. Park. 2015. HPTLC densitometry method for simultaneous determination of flavonoids in selected medicinal plants. *Frontiers in Life Science* 8: 97–103.

Niraj, S., and S. Varsha. 2020. A review on scope of immuno-modulatory drugs in Ayurveda for prevention and treatment of Covid-19. *Plant Science Today* 7: 417–423.

Pandith, S., R. Dar, S. Lattoo, M. Shah, and Z. Reshi. 2018. *Rheum australe*, an endangered high-value medicinal herb of North Western Himalayas: a review of its botany, ethnomedical uses, phytochemistry and pharmacology. *Phytochemistry Reviews* 17. 10.1007/s11101-018-9551-7.

Pant, S., and T. Rinchen. 2012. *Dactylorhiza hatagirea*: a high value medicinal orchid. *Journal of Medicinal Plant Research* 6: 3522–3524.

Patil, R., M. Mohan, V. Kasture, and S. Kasture. 2009. *Rubia cordifolia*: a review. *Oriental Pharmacy and Experimental Medicine* 9: 1–13.

Paul, A., A. Kumar, G. Singh, and A. Choudhary. 2018. Medicinal, pharmaceutical and pharmacological properties of *Zanthoxylum armatum*: a review. *Journal of Pharmacognosy and Phytochemistry* 7: 892–900.

Paul, A., A. Kumar, and N. Kaur. 2018. Chemical constituents, therapeutic uses, benefits and side effects of *Bistorta vivipara*: a review. *Plantica* 2: 180–199.

Rai R. 2017. Promising medicinal plants their parts and formulations prevalent in folk medicines among ethnic communities in Madhya Pradesh, *India. Pharmacy and Pharmacology International Journal* 5: 99–106.

Raj, J., O. Chaurasia, P. Bajpai, P. Muthaiah, and S. Bala. 2009. Antioxidative activity and phytochemical investigation on a high altitude medicinal plant *Dracocephalum* heterophyllum Benth. *Pharmacognosy Journal* 1: 246–251.

Rana, M.S., and S.S. Samant. 2011. Diversity, indigenous uses and conservation status of medicinal plants in Manali wildlife sanctuary, north western Himalayas. *Indian journal of traditional knowledge* 10: 439–459.

Rastogi, S., D. Pandey, and R. Singh. 2020. COVID-19 Pandemic: a pragmatic plan for Ayurveda Intervention. *Journal of Ayurveda and Integrative Medicine*. 10.1016/j.jaim.2020.04.002.

Rawat, S., I. Bhatt, R. Rawal, and S. Nandi. 2016. Geographical and environmental variation in chemical constituents and antioxidant properties in *Roscoea procera* Wall. *Journal of Food Biochemistry* 41: e12302.

Riaz, M., N.U. Rahman, M. Zia-Ul-Haq, H.Z.E. Jaar, and R. Manea. 2019. Ginseng: A dietary supplement as immune-modulator in various diseases. *Trends in Food Science and Technology* 83: 12–30.

Ridley, J., A. Wiltshire, and C. Mathison. 2013. More frequent occurrence of westerly disturbances in Karakoram up to 2100. *Science of The Total Environment* 468–469 Supplement: S31–S35.

Rios, J. 2010. Effects of triterpenes on the immune system. *Journal of Ethnopharmacology* 128: 1–14.

Sahu, P., D. Giri, R. Singh, P. Pandey, S. Gupta, A. Shrivastava, A. Kumar, and K. Pandey. 2013. Therapeutic and medicinal uses of *Aloe vera*: a review. *Pharmacology and Pharmacy* 4: 599–610.

Samal, P.K., and P.P. Dhyani. 2006. Indegenous soil-fertility maintenance and insecticides practices in traditional agriculture in Indian central Himalaya: emperical evidence and issues. *Outlook Agriculture* 36:49–56.

Shaheen, S., Y. Bibi, M. Hussain, M. Iqbal, H. Saira, I. Safdar, H. Mehboob, Q. Ain, K. Naseem, and S. Laraib. 2017. A review on *Geranium wallichianum* D-Don Ex-Sweet: an endangered medicinal herb from Himalaya Region. *Medicinal and Aromatic Plants* 6: 288–293.

Sharma, P., M.M.M. Sharma, A. Patra, M. Vashisth, S. Mehta, B. Singh, M. Tiwari, and V. Pandey. 2020. The role of key transcription factors for cold tolerance in plants. In: *Transcription Factors for Abiotic Stress Tolerance in Plants*. Ed. S.H. Wani, Academic Press, pp. 123–152.

Sharma, P., P. Kumar, R. Sharma, G. Gupta, and A. Chaudhary. 2017. Immunomodulators: role of medicinal plants in immune system. *National Journal of Physiology Pharmacy and Pharmacology* 7: 552–556.

Sharma, P.K., N.S. Chauhan, B. Lal, A.M. Husain, and A. Jaime. Conservation of Phytodiversity of Parvati Valley in Northwestern Himalayas of Himachal Pradesh, India (2010) Medicinal Plants of the Himalayas: Advances and Insights. Global Science Books, UK, pp. 47–63.

Singh, L., A. Kumar, and A. Paul. 2018. *Bergenia ciliata*: the medicinal herb of cold desert. *International Journal of Chemical Studies* 6: 3609–3613.

Singh, N., M. Tailang, and S.C. Mehta. 2016. A review on herbal plants as immunomodulators. *International Journal of Pharmacy Science and Research* 7: 3602–3610.

Singh, S.K., and G.S. Rawat. 2000. Flora of Great Himalayan National Park, Himachal Pradesh. In: *The Great Himalayas*. Eds. Singh B., Singh M.P. Jaipal Publications, Dehradun, pp. 105–109.

Smit, H. 2020. *Picrorhiza scrophulariiflora*, from traditional use to immunomodulatory activity.

Sotto, A.D., A. Vitalone, and S.D. Giacom. 2020. Plant-derived nutraceuticals and immune system modulation: an evidence-based overview. *Vaccines* 468: 1–34.

Sourabh, P., J. Thakur, P. Uniyal, and A. Pandey. 2015. Biology of *Lilium polyphyllum* - a threatened medicinal plant. *Medicinal Plants. International Journal of Phytomedicines and Related Industries* 7: 158.

Spelman, K., J. Burns, D. Nichols, N. Winters, S. Ottersberg, and M. Tenborg. 2006. Modulation of cytokine expression by traditional medicines: a review of herbal immunomodulators. *Alternate Medicinal Reviews* 11: 128–150.

Sun, Y.; S. Chen, R. Wei, X. Xei, C. Wang, S. Fan, X. Zhang, J. Su, J. Liu, and W. Jia. 2018. Metabolome and gut microbiota variation with long-term intake of *Panax ginseng* extracts on rats. *Food Functions* 9: 3547–3556.

Surya, M.I., S. Suhartati, and L. Ismaini. 2017. Fruit nutrients of five species of wild Raspberries (Rubus spp.) from Indonesian Mountain's Forests. *Journal of Tropical Life Science* 8: 75–80.

Thangadurai, K., R. Savitha, S. Rengasundari, K. Suresh, and V. Banumathi. 2018. Immunomodulatory action of traditional herbs for the management of acquired immunodeficiency syndrome: a review. *International Journal of Herbal Medicine* 6: 10–14.

Tripathi, R., A. Kumar, S. Kumar, S. Prakash, and A. Singh. 2019. *Ficus benghalensis* Linn.: a tribal medicine with vast commercial potential. *Indian Journal of Agriculture and Allied Sciences* 2015: 95–102.

Utami, S.H., R. Dwi, Y.S. Ria, D.F. Rizka, and M.A. Putri. 2018. Antimicrobial activity of endophytic fungi isolated from a medicinal plant, *Hedychium acuminatum* Roscoe. *AIP Conference Proceedings*, 050002.

Verma, S. 2011. Therapeutic uses of *Withania somnifera* (Ashwagandha) with a note on withanolides and its pharmacological actions. *Asian Journal of Pharmaceutical and Clinical Research* 4: 1.

Villinger, F. 2003. Cytokines as clinical adjuvants: how far are we?. *Expert Review of Vaccines* 2: 317–326.

Viste, E., and A. Sorteberg. 2015. Snowfall in the Himalayas: an uncertain future from alittle-known past. *The Cryosphere* 9: 1147–1167.

Wangchuk, P., H. Simon, J. Michael, P.L. Groves, A. Loukas, and D.L. Doolan. 2018. Defined small molecules produced by himalayan medicinal plants display immunomodulatory properties. *International Journal of Molecular Science* 19: 1–21.

Wani, P., K. Ganaie, A. Irshad, Nawchoo, and B.A. Wafai. 2006. Phenological Episodes and Reproductive Strategies of *Inula racemosa* (Asteraceae)-a Critically Endangered Medicinal Herb of North West Himalaya. *International Journal of Botany* 2: 388–394.

Wu, J.Y., Q.X. Zhang, and P.O. Leung. 2007. Inhibitory effect of ethyl acetate extract of *Cordyceps sinensis* mycelium on various cancer cells in culture and B16 melanoma in C57BL/6 mice. *Phytomedicine* 14: 43–49.

Yadav, R., R.K. Khare, and A. Singhal. 2017. Qualitative phytochemical screening of some selected medicinal plants of shivpuri district (mp). *The International Journal of Life Sciences Scientific Research* 3: 844–847.

Zheng, Y., W. Ren, L. Zhang, Y. Zhang, D. Liu, and Y. Liu. 2020. A review of the pharmacological action of *Astragalus* polysaccharide. *Frontiers in Pharmacology* 11: 349.

9 Traditional South Indian Herbal Plants for a Strong Immune System

Mani Divya and Sekar Vijayakumar

CONTENTS

9.1 INTRODUCTION

In recent times, the World Health Organization (WHO) estimated that approximately 80% of people globally depended on herbal medicines for primary health care requirements (WHO 1993). Approximately 21,000 plant species have potential for use as medicinal plants. The use of plants is mankind's oldest approach to health care. Herbal remedies are occasionally called traditional medicines. Various herbal plants which are recognized in the traditional structure of medicine contain a large number of pharmacologically active chemicals bioactives (Ford and Roach, 2009). In the period of globalization, health-conscious individuals around the world began to emphasize the use of medicinal herbs of Indian origin (Sarkar et al. 2015). Increasingly, herbal plants have gained a good reputation as a result largely of the work of local traditional herbal practitioners. It is noteworthy to point out here that the majority of the Indian herbal plants are found throughout South India (Rajan et al. 2005). In light of the significance of traditional herbal medicinal plants of southern India as a resource to fight against infectious diseases, there is the likelihood that some function by stimulating the immune response of the host. As a consequence, plant extracts used in traditional herbal remedies should be assessed for immunomodulatory activities (Upadhyay, 1997).

DOI: 10.1201/9781003137955-9

The basic structural design of the immune system is multifaceted, with fortifications at several different stages (Kumar et al. 2012). If pathogens have effectively entered the body of the host, then they are faced with the rapid but short-lived non-specific innate immune response or the slower-acting but longer-lasting specific adaptive immune response (Hofmeyr, 2001). It should be obvious that there are many healing plants that make use of immunomodulatory activity. The range of phytochemicals in herbal formulations may lead to a cooperative effect in achieving greater defence through inducing both innate and adaptive immunities, with both defensive antibodies and the development of effective cell-mediated immune responses (Vimalanathan et al. 2009). There are a large number of herbal products with prospective therapeutic applications because of their high effectiveness, low cost, and low toxicity. Such herbal formulations may consequently be recommended as a positive immunomodulator. The exhibition of increased immunity by the use of herbal plants and their extracts or derivatives shows potential as a promising health care strategy for the future (Singh et al. 2016).

9.2   HERBAL PLANTS

'Herbs' refer to the use of some or all parts of the plant, such as seed, bark, stem, leaf, stigma, flower, fruit, root, or whole plant. Over the past two decades, there has been a marked increase in the use of herbal medicines. Consequently, since 1999, WHO has published three volumes of monographs on herbal plants (http://WHO). Treatment with preparations of confirmed medicinal herbs increases the resistance of the patient to disease and other conditions. Plant-based herbal therapies are potent, with low toxicity and low cost, and are accessible to the local community. Problems of traditional herbal medications are often associated with the presence of natural or man-made contaminants, which may result in poor response by the patient and even death (van Wyk and Prinsloo, 2020). Studies on traditional healing plants have turned out to be even more valuable with respect to the expansion of healthcare programmes throughout the world (Shil et al. 2014). Traditional medicine systems are based on plant-derived bioactive molecules with pharmaceutical activities (Rehechoa et al. 2011). Treatment of some diseases by means of herbal plant preparations is considered to be superior to conventional medicines because of the negligible side effects. Medicinal herbs can show therapeutic superiority over conventional single-compound medicines, especially with respect to hard-to-treat or chronic diseases. Numerous modern pharmaceutical drugs are derived in some way from phytochemicals. The use of conventional herbal medicines occurs predominantly in developing countries (UNESCO, 1996), though their adoption in the developed countries is increasing markedly. Current estimates list more than 9,000 plants with recognized therapeutic relevance in different traditions and countries.

9.3   IMMUNE SYSTEM

In recent times, there has been steady progress in our understanding of the immune system, and its ability to defend the body from infection, identifying each phase of

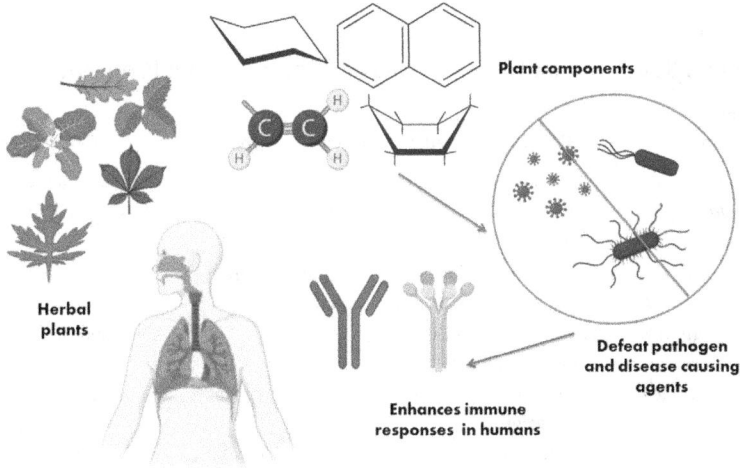

FIGURE 9.1 Traditional herbal plants which suppress disease-causing pathogens and stimulate the human immune system.

immunology (Murphy et al. 2007). The immune system involves a network of genes, molecules, cells, and pathways to defend the membrane, intestinal tract, respiratory channel, and other parts from antigens from the attacker (Figure 9.1).

The innate and adaptive immune systems are expressed *via* different pathways, though they typically perform as one. The innate reaction reflects the initial barrier of the host defence, with the adaptive immune reaction peaking later, by which time antigen-specific T and B cells have undergone clonal extension (Huston, 1997). The innate immune system uses receptors that are encoded by intact genes inherited through the germline, whereas the adaptive immune system uses antigen receptors encoded by genes that are assembled from individual gene segments during lymphocyte development, a process that leads to each individual cell expressing a receptor of unique specificity (Holmskov et al. 2003). A major problem faced with the immune classification involves recognition of host cells that have been contaminated by microorganisms (Chaplin, 2010). Innate and adaptive immunities are not reciprocally elite methods of host defence, although they can quite harmonize together. Innate immunity is the initial immunological, non-specific means for defending against a pathogen (Turvey and Broide, 2010). This resistant reaction is rapid and is carried out between numerous cells, including eosinophils, phagocytes, basophils, and the complement system. Adaptive immunity expands through innate immunity to eradicate transferable agents (Bonilla and Oettgen, 2010).

9.4 TRADITIONAL SOUTH INDIAN HERBAL PLANTS AND THE IMMUNE SYSTEM

Some of the important traditional herbal plants distributed within India, and particularly in India, are listed in Table 9.1. The plants are recognized to exhibit several

TABLE 9.1

Traditional South Indian Herbal Plants and their Healing Properties

South Indian Herbal Plant	Diseases Treated and Activities Exhibited	References
Andrographis paniculata	Anti-inflammatory, immunostimulant, antiparasitic, hepatoprotective, antihyperglycaemic and antihypoglycaemic	Sagadevan and Suresh, (2015)
Acalypha indica	Anthelmintic, antibacterial, anti-ulcer, to treat wounds, asthma, and bronchitis	Zahidin et al. (2017)
Cassia auriculata	Anti-tumour, anti-diabetic, and immunomodulatory	Chakraborthy, (2009)
Calotropis gigantea	Antifertility, vermicidal activity, and pregnancy interceptive	Kumar et al. (2013)
Cardiospermum halicacabum	Immunomodulatory and anti-arthritic activities	Saravandaa et al. (2018)
Catharanthus roseus	Anti-helmintic, pesticidal, and antidiabetic activities	Kaushik et al. (2017)
Cynodon dactylon	Immunomodulatory effects	Mangathayan et al. (2009)
Datura metel	Antimicrobial, antipyretic, anti-asthmatic, analgesic, and nephroprotective activities	Alam et al. (2020)
Euphorbia susanholmesiae	To treat skin cancer and actinic keratosis	Ernst et al. (2015)
Gloriosa superba	Antidote for snake bite, as a laxative, to treat ulcers, arthritis, cholera, colic, kidney problems, and typhus	Zahir et al. (2012); Kavithamani et al. (2013)
Lufa acutangula	Immunomodulatory, analgesic, and gastroprotective effects	Al- Snafi, (2019)
Lyngodium flexuosum	Jaundice, wound healing, and eczema	Esha et al. (2011)
Morinda pubescens	Antimicrobial activity	Ravikumar et al. (2012); Tyagi et al. (2015)
Myrtus communis	Immunostimulant	Taee et al. (2017)
Opuntia ficus-indica	Anti-inflammatory and hypoglycaemic effects, delay of stomach ulceration, and neuroprotective effects	Kaur et al. (2012)
Phyllanthus emblica	Antiviral, antimicrobial, anticancer, hepatoprotective, and antidiabetic properties	Khan (2009)
Phyllanthus niruri	Antispasmodic, analgesic, anticonvulsant, aphrodisiac, and contraceptive activities	Kamruzzaman and Hoq (2016);
Physalis angulata	Antitumour and immunomodulatory effects	Chiang et al. (1992); Lin et al. (1992)
Piper longum	To treat cough, stomach-ache, diseases of the spleen, bronchitis, and tumours	Kumar et al. (2011)
Ruellia tuberose	To treat stomach cancer, gonorrhoea, and bladder diseases	Chothani et al. (2010)

(Continued)

TABLE 9.1 (CONTINUED)
Traditional South Indian Herbal Plants and their Healing Properties

South Indian Herbal Plant	Diseases Treated and Activities Exhibited	References
Thevetia peruviana	Larvicidal, antidiabetic, antifertility, antimicrobial, and anticancer properties	Ahmad et al. (2017)
Tridax procumbens	Immunomodulatory effects	Tiwari et al. (2004)
Vitex negundo	Anti-inflammatory and antioxidant activities	Utpalendu et al. (1999); Tiwari (2007)
Withania somnifera	Chemopreventive, used to treat Alzheimer's disease and Parkinson's disease, as a memory enhancer and an immunomodulator	Umadevi et al. (2012)

activities which enables them to treat human diseases, including stimulation of the immune system (Nath et al. 2011). The goal of this study was to screen the methanol or acetone extracts of four plant species from South India for antileishmanial activity. This provided the primary details on the *in-vitro* activity of certain plants towards the intracellular human parasite *Leishmania donovani*. The effectiveness of the effective herbal plants will be further explored extensively with regard to a number of activities, because it is obligatory to follow up these findings with pharmacological and phytochemical analysis of the traditional herbal plants. The major focus of these traditional herbal plants on the immune system highlights the need to evaluate the potential of South Indian herbal plants to offset the side effects of modern therapies by stimulating the immune systems of the host.

9.4.1 MEDICINAL VALUE OF HERBAL PLANTS

Medicinal plants have been used since ancient times to treat a wide range of diseases, ailments and conditions. Herbal medicinal plants are gaining a positive reputation among individuals in both urban and rural areas (Katic, 1980). The most famous author on plant drugs was Dioscorides, "the father of pharmacognosy," who, as an army doctor and pharmacognosist with Nero's army, studied medicinal plants everywhere he travelled with the Roman Army (Nikolovski, 1961). Subsequently, as society and cultures evolved, the curative properties of confirmed herbal plants were noted, recognized, and directed towards the appropriate age group (Petrovska, 2012).

The significance of the contribution of herbal plants to human health cannot be overestimated. These plants contain curative phytochemicals in individual organs or in several of them. The use of these plants is increasing globally in terms of the expansion of established medicine and the increasing interest in herbal medicine. Plants are used as a source of natural drugs to sustain and expand the patient's physical and mental condition (Idu, 2009). For instance, the use of herbal medicine to treat

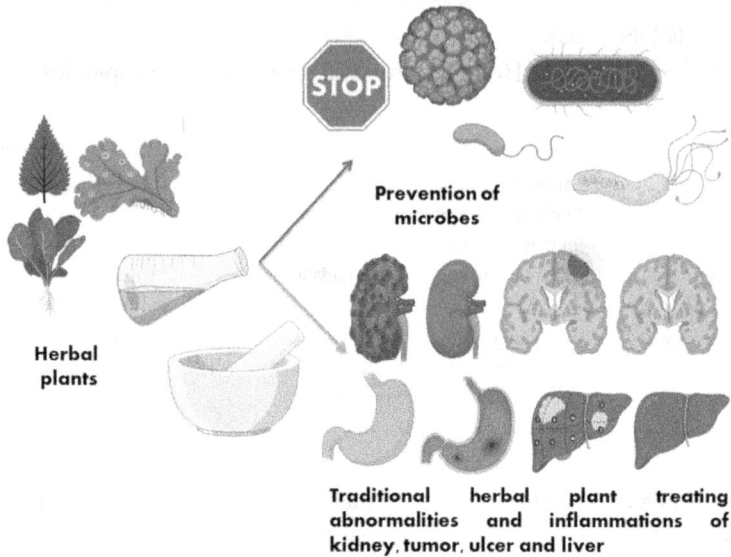

FIGURE 9.2 Herbal plants which helps to inhibit the pathogen and combat several diseases.

diseases related to asthma, cancer, neurological and hepatic diseases is estimated to be approximately 80%, 55%, 42%, and 90% of people, respectively (Al-Moamary, 2008; Jazieh et al. 2012; Mohammad et al. 2015) (Figure 9.2). Each part of the medicinal plant possesses healing properties, including activities, such as anti-inflammatory, anti-insecticidal, antioxidant, antibiotic, antiparasitic, and antihaemolytic properties, and so on (Neelam Bamola et al. 2018). The medicinal value of plants lies in their secondary plant metabolites for treatment of numerous illnesses (Modak et al. 2007).

Phytochemicals are pharmacologically active compounds of several different types: terpenoids, which are recognized for their antihelmintic, antiviral, anticancer, antibacterial, anti-inflammatory, and antimalarial properties; alkaloids, which have antispasmodic, analgesic, antimalarial, and diuretic activities; and phenolics and flavonoids, which have antioxidant, antibacterial, and antiallergic properties (Maurya et al. 2008). In addition, saponins (a type of terpenoid) are known to exhibit anti-inflammatory, antiviral, and plant defence activities, whereas glycosides of other groups of secondary metabolites can show antifungal and antibacterial properties (Chopra et al. 2002). Thus, traditional knowledge of herbal plants assists the pharmaceutical industries in developing novel drugs and to employ them to achieve the treatment of different diseases (Forouzan et al. 2012; Bahmani et al. 2013; Divya et al. 2020).

9.5 CONCLUSION

As our way of life becomes increasingly dominated by technology, we are becoming more widely separated from the natural world. As herbs are natural products, their availability is reasonably secure, recyclable, and accessible. By tradition, there are groups of herbs used for treating particular disorders during a specific season of the year. Herbs had been exploited for flavouring, medicinal, and scented characteristics for centuries, but the synthetic chemicals used for the same ends in the modern age have become predominant. This chapter deals only with the traditional knowledge of medicinal plants from the South Indian region, as directly related to medicinal research with respect to the practice of traditional medicines in that region as well as in neighbouring areas. To conclude, this book chapter focuses on a range of natural traditional herbal medicines to stimulate the immune system of humans. This also emphasizes the progress achieved in medicinal innovation dealing with the medicinal plants of South India, with a number of suggestions, recommendations, and future goals for this aspect of herbal medicine.

ACKNOWLEDGEMENTS

The corresponding author, Dr. Sekar Vijayakumar, is grateful to Shandong University, Weihai, P.R. China, for providing a post-doctoral research fellowship.

REFERENCES

Ahmad, T., A.T. Hamid, A. Sharma, U. Bhardwaj. 2017. *Thevetia peruviana*: a multipurpose medicinal plant. *International Journal of Advanced Research* 8:486–93.

Alam, W., H. Khan, S.A. Khan, S. Nazir, E.K. Akkol. Datura metel: 2020. A review on chemical constituents, traditional uses and pharmacological activities. *Current Pharmaceutical Design*.

Al Moamary, M.S. 2008. Unconventional therapy use among asthma patients in a tertiary care center in Riyadh, Saudi Arabia. *Annals of Thoracic Medicine* 3(2):48.

Al-Snafi, AE. 2019. A review on *Luffa acutangula*: a potential medicinal plant. *Magnesium* 52:53.

Bahmani, M., H. Golshahi, A. Mohsenzadegan, M.G. Ahangarani, E. Ghasemi. 2013. Comparative assessment of the anti-Limnatis nilotica activities of *Zingiber officinale* methanolic extract with levamisole. *Comparative Clinical Pathology* 22(4):667–70.

Bamola, N., P. Verma, C. Negi. 2018. A review on some traditional medicinal plants. *International Journal of Life-Sciences Scientific Research* 4(1):1550–6.

Bonilla, F.A., H.C. Oettgen. 2010. Adaptive immunity. *Journal of Allergy and Clinical Immunology*. 125(2):S33–40.

Chakraborthy, GS. 2009. Evaluation of immunomodulatory activity of *Cassia auriculata* Linn. *Journal of Herbal Medicine and Toxicology* 3(2):111–3.

Chaplin, D.D. 2010. Overview of the immune response. *Journal of Allergy in Clinical Immunology* 125 Supplement 2: S3–23.

Chiang, H.C., S.M. Jaw, C.F. Chen, W.S. Kan. 1992. Antitumor agent, physalin F from *Physalis angulata* L. *Anticancer Research* 12(3):837–43.

Chopra, A., V. Doiphode. 2002. Ayurvedic medicine: core concept, therapeutic principles and current relevance. *Medical Clinics of North America* 86:75–89.

Chothani, D.L., M.B. Patel, S.H. Mishra, H.U. Vaghasiya. 2010. Review on *Ruellia tuberosa* (Cracker plant). *Pharmacognosy Journal* 2(12):506–12.

Divya, M., S. Vijayakumar, J. Chen, B. Vaseeharan, E.F. Durán-Lara. 2020. South Indian medicinal plants can combat deadly viruses along with COVID-19? - a review. *Microbial Pathogenesis* 28:104277.

Esha, Y., M. Munesh. 2011. Pharmacognostic and phytochemical investigation on the leaves of *Lygodium flexuosum* Linn. *International Journal of Research in Ayurveda and Pharmacy* 2(5):1588–92.

Ernst, M., O.M. Grace, C.H. Saslis-Lagoudakis, N. Nilsson, H.T. Simonsen, N. Rønsted. 2015. Global medicinal uses of *Euphorbia* L.(Euphorbiaceae). *Journal of Ethnopharmacology* 176:90–101.

Ford, M.S., and S.S. Roach. 2009. *Introductory Clinical Pharmacology*. 27th ed. USA: Lippincott Williams and Wilkins; 567–568.

Forouzan, S., M. Bahmani, P. Parsaei, A. Mohsenzadegan, M. Gholami Ahangaran, E. Sadeghi, K. Saki, M. Delirrad. 2012. Anti-parasitic activites of *Zingiber officinale* methanolic extract on *Limnatis nilotica*. *Global Veterinaria* 9(2):144–8.

Hemapriya, V.S., S.M. Logambal, R.D. Michael. 1997. Immunostimulation by leaf extracts of a few south Indian medicinal plants in *Oreochromis mossambicus* (Peters). *Developmental and Comparative Immunology* 2(21):175.

Hofmeyr, S.A. 2001. An interpretative introduction to the immune system. In: Cohen I, Segel L, editors. Design principles for the immune system and other distributed autonomous systems. NY, USA: Oxford University Press, Inc; pp. 3–24.

Holmskov, U., S. Thiel, J.C. Jensenius. 2003. Collectins and ficolins: humoral lectins of the innate immune defense. *Annual Review of Immunology* 21:547–578. http://www.who.int/medicines/areas/traditional/SelectMonoVol4.pdf

Huston, D.P. 1997. The biology of the immune system. *Journal of American Medical Association* 278:1804–1814.

Idu, M. 2009. The plant called medicine: the 104th Inaugural Lecture Series of University of Benin City, Nigeria: Calameo.

Jazieh, A.R., R. Al Sudairy, O. Abulkhair, A. Alaskar, F. Al Safi, N. Sheblaq. 2012. Young S, Issa M, Tamim H. Use of complementary and alternative medicine by patients with cancer in Saudi Arabia. *The Journal of Alternative and Complementary Medicine* 18(11):1045–9.

Kamruzzaman, H.M., O. Hoq. 2016. A review on ethnomedicinal, phytochemical and pharmacological properties of *Phyllanthus niruri*. *Journal of Medicinal Plants Studies* 4(6):173–80.

Katic, R. 1980. In: The Chilandar medical codex N. 517. Milincevic V., editor. Beograd: National library from Srbija; pp. 9–80.

Kaur, M., A. Kaur, R. Sharma. 2012. Pharmacological actions of *Opuntia ficus indica*: a review. *Journal of Applied Pharmaceutical Science* 2(7):15–8.

Kaushik, S.H., R.S. Tomar, M. Gupta, R.K. Mishra. 2017. An overview of *Catharanthus roseus* and medicinal properties of their metabolites against important diseases. *European Academic Research* 2:123–47.

Kavithamani, D., M. Umadevi, S. Geetha. 2013. A review on *Gloriosa superba* L as a medicinal plant. *Indian Journal of Research in Pharmacy and Biotechnology* 1(4):554.

Khan, K.H. 2009. Roles of *Emblica officinalis* in medicine - a review. *Botany Research International* 2(4):218–228.

Kumar, D., V. Arya, R. Kaur, Z.A. Bhat, V.K. Gupta, V. Kumar. 2012. A review of immunomodulators in the Indian traditional health care system. *Journal of Microbiology, Immunology and Infection* 45(3):165–84.

Kumar, P.S., E. Suresh, S. Kalavathy. 2013. Review on a potential herb *Calotropis gigantea (L.) R. Br. Scholars Academic Journal of Pharmacy* 2(2):135–43.

Kumar, S., J. Kamboj, Suman, S. Sharma. 2011. Overview for various aspects of the health benefits of *Piper longum* linn. fruit. *Journal of Acupuncture Meridian Studies* 4(2):134–40.

Lin, Y.S., H.C. Chiang, W.S. Kan, E. Hone, S.J. Shih, M.H. Won. 1992. Immunomodulatory activity of various fractions derived from *Physalis angulata* L extract. *The American Journal of Chinese Medicine* 20(03n04):233–43.

Mangathayaru, K., M. Umadevi, C.U. Reddy. 2009. Evaluation of the immunomodulatory and DNA protective activities of the shoots of *Cynodon dactylon*. *Journal of Ethnopharmacology* 123(1):181–4.

Maurya, R., G. Singh, P.P. Yadav. 2008. Antiosteoporotic agents from natural sources. In: Atta-ur-Rahman (Ed.) *Studies in Natural Products Chemistry* 35:517–545.

Modak, M., P. Dixit, J. Londhe, S. Ghaskadbi, T. Paul, A. Devasagayam. 2007. Indian herbs and herbal drugs used for the treatment of diabetes. *Journal of Clinical Biochemistry & Nutrition* 40(3):163–173.

Mohammad, Y., A. Al-Ahmari, F. Al-Dashash, F. Al-Hussain, F. Al-Masnour, A. Masoud, H. Jradi. 2015. Pattern of traditional medicine use by adult Saudi patients with neurological disorders. *BMC Complementary and Alternative Medicine* 15(1):102.

Murphy, K.M., P. Travers, M. Walport. 2007. *Janeway's Immunobiology*. 7th ed. New York: Garland Science.

Nath, S., D.C. Manabendra, R.C. Shubhadeep, A.T. Das, A.V. Sirotkin, B. Zuzana, A. Kádasi, M. Nora, K. Adriana. 2011. Restorative aspect of castor plant on mammalian physiology: a review. *Journal of Microbiology, Biotechnology and Food Sciences* 1: 236–246.

Nikolovski, B. 1961. Arab pharmacy in Macedonia. Bulletin 1:20–7.

Petrovska, B.B. 2012. Historical review of medicinal plants' usage. *Pharmacognosy Reviews* 6(11):1.

Rajan, S., M. Jayendran, M. Sethuraman. 2005. Folk herbal practices among Toda tribe of the Nilgiri Hills in Tamil Nadu, India. *Journal of Natural Remedies* 5(1):52–8.

Ravikumar, S., S.J. Inbaneson, P. Suganthi. 2012. In vitro antiplasmodial activity of ethanolic extracts of South Indian medicinal plants against *Plasmodium falciparum*. *Asian Pacific Journal of Tropical Disease*. 2(3):180–3.

Rehecho, S., I. Uriarte-Pueyo, J. Calvo, L.A. Vivas, M.I. Calvo. 2011. Ethnopharmacological survey of medicinal plants in Nor-Yauyos, a part of the Landscape Reserve Nor-Yauyos-Cochas, Peru. *Journal of Ethnopharmacology* 133(1):75–85.

Sagadevan, P., S.N. Suresh. 2015. In vitro antifungal and anticancer efficacy of methanolic leaf extract of *Andrographis paniculata* (nees). *Internatonal Journal of Pharm Tech Research* 7(1):148–55.

Sarvanandaa, L., A.D. Premarathna, S.C. Karunarathnad. 2018. Immunomodulatory effect of *Cardiospermum Halicacabum* against cancer. *Biomedical Journal* 1:4.

Sarkar, P., L.K. DH, C. Dhumal, S.S. Panigrahi, R. Choudhary. 2015. Traditional and ayurvedic foods of Indian origin. *Journal of Ethnic Foods* 2(3): 97–109.

Shil, S., M.D. Choudhury, S. Das. 2014. Indigenous knowledge of medicinal plants used by the Reang tribe of Tripura state of India. *Journal of Ethnopharmacology* 152(1):135–41.

Singh, N., M. Tailang, S.C. Mehta. 2016. A review on herbal plants as immunomodulators. *International Journal of Pharmaceutical Sciences and Research* 7(9):3602.

Taee, H.M., A. Hajimoradloo, S.H. Hoseinifar, H. Ahmadvand. 2017. Dietary Myrtle (*Myrtus communis* L.) improved non-specific immune parameters and bactericidal activity of skin mucus in rainbow trout (*Oncorhynchus mykiss*) fingerlings. *Fish & Shellfish Immunology* 64:320–4.

Tiwari, U., B. Rastogi, P. Singh, D.K. Saraf, S.P. Vyas. 2004. Immunomodulatory effects of aqueous extract of *Tridax procumbens* in experimental animals. *Journal of Ethnopharmacology* 92(1):113–9.

Tiwari, O.P., Y.B. Tripathi. 2007. Antioxidant properties of different fractions of *Vitex negundo* Linn. *Food Chemistry* 100(3):1170–6.

Turvey, S.E., D.H. Broide. 2010. Innate immunity. *Journal of Allergy in Clinical Immunology* 125(Suppl 2):S24–32.

Tyagi, B.K., R.K. Goyal, P. Chauhan. 2015. *Morinda pubescens* bark extracts shows antimicrobial activity. *International Journal of Pharmaceutical Sciences and Research.* 6(1):345.

Umadevi, M., R. Rajeswari, C. Sharmila Rahale, S. Selvavenkadesh, R. Pushpa, K.P. Sampath, et al. 2012. Traditional and medicinal uses of *Withania somnifera. The Pharma Innovation* 1(9):102–110.

UNESCO. Culture and Health, Orientation Texts – World Decade for Cultural Development 1988 – 1997, Document CLT/DEC/PRO – 1996, Paris, France, pgs. 129,1996.

Upadhyay, S.N., "Plant products as immune response modulators". In: *Proceedings of the International ayurveda conference, Sanjay Gandhi post graduate institute of medical sciences,* Lucknow. 1997, pp. 10

Utpalendu, J., R.N. Chattopadhyay, P.S. Badri. 1999. Preliminary studies on anti-inflammatory activity of *Zingiber officinale* Rosc., *Vitex negundo* Linn and *Tinospora cordifolia* (willid) Miers in albino rats. *Indian journal of pharmacology* 31(3):232.

Vimalanathan S, S. Ignacimuthu, J.B. Hudson. 2009. Medicinal plants of Tamil Nadu (Southern India) are a rich source of antiviral activities. *Pharmaceutical Biology* 47(5):422–9.

van Wyk, A.S., G. Prinsloo. 2020. Health, safety and quality concerns of plant-based traditional medicines and herbal remedies. *South African Journal of Botany* 133:54–62.

WHO. 1993. *Research Guidelines for Evaluating the Safety and Efficacy of Herbal Medicines.* Manila.

Zahir, A.A., A.A. Rahuman, S. Pakrashi, D. Ghosh, A. Bagavan, C. Kamaraj, G. Elango, M. Chatterjee. 2012. Evaluation of antileishmanial activity of South Indian medicinal plants against *Leishmania donovani. Experimental parasitology* 132(2):180–4.

Zahidin, N.S., S. Saidin, R.M. Zulkifli, et al. 2017. A review of *Acalypha indica* L. (Euphorbiaceae) as traditional medicinal plant and its therapeutic potential. *Journal of Ethnopharmacology* 207:146–173.

10 Sacred Medicinal Plants and their Use by Indigenous People for Strengthening the Immune System

Jamal Akhtar and Fouzia Bashir

CONTENTS

DOI: 10.1201/9781003137955-10

10.1 INTRODUCTION

India, the second most heavily populated country in the world, with twenty-eight states and eight Union territories, is also one of the most diverse nations in the world in terms of religions and cultures. Religion plays a vital and absolute role in the life of many of its people. Although India is a secular country, it has several different religions, i.e., Hindus, Muslims, Christians, Sikhs, Buddhists, Jains, and various tribal populations in India. According to the census of India (2011), the Indian population comprises 79.80% Hindus, 14.23% Muslims, 2.3% Christians, 1.72% Sikhs, 0.70% Buddhists, 0.4% Jains, and 0.9% others (Anonymous 2004). Every religion has their 'Sacred' books and places, which demand deep respect and are 'set aside' for purposes of the spiritual or religious.

In the Qur'an, the holy book of Muslims, many plants, like Teen (*Ficus carica*), Zaitoon (*Olea europaea*), Khurma (*Phoenix dactylifera*), Munaqqa (*Vitis vinifera*), Anar (*Punica granatum*), Kafoor (*Cinnamomum camphora*), Ber (*Zizyphus jujuba*), Mauz (*Musa paradisiaca*), and Kalonji (*Nigella sativa*), etc., are quoted as being part of a diet for the preservation of health and the management of diseases. According to Vedas in Hindu mythology, various 'Sacred' plants are described for improving health and for curing diseases, such as Tulsi (*Ocimum sanctum*), Peepal (*Ficus religiosa*), Bael (*Aegle marmelos*), Neem (*Azadirachta indica*), Sandal (*Santalum album*), Bhang (*Cannabis sativa*), and Ashok (*Saraca asoca*), etc. Similarly, in the Bible, the holy book of Christians, Teen (*Ficus carica*), Nard/Sumbul-ut-Teeb

(*Nardostachys jatamansi*), Zoofa (*Hyssopus officinalis*), Foful (*Areca catechu*), and Nilofar (*Nymphaea alba*), etc. are mentioned for the maintenance of health.

These medicinal plants have been given so much importance for health maintenance that people even worship them, an act which attracted scientists from different fields, namely botanists, pharmacologists, biochemists, and pharmacognosists, to determine the science behind these sacred medicinal plants. They tried to identify the active ingredients and the molecular mechanisms between these phytochemicals and health issues, which not only cause the health benefits and health-promoting effects but which are also used in the management of diseases. This chapter highlights some of the readily accessible sacred plants mentioned in the holy Qur'an/Ahadith and other religious books to identify established immunomodulatory and other medicinal effects.

10.2 PLANTS MENTIONED IN SACRED BOOKS

The sacred book of Islam, the Qur'an, is the Word of God, as it was revealed to Prophet Muhammad (PBUH). With its unique composition and style, the Qur'an is also considered to be the pre-eminent literary masterpiece of the Arabic language. Its contents provide the basics of the doctrinal tenets and principles of Islam. The Qur'an comprises 6,236 verses (ayahs) which are divided into 114 chapters or surahs, each of which takes its name from a prominent event, theme, or topic relevant to the chapter. A report of the sayings or actions of Muhammad or his companions, together with the tradition of its chain of transmission, is called Ahadith.

The Hindu sacred text has been divided into the revealed and the remembered texts, and the original language of the early Hindu sacred books is Sanskrit. The revealed texts are found in the Veda, which may be divided into four parts, the Rig Veda, the Yajur Veda, the Sama Veda, and the Atharva Veda, while the remembered texts consist of post-Vedic texts, including two epics, the Mahabharata and the Ramayana; the Bhagavad Gita, based on the god Krishna, a script inserted into the Mahabharata, and the Dharam sastras based on dharma. The Bible for Christians, the Guru Granth Sahib for the Sikhs, the Tipitaka for the Buddhists, and the Agam Sutras for the Jains are the sacred books of different religions practised in India.

In Islam, according to the Qu'ran and Ahadith, the importance of various plants is mentioned, e.g., Teen (*Ficus carica*), Zaitoon (*Olea europoea*), Khurma (*Phoenix dactylifera*), Maweez (*Vitis vinifera*), Anar/Rumman (*Punica granatum*), Balsan (*Ocimum basilicum*), Kafoor (*Cinnamomum camphora*), Miswak (*Salvadora persica*), Khardal (*Brassica nigra*), Ber (*Zizyphus jujuba* Lam.), Hanzal (*Citrulus colocynthis*), Mauz (*Musa paradisiaca*), and Kalonji (*Nigella sativa*).

The Qur'anic verses which contain description of plants and their parts are to inspire people to think about Allah's creation and to aid them to reach a level of faith based on conviction. These verses also remind people of Allah's blessings and the need to thank Him for what He has offered them.

وَمِن ثَمَرَٰتِ ٱلنَّخِيلِ وَٱلۡأَعۡنَٰبِ تَتَّخِذُونَ مِنۡهُ سَكَرًا وَرِزۡقًا حَسَنًا إِنَّ فِى ذَٰلِكَ لَءَايَةً لِّقَوۡمٖ

يَعۡقِلُونَ ﴿٦٧﴾

'And from the fruits of the palm trees and grapevines you take intoxicant and good provision. Indeed, in that is a sign for a people who reason'. (Qur'anic Verse, 16:67)

وَٱلتِّينِ وَٱلزَّيْتُونِ ﴿١﴾

'By the fig and the olive' (Qur'anic Verse, 95:1)

وَإِذْ قُلْتُمْ يَٰمُوسَىٰ لَن نَّصْبِرَ عَلَىٰ طَعَامٍ وَٰحِدٍ فَٱدْعُ لَنَا رَبَّكَ يُخْرِجْ لَنَا مِمَّا تُنۢبِتُ ٱلْأَرْضُ مِنۢ بَقْلِهَا وَقِثَّآئِهَا وَفُومِهَا وَعَدَسِهَا وَبَصَلِهَا قَالَ أَتَسْتَبْدِلُونَ ٱلَّذِى هُوَ أَدْنَىٰ بِٱلَّذِى هُوَ خَيْرٌ ٱهْبِطُواْ مِصْرًا فَإِنَّ لَكُم مَّا سَأَلْتُمْ وَضُرِبَتْ عَلَيْهِمُ ٱلذِّلَّةُ وَٱلْمَسْكَنَةُ وَبَآءُو بِغَضَبٍ مِّنَ ٱللَّهِ ذَٰلِكَ بِأَنَّهُمْ كَانُواْ يَكْفُرُونَ بِـَٔايَٰتِ ٱللَّهِ وَيَقْتُلُونَ ٱلنَّبِيِّـۧنَ بِغَيْرِ ٱلْحَقِّ ذَٰلِكَ بِمَا عَصَواْ وَّكَانُواْ يَعْتَدُونَ ﴿٦١﴾

'And [recall] when you said, "O Moses, we can never endure one [kind of] food. So, call upon your Lord to bring forth for us from the earth its green herbs and its cucumbers and its garlic and its lentils and its onions". [Moses] said, "Would you exchange what is better for what is less? Go into [any] settlement and indeed, you will have what you have asked". And they were covered with humiliation and poverty and returned with anger from Allah [upon them]. That was because they [repeatedly] disbelieved in the signs of Allah and killed the prophets without right. That was because they disobeyed and were [habitually] transgressing'. (Qur'anic Verse, 2:61)

وَهُوَ ٱلَّذِىٓ أَنزَلَ مِنَ ٱلسَّمَآءِ مَآءً فَأَخْرَجْنَا بِهِۦ نَبَاتَ كُلِّ شَىْءٍ فَأَخْرَجْنَا مِنْهُ خَضِرًا نُّخْرِجُ مِنْهُ حَبًّا مُّتَرَاكِبًا وَمِنَ ٱلنَّخْلِ مِن طَلْعِهَا قِنْوَانٌ دَانِيَةٌ وَجَنَّٰتٍ مِّنْ أَعْنَابٍ وَٱلزَّيْتُونَ وَٱلرُّمَّانَ مُشْتَبِهًا وَغَيْرَ مُتَشَٰبِهٍ ٱنظُرُوٓاْ إِلَىٰ ثَمَرِهِۦٓ إِذَآ أَثْمَرَ وَيَنْعِهِۦٓ إِنَّ فِى ذَٰلِكُمْ لَءَايَٰتٍ لِّقَوْمٍ يُؤْمِنُونَ ﴿٩٩﴾

'It is He Who sends down water [rain] from the sky, and with it We bring forth vegetation of all kinds, and out of it We bring forth green stalks, from which We bring forth thick clustered grain. And out of the date palm and its spathe come forth clusters of dates hanging low and near, and gardens of grapes, olives, and pomegranates, each similar (in kind) yet different (in variety and taste). Look at their fruits when they begin to bear, and the ripeness thereof. Verily! In these things there are signs for people who believe'. (Qur'anic Verse, 6:99)

وَهُوَ ٱلَّذِىٓ أَنشَأَ جَنَّٰتٍ مَّعْرُوشَٰتٍ وَغَيْرَ مَعْرُوشَٰتٍ وَٱلنَّخْلَ وَٱلزَّرْعَ مُخْتَلِفًا أُكُلُهُۥ وَٱلزَّيْتُونَ وَٱلرُّمَّانَ مُتَشَٰبِهًا وَغَيْرَ مُتَشَٰبِهٍ كُلُواْ مِن ثَمَرِهِۦٓ إِذَآ أَثْمَرَ وَءَاتُواْ حَقَّهُۥ يَوْمَ حَصَادِهِۦ وَلَا تُسْرِفُوٓاْ إِنَّهُۥ لَا يُحِبُّ ٱلْمُسْرِفِينَ ﴿١٤١﴾

'And He it is who causes gardens to grow, [both] trellised and untrellised, and palm trees and crops of different [kinds of] food and olives and pomegranates, similar and dissimilar. Eat of [each of] its fruit when it yields and give its due [zakah] on the day of its harvest. And be not excessive. Indeed, He does not like those who commit excess'. (Qur'anic Verse 6:141)

According to Hindu mythology, various 'Sacred' plants and herbs are described for improving health and for curing diseases, e.g., Tulsi (*Ocimum sanctum*), Peepal (*Ficus religiosa*), Bael (*Aegle marmelos*), Neem (*Azadirachta indica*), Sandal (*Santalum album*), Bhang (*Cannabis sativa*), Ashok (*Saraca asoca*), and Coconut (*Cocos nucifera*).

क्षुधामारं तृष्णामारमगोतांमनपुत्यतांम् । अपांमार्गं त्वयां वुयं सर्वं तदपं मृज्महे ॥

'We cleanse and wipe away, through Apamarga, the harm caused by hunger, harm caused by thirst, debility of limbs, and childlessness'. (Atharvaveda, 4, 17, 6)

शतवांरो अनीनशुद्यक्ष्मात्रक्षांसि तेजंसा । आरोहन्वर्चसा सह मुणिद्विर्णामुचातॅनः ॥

'The praiseworthy germicidal shatavara [the name of herb which prevents one hundred diseases] mounting over the disease with splendour vanishes the tuberculosis and its germs with power'. (Atharvaveda, 19, 36, 1)

पिप्पुल्यं1 समंवदन्तायुतीर्जनंनादधिं । यं जीवमृश्ववांमहे न स रिष्यांति पूरुषः ॥

'These *Piper longum*, as if confabulating mutually tell them that from their origin, the alive man whom they were applied to, does not feel troubled by rheumatic pain'. (Atharvaveda, 6, 109, 2)

यथाह्युल्पेनयत्नेनच्छिद्यतेतरुणस्तरुः।

सएवाऽतिप्रवृद्धस्तुच्चृछिद्यतेऽतिप्रयन्नतः॥

एवमेवविकारोऽपितरुणःसाध्यतेसुखम्।

विवृद्धःसाध्यतेकृच्छ्रादसाध्योवाऽपिजायते॥

'Just as a tender plant is easy to cut down, the same requires much more effort when fully grown. Likewise, any disease is manageable in the early stage; it becomes almost incurable when it grows' (Charak Nidaan 5/13–16).

Some plants with medicinal value are mentioned in the Bible, such as Teen (*Ficus carica*), Nard/Sumbul-ut-Teeb (*Nardostachys jatamansi*), Zoofa (*Hyssopus offi-cinalis*), Ood Balsan (*Commiphora opobalsamum*), and Foful (*Areca catechu*). In Buddhism, some flowers, like Nilofar (*Nymphaea alba*), Champa (*Michelia champaca*), and Chameli (*Plumeria rubra*), are also said to have medicinal value.

'Now Isaiah had said, "Let them take a cake of figs and apply it to the boil that he may recover'. (Isaiah 38:21 ESV/157)

'Mary therefore took a pound of expensive ointment made from pure nard and anointed the feet of Jesus and wiped his feet with her hair. The house was filled with the fragrance of the perfume'. (John 12:3 ESV/9)

'Purge me with hyssop, and I shall be clean; wash me, and I shall be whiter than snow'. (Psalm 51:7 ESV/39).

The different parts of these sacred plants have been used medicinally by indigenous people to treat different ailments. These plants have also been mentioned by the ancient Hakims and Vaids for the treatment of several diseases, as well as to improve immunity or to act as a tonic. While centuries of use of these sacred medicinal plants is the basis of the testimony, nowadays, more specific and reproducible results are needed to certify the quality, safety, and reliability of the phytomedicines, as well as scientific evidence in relation to health claims, according to international guidelines. These plants have been scientifically evaluated for different activities, e.g., immunostimulant, cardioprotective, anti-arrhythmic, spasmolytic, hypotensive, antihyperglycaemic, antimicrobial, and anti-inflammatory effects.

According to the World Health Organization (WHO), 80% of the world's population still relies on botanical medicines for primary health care (Mukherjee et al. 1998a; Mukherjee 2002a). There is a need for experimental data, proper documentation on mechanisms of action, standardization and fractionation by modern techniques, and *in-vitro* and *in-vivo* studies to check safety and efficacy assurance and to identify the molecular mechanism behind the medicinal effects of these sacred plants. Therefore, evidence for the potential immunomodulatory effects of these sacred medicinal plants, based on research demonstrating a biological activity in relevant *in-vitro* and/or *in-vivo* bioassays, using animal models, is necessary. These plants have been studied scientifically to establish the link between traditional knowledge and modern science. Various investigations on these sacred plants have confirmed the immunomodulatory effects of these plants.

10.2.1 KHAJOOR

Botanical Name *Phoenix dactylifera* L.

Kingdom/Subkingdom – Plantae/Tracheobionta
Super division/Division – Spermatophyta/Magnoliophyta
Class/Subclass – Liliopsida/Arecidae
Order/Family – Arecales/Arecaceae
Genus/Species – *Phoenix/dactylifera*

Vernacular Names

Arabic – Tammar, Nahal, Balah, Rutab
Urdu – Khajur
Hindi – Khajoor
English – Date palm
Persian – Khurma

Khajoor (*P. dactylifera*) is one of the sacred plants mentioned in the Holy Qur'an and belongs to the Arecaceae family. It has been cultivated in the deserts of Iraq, the Arab world, North Africa, Pakistan, and India. The fruit is commonly available and is a rich source of dietary fibre, and also contains large amounts of lipids, minerals, protein, and certain essential vitamins (Figure 10.1a). It is used in the diet to improve health. The dates have also been used to treat a variety of ailments in the various traditional systems of medicine, e.g., heart diseases, skin diseases, as an antidote, to treat intestinal colic, as a wound healer, to treat diarrhoea, stomach-ache, sexual weakness, piles, physical debility, a shrill voice, and liver disorders (Anonymous 1986; Qarshi 2011).

10.2.1.1 Evidence-based Research

Khajoor (*P. dactylifera*) were evaluated scientifically for immunomodulatory effects. Polyphenols, identified as chlorogenic acid, caffeic acid, pelargonin, and ferulic

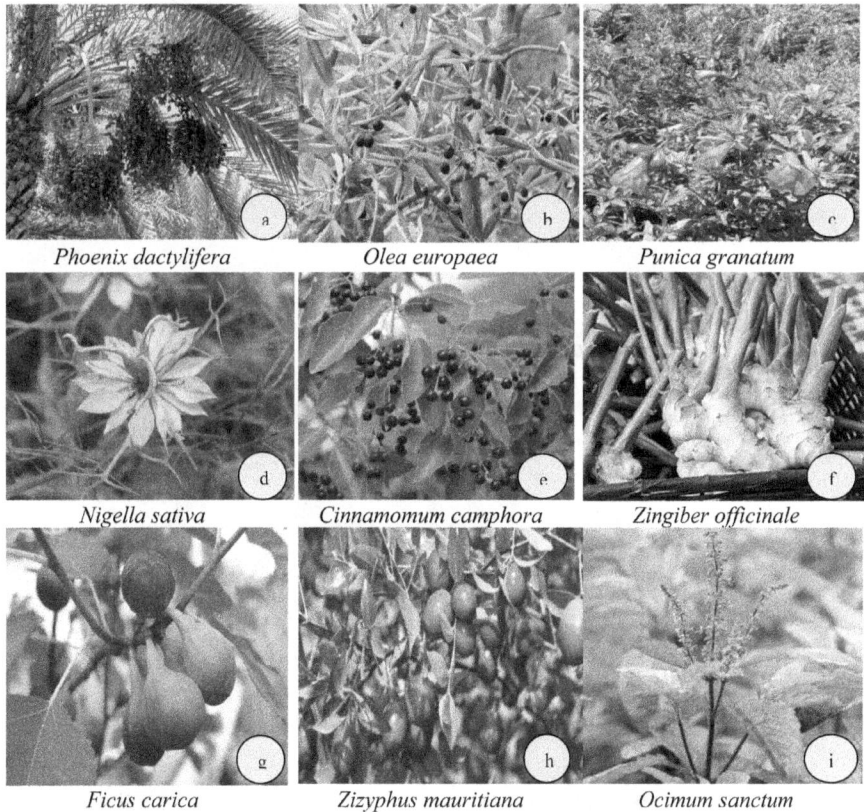

Phoenix dactylifera   *Olea europaea*   *Punica granatum*

Nigella sativa   *Cinnamomum camphora*   *Zingiber officinale*

Ficus carica   *Zizyphus mauritiana*   *Ocimum sanctum*

FIGURE 10.1 Sacred medicinal plants for a strong immune system: (a) *Phoenix dactylifera* – Khajoor, (b) *Olea europaea* – Zaitoon, (c) *Punica granatum* – Rumman, (d) *Nigella sativa* – Kalonji, (e) *Cinnamomum camphora* – Kafoor, (f) *Zingiber officinale* – Zanjabeel, (g) *Ficus carica* – Anjeer, (h) *Zizyphus mauritiana* – Ber, and (i) *Ocimum sanctum* – Rehan.

acid, from the hot water extract of matured fruit of the date palm tree, stimulated the expression of interferon IFN-γ mRNA significantly in experimental animals by stimulating the cell-mediated immune mechanism (Koji 2011). Similarly, the immunomodulatory effects of hot water extracts of date, prune, or fig were investigated, and it was observed that date extract stimulated the cellular system more than did the prune or fig extracts (Mansouri 2005). Khajoor extract at a dosage of 50 mg/kg bodyweight showed an immunostimulatory effect on the reticulo-endothelial system and antioxidant activity (Eddine 2014). It was also observed that Khajoor extract normalized the level of circulatory CD161 natural killer (NK) cells, and breast tissue TNF-alpha, cell size, and proliferation, and improved overall survival rates (Elhemeidy 2018). Tahneeq is a traditional method in which premasticated Ajwa palm dates are rubbed manually onto the palatal mucosa of newborn babies. A study was conducted to investigate the effects of Ajwa palm dates on interleukin IL-12 expression in dendritic cells and blood T lymphocytes expressing CD8$^+$ in experimental rats. They were divided into three groups of neonatal Wistar rats immediately after birth: the control group received breastmilk, the first treatment group (T1) received breast milk and mild-scratched intensity of tahneeq, whereas the second treatment group (T2) received breast milk and strong-scratched intensity of tahneeq on the palatal and gingival mucosa. It was observed that treatment groups 1 and 2 had significantly higher interleukin-12 (IL-12) expression than the control group. The increased IL-12 expression in T2 group was significantly higher than IL-12 expression in the T1 and control groups.

10.2.2 ZAITOON

Botanical Name *Olea europaea* L.

Kingdom/Subkingdom – Plantae/Tracheobionta
Superdivision/Division – Spermatophyta/Magnoliophyta
Class/ Subclass – Magnoliopsida/Asteridae
Order/Family – Scrophulariales/Oleaceae
Genus/Species – *Olea/europaea*

Vernacular Names

English – Olive
Hindi – Jaitoon
Urdu – Zaitoon
Arabic – Zaitoon
Persian – Zaitoon

Zaitoon (*O. europaea*) plants have religious importance and are usually found in northern Iran, coastal areas of the eastern Mediterranean region, south-eastern Europe, the western part of Asia, and northern Africa (Ali 2004). Olives are mentioned many times in the Bible, both in the New and Old Testaments. The olive tree has also been praised as a blessed tree and fruit in the Holy Qur'an. The Prophet

Muhammad (PBUH) recommended various plants e.g., dates, black seed, and olive, for the management of different diseases (Anonymous 2000; Maryam et al. 2009). The plant has laxative, mouth cleanser, tonic, and vasodilator properties, and is known to reduce blood sugar, cholesterol, and uric acid levels (Figure 10.1b). It has also been used to treat various disorders, e.g., hypertension, diabetes, inflammation, haemorrhoids, diarrhoea, respiratory diseases (including bronchial asthma), urinary tract infections, gastrointestinal disorders, and musculo-skeletal disorders (Nadkarni 1986; Anonymous 1999; Nigrami 2009).

10.2.2.1   Evidence-based Research

Leaves, fruits, and oil of Zaitoon play an important role in the management of different diseases, which may be due to the presence of simple phenolics (hydroxytyrosol, tyrosol) and polyphenols. Different research studies conducted on *in-vitro* and *ex-vivo* models have revealed that phenolics present in olive oil have antioxidant activity towards lipids and DNA oxidation greater than the industrial standard, vitamin E (Owen 2000). Extracts of leaves collected from three olive cultivars were investigated for phenolic compounds, using a high-performance liquid chromatography system coupled to a diode array detector time-of-flight mass spectrometer (HPLC-DAD-TOF-MS). Thereafter, an *in-vitro* study was carried out on RAW 264.7 mouse macrophages to investigate the immunomodulatory properties of the crude phenolic extracts. A total number of 28 phenolic compounds were identified in the olive leaf extracts. It was also observed that all olive leaf extracts exhibited immunomodulatory properties, as they inhibited the release of nitric oxide from RAW 264.7 cells treated with lipopolysaccharide (LPS), which is a pro-inflammatory mediator. It may be concluded that the inhibition of nitric oxide by the leaf extracts of Zaitoon depends more on the type of phenolic compounds present in the extract than on the total phenolic concentration (Talhaoui 2015).

10.2.3   MAWEEZ

Botanical Name *Vitis vinifera* L.

   Kingdom/Subkingdom – Plantae/Tracheobionta
   Superdivision/Division – Spermatophyta/Magnoliophyta
   Class/Subclass – Magnoliopsida/Rosidae
   Order/Family – Rhamnales/Vitaceae
   Genus/species – *Vitis/vinifera*

Vernacular Names

   Arabic – lnab
   Persian – Kishmish
   Urdu – Maweez, Zabeeb, Munaqqaa, Kishmish
   Hindi – Angur
   English – Grape
   Sanskrit – Draksha

Maweez (*V. vinifera*) is a woody and shrubby climber, which is usually found in Southeastern Europe, but nowadays is widely cultivated in Europe, Australia, California, and other parts of North America. It is cultivated for agricultural purposes in many states across India, e.g., Punjab, Rajasthan, Delhi, Uttar Pradesh, Maharashtra, Karnataka, Andhra Pradesh, and Tamil Nadu. The flowers are small, pale, and green in colour which appear in the summer season, followed by bunches of green to purple-black berry fruits. Ripe berries are often used as a mild laxative and nutrient, while unripe berries are used to neutralize excessive bile and thus improve ailments of the gastro-intestinal system. Dried berries have stomachic, antiemetic, hepatoprotective and blood-purifying properties. Maweez is used to treat coughs and other respiratory tract diseases. It is also beneficial in the treatment of liver disorders, gastro-intestinal problems, haemorrhagic diseases, and gout, as well as dyspnoea (Ghani YNM; Gruner 1970; Nadkarni 1976, 1982).

10.2.3.1 Evidence-based Research

An *in-vivo* and an *in-vitro* study were conducted to explain the molecular mechanisms involved in the immunomodulation effects and antitumour therapeutic effect of grape seed proanthocyanidins (GSPs). The *in-vivo* study revealed that GSPs inhibit the growth of Sarcoma 180 tumour cells significantly and increase the thymus and spleen weight of Sarcoma 180-bearing mice remarkably, elevating the secretion level of serum Tumour Necrosis Factor-α (TNF-α). It was also observed that exposure to GSPs could increase the lysosomal enzyme activity, stimulate the lymphocyte transformation and the phagocytic capability of peritoneal macrophages, and markedly promote the production of TNF-α. The results of this study suggest that GSPs improve the immune system (Tong 2011).

10.2.4 Rumman

Botanical Name *Punica granatum* L.
Kingdom – Plantae
Division – Spermatophytina
Class – Magnoliopsida
Superorder/Order – Rosanae/Myrtales
Family – Lythraceae
Genus/species – *Punica/granatum*

Vernacular Names
Arabic – Rummän, Shajarätur-Rummän
Urdu – Anar Mitha
English – Pomegranate tree
Hindi – Anaar, Dhalim
Persian – Darakht-e-Anar, Gulnar, Anar
Sanskrit – Bijapura, Dadima, Shuka-dana, Kuchaphala

Anar/Rumman (*P. granatum*) is an ancient, mystic, distinctive fruit, borne on the long-lived pomegranate tree. It is a large, deciduous shrub or small tree, having smooth grey bark, and is often armed with small axillary or terminal thorns. It is found throughout India from the Balkans to the Himalayas. Nowadays, it is cultivated in most regions of the world, e.g., Iran, Spain, Italy, Afghanistan, USA, India, China, Russia, Uzbekistan, Morocco, and Greece (Figure 10.1c). Pomegranate is used to treat various ailments in the Unani system of medicine. Extract of pomegranate flowers acts as an astringent, checking haemorrhage from all internal organs. Its desiccant properties dry up morbid bodily secretions. Application of the powder or its decoction is useful in treating stomatitis, and also prevents various oro-dental disorders, like bleeding gums, shaky teeth, bad odour, mouth ulcer, etc. The ointment is effective in wound healing because of its cicatrizing (scar development) properties. It is also effective in the treatment of diarrhoea and dysentery. The flower extract is also beneficial in treating skin diseases, such as scabies, pruritus, etc. Either root or stem bark, being anthelmintic in action, expel intestinal worms when administered in the form of decoction. Whole fruit is used as a cardiac and liver tonic and as an aphrodisiac in cases of sexual debility. Seeds are anti-emetic and diuretic in action (Ghani 1921; Momin YNM; Baitar YNM; Hamdani 2001).

10.2.4.1 Evidence-based Research

Investigations on fruit rind powder were carried out to evaluate the immunomodulatory activity of Rumman. An aqueous suspension of fruit rind powder in a dose of 100 mg/kg bodyweight was administered orally, which stimulated the cell-mediated and humoral components of the immune system. Antibody titre to the typhoid-H antigen (HA) was also increased (Ross et al. 2001). An *in-vitro* assay, using four separate antioxidant testing methods, demonstrated that extracts of pomegranate juice and seed exhibited two to three times the antioxidant activity (Gil et al. 2000). The immunomodulatory effect on cell-mediated immunity of an ethanolic extract of the peel and fruit juice of *P. granatum* was evaluated. The neutrophil adhesion test and cyclophosphamide-induced myelosuppression activity assay were also used as testing methods. HA titres were used to determine the effect on antibody-mediated immunity. It was observed that the effects of the extract on the percentage neutrophil adhesion, cyclophosphamide-induced myelosuppression, and HA titre were significant, when compared to the standard (Levamisole) group. The study revealed that the peel extract and the fruit juice had significant effects on cell-mediated and humoral immunity (Ittiyavirah 2014). *In-vitro* studies were conducted to investigate the radical scavenging and antitumour activities of polysaccharides (PSP001) isolated from *P. granatum*. It was shown that an *in-vitro* growth stimulatory effect on isolated normal lymphocytes, and a proliferative index of 1.21 ± 0.01 at a concentration of 1000 µg/ml was obtained, indicating immunomodulatory activity. The results of this study indicated that further studies are required on PSP001 in order to use this compound as an antitumour agent (Joseph et al. 2012).

10.2.5 Kalonji

Botanical Name – *Nigella sativa* L.

Kingdom/Subkingdom – Plantae/Tracheobionta
Superdivision/Division – Spermatophyta/Magnoliophyta

Class/Subclass – Magnoliopsida/Magnoliidae
Order/Family – Ranunculales/Ranunculaceae
Genus/Species – *Nigella/sativa*

Vernacular Names

Arabic – Kamun Aswad, Habbatussauda
Persian – Shooneez
Hindi – Kalonji, Mungrela
Urdu – Kalonji
English – Black Cumin, Small Fennel, Nigella Seed

Kalonji (*N. sativa*) is an annual flowering plant which grows to 20–90 cm tall. It is commonly grown in Saudi Arabia, northern Africa, and Asia. Kalonji seeds are widely used as spices and food preservatives, as well as being used as medicine for centuries around the world. The leaves are finely divided. The flowers have 5–10 petals and are yellow, white, pale blue, or pale purple in colour (Figure 10.1d). Seeds are dark, thin, and crescent shaped, with a pungent smell and a bitter taste. Prophet Muhammad (PBUH) stated that Habbatus sauda/Kalonji (Nigella seeds) can cure every disease except death. Seeds were prescribed by ancient Unani physicians to treat headache, nasal congestion, toothache, and intestinal worms, as well as acting as a diuretic, to regulate menstruation, and to promote milk production (Maseehi 2008; Husain 2010; Bashir et al. 2018).

10.2.5.1 Evidence-based Research

Methanolic extracts of the shoots, roots, or seeds of Kalonji were assessed for antioxidant, anti-inflammatory, anticancer and antibacterial activities. The results showed that all these extracts exhibited strong antioxidant activity (Bourgou et al. 2008). It was also observed that Kalonji powder inhibited the oxidative stress caused by administration of oxidized corn oil to experimental animals (Al-Othman et al. 2006). Thymoquinone (TQ) is one of the major bioactive components extracted from the volatile oil of *N. sativa* seeds. It was evaluated for antioxidant and anti-arthritic activity in collagen-induced arthritis. It was found that oral administration of TQ reduced the levels of pro-inflammatory mediators [IL-1β, IL-6, TNF-α, IFN-γ and PGE (2)] and increased the IL-10 level (Umar et al. 2012). It was also observed that treatment with Nigella seed for six weeks protected the liver of broiler chicks from oxidative stress by increasing the activities of enzymes such as glutathione-S-transferase, myeloperoxidase, adenosine deaminase, and catalase and by decreasing hepatic lipid peroxidation (Sogut 2008). The crude methanolic extract of Nigella seed cake was found to exhibit significant antioxidant properties under an *in-vitro* system (Mariod 2009). The effect of *N. sativa* oil on the selected T cell subset percentage in females with rheumatoid arthritis (RA) was investigated. A significant decrease was observed in serum high-sensitivity C-reactive protein (hs-CRP) level and DAS-28 score and there was a decreased number of swollen joints compared with baseline and placebo groups. A comparable CD4+T-cell percentage was observed in the *N. sativa* and placebo groups either in the baseline or at the end of the study. The treatment also resulted in a reduction in CD8+, and an increase in CD4+CD25+T cell percentage, with the CD4+/CD8+ ratio being observed in the treatment group as compared with the placebo (Kheirouri et al. 2016). The effects of three different concentrations of each of the ethanolic extract of *N. sativa*, thymoquinone (TQ), dexamethasone, and saline were investigated, and it was observed that the ethanolic extract of *N. sativa* and TQ had cytotoxic activity and immunomodulatory effects, especially at the higher concentrations. The highest concentration of *N. sativa* extract increased the IFNγ/IL-4 ratio in both non-stimulated and stimulated cells, while the higher concentrations of TQ increased the IFNγ/IL-4 ratio in stimulated cells only (Gholamnezhad et al. 2015). The immunomodulatory effect of *N. sativa* was studied, and it was observed that extracts of *N. sativa* had an immunostimulating effect on non-PHA (Phytohaemagglutinin)-stimulated proliferation of human PBMCs (Peripheral blood mononuclear cells) (Alshatwi 2014).

10.2.6 KAFOOR

Botanical Name *Cinnamomum camphora* L.

Kingdom/Subkingdom – Plantae/Tracheobionta
Superdivision/Division – Spermatophyta/Magnoliophyta
Class/Subclass – Magnoliopsida/Magnoliidae
Order/Family – Laurales/Lauraceae
Genus/species – *Cinnamomum/camphora*

Vernacular Names

Arabic – Kafoor
Urdu – Kafoor
English – Camphor tree
Hind – Kapoor

Kafoor or camphor is a white, crystalline substance with a strong odour and a pungent taste. It is obtained from the wood of camphor laurel and other related trees of the laurel family. The Kafoor tree (*C. camphora*) is found in India, China, Mongolia, Taiwan, and Japan, with a variety of this fragrant, evergreen tree being grown in the southern United States, especially in Florida (Figure 10.1e) (Frizzo 2000). Kafoor is obtained by steam distillation, purification, and sublimation of wood, twigs, and bark of the tree (Zuccarini 2009). There are many pharmaceutical activities of Kafoor, such as a topical analgesic, and anti-inflammatory, antispasmodic, antiseptic, antipruritic, anti-infective, contraceptive, rubefacient, nasal decongestant, mild expectorant, cough suppressant activities, etc. (Chelliah 2008; Zuccarini 2009). Kafoor is easily absorbed through the skin and can also be administered by injection, inhalation, or ingestion (Sydney 1978; Zuccarini 2009). It is used in medicine in preparations of toothpaste, powder, as a diaphoretic or antiseptic, and to treat hysteria and dysmenorrhoea (Kabeeruddin 2009; Jurjani 2010; Lone 2012).

10.2.6.1 Evidence-based Research

Immunomodulatory effects of Kafoor and Kakuti (*Ziziphora tenuior*) were studied, and it was found that the extracts had a non-significant macrophage cytotoxicity in the dimethylthiazol-diphenyltetrazolium bromide (MTT) cell metabolic activity assay (Kanan 2020).

10.2.7 ZANJABEEL

Botanical Name *Zingiber officinale* Roscoe

Kingdom – Plantae
Division – Magnoliophyta
Class/Sub Class – Liopsida/Zingiberidae
Order – Zingiberales
Family – Zingiberaceae
Genus/species – *Zingiber/officinale*

Vernacular Names

Arabic – Qafeer, Zanjabeel
Urdu – Sonth, Zanjabeel
Persian – Sahangrez, Zanjabil
English – Ginger
Hindi – Sonth, Adrak
Sanskrit – Naara, Visva, Adraka, Anupama

Zanjabeel (*Z. officinale*) is an important medicinal plant which is cultivated on a large scale in different parts of India, especially in the warm, moist regions, e.g., Chennai, Cochin, and Travancore, and, to a somewhat lesser extent, in Bengal and Punjab. It is also found at some places in the western Ghats. Ginger requires a warm and humid climate. The plant thrives well from sea level up to an altitude of 1500 m in the Himalayas, the optimum elevation being between 300 and 900 m. The crop needs adequate rainfall and high temperatures during the growing period (Figure 10.1f). According to Unani literature, ginger acts as carminative, digestive, expectorant, and detergent (Ghani 1921). Many commentators have said that Arabs were pleased with drinking wine mixed with ginger, because it made the wine tastier. Now, the Holy Qur'an speaks about 'a cup (of pure drink)' which is mixed with Zanjabeel, but it is obvious that this mixed drink is completely different from that of wine. In other words, the difference between these two kinds of drink is as far as the distance between this world and the next world (Kabeeruddin 1954, 1994).

10.2.7.1 Evidence-based Research

Z. officinale has antioxidant activities as it scavenges peroxide and hydroxyl ions, as well as suppressing lipid peroxidation (Kabuto 2005). The immunomodulatory effects of *Z. officinale* and some other plant oils were evaluated by studying humoral and cell-mediated immune responses, and it was found that ginger essential oil recovered the humoral immune response in immunosuppressed mice (Carrasco et al. 2009). An *in-vitro* study was conducted to determine the immunomodulatory effect of *Z. officinale* and it was found that the plant extract inhibited lymphocyte proliferation, which was mediated by reductions in IL-2 and IL-10 production (Wilasrusmee et al. 2002). An aqueous extract of ginger was investigated for immunomodulatory effects, and significant increases in the production of IL-1β, IL-6, and TNF-α were observed in activated peritoneal mouse macrophages, and increases occurred with respect to splenocyte proliferation and cytokine production (Ryu and Kim 2004). Ginger rhizome powder was found to be capable of improving non-specific immune response in rainbow trout (Haghighi and Rohani 2013). The therapeutic efficacy and mechanisms of action of ginger on key immunopathogenic mechanisms was relevant to psoriasis treatment (Nurul et al. 2013). The successful isolation of pure bioactive compounds from *Z. officinale* confirmed the traditional use of the plant to stimulate the immune system (Tan and Vanitha 2004).

10.2.8 ANJEER

Botanical Name *Ficus carica* L.

Kingdom – Plantae
Division – Magnoliophyta
Class – Magnoliopsida
Order – Urticales
Family – Moraceae
Genus – *Ficus*

Vernacular Names

Arabic – Teen
English – Common Fig, Fig
Indian – Anjir

Anjeer (*F. carica*) is a large tree or shrub 4.5–9.0 m high, which has been cultivated throughout the world since ancient times, both for its decorative purposes as well as for the usefulness of its fruit. The plant produces several branches from the trunk, and the bark of the tree is grey or dull white, smooth or hairy. The leaves are broad, lobed, ovate or nearly orbicular, with a blade 10–20 cm long and petioles 5.0–7.5 cm long with a rough surface (Figure 10.1g). In classical Unani literature, it has been mentioned that fruits of Anjeer can be eaten fresh as well as dried and used as jam. It has a high nutrititive value and provides energy to the human body. Pharmacologically, Anjeer fruit has diuretic, detergent, laxative, de-obstruent, and anti-inflammatory properties, and it can be used in the treatment of chickenpox, measles, respiratory diseases, palpitations, etc. (Kabeeruddin 2006; Qamri 2010; Khan 2011).

10.2.8.1   Evidence-based Research

An ethanolic extract of the leaves of *F. carica* was assessed for immunomodulatory effect and it was revealed that the extract of the leaves had significantly ameliorated the cell-mediated and humoral antibody response. The results indicated that the extract possessed immunostimulant properties (Patil 2010). Anjeer fruits from six commercial fig varieties of different colours (black, red, yellow, or green) were evaluated for total polyphenols, total flavonoids, antioxidant capacity, and profile of anthocyanins, and it was found that the fruits contained the highest levels of polyphenols, flavonoids, and anthocyanins, and exhibited the highest antioxidant capacity (Çalişkan 2011). The antioxidant potential of fig extract was determined by the ABTS assay and it was found to be very high (19.8 mg/ml) (Soni et al. 2014). A novel polysaccharide (FCPW80-2) was isolated from *F. carica* through hot water extraction and several chromatographic methods. The results showed that MAPK and NF-κB signalling pathways contributed to FCPW80-2-induced macrophage activation, so that FCPW80-2 has potential to be used as an immunomodulating functional food (Du et al. 2018). Antioxidant activity and the effect on the immune response by fermented fig extracts were investigated in mice. It was observed that the extracts enhanced immune organ indexes, improved immune organ injuries, helped in the production of immune-related cytokines, and improved the histopathological state of immune organs (Zhao et al. 2020).

10.2.9   Mauz

Botanical Name *Musa paradisiaca* L.

Kingdom/Subkingdom – Plantae/Tracheobionta
Superdivision/Division – Spermatophyta/Magnoliophyta
Class/ Subclass – Liliopsida/Zingiberidae
Order/Family – Zingiberales/Musaceae
Genus/Species – *Musa/paradisiaca*

Banana (*M. paradisia ca*) is a very important fruit crop in India. Its accessibility, affordability, taste, range, nutritional, and medicinal values make it the favourite fruit among all classes of people. Bananas are spread over almost the entire world. In India, it is cultivated in particular in Andhra Pradesh, Assam, Gujarat, Jharkhand, Karnataka, Kerala, Madhya Pradesh, Maharashtra, Orissa, Tamil Nadu, and West Bengal. It is used as food, medicine (*Ilaj Bil Ghiza*) for treatment of several diseases, like diarrhoea, dysentery, constipation, etc. The fruit is a very rich source of valuable phytochemicals, including phenolic compounds and vitamins. (Khare 2007; Imam 2011; Deepthi 2012; Sampath 2012).

10.2.9.1   Evidence-based Research

A study was carried out on powdered CandI banana (*M.* × *paradisiaca*) extracted with ethanol or ethyl acetate in an ultrasonic bath and it was observed that these extracts had antioxidant activities which were higher in the ethanolic extract than in the ethyl acetate extract (Laeliocattleya 2018). Flavonoids isolated from peels of *M.* × *paradisiaca* were investigated for immunomodulatory properties. It was revealed that these flavonoids showed dose-dependent increases in antibody titre at higher doses, which confirmed the immunomodulatory activities of these flavonoids isolated (Abhijit et al. 2017).

10.2.10 BER

Botanical Name *Ziziphus mauritiana* (Lamk.)

Kingdom – Plantae
Division/Subdivision – Magnoliophyta/Angiosperm
Class – Magnoliopsida
Order/ Family – Rosales/Rhamnaceae
Genus – *Ziziphus*/*mauritiana*

Vernacular Names

Urdu – Annab, Baer, Ber, Unab, Unnab
Arabic – Annab, Aunnab e hindi, Nabig, Nabiq
Persian – Kanar, Kunar
English – Chinese Apple, Cottony Jujube, Indian Cherry, Indian Jujube
Hindi – Ber
Sanskrit – Ajapriya, Badara, Karkandhu

Ber (*Z. mauritiana*) is a very common plant, which is cultivated throughout India and other countries on the Indian subcontinent. It is a spiny, evergreen shrub or small tree with a height up to 15 m, with a trunk diameter of 40 cm or more, a spreading crown, stipular spines, and many drooping branches. It is a multi-purpose tree grown mainly for its fruits. Bearing of fruits starts after 6–8 years of growth. The fruit can be eaten fresh or dried like dates, candied, salted, or pickled (Figure 10.1h). It can also be used as flour meal, paste, juice, syrup, or as a beverage. It may be used in the treatment of insomnia, chronic bronchitis, constipation, liver diseases, fever, bronchial asthma, urinary diseases, and gastro-intestinal disorders (Mediratta 2002; Tabri 2003; Akassh 2020).

10.2.10.1 Evidence-based Research

Root of *Z. mauritiana* were investigated and it was found that the root extract, particularly that extracted in dichloromethane, had immunomodulatory, cytotoxic, and antioxidant activities (Afzal 2017). Twenty-eight varieties of Indian jujube were investigated for different compounds, e.g., ascorbic acid, total phenolics, flavanols, total flavonoids, and dihydric phenol. It was observed that cv. ZG_3 was found to exhibit the highest DPPH free radical scavenging activity, followed by 'Katha Phal' and 'Thar Sevika'. Variation in relation to their phenolic content and antioxidant activity among the genotypes was also observed (Krishna 2013). *Ficus religiosa* (sacred fig) and *Z. mauritiana* were investigated for immunostimulatory effect and it was found that both extracts in higher doses increased paw oedema in comparison with the control group. This revealed the immunostimulatory effect of the selected plant extracts on the cell-mediated immune response (Maity et al. 2012). The aqueous or ethanolic extracts of *Z. mauritiana* seed were studied for immunomodulatory activities, with results indicating that up-regulation of cell-mediated humoral immune response, as well as in Th-1-mediated cytokine IFN-gamma levels, and decreases in Th-2-mediated cytokine IL-4 were the most significant changes (Mishra 2010).

10.2.11 REHAN

Botanical Name *Ocimum sanctum* L.
Kingdom/ Subkingdom – Plantae/Tracheobionta
Superdivision/Division – Spermatophyta/Magnoliophyta
Class/Subclass – Magnoliopsida/Asteridae
Order/Family – Lamiales/Lamiaceae
Genus/species – *Ocimum/sanctum*

Vernacular Names
Urdu – Rehaan
Arabic – Rehan
Persian – Jasaspermum
English – Holy Basil, Sweet Basil
Hindi – Tulsi
Sanskrit – Tulsipatr, Tulsidal, Vrinda

Rehan (*O. sanctum*) is a tropical plant which grows as a weed or is cultivated. Rehan or Tulsi is worshipped by Hindus and is considered to be very important in the Hindu faith. It is a branched, fragrant, and erect herb which has hairs all over. Mature plants may grow up to a height of 75–90 cm (Figure 10.1i). Different parts (leaves, stems, flowers, roots, seeds, and even whole plants) of Tulsi have been used widely by the traditional medical practitioners for the treatment of various diseases in their day-to-day practice, such as malaria, bronchial asthma, bronchitis, diarrhoea, chronic fever, dysentery, arthritis, skin diseases, painful eye diseases, insect bite, etc. (Anonymous 1989; Hakeem 2002; Zaidi 2011; Gupta 2018).

10.2.11.1 Evidence-based Research

O. sanctum seed oil was evaluated for immunomodulatory activity in both non-stressed and stressed animals, and it was revealed that *O. sanctum* seed oil modulated humoral and cell-mediated immune sensitivity (Mediratta 2002). An aqueous extract of *O. sanctum* leaves has shown immunotherapeutic potential in sub-clinical trials, and there was a reduction in the total bacterial count, and an increase in neutrophils and lymphocytes with good phagocytic activity (Mukherjee 2005). Aqueous and ethanolic extracts of *O. sanctum* leaves were evaluated for immunomodulatory activity, which stimulated both specific and non-specific responses assessed by the Haemagglutination Antibody (HA) titre assay, the neutrophil adhesion test, and the Delayed Type Hypersensitivity (DTH) test (Das et al. 2015). The aqueous or methanolic extracts of *O. sanctum* leaves produced clinically significant immunostimulation of the humoral immunological response (Godhwani 1988). Methanolic and aqueous extracts of *O. sanctum* leaves exhibited immunoregulatory activity (Kelm 2000; Dashputre 2010). Aqueous leaf extracts of *O. sanctum* were investigated *in vitro* and *in vivo* for immunomodulatory activity and it was observed that the extract increased the DTH response, the TLC (Total Leukocyte Count) and the DLC (Differential Leukocyte Count) count significantly, with the extract at 200 mg/kg bodyweight showing only a significant effect but a dose of 400 mg/kg and the standard treatment showing highly significant effects, compared with the control group (Venkatachalam 2013). A study was conducted to compare the immunomodulatory effects of *O. sanctum* with those of *Ocimum basilicum* in mice and it was observed that neither preparation caused any mortality or any signs of behavioural changes or toxicity at the dose level of 2000 mg/kg bodyweight in mice, but *O. sanctum* improved the DTH reaction in mice in T cell-dependent antigen response, which may be due to the stimulatory effect of *O. sanctum* on T cells (Jeba 2013).

10.2.12 PEEPAL

Botanical name *Ficus religiosa* L.

Kingdom/Subkingdom – Plantae/Viridaeplantae
Class/Subclass – Magnoliopsida/Dilleniidae
Order/Family – Urticales/Moraceae
Genus/species – *Ficus/religiosa*

Vernacular Names

Hindi – Pipli, Papal, Pipar
Sanskrit – Asvattha
English – Peepal Tree, Sacred Fig

Peepal (*F. religiosa*) is one of the oldest trees mentioned in Indian literature. The tree is described in the holy books of Hinduism, such as Arthasastra, Puranas, Upanishads, Ramayana, Mahabharata, and Bhagavad Geeta, and in Buddhist literature. The tree is native to India and is believed to have originated mainly in northern and eastern India. It is also grown in neighbouring countries, like Bangladesh, Pakistan, Nepal, Sri Lanka, and China. The tree grows very large, with wide spreading branches and brown-coloured bark. The plant has thin shiny leaves and the fruit is flattened and circular in shape (Figure 10.2a). Young immature leaves are reddish-pink in colour, turning deep green on maturity. Fruits are known to cure various diseases, such as bronchial asthma and digestive disorders. The leaves are effective in the treatment of different diseases like hiccoughs, vomiting, gonorrhoea etc. The bark also shows beneficial effects with respect to diseases such as diarrhoea, dysentery, inflammation, bacterial infections, paralysis, and bleeding (Azmi 1995; Anonymous 2006).

10.2.12.1 Evidence-based Research

An alcoholic extract of the bark of *F. religiosa* was investigated for immunomodulatory activity and it was observed that the extract ameliorated both the cell-mediated and the humoral antibody response to a great degree. It was concluded that the extract possessed promising immunostimulant properties (Mallurvar 2008). The

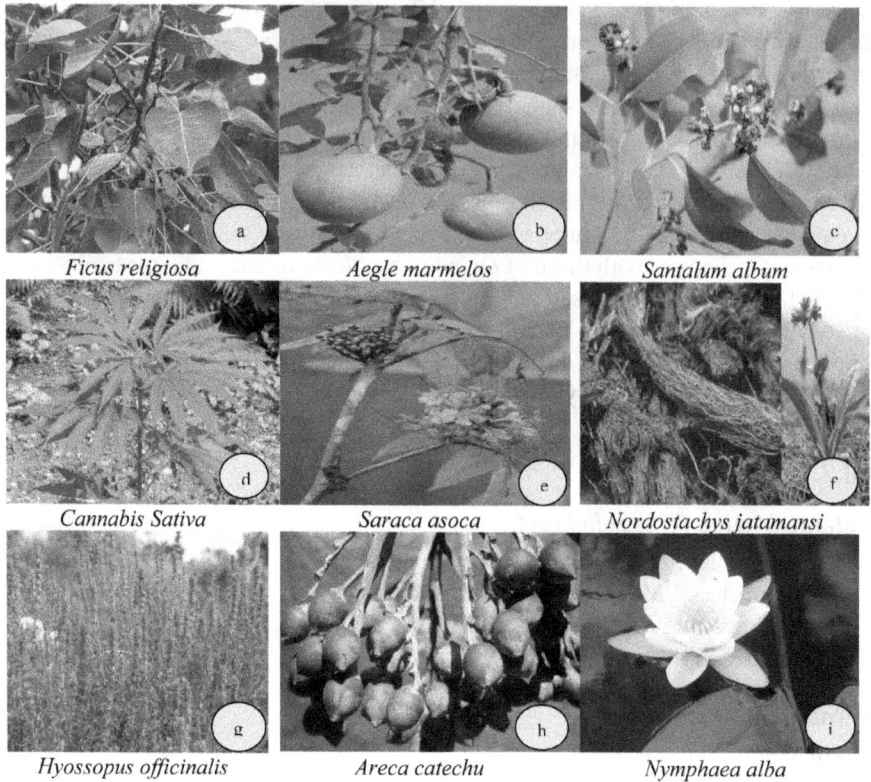

FIGURE 10.2   Sacred medicinal plants for a strong immune system: (a) *Ficus religiosa* – Peepal, (b) *Aegle marmelos* – Bael, (c) *Santalum album* – Sandal, (d) *Cannabis sativa* – Qinnab, (e) *Saraca asoca* – Ashok, (f) *Nordostachys jatamansi* – Sumbul ut Teeb, (g) *Hyossopus officinalis* – Zoofa, (h) *Areca catechu* – Foful, and (i) *Nymphaea alba* – Nilofar.

aqueous extract of *F. religiosa* reduced oxidative stress in rats with experimentally induced type 2 diabetes (You 2006).

10.2.13 BAEL

Botanical Name *Aegle marmelos* (L.) Correa
Kingdom/Subkingdom – Plantae/Tracheobionta
Superdivision/Division – Spermatophyta/Magnoliophyta
Class/Subclass – Magnoliopsida/Rosidae
Order/Family – Sapindales/Rutaceae
Genus/Species – *Aegle/marmelos*

Vernacular Names
Urdu – Bel
English – Apple wood, Bengal Quince, Golden Apple, Japanese Orange

Hindi – Sir Phal, Bel
Sanskrit – Shree Phal, Bilva, Asholam
Gujrati – Billi (Baghdadi 2005)

Bael (*A. marmelos*) is a very common spiritual and religious plant, which is a native of India and Bangladesh but is cultivated throughout SouthEast Asia. Bael is sweet, aromatic, and astringent in nature (Bashir et al. 2018). It is one of the few Unani plants where all the different parts, from roots to leaves, are used for medicinal purposes against different diseases (Figure 10.2b). Due to its digestive and carminative properties, it is used for curing chronic diarrhoea and dysentery. It is also used to treat intermittent fevers and heart disorders (Bashir et al. 2018; Bhar et al. 2019).

10.2.13.1 Evidence-based Research

A study was carried out to assess the immunomodulatory activity of a methanolic extract of *A. marmelos* fruit in an experimental model of immunity. The results showed that the fruit extract at 100 and 500 mg/kg bodyweight produced significant increases in adhesion of neutrophils and an increase in phagocytic index in the carbon clearance assay in the test animals (Patel et al. 2010). Pratheepa and colleagues carried out a study where fish were challenged with pathogens through the water medium for thirty days and the immunomodulatory effect of the *A. marmelos* leaf extract was evaluated on blood samples every five days until fifteen days after infection. The results obtained from the study showed that the dosage of 25 g leaf extract/kg of feed was found to be capable of achieving the optimum immune response (Pratheepa et al. 2011).

10.2.14 Neem

Botanical Name *Azadirachta indica*

Kingdom/Subkingdom – Plantae/Tracheobionta
Order/Suborder – Rutales/Rutinae
Family/Subfamily – Meliaceae/Melioideae
Genus/Species – *Azadirachta/indica*

Vernacular Names

Urdu – Neem
Sanskrit – Nimbah, Arista, Arkapadapa
English – Indian lilac, Margosa tree
Tamil – Vepamaram, Vemu, Vembu
Hindi – Balnimb, Nim, Neem, Nimb
Persian – Azad Darakth-e-Hind, Nib, Neeb

Neem (*A. indica*) is a popular, evergreen tree, which is found commonly in India, Africa, and USA. It grows to a height of 12–18 m, with a girth of 1.8–2.4 m. Its straight, long, and spreading branches form a broad crown. (Brahmachari 2004) The leaves are alternate, imparipinnate, and 20–38 cm long. The leaflets are 8–19 cm long, alternate or opposite, and the fruit is one seeded. Neem is used in Ayurveda,

Unani, homoeopathy, and modern medicine for the treatment of many infectious, metabolic, or cancer diseases. It is a multipurpose tree with immense potential. It possesses more useful non-wood products (leaves, bark, flowers, fruits, seed, gum, oil, and neem cake) than any other tree in India. Various properties of Neem have been mentioned in classical Unani literature, such as antiseptic, antipyretic, antitussive, cicatrizant, carminative, etc., which can be used to treat skin diseases, arthritis, dropsy, earache, and other diseases (Ahmedullah 1999).

10.2.14.1   Evidence-based Research

An aqueous extract of the flowers of *A. indica* was evaluated for immunomodulatory activity on humoral and cell-mediated immune response to ovalbumin. Treatment with the extract showed a significant increase in phagocytic index, which reflects activation of the reticulo-endothelial system through release of the mediators. The extract also resulted in an increase in antibody titre against ovalbumin, with a significant effect on stimulation of T cells at the dose of 400 mg/kg bodyweight (Abhishek 2009). It was confirmed that a methanolic extract of the leaves of *A. indica* exhibited antioxidant activity (Pokhrel 2015). A study was conducted to evaluate the immunomodulatory effects of Neem oil in experimental animals, which revealed that Neem oil works as a non-specific immunostimulant by selectively activating the CMI (Cell-Mediated Immunity) mechanisms (Upadhyay et al. 1992). NIM-76, a volatile fraction from Neem oil, was assessed for its immunomodulatory properties and it was found that NIM-76 acts through cell-mediated mechanisms by activating macrophages and lymphocytes (Ram et al. 1997). An aqueous extract of the stem bark of *A. indica* showed strong anticomplement effects, which were dose- and time-dependent and most pronounced in the classical complement pathway assay (Van der Nat et al. 1987). The growth-promoting and immunomodulatory effect of a Neem leaf infusion was evaluated on broilers and it was observed that the Neem infusion significantly increased antibody titre, growth performance, and gross return (Durrani et al. 2008).

10.2.15   SANDAL

Botanical Name *Santalum album*
> Kingdom/Subkingdom – Plantae/Tracheobionta
> Superdivision/Division – Spermatophyta/Magnoliophyta
> Class/Subclass – Magnoliopsida/Rosidae
> Order/Family – Santalales/Santalaceae
> Genus/species – *Santalum/album*

Vernacular Names
> Arabic – Khashab ul Sandal
> English – Sandalwood
> Hindi – Chandan
> Persian – Chob Sandal
> Sanskrit – Shrigandha
> Urdu – Sandal

Sandal (*S. album*) is one of the most precious trees in the world, with great sacred value. Ancient history reveals that sandalwood has been referred to in Indian mythology, folklore, and ancient scriptures. The finest sandalwood grows in the driest regions, mainly on red or stony ground; on rocky ground, the tree often remains small but gives the highest yield of oil. It is an evergreen tree that grows up to 20 m, attaining a girth of up to 2.4 m, with slender drooping branchlets (Figure 10.2c). A wide range of articles, such as boxes, jewel cases, picture frames, combs, pen holders, card cases, hand fans, and bookmarks, are made from sandalwood. As medicine, sandalwood is regarded as a coolant, sedative, astringent, and disinfectant in the genitourinary and bronchial tracts, and as a diuretic, expectorant, and stimulant. The wood, root, bark, and leaves of the tree are used to treat liver diseases, such as jaundice, by the tribal healers (Duke 2002). It is used by the Jews, the Buddhists, and the Hindus, as well as adherents to almost every other belief system for its vast diversity of attributes (Joshi 2003; Sina 2010; Arun 2012).

10.2.15.1 Evidence-based Research

The FRAP (Ferric Reducing Antioxidant Power Assay) antioxidant assay of an aqueous extract of *S. album* confirmed the antioxidant activity of the plant (Shamsi et al. 2014).

10.2.16   QINNAB

Botanical Name *Cannabis sativa*

Kingdom/Subkingdom – Plantae/Tracheobionta
Superdivision/Division – Spermatophyta/Magnoliophyta
Class/Subclass – Magnoliopsida/Hamamelididae
Order/Family – Rosales/Cannabaceae
Genus/Species – *Cannabis*/*sativa*

Vernacular Names (Kalam 2020)

Arabic – Banj, Qinnab, Warq al-Khiyal
Persian – Bang, Hashish, Falaksair, Arshnuma, Falaktaz, Kinnab
Bengali – Bhang
English – Indian hemp.
Gujarati – Bhang, Gajna
Hindi – Bhang, Bhanga, Ganja, Charas, Shiv Booti

Qinnab (*C. sativa*) is a native of Persia, western and Central Asia. Nowadays, it is cultivated all over India and is wild in the western Himalayas from Kashmir to East of Assam. The drug is mentioned in early Hindu and Chinese works on medicine. It is an erect, much-branched 40–75 cm tall herb, which commonly grows along roadsides and on waste ground. The leaves have a strong, characteristic odour, with a somewhat acrid and pungent taste (Figure 10.2d). Because of its soothing properties, it is effectively used for the treatment of diseases related to the brain and nerves (Samarqandi 1906; Killestein 2003).

10.2.16.1 Evidence-based Research

Cannabidiol is one of the key pharmacologically active compounds of *C. sativa*. It was clinically tested on patients suffering from multiple sclerosis, and a modest increase in TNF-alpha in lipopolysaccharide (LPS)-stimulated whole blood was found in the treatment group, although no changes in other cytokines were observed (Killestein 2003). Cannabidiol protects lipids and proteins against oxidative stress damage by modulating the level of oxidative stress, by participating in cell signalling pathways (Atalay 2019).

10.2.17 ASHOK

Botanical Name *Saraca asoca* L.
 Kingdom/Subkingdom – Plantae/Tracheophyta
 Superdivision/Division – Spermatophyta/Magnoliophyta
 Class – Magnoliopsida
 Order/Family – Fabales/Fabaceae
 Genus/Species – *Saraca*/*asoca*

Vernacular Names
 Urdu – Ashok Chaal
 Bengali – Asok, Asoka
 English – Asoka Tree.
 Gujarati – Ashopalava
 Hindi – Ashok, Asok
 Sanskrit – Apashoka, Ashok, Chitra, Doshahari, Gandhapushpa

Ashok (*S. asoca*) is a medium-sized, evergreen tree with glabrous branches. It is generally found in hilly areas of Assam, West Bengal, and the western Ghats of Maharashtra in India. The leaves are pinnate and rigidly coracious (Figure 10.2e). Moist and well-drained soil is very suitable for the growth of the plant. It is a moderately shade-loving tree. The bark of the plant has been described in classical Unani literature as a uterine tonic, antimenorrhagic, refrigerant, vermicidal, nervine tonic, and anti-inflammatory, which may be used in uterine debility, leucorrhoea, etc. (Kabiruddin YNM; Kirtikar 1991; Rushd 1997; Tariq 2010).

10.2.17.1 Evidence-based Research

A methanol extract of the bark of *S. asoca* showed the highest radical scavenging activity, using the DPPH assay, at a concentration of 200 µg/µl, which confirms the antioxidant activity of plant extracts of *S. asoca* (Mohan 2016). The antioxidant potential of the petroleum ether, ethyl acetate, benzene, ethanol, and methanol extracts of the flowers of *S. asoca* was also evaluated. The results showed that ethanol extract of the flowers of the plant exhibited the highest antioxidant activity (Tresina et al. 2018).

10.2.18 Sumbul-ut Teeb

Botanical name *Nardostachys jatamansi* (D. Don) DC

Kingdom – Plantae
Division – Mangnoliophyta
Class – Mangnoliopsida
Order – Dipsacales
Family – Caprifoliaceae
Genus – *Nardostachys*

Vernacular Names

Urdu – Sumbul-ut-teeb, Balchar
Arabic – Sumbul-ut-teeb
Persian – Sumbul-ut Teeb
English – Muskroot, Indian Spikenard, Spikenard
Hindi – Balchar, Balchir, Jatamansi
Sanskrit – Mansi, jati, jatila Jatamansi, Janani Jatamansi

Sumbul-ut Teeb (*N. jatamansi*) is a perennial plant commonly cultivated in the hilly regions of Himachal Pradesh, Sikkim, Uttaranchal, and Jammu and Kashmir. The plant is up to 60 cm in height, with long woody rootstocks. Dark grey rhizomes are crowned with reddish brown tufted fibres internally. These rhizomes are elongated and cylindrical in shape, from 2.5 to 7.5 cm in length (Muzafar 2017). The radical and elongated leaves are sessile, oblong, or sub-ovate (Figure 10.2f). Flowers are pale pink or blue in colour. According to classical Unani literature, Sumbul-ut Teeb acts as an emmenogogue, carminative, diuretic, cardiotonic, and brain tonic and can be used to treat insomnia, hypertension, asthma, and epilepsy (Razi 1991; Rizwan 2010).

10.2.18.1 Evidence-based Research

A methanolic extract of Sumbul-ut Teeb exhibited antioxidant activity, using the FRAP (10.18 mg ascorbic acid equivalent (AAE)/100 g dry weight, DW) and ABTS assays (4.87 mg AAE/100 g DW); on the other hand, the 2,2-diphenyl-1-picrylhydra-zyl (DPPH) assay showed significantly higher antioxidant activity (5.84 mg AAE/100 g DW; Bhatt et al. 2012). The antioxidant activity of the essential oil and of differ-ent extracts of *N. jatamansi* roots, measured by DPPH radical scavenging and the chelation power assay, showed that the methanolic extract had definite antioxidant properties, which may be due to the presence of high concentrations of polyphenols and flavonoids (Sakshima et al. 2014).

10.2.19 Zoofa

Botanical Name *Hyssopus officinalis* L.

Kingdom/Subkingdom – Plantae/Tracheobionta
Superdivision/Division – Spermatophyta/Magnoliophyta

Class/Subclass – Magnoliopsida/Asteridae
Order/Family – Lamiales/Lamiaceae
Genus/Species – *Hyssopus/officinalis*

Vernacular Names

Urdu – Zufa khushk
Sanskrit – Jupha
Persian – Ushnan-e Dawood
Hindi – Zupha
English – Hyssop, Holy herb

Zoofa (*H. officinalis*) is an aromatic perennial plant which is found in the western Himalayan region from Kashmir to Kumaun. It grows to a height of 120 cm. The plant has been used for culinary and medicinal purposes since ancient times. The plant leaves are often used for their minty flavour and as a condiment in the food industry (Figure 10.2g). The oil extracted from the aerial part of the plant is used as a flavouring agent for alcoholic beverages and meat products. The benefits of Hyssop have been documented in the primary texts of Christianity and Judaism. Medicinally, it is used as a carminative, tonic, antiseptic, expectorant, and cough reliever (Rafeequddin 1985; Fathiazad 2011).

10.2.19.1   Evidence-based Research

The antioxidant activity of an ethanolic extract of Zoofa (*H. officinalis*) was determined and it was found that appreciable antioxidant activity was present in the extract as assayed by DPPH radical scavenging test, the Trolox equivalent antioxidant capacity assay, the electron paramagnetic resonance radical detection assay, and the haemoglobin ascorbate peroxidase activity inhibition assay (Vlase et al. 2014).

10.2.20   Foful

Botanical Name *Areca catechu* L.

Kingdom/Subkingdom – Plantae/Tracheobionta
Superdivision/Division – Spermatophyta/Magnoliophyta
Class/Subclass – Liliopsida/Arecidae
Order/Family – Arecales/Arecaceae
Genus/species – *Areca/catechu*

Vernacular Names

Urdu – Chalia, Supari
Arabic – Fufal, Fofal
English – Betel Palm
Hindi – Supari

Persian – Popal
Sanskrit – Ghonta, Kramuka, Gubak, Poogaphalam
Unani – Fufal, Chhalia, Supari (Anonymous 2007)

Foful (*A. catechu*) is a tree of up to 20 m in height, found on plains and hilly regions. In India, it is commercially cultivated on the western Coast, West Bengal, and Assam. The nut has a rounded cone-shape, 2–3 cm in height (Figure 10.2h). Its seeds can be used to strengthen the teeth and gums, can act as an anthelmintic, and improves the digestive system as it is both a digestive and a stimulant (Anonymous 2007; Rashid et al. 2015).

10.2.20.1 Evidence-based Research

An experimental study conducted on rats showed that areca nut extract increased the number of while blood cells (WBCs) and improved the activity and capacity of macrophages in rats infected with the bacterium *Staphylococcus aureus*. The immunomodulatory ability may be due to the presence of phytochemicals in the areca nut (Sari et al. 2020).

10.2.21 NILOFAR

Botanical Name *Nymphaea alba* L.

Kingdom/Subkingdom – Plantae/Tracheobionta
Superdivision/Division – Spermatophyta/Magnoliophyta
Class/Subclass – Magnoliopsida/Magnoliidae
Order/Family – Nymphaeales/Nymphaeaceae
Genus/Species – *Nymphaea/alba*

Vernacular Names

Urdu – Nilofar
Hindi – Nilkamal, Nilpadma
English – European White Water lily, White lotus
Tamil – Karuneythal
Bengali – Nilshapla, Nilpadma
Gujarati – Nilkamal
Tamil – Karuneythal

Nilofar (*N. alba*) is a perennial aquatic plant which is found in ponds and lakes in Bangladesh, Africa, and warmer parts of India (Figure 10.2i). It is an important and well-known medicinal plant, which has been advocated by various systems of medicine, like Unani, Ayurveda, and Siddha, for the treatment of diabetes, inflammation, liver disorders, urinary disorders, menorrhagia, menstrual problems, and as an aphrodisiac, brain tonic, and cardiotonic (Doli et al. 2012; Lakshmi 2013).

10.2.21.1 Evidence-based Research

An ethanolic extract of the rhizomes of Nilofar (*N. alba*) has shown significant anti-oxidant activity, which may be due to the presence of tannins and other phenolic compounds (Bose 2012). Aqueous and ethanolic extracts of the flowers of *N. alba* were investigated for antioxidant ability by performing the DPPH radical scavenging assay, the hydroxyl radical scavenging assay, and the nitric oxide scavenging assay. The results of all three assays concluded that ethanolic extract of *N. alba* had significant antioxidant activity in comparison with the aqueous extract (Madhusudhanan et al. 2011).

More information related to sacred medicinal plants is presented in Table 10.1.

10.4   CONCLUSION AND FUTURE PERSPECTIVES

Different plants have long been believed to be sacred by communities all over the world. Various religions have different religious books, describing plants for the maintenance and the preservation of health. India has a very extensive and diverse flora, which has a special place in our rituals, worship, myths, epics, and daily life. Diseases are cured in two ways in Islam: cure of the soul through prayers and cure of ailments through medicines. The Holy Qur'an described the importance of different plants for treating various ailments. Khajoor (*P. dactylifera*) has the greatest number of references in The Holy Book. Many food products are prepared from dates these days. Zaitoon (*O. europaea*) also has many references in the Holy Qur'an and Ahadith. In the Holy Qur'an it is mentioned: 'Your God is that who has made different kinds of orchids and gardens for you, those have colourful crops of Khajoor, Zaitoon and Anar/Rumman. Eat these fruits when ripe but keep the share for poor relatives and the needy and do not waste them'. (Holy Qur'an: 141, Surah- Al-Anam). Lord Buddha meditated on the path to enlightenment under Peepal (*F. religiosa*); Sita sheltered in a grove of Ashok (*S. asoca*), when she was detained by Ravana, and no Hindu household is considered complete without Tulsi (*O. sanctum*), with the leaves of Bael (*A. marmelos*) being used for the worship of Shiva.

The need for exploration of such useful data from the Holy Qur'an, Ahadith, Vedas, and the Bible has long been felt, with the increasing need for drugs, medicines, and other useful products. This approach was adopted to record the medicinal uses of sacred plants for the welfare of human beings.

This chapter may supply the scientific knowledge of the medicinal plants mentioned in the Holy Qur'an, Vedas, and other religious books to the botanists practising both basic and applied aspects of plant research. This may ensure essential ethno-pharmacological investigations of most of these plants and may correlate botanical clarification with the unique sacred books or may denote an additional biological theme to the list of important independent subjects learned from the Holy book.

Various uses of sacred plants for food and animal feed, folk medicine, and for normal life are reported in more than one verse in the Holy Qur'an and other religious

TABLE 10.1
Medicinal Activities of Sacred Medicinal Plants

Common Name	Scientific Name	Proven Medicinal Activities	References
Khajoor	Phoenix dactylifera	Anti-inflammatory, antioxidant, antitumour, antimicrobial, antidiabetic, nephroprotective, and for labour relaxation	Michael et al. (2013), Eddine (2013), and Badreldin et al. (2008)
Zaitoon	Olea europaea	Hypoglycaemic, hypotensive, diuretic, antipyretic, anti-inflammatory, general tonic, cleanser, and laxative	Amel (2013), Ali-Shtayeh (2012), Vardanian (1978), Fujita (1995), Gastaldo (1974), Ribeiro (1986), and Khalil (1995)
Maweez	Vitis vinifera	Skin protective, antibacterial, anticancer, anti-inflammatory, antidiabetic, hepatoprotective, and neuroprotective	Saada et al. (2009), Lakshmi et al. (2013), Silva et al. (2015), Kang et al. (2012), Yanni et al. (2015), Porquet et al. (2013), and Giribabu et al. (2015)
Kalonji	Nigella sativa	Antihypertensive, liver tonic, diuretic, digestive, anti-diarrhoeal, appetite stimulant, analgesic, antibacterial, antidiabetic, anticancer, immunomodulator, and antioxidant	Abedi (2017), Adam et al. (2016), Ahmad et al. (2013), Aljabre et al. (2015), and Malik et al. (2016)
Rumman	Punica granatum	Anti-inflammatory, anticancer, antidiabetic, cardioprotective, and hepatoprotective	Murthy (2004), Schubert (1999), Esmaillzadeh (2006), Adhami (2009), Sumner (2005), and Xu (2009)
Kafoor	Cinnamomum camphora	Antioxidant, anti-inflammatory, antitumour, antifungal, antimicrobial, and antihyperglycaemic	ChenLung (2009), Edris (2007), Ngadiman (2005), Agarwal (2012), Satyal (2013), Inouye (2001) and Lin (2015)
Zanjabeel	Zingiber officinale	Cardiotonic, powerful antioxidant, anticancer, anticoagulant, anti-inflammatory, anti-atherosclerotic, antacid, antiviral, antimicrobial, and antitussive	Khare (2007), Nadkarni (2009), Rehman (2010), Lantz (2007), and Mahmoud (2012)
Anjeer	Ficus carica	Anticancer, hepatoprotective, hypoglycaemic, hypolipidaemic, antipyretic, antispasmodic, antiplatelet and antihelmintic	Yancheva et al. (2005), Rubnov (2001), Gond (2008), Perez (1998), Asadi (2006), Patil (2010), Mohamad (2011), and Amorin (1999)
Mauz	Musa × paradisiaca	Antidiarrhoeal, anti-ulcerative, hypoglycaemic, antihypertensive, diuretic, antioxidant, and wound healer	Rabbani et al. (1999), Rabbani et al. (2001), Jain et al. (2007), Singh et al. (2007), Orie (1997), and Yin et al. (2008)

(Continued)

TABLE 10.1 (CONTINUED)
Medicinal Activities of Sacred Medicinal Plants

Common Name	Scientific Name	Proven Medicinal Activities	References
Baer	*Ziziphus mauritiana*	Anticancer, antioxidant, antihyperglycaemic, antidiarrhoeal, hepatoprotective, and antimicrobial	Mishra et al. (2011) and Jarald (2009)
Rehan	*Ocimum sanctum*	Antibacterial, antifungal, antiviral, analgesic, antipyretic, and anti-inflammatory	Joshi et al. (2011), Amadi et al. (2010), Sharma et al. (2002), Vogel (2002), and Mahima et al. (2012)
Peepal	*Ficus religiosa*	Antimicrobial, antiparasitic, anticonvulsant, hepatoprotective, nephroprotective, antidiabetic, anti-inflammatory, analgesic, anti-ulcer, and wound healer	Rahman (2014), De Amorin (1999), Singh (2014), Parameswari et al. (2013), Yadav (2015), Kirana (2009), Viswanathan et al. (1990), Gulecha (2011), Gregory et al. (2013), and Murti et al. (2011)
Bael	*Aegle marmelos*	Antidiabetic, hepatoprotective, antimicrobial, analgesic, anti-inflammatory, antipyretic, antifungal, anticancer, anti-ulcer, and antithyroid	Singanan et al. (2007), Maheshwari et al. (2009), Arul et al. (2005), Patil (2009), Leticia (2005), Goel (1997), and Panda (2006)
Neem	*Azadirachta indica*	Antioxidant, anticancer, anti-inflammatory, hepatoprotective, wound healing, antidiabetic, antimicrobial, antimalarial, and antinephrotoxic	Ghimeray et al. (2009), Harish (2009), Naik. (2014), Baligar et al. (2014), Osunwoke et al. (2013), and Joshi et al. (2011)
Sandal	*Santalum album*	Hepatoprotective, memory enhancement, anti-ulcer, antibacterial, antifungal, antiviral, anticancer, antihypertensive, antipyretic, sedative, cardioprotective, anti-inflammatory, and antihyperlipidaemic	Hegde (2014), Papaiah et al. (2010), Okugawa et al. (1995), Ahmed et al. (2013), Viollon (1994), and Kulkarni et al. (2012)
Qinnab	*Cannabis sativa*	Anticancer and antidiabetic	Levendal (2006) and Ramer (2015)

(Continued)

TABLE 10.1 (CONTINUED)
Medicinal Activities of Sacred Medicinal Plants

Common Name	Scientific Name	Proven Medicinal Activities	References
Ashok	*Saraca asoca*	Antimenorrhagic, antimicrobial, uterine tonic, larvicidal, anticancer, anti-oxytocic, anti-inflammatory, anti-arthritic, cardioprotective, analgesic, anti-ulcer, and antihelmintic	Teunisdie et al. (1983), Pal et al. (1985), Mitra et al. (1999), Mathew et al. (2008), Bhandary et al. (1995), Ghosh et al. (1999), Joseph et al. (2009), Verma et al. (2010), Preethi (2011), Lakshmi et al. (2013)
Sumbul ut Teeb	*Nordostachys jatamansi*	Antifungal, hepatoprotective, anticonvulsant, antidiabetic, neuroprotective, and antioxidant	Mishra et al. (1995), Ali et al. (2007), Rao (2005), and Salim et al. (2003)
Zoofa	*Hyssopus oficinalis*	Antiviral, antimicrobial, and antioxidant	Gollapudi et al. (1995), Hong et al. (2005), and Ozer et al. (2006)
Foful	*Areca catechu*	Antioxidant, anti-inflammatory, hypolipidaemic, hypoglycaemic, antihypertensive, vascular relaxant, antidepressant, anti-allergenic, and anticonvulsant	Koleva et al. (2002), Chempakam (1993), Byun et al. (2001), Inokuchi et al. (1986), Hirozo et al. (1997), Kumarnsit et al. (2005), Lee et al. (2004), and Lodge et al. (1977)
Nilofar	*Nymphaea alba*	Anxiolytic, antifungal, antitumour, and antioxidant	Thippeswamy et al. (2011) and Cudalbeanu et al. (2020)

books. The scientific studies of these sacred plants have shown the promising effect in many cases to be immunomodulatory, antioxidant, and tonic in nature. In addition, these sacred plants also possess other properties, such as anti-inflammatory, analgesic, antipyretic, blood purifier, haemopoietic, wound healing, antifungal activity, anticancer, and antidiabetic, etc., which have been confirmed by modern scientific research.

Although the research data of many eminent researchers have been included in this document, many gaps still remain to be filled, but we hope that this chapter will inspire future scientists and research scholars to take up the task of preserving, documenting, and re-establishing sacred groves to a new level, supported by scientific evidence. These findings may reach the great masses living in the Urban areas. This will also benefit the underprivileged persons residing in the remote areas of the world where it is difficult to buy expensive medicines.

ACKNOWLEDGEMENTS

Special gratitude is expressed to Dr. Sana Nafees, Aligarh Muslim University, Aligarh, Dr. Nighat Anjum and Dr. Mokhtar Alam, Research Officers, Central Council for Research in Unani Medicine, New Delhi, and Dr. Salma Jamal, Jamia Tibbiya, Deoband, for their moral support and prolific suggestions after reading earlier drafts of this manuscript.

BIBLIOGRAPHY

Abedi, A.S., M. Rismanchi, M. Shahdoostkhany, et al. 2017. Microwave-assisted extraction of *Nigella sativa* L. essential oil and evaluation of its antioxidant activity. *Journal of Food Science and Technology* 54:3779–3790.

Abhijit, B.P., A. Gupta, S. Kamble, and B. Shinde. 2017. Immuno-modulatory effect of Flavonoid from *Musa Paradisiaca* on human whole blood against specific Protein Antigen. *European Journal of Biomedical and Pharmaceutical Sciences* 4(2): 376–379.

Abhishek, S.S., M.A. Gunjal, and A.R. Juvekar. 2009. Immunostimulatory activity of aqueous extract of *Azadirachta indica* flowers on specific and nonspecific immune response. *Journal of Natural Remedies* 9(1): 35–42.

Adam, G.O., M.M. Rahman, S.J. Lee, et al. 2016. Hepatoprotective effects of *Nigella sativa* seed extract against acetaminophen-induced oxidative stress. *Asian Pacific Journal of Tropical Medicine* 9:221–227.

Adhami, V.Q., N. Khan, and H. Mukhtar. 2009. Cancer chemoprevention by pomegranate: laboratory and clinical evidence. *Nutrition and Cancer* 6: 811–815.

Afzal, S., M. Batool, A. Ahmad, et al. 2017. Immunomodulatory, cytotoxicity, and antioxidant activities of roots of Ziziphus mauritiana. *Pharmacognosy Magazine* 13(2): S262–S265.

Agarwal, R., A.K. Pant, and O. Prakash. 2012. Chemical composition and biological activities of essential oils of *Cinnamomum tamala, Cinnamomum zeylenicum* and *Cinnamomum camphora* growing in Uttarakhand. *Chemistry of Phytopotentials: Health, Energy and Environmental Perspectives*, p. 87–92.

Ahmad, A., A. Husain, M. Mujeeb, et al. 2013. A review on therapeutic potential on *Nigella sativa*: a miracle herb. *Asian Pacific Journal of Tropical Biomedicine* 3:337–352.

Ahmed, N.S., A. Khan, M.M. Jais, et al. 2013. Anti-ulcer activity of Sandalwood (*Santalum album* L.) stem hydroalcoholic extract in three gastric-ulceration models of wistar rats. *Boletín Latinoamericano y del Caribe de Plantas Medicinales y Aromáticas* 12(1): 81–91.

Ahmedullah, M., and M.P. Nayar. 1999. Red data book of Indian plants, Vol. 4. Peninsular India, Calcutta: Botanical Survey India.

Akassh, M., T. Fathima, and K. Mruthunjaya. 2020. Health promoting effects of *Ziziphus mauritiana*: an overview. *International Journal of Research in Pharmaceutical Sciences.* 11(1): 1067–1072.

Alam, S., N. Anjum, J. Akhtar, et al. 2018. Phytochemical and pharmacological investigations on Rummän (*Punica granatum* L.). *Hippocratic Journal of Unani Medicine* 13(4): 13–23.

Ali, S.S. 2004. Unani Advia-e-Mufrida. *Qaumi Council Bara-e-Faroogh Urdu Zabaan, New Delhi.* pp -177.

Ali, S., K.A. Ansari, M.A. Jafry, et al. 2007. Jatamansi protects against liver damage by induced by thioacetamide in rats. *Journal of Ethonopharmacology* (72): 359–363.

Ali-Shtayeh, M.S., and R.M. Jamous. 2012. Complementary and alternative medicine use amongst Palestinian diabetic patients. *Complementary Therapies in Clinical Practice* 18(1):16–21.

Aljabre, S.H.M., O.M. Alakloby, and M.A. Randhawa. 2015. Dermatological effects of *Nigella sativa. Journal of Dermatology & Dermatologic Surgery* 19:92–98.

Al-Khalil, S. 1995. A survey of plants used in Jordanian traditional medicine. *Pharmaceutical Biology* 33(4): 317–323.

Al-Othman, A.M., F. Ahmad, S. Al-Orf, et al. 2006. Effect of dietary supplementation of *Ellateria cardamum* and *Nigella sativa* on the toxicity of rancid corn oil in rats. *International Journal of Pharmocology* 2(1): 60–65.

Alshatwi, A.A. 2014. Bioactivity-guided identification to delineate the immunomodulatory effects of methanolic extract of *Nigella sativa* seed on human peripheral blood mononuclear cells. *Chinese Journal of Integrative Medicine.* https://Doi.org/10.1007/s11655-013-1534-3.

Amadi, J.E., S.O. Salami, and C.S. Eze. 2010. Antifungal properties and phytochemical screening of extracts of African Basil (*Ocimum gratissimum* L.) *Agriculture and Biology Journal of North America* 1(2):163–166.

Amel, B. 2013. Traditional treatment of high blood pressure and diabetes in Souk Ahras district. *Journal of Pharmacognosy and Phytotherapy* 5(1): 12–20.

Amorin, A.D., H.R. Borba, J.P. Carauta, et al. 1999. Anthelmintic activity of the latex of *Ficus* species. *Journal of Ethnopharmacology* 64(3): 255–258.

Anonymous. 1986. Qarabadeene Majidi. Hamdard Wakf Laboratory: New Delhi. p- 297, 302–305, 310, 387.

Anonymous. 1989. The Wealth of India (Raw material). Council of Industrial and Scientific Research, New Delhi.Vol XI: X-Z. p-111-124.

Anonymous. 1999. The Unani Pharmacopoeia of India. Govt.of India Ministry of Health & Family Welfare (Dept. of AYUSH New Delhi). 1(2): 8, 73.

Anonymous. 2000. Dar-ul-Iman Healing. Food of the Prophet (PBUH).

Anonymous. 2012. Census of India 2011 - The First Report on Religion Data https://censusindia.gov.in/Census_And_You/religion.aspx.

Anonymous. 2006. National Formulary of Unani Medicine. Govt.of India Ministry of Health & Family Welfare (Dept. of AYUSH-New Delhi). 1(1): 71,132.

Anonymous. 2007. Unani Pharmacopoeia of India New Delhi. (AYUSH), Ministry of Health & Family Welfare, Government of India. 1(1): 28–29.

Arul, V., S. Miyazaki, and R. Dhananjayan. 2005. Studies on the anti-inflammatory, antipyretic and analgesic properties of the leaves of *Aegle marmelos* Corr. *Journal of Ethnopharmacology* 96(4):159–163.

Arun, K.A.N., G. Joshi, and H.Y.M. Ram. 2012. Sandalwood: history, uses, present status and the future. *Current Science* 103(12): 1408–1416.

Asadi, F., P. Malihe, M. Robin, et al. 2006. Alterations to lipid parameters in response to fig tree (*Ficus carica*) leaf extract in chicken liver slices. *Turkish Journal of Veterinary and Animal Sciences* 30(3): 315–318.

Atalay, S., I.J. Karpowicz and E. Skrzydlewska. 2019. Antioxidative and anti-inflammatory properties of cannabidiol. *Antioxidants (Basel)* 9(1): 21.

Azmi, A.A. 1995. Basic concepts of Unani Medicine. Jamia hamdard: New Delhi. P-135–136.

Badreldin, H.A., G.M. Blunden, and O. Tanira. 2008. Some phytochemical, pharmacological and toxicological properties of ginger (*Zingiber officinale* Roscoe): a review of recent research. *Food and Chemical Toxicology* 46(2): 409–420.

Baghdadi, A.I.H. 2005. Kitab ul Mukhtarat Fit Tibb, Vol. II (Urdu Translation): Central Council for Research in Unani Medicine. New Delhi. p-226.

Baitar, I. YNM. Jame-ul-Mufaradat Advia-wa-al-Aghzia, (Urdu Translation) Vol. I, CCRUM, New Delhi. pp. 410–412.

Baligar, N.S., R.H. Aladakatti, M. Ahmed, et al. 2014. Hepatoprotective activity of the neem-based constituent azadirachtin-A in carbon tetrachloride intoxicated Wistar rats. *Canadian Journal of Physiology and Pharmacology.* 92(4): 267–77.

Bashir, F., J. Akhtar, N. Anjum, et al. 2018. Kalonji (*Nigella sativa*): transformation from herb to multifunctional medicine. *Journal of Emerging Technologies and Innovative Research* 5(8):132–141.

Bashir, F., J. Akhtar, N. Anjum, et al. 2018. Pharmacological investigations on bael (*Aegle marmelos* Linn.): a Unani medicinal plant. *European Journal of Pharmaceutical and Medical Research* 5(5): 214–219.

Bhandary, M.J., K. Chandrashekar, and K.M. Kaveriappa. 1995. Medical ethnobotany of the Siddis of Uttara Kannada district, Karnataka, India. *Journal of Ethnopharmacology* 47(3):149–58.

Bhar, K., S. Mondal, and P. Suresh. 2019. An eye-catching review of *Aegle marmelos* L. (Golden Apple). *Pharmacognosy Journal* 11(2): 207–24.

Bhat, M., K. Sandeepkumar, R. Amruta, et al. 2011. Antidiabetic properties of *Azardiracta indica* and *Bougainvillea spectabilis*: *In vivo* studies in murine diabetes model. *Evidence-Based Complementary and Alternative Medicine.* Article ID 561625.

Bose, A., S.D. Ray, and M. Sahoo. 2012. Evaluation of analgesic and antioxidant potential of ethanolic extract of *Nymphaea alba* rhizome. *Oxidants and Antioxidants in Medical Science* 1(3): 217–223.

Bourgou, S., R. Ksouri, A. Bellila, et al. 2008. Phenolic composition and biological activities of Tunisian *Nigella sativa* L. shoots and roots. *C R Biology* 331(1): 48–55.

Brahmachari, G. 2004. Neem—an omnipotent plant: a retrospection. *Chem Bio Chem* 5(4): 408–421.

Byun, S.J., H.S. Kim, S.M. Jeon, et al. 2001. Supplementation of *Areca catechu* L. extract alters triglyceride absorption and cholesterol metabolism in rats. *Annals of Nutrition and Metabolism* 45(6): 279–84.

Çalişkan, O., and A.A. Polat. 2011. Phytochemical and antioxidant properties of selected fig (*Ficus carica* L.) accessions from the eastern Mediterranean region of Turkey. *Scientia Horticulturae* 128(4): 473–478.

Carrasco, F.R., G. Schmidt, A.L. Romero, et al. 2009. Immunomodulatory activity of *Zingiber officinale* Roscoe, *Salvia officinalis* L. and *Syzygium aromaticum* L. essential oils: evidence for humor- and cell-mediated responses. *Journal of Pharmacy and Pharmacology* 61(7): 961–7. Doi: 10.1211/jpp/61.07.0017. PMID: 19589240.

Chelliah, A.D. 2008. Biological activity prediction of an ethnomedicinal plant *Cinnamomum Camphora* through bio-informatics. *Ethnobotanical Leaflets* 12:18190.

Chempakam, B. 1993. Hypoglycemic activity of arecoline in betel nut *Areca catechu* L. *Indian Journal of Experimental Biology* 31(5): 474–475.

ChenLung, H., E.I. ChenWang, and Y. Su. 2009. Essential oil compositions and bioactivities of the various parts of *Cinnamomum Camphora* Sieb.Var. *Linaloolifera Fujuta* 31(2):779.

Cudalbeanu, M., B. Furdui, V. Barbu, et al. 2020. Antifungal, antitumoral and antioxidant potential of the danube delta *Nymphaea alba* extracts. *Antibiotics* 9(1): 7.

Dahiru, D, J.M. Sini. 2006. Antidiarrhoeal activity of *Ziziphus mauritiana* root extract in rodents. *African Journal of Biotechnology* 5:941–5.

Dahiru, D., D.N. Mamman, and H.Y. Wakawa. 2010. *Ziziphus mauritiana* fruit extract inhibits carbon tetrachloride-induced hepatotoxicity in male rats. *Pakistan Journal of Nutrition* 9:990–3.

Das, R., R.P. Raman, H. Saha, and R. Singh. 2015. Effect of *Ocimum sanctum* Linn. (Tulsi) extract on the immunity and survival of Labeorohita(Hamilton) infected with Aeromonas hydrophila. *Aquaculture Research* 46(5): 1111–1121.

Dashputre, N.L., and N.S. Naikwade. 2010. Preliminary immunomodulatory activity of aqueous and ethanolic leaves extracts of *Ocimum basilicum* Linn in mice. *International Journal of PharmTech Research* 2(2): 1342–1349.

De Amorin, A., H.R. Borba, J.P. Carauta, et al. 1999. Anthelmintic activity of the latex of Ficus species. *Journal of Ethnopharmacology* 64(3): 255–258.

De, L.P.R., V.R. Gutierrez, and J.R. Hoult. 1999. Inhibition of leukocyte 5-lipooxigenase by phenolics from virgin olive oil. *Biochemical Pharmacology* 157:445–9.

Deepthi, R., and K. Asha. 2012. Fast foods and their impact on health. *Journal of Krishna Institute of Medical Sciences University* 1(2): 7–15.

Doli, D., A. Sachan, S. Mohd, et. al. 2012. *Nymphaea Stellata*: a potential herb and its medicinal importance. *Journal of Drug Delivery & Therapeutics* 2(3): 41–44.

Du, J., L. Jingjing, Z. Jianhua et al. 2018. Structural characterization and immunomodulatory activity of a novel polysaccharide from *Ficus carica*. *Food and Function* 9: 3930. DOI: 10.1039/C8FO00603B.

Duke, J. A., M. J. B. Godwin, J. Ducellier, et al. 2002. Handbook of Medicinal Herbs. 2(1): 646–647.

Durrani F.R., N. Chand, M. Jan, et al. 2008. Immunomodulatory and growth promoting effects of neem (*Azadirachta indica*) leaves infusion in broiler chicks. *Sarhad Journal of Agriculture* 24(4): 655–659.

Eddine, K.H., S. Zerizer, and Z. Kabouche. 2014. Immunostimulatory activity of *Phoenix dactylifera*. *International Journal of Pharm Pharm Science* 6(3): 73–76.

Eddine, L.S., L. Segni, G. Noureddine, et al. 2013. Antioxidant, anti-inflammatory and diabetes related enzyme inhibition properties of leaves extract from selected varieties of *Phoenyx dactylifera* L. *Innovare Journal of Life Sciences*. (1):14–18.

Edris A.E. 2007. Pharmaceutical and therapeutic potentials of essential oils and their individual volatile constituents: a review: *Phytotherapy Research* 21(4): 308–23. doi: 10.1002/ptr.2072.

Elhemeidy, R.M.M., L. Diana, and E. Widjajanto. 2018. Date fruit extract (*Phoenix dactylifera*, Ajwa) modulates NK cells and TNF Alpha in DMBA-induced mammary cancer Sprague-Dawley rats. *Journal of Tropical Life Science* 8(3): 227–235.

Esmaillzadeh, A., F. Tahbaz, I. Gaieni, et al. 2006. Cholesterol-lowering effect of concentrated pomegranate juice consumption in type II diabetic patients with hyperlipidemia. *International Journal of Vitamin and Nutritional Resources* 76(3): 147–51.

Fathiazad, F., and S. Hamedeyazdan. 2011. A review on *Hyssopus officinalis* L.: composition and biological activities. *African Journal of Pharmacy and Pharmacology* 5(17): 1959–1966.

Frizzo, C.D., A.C. Santos, P. Natalia, S.A. Luciana, and L. Daniel. 2000. Essential oils of camphor tree (*Cinnamomum Camphora* Nees & Eberm) cultivated in Southern Brazil. *B. of Biology and Technology* 43(3).

Fujita, T., E. Sezik, and M. Tabata. 1995. Traditional medicine in Turkey VII. Folk medicine in middle and west Black Sea regions. *Economic Botany* 49(4): 406–422.

Gastaldo, P. 1974. Official compendium of the Italian flora. XVI. *Fitoterapia*, 45(1): 199–217.

Ghani, N.M. 1921. Khazain ul Adviya, Vol. III. Sheikh Mohammad Basheer and Sons, Urdu Bazar, Lahore, p-568.

Ghani, N.M. YNM. Khazain ul Adviya, part 1 to 4, Idara-kitab-ul-Shifa, New Delhi. P-332, 333, 549, 550, 551, 761, 762, 763, 869, 870, 918, 919, 920, 1191, 1192, 1193, 1248, 1249, 1284.

Ghimeray, A.K., C. Jin, B.K. Ghimire, et al. 2009. Antioxidant activity and quantitative estimation of azadirachtin and nimbin in *Azadirachta indica* A. Juss grown in foothills of Nepal. *African Journal of Biotechnology.* 8(13): 3084–3091.

Gholamnezhad, Z., H. Rafatpanah, H.R. Sadeghnia, et al. 2015. Immunomodulatory and cytotoxic effects of *Nigella sativa* and thymoquinone on rat splenocytes. *Food and Chemical Toxicology* 86: 72–80.

Ghosh, S., M. Majumder, S. Majumder, et al. 1999. Saracin: a Lactin from *Saraca indica* seed integument induces apoptosis in Human T-Lymphocytes. *Archives of Biochemistry and Biophysics* (371):163–68.

Gil, M.I., D.M. Holcroft, A.A. Kader, et al. 2000. Antioxidant activity of pomegranate juice and its relationship with phenolic composition and processing. *Journal of Agricultural and Food Chemistry* 48(10):4581–9.

Giribabu, N., K.E. Kumar, S.S. Rekha et al. 2015. *Vitis vinifera* (Muscat Variety) seed ethanolic extract preserves activity levels of enzymes and histology of the liver in adult male rats with diabetes. *Evidence Based Complementary and Alternative Medicine*: 542026.

Godhwani, S., J.L. Godhwani, and D.S. Vyas. 1988. *Ocimum sanctum*-a preliminary study evaluating its immunoregulatory profile in albino rats. *Journal of Ethnopharmacology* 24(2–3): 193–198.

Goel, R.K., R.N. Maiti, and A.B. Ray. 1997. Antiulcer activity of naturally occurring pyrano cumarin and isocoumarins and their effect on prostanoid synthesis using human colonic mucosa. *Indian Journal of Experimental Biology* 35(1): 1080–83.

Gollapudi, S.A., 1995. Isolation of a previously unidentified polysaccharide (MAR-10) from Hyssop officinalis that exhibits strong activity against human immunodeficiency virus type 1. *Biochemical and Biophysical Research Communications* (210): 145–151.

Gond, N.Y. and S.S. Khadabadi. 2008. Hepatoprotective activity of *Ficus carica* leaf extract on rifampicin-induced hepatic damage in rats. *Indian Journal of Pharmaceutical Sciences* 70(3): 364–366.

Gregory, M., B. Divya, A.M. Revina, et al. 2013. Anti-ulcer activity of *Ficus religiosa* leaf ethanolic extract. *Asian Pacific Journal of Tropical Biomedicine* 3(7): 554–556.

Gruner O.C. 1970. A Treatise on the Canon of Medicine of Avicenna (Incorporating a translation of the first Book.) Luzac and Co. London. p-416.

Gulecha, V., T. Sivakumar, A. Upaganlawar, et al. 2011. Screening of *Ficus religiosa* leaves fractions for analgesic and anti-inflammatory activities. *Indian Journal of Pharmacology* 43(6):662–666.

Gupta, B.M., R. Gupta, A. Agarwal, and S. Goel. 2018. *Ocimum Sanctum* (medicinal plant) research: A scientometric assessment of global publications output during 2008–17. *International Journal of Information Dissemination and Technology* 8(2): 67–73.

Haghighi, M., and M.S. Rohani. 2013. The effects of powdered ginger (*Zingiber officinale*) on the haematological and immunological parameters of rainbow trout Oncorhynchus mykiss. *Journal of Medicinal Plant and Herbal Therapy Research* 1:8–12.

Hakeem, M.A. 2002. Bustan-ul-Mufradat. Idara Kitab-us-Shifa, Koocha Chelan, Darya Ganj, New Delhi. pp 71, 83, 84, 108, 110, 121, 141, 195, 230, 256, 371, 416, 417, 439, 489.

Hamdani, K.H. 2001. Usoole-Tibb. New Delhi: Qaumi council baraye farogh urdu zaban. p- 400–80.

Harish, K.G., K.V.C. Mohan, A.J. Rao, et al. 2009. Nimbolide a limonoid from *Azadirachta indica* inhibits proliferation and induces apoptosis of human choriocarcinoma (BeWo) cells. *Investigational New Drugs*. 27(3): 246–52.

Hegde, K., T.K. Deepak, and K.K. Kabitha. 2014. Hepatoprotective potential of hydroalcoholic extract of *Santalum album* Linn. leaves. *International Journal of Pharmaceutical Sciences and Drug Research* 6(3): 224–228.

Hirozo, M. 1997. Endothelium -dependent vasodilator effect of extract prepared from the seeds of *Areca catechu* on isolated rat aorta. *Phytotherapy Research* 11(6): 457–459.

Hong, J., L.K. Seok, I.K. Soon, et al. 2005. Anti-acne composition containing plant oil, especially related to composition containing plant essential oil with excellent anti-bacterial activity to propionibacterium acnes and skin safety. R.K.K.T. Kongbo. Korea. KR 2005073080.

Husain, A., G. Sofi, R. Dang, et al. 2010. Unani system of medicine-Introduction and Challenges. *Medical Journal of Islamic World Academy of Sciences* 18(1): 27–30.

Imam, M.Z., and S. Akter. 2011. *Musa paradisiaca* L. and *Musa sapientum* L.: A phytochemical and pharmacological review. *Journal of Applied Pharmaceutical Science* 01(05): 14–20.

Indra, D., P. Dauthala, S. Rawata, et al. 2012. Characterization of essential oil composition, phenolic content, and antioxidant properties in wild and planted individuals of *Valeriana jatamansi* Jones. *Scientia Horticulturae* (136): 61–68.

Indra, D.B., D. Preeti, R. Sandeep, S.G. Kailash, J. Arun, S.R. Ranbeer, and D. Uppeandra. 2012. Characterization of essential oil composition, phenolic content, and antioxidant properties in wild and planted individuals of *Valeriana jatamansi* Jones. *Scientia Horticulturae* 136: 61–68.

Inokuchi, J., H. Okabe, T. Yamauchi, et al. 1986. Antihypertensive substance in seeds of *Areca catechu* L. *Life Sciences* 38(15): 1375–82710.

Inouye, S., H. Yamaguchi, and T. Takizawa. 2001. Screening of the antibacterial effects of a variety of essential oils on respiratory tract pathogens, using a modified dilution assay method. *Journal of Infection and Chemotherapy* 7(4):251–254.

Ittiyavirah, S.P. and P. Varghese. 2014. Evaluation of in vivo immunomodulatory activity of *Punica granatum* Linn. *International Journal of Research in Ayurveda and Pharmacy* 5(2):175–178.

Jain, D.L., A.M. Baheti, S.R. Parakh, et al. 2007. Study of antacid and diuretic activity of ash and extracts of *Musa sapientum* L. fruit peel. *Pharmacognosy Magazine* 3(10): 116–119.

Jarald, E.E., S.B. Joshi, and D.C. Jain. 2009. Antidiabetic activity of extracts and fraction of *Zizyphus mauritiana*. *Pharmaceutical Biology* 47: 328–34.

Jeba, R.C., and G. Rameshkumar. 2013. Comparative study of immuno-modulatory activity of Ocimum species in mice. *International Journal of Pharmaceutical Sciences and Research* 4(9): 3518–3523.

Joseph, L., V. Gupta, R. Chulet, et al. 2009. *Saraca asoca* (Ashoka): a review. *Journal of Chemical and Pharmaceutical Research* 1(1): 62–71.

Joseph, M.M., S.R. Aravind, S. Varghese, et al. 2012. Evaluation of antioxidant, antitumor and immunomodulatory properties of polysaccharide isolated from fruit rind of *Punica granatum*. *Molecular Medicine Reports* 5(2): 489–496.

Joshi, B., S.G. Prasad, B.B. Basnet, et al. 2011. Photochemical extraction and antimicrobial properties of different medicinal plants: *Ocimum sanctum* (Tulsi), *Eugenia caryophyllata* (Clove), *Achyranthes bidentata* (Datiwan) and *Azadirachta indica* (Neem). Journal of Microbiology Antimicrobials 3(1): 1–7.

Joshi, S.G. 2003. *Medicinal Plants*, Oxford & IBH Publishing Co. Pvt. Ltd. New Delhi, 157–158.

Jurjani, I. 2010. Zakheera khwarzam shahi (Urdu Translation). New Delhi: Idara kitab ul shifa. p-18-21, 414–16.

Kabeeruddin, A.M. 1954. Kulliyat-e-Nafisi. New Delhi: Idara kitab ul shifa. p-404-415.

Kabeeruddin, A.M. 1994. Makhzan al-Mufradat. New Delhi: Aijaz Publishing House. p-53.

Kabeeruddin, A.M. 2006. Kulliyat e Qanoon. Aijaz Publishing House, New Delhi. p-239-240.

Kabeeruddin, A.M. 2009. Tarjuma wa Shrah Kulliyat e Nafeesi. New Delhi: Idare Kitab ul Shifa. p-278: 424–427.

Kabeeruddin, H. YNM. Makhzan-ul Mufradaat ba Khawas-ul Advia. Published by Shaikh Mohammad Bashir & Sons, Lahore. PP. 78–79.

Kabuto, H., M. Nishizawa, M. Tada, C. Higashio, T. Shishibori, and M. Kohno. 2005. Zingerone [4-(4- hydroxy-3-methoxyphenyl)-2-butanone] prevents 6-hydroxydopamine depression in mouse striatum and increases superoxide scavenging activity in Serum. *Neurochemical Research* 30(3): 325–332.

Kalam, M.A., Y. Siddique, and A. Ahmad. 2020. Bhang (*Cannabis sativus*): a review of the drug with special emphasis on single use and compound formulations and its pharmacological studies relevant to Unani system of medicine. *World Journal of Pharmaceutical Research* 9(6): 828–841.

Kanaan, M.H., G. Anah, A. Sadiya, et al. 2020. In- vitro protoscolicidal and immunomodulatory effects of *Cinnamomum camphora* and *Ziziphora tenuior* against Echinococcus granulosus protoscolices. *Reviews in Medical Microbiology* July 20

Kang, J.W., S.J. Kim, H.Y. Kim, et al. 2012. Protective effects of HV-P411 complex against D-galactosamine-induced hepatotoxic-ity in rats. *The American Journal of Chinese Medicine* 40(3): 467–480.

Kayser, O., and S.K. Arndt. 2000. Antimicrobial activity of some Ziziphus species used in traditional medicine. *Pharma Pharmacolo Lett.* 10:38–40.

Kelm, M.A., M.G. Nair, G.M. Strasburg, and D.L. DeWitt. 2000. Antioxidant and cyclooxygenase inhibitory phenolic compounds from *Ocimum sanctum* Linn. *Phytomedicine* 7(1): 7–13.

Khan, H.A. 2011. Al-Akseer. Urdu translation, by Hkm. Kabiruddin. New Delhi, Published by Idara Kitab-Us-Shifa. p-519–22.

Khare, C.P. 2007. Indian Medicinal Plants: an illustrated dictionary. New Delhi: Springer (India) Private Limited, pp- 238, 400, 652, 653, 735, 150–151, 711–12, 492, 491, 501, 363–64, 163–64, 488, 452.

Khare, C.P. 2007. Indian Medicinal Plants: An Illustrated Dictionary. Springer India (P) Ltd. New Delhi. p-122, 154–155, 157, 175–76, 265, 396–97, 423, 448, 519, 521.

Kheirouri, S., H. Vahid, and M. Alizadeh. 2016. Immunomodulatory effect of *Nigella sativa* oil on T Lymphocytes in patients with Rheumatoid Arthritis. *Immunological Investigations* 45(4): 271–283.

Killestein, J., E. Hoogervorst, M. Reif, M. Smits, B.M.J. Uitdehag, and C.H. Polman. 2003. Immunomodulatory effects of orally administered cannabinoids in multiple sclerosis. *Journal of Neuroimmunology* 137(1–2):140–3.

Kirana, H., S.S. Agrawal and B.P. Srinivasan. 2009. Aqueous extract of Ficus religiosa Linn. reduces oxidative stress in experimentally induced type 2 diabetic rats. *Indian Journal of Experimental Biology* 47(10): 822–826.

Kirtikar, K.R., and B.D. Basu. 1991. Indian Medicinal Plants. Published by Bishen Singh Mahendra Pal Singh, Dehradun. 2nd edition, pp. 883–884.

Koji, K., U. Yuji, H. Mitsuru, and O. Hajime. 2011. A matured fruit extract of date palm tree (*Phoenix dactylifera* Linn.) stimulates cellular immunity in mice. *Journal of Agricultural and Food Chemistry* 59(20): 11287–11293.

Koleva, T.A., V. Beek, P.H. Linssen, et al. 2002. Screening of plant extracts for antioxidant activity: a comparative study on three testing methods. *Phytochemical Analysis* (13): 8–17.

Krishna, H., and A. Parashar. 2013. Phytochemical constituents and antioxidant activities of some indian jujube (*Ziziphus mauritiana* Lamk.) cultivars. *Journal of Food Biochemistry* 37(5): 571–577.

Kulkarni, C.R., M.M. Joglekar, S.B. Patil, et al. 2012. Antihyperglycemic and antihyperlipidemic effect of *Santalum album* in streptozotocin induced diabetic rats. *Pharmaceutical Biology* 50(3): 360–365.

Kumarnsit, E., N. Keawpradub, U Vongvatcharanon, et al. 2005. Suppressive effects of dichloromethane fraction from the *Areca catechu* nut on naloxone-precipitated morphine withdrawal in mice. *Fitoterapia*. 76(6): 534–9.

Laeliocattleya, R.A., V. Estiasih, G. Griselda, and J. Muchlisyiyah. 2018. The bioactive compounds and antioxidant activity of ethanol and ethyl acetate extracts of Candi banana (*Musa paradisiaca*). In: Proceedings of the International Conference on Green Agro-industry and Bioeconomy. IOP Publishing; IOP Conference Series: Earth and Environmental Science.

Lakshmi C., M. Madhuri, S. Anwar, et al. 2013. Evaluation of antiulcerogenic activity of various extracts of *Saraca indica* bark on aspirin induced gastric ulcers in albino rats. *International Journal of Research in Pharmacy and Chemistry* (3). 753–58.

Lakshmi, B.V., M. Sudhakar and M Aparna. 2013. Protective potential of Black grapes against lead induced oxidative stress in rats. *Environmental Toxicology and Pharmacology* 35: 361–368.

Lakshmi, T., N. Madhusudhanan, R. Rajendran. 2013. *Nymphaea alba* Linn- an overview. *Research Journal of Pharmacy and Technology* 6(9): 974–977.

Lantz, R.C., G.J. Chen, M. Sarihan, et al. 2007. The effect of extracts from ginger rhizome on inflammatory mediator production. *Phytomedicine* 14:123–128.

Latica, V., and L. Costa. 2005. Evaluation of anticancer potential used in Bangladeshi folk medicine. *Journal of Ethnopharmacology* 99(1): 21–38.

Lee, K.K. and J.D. Choi 1999. The effects of *Areca Catechu* L extract on anti-inflammation and anti-melanogenesis. *International Journal of Cosmetic Science* 21(4): 275.

Lee, V. 2004. *In-vitro* and *in-vivo* anti-allergic actions of Arecae semen. *Journal of Pharmaceutics and Pharmacology* 56(7): 927.

Levendal, R.A., and C.L. Frost. 2006. In vivo effects of *Cannabis sativa* L. extract on blood coagulation, fat and glucose metabolism in normal and Streptozocin-induced diabetic rats. *African Journal of Traditional, Complementary and Alternative Medicines* 3(4): 1–12.

Lin, G.M., Y. Chen, P. Yen, et al. 2015. Antihyperglycemic and antioxidant activities of twig extract from *Cinnamomum osmophloeum*. *African Journal of Traditional, Complementary and Alternative Medicines* 6: 281–8.

Liza, M.S. 2020. Analysis of phenolic compounds and immunomodulatory activity of areca nut extract from Aceh, Indonesia, against Staphylococcus aureus infection in Sprague-Dawley rats. *Veterinary World* 13(1): 134–140.

Lodge, M. 1977. Brand: Effects of the Areca nut constituents arecaidine and guvacine on the action of GABA in the cat central nervous system. *Brain Research* 136 (3): 513–522.

Lone A.H., T. Ahmed, M. Anwar, et al. 2012. Perception of health promotion in Unani herbal medicine. *Medical Journal of Islamic World Academy of Sciences* 20(1): 1–5.

Madhusudhanan, P. 2011. Invitro antioxidant and free radical scavenging activity of aqueous and ethanolic flower extract of *Nymphaea Alba*. *International Journal of Drug Development and Research* 3(3): 252–258.

Maheshwari, V.L., P.V. Joshi, and R.H. Patil. 2009. In vitro anti-diarrhoeal activity and toxicity profile of *Aegle marmelos* Correa ex. Roxb. dried fruit pulp. *Natural Product Radiance* 8 (5): 498–502.

Mahima, F. 2012. Immunomodulatory and therapeutic potentials of herbal, traditional / indigenous and ethno veterinary medicines. *Pakistan Journal of Biological Sciences* 15(16): 754–774.

Mahmoud, M.F., A.A. Diaai, and F. Ahmed. 2012. Evaluation of the efficacy of ginger, Arabic gum, and Boswellia in acute and chronic renal failure. *Renal Failure* 34:73–82.

Maity, S. 2012. Immuno-modulatory effect of *Ficus religiosa* and *ziziphus mauritiana* leaf extracts in broiler birds. *Indian Journal of Field Veterinarians* 7(4): 39–41.

Malik, M.S., S.K. Jaouni, and M.F. Malik. 2016. Review-therapeutic implications of *Nigella sativa* against cancer metastasis. *Pakistan Journal of Pharmaceutical Science* 29:1881–1884.

Mallurvar, V. and A.K. Pathak. 2008. Studies on immunomodulatory activity of *Ficus religiosa*. *Indian Journal of Pharmaceutical Education and Research* 42(4): 343–347.

Mansouri, A., G. Embarek, E. Kokkalou, and P. Kefalas. 2005. Phenolic profile and antioxidant activity of the Algerian ripe date palm fruit (*Phoenix dactylifera*). *Food Chemistry* 89:411–420.

Mariod, A.A., R.M. Ibrahim, M. Ismail, and N. Ismail. 2009. Antioxidant activity and phenolic content of phenolic rich fractions obtained from black cumin (*Nigella sativa*) seedcake. *Food Chemistry* 116(1): 306–312.

Marwat, S.K., M.A. Khan, F. Rehman, I.U. Bhatti. 2009. Aromatic plant species mentioned in the Holy Qura'n and Ahadith and their ethnomedicinal importance. *Pakistan Journal of Nutrition* 8:1472–1479.

Maseehi A.S. 2008. Kitab-ul-Mia. Central Council for Research In Unani Medicine New Delhi. Ministry of Health & Family Welfare, Govt. of India. 1: 257–293.

Mathew, L. 2008. Larvicidal activity of Saraca indica, Nyctanthes arbor-tristis, and Clitoria ternatea extracts against three mosquito vector species. *Parasitology Research.* (104): 1017–25.

Mediratta, P.K., K.K. Sharma, and S. Singh. 2002. Evaluation of immunomodulatory potential of *Ocimum sanctum* seed oil and its possible mechanism of action. *Journal of Ethnopharmacology* 80(1): 15–20.

Michael, H.N., J.Y. Salib, and E.F. Eskander. 2013. Bioactivity of diosmetin glycosides isolated from the epicarp of date fruits, *Phoenix dactylifera*, on the biochemical profile of alloxan diabetic male rats. *Phytotherapy Research* 27:699–704.

Mishra et al. 1995. The fungitoxic effect of the essential oil of the herb *N. jatamansi* DC, *Tropical Agriculture* (72): 48–52.

Mishra, T., and A. Bhatia. 2010. Augmentation of expression of immunocytes functions by seed extract of *Ziziphus mauritiana* (Lamk.). *Journal of Ethnopharmacology* 127: 341–5.

Mishra, T., M. Khullar, and A. Bhatia. 2011. Anticancer potential of aqueous ethanol seed extract of *Ziziphus mauritiana* against cancer cell lines and Ehrlich ascites carcinoma. *Evidence based Complementary and Alternative Medicine.* 765029.

Mitra, S. 1999. Uterine tonic activity of U-3107(even care), a herbal preparation in rats. *Indian Journal of Pharmacology* (31): 200–203.

Mohamad, S., N.M. Zin, and H.A. Wahab. 2011. Anti-tuberculosis potential of some ethno botanically selected Malaysian plants. *Journal of Ethnopharmacology* 133(3): 1021–1026.

Mohan, C., S. Kistamma, P. Vani, N.A. Reddy. 2016. Biological Activities of Different Parts of *Saraca asoca* an Endangered Valuable Medicinal Plant. *International Journal of Current Microbiology and Applied Sciences.* 5(3): 300–308.

Momin, H., Y.N.M. Tohfatul Momineen, Matba Hasni (Persian version). P- 128.

Mukherjee, R., P.K. Dash, and G.C. Ram. 2005. Immunotherapeutic potential of *Ocimum sanctum* (L.) in bovine subclinical mastitis. *Research in Veterinary Science* 79(1): 37–43.

Mukherjee, P.K., M. Sahu, and B. Suresh. 1998a. Indian herbal medicines – a global approach. *Eastern Pharmacist* 21–23.

Mukherjee, P.K. 2002a. Problems and prospects for the GMP in herbal drugs in Indian Systems of Medicine. *Journal of Drug Information* USA 63: 635–644.

Murthy, K.N., V.K. Reddy, and J.M. Veigas. 2004. Study on wound healing activity of Punica granatum peel. *Journal of Medicinal Food*. 7:256–9.

Murti, K. 2011. Exploration of healing promoting potentials of roots of *Ficus religiosa*. *Pharmacologia* 2: 374–378.

Muzafar, D., A. Bhat, and R. Malik. 2017. Pharmacological profile and uses of Sumbul-ut-teeb (*Nardostachys jatamansi*) in unani system of medicine. *International Journal of Advanced Complementary and Traditional Medicine* 3(1): 51–58.

Nadkarni A.K. 2009. Indian Materia Medica with Ayurvedic, Unani-Tibbi, Siddha, Allopathic, Homeopathic, Naturopathic and Home remedies. Bombay: Popular Prakashan Private Ltd, 1st Volume. pp -480, 772, 1203, 1309, 333, 1285–86, 969–72, 965, 140, 991–92, 957, 873–74.

Nadkarni K.M. 1976. Indian materia medica. 3rd edition. Bombay Popular Prakashan. p- 1038.

Nadkarni K.M. 1982. Indian materia medica, Vol. 1. Popular Book Depot, Bombay-India. p- 545–547.

Nadkarni, K.M. 1986. Indian Materia Medica. Popular Prakashan, Bombay. p- 1315–1319.

Naik, L. 2014. Study of anti-inflammatory effect of neem seed oil (*Azadirachta indica*) on infected albino rats. *Journal of Health Research and Reviews*. 1(3): 66–69.

Ndhlala, A.R. 2008. Antioxidant properties of methanolic extracts from *Diospyros mespiliformis* (jackal berry), *Flacourtia indica* (Batoka plum), *Uapaca kirkiana* (wild loquat) and *Ziziphus mauritiana* (yellow berry) fruits. *International Journal of Food Science and Technology* 43:284–8.

Ngadiman, H.S. 2005. Distribution of Camphor Mono oxygenase in Soil Bacteria. *Indonesian Journal of Biotechnology* 10(2): 84853.

Nigrami H. 2009. Tarikh e Tibb. New Delhi: Qaumi council baraye farogh urdu zaban. p- 345–50.

Nurul, H. 2013. Immunomodulatory effects of *Zingiber Officinale* Roscoe var. Rubrum (Halia Bara) on Inflammatory Responses Relevant to Psoriasis. *The Open Conference Proceedings Journal* 4: 76.

Okugawa, N. 1995. Effect of α- santalol and β- santalol from sandalwood on the central nervous system in mice. *Phytomedicine*. 2(2): 119–126.

Orie, N.N. 1997. Direct vascular effects of plantain extract in rats. *Exploratory Physiology* 82: 501–506.

Osunwoke, D. 2013.The wound healing effects of aqueous leave extracts of *Azadirachta indica* on wistar rats. *Journal of Natural Science and Research*. 3(6): 181–186.

Owen, R.W., W. Mier, A. Giacosa, W.E. Hule, B. Spiegelhalder, and H. Bartsch. 2000. Phenolic compounds and squalene in olive oils: the concentration and antioxidant potential of total phenols, simple phenols, secoroids, lignans and squalene. *Food and Chemical Toxicology* 38:647–59.

Ozer, M.H.S.H. Itihad, N.M.Al Bashr, et al. 2006. In vitro antimicrobial and antioxidant activities of the essential oils and methanol extracts of *Hyssopus officinalis* L. ssp. Angustifolius. *Italian Journal of Food Sciences* 18: 73–83.

Pal, J. 1985. Plant profile, phytochemistry and pharmacology of Ashoka (*Saraca asoca* (Roxb.), De. Wilde) – a comprehensive review. *Indian Journal of Medicinal Research* 82(2):188–189.

Panda, S., A. Kar. 2006. Evaluation of the antithyroid, antioxidative and antihyperglycemic activity of scopoletin from *Aegle marmelos* leaves in hyperthyroid rats. *Phytotherapy Research* 20(12): 1103–5.

Papaiah, S. 2010. Memory enhancing property of *Santalum album* L. on mice. *Research J. Pharmacology and Pharmacodynamics* 2(1): 94–96.

Parameswari, S.A., C.M. Chetty and K.B. Chandrasekhar. 2013. Hepatoprotective activity of *Ficus religiosa* leaves against isoniazid + rifampicin and paracetamol induced hepatotoxicity. *Pharmacognosy Research* 5(4): 271–276.

Patel, P., S. Mohammed, A. Basheeruddin. 2010. Immunomodulatory activity of methanolic fruit extract of *Aegle marmelos* in experimental animals. *Saudi Pharmaceutical Journal* 18(3): 161–165.

Patil, R.H., B. Chaudhary, and S. Settipalli. 2009. Antifungal and Anti aflatoxigenic activity of *Aegle marmelos* Linn. *Pharmacognosy Journal* 1(4): 298–301.

Patil, V.V., S.C. Bhangale, and V.R. Patil. 2010. Evaluation of anti-pyretic potential of *Ficus carica* leaves. *International Journal of Pharmaceutical Sciences Review and Research*, 2(2): 48–50.

Patil, V.V., S.C. Bhangale, and V.R. Patil. 2010. Studies on immunomodulatory activity of *Ficus carica*. *International Journal of Pharmacy and Pharmaceutical Sciences* 2(4): 97–99.

Perez, C. 1998. A study on the glycaemic balance in streptozotocin-diabetic rats treated with an aqueous extract of *Ficus carica* (fig tree) leaves *Phytotherapy Research*, 10(1): 82–83.

Pokhrel, B., S. Rijal, S. Raut, and A. Pandeya. 2015. Investigations of antioxidant and antibacterial activity of leaf extracts of *Azadirachta indica*. *African Journal of Biotechnology* 14(46): 3159–3163.

Porquet, D., G. Casadesús, S. Bayod, et al. 2013. Dietary resveratrol prevents Alzheimer's markers and increases life span in SAMP8. Age (Dordr) 35: 1851–1865.

Pratheepa, V., D. Madasamy, and N. Sukumaran. 2011. Immunomodulatory activity of *Aegle marmelos* in freshwater fish (Catla catla) by non-specific protection. *Pharmaceutical Biology* 49(1): 73–7.

Preethi, F. and K. Krishnakumar. 2011. Anti-inflammatory activity of the barks of *Saraca indica* Linn. *Pharmacology Online*. (2): 657–62.

Preeti, B., A. Bharti, A. Sharma, et al. 2012. A review on *Saraca indica* plant. *International Research Journal of Pharmaceutics* (3): 80–84.

Qamri, A.A. 2008. Ghana Mana. Urdu Translation. Central Council for Research In Unani Medicine New Delhi. Ministry of Health & Family Welfare, Govt. of India. p- 331, 451.

Qarshi, A.A. 2010. Ifada e Kabeer (Majmal) (Urdu translation By Mohd Kabeeruddin). New Delhi: Idara e Kitab us Shifa. p- 83, 88,135,136.

Qarshi, M.H. 2011. Jamiul Hikmat. Volume 2. New Delhi: Aijaz Publishing House. P-797–800.

Rabbani, G.H. 1999. Short chain fatty acids inhibit fluid and electrolyte loss induced by cholera toxin in proximal colon of Rabbit *in vivo*. *Digestive Diseases and Sciences* 44: 1547–1553.

Rabbani, G.H. 2001. Clinical studies in persistent diarrhoea: Dietary management with green banana or pectin in Bangladeshi children. *Gastroenterology*. 121: 554–560.

Rafeequddin, M. 1985. Kanzul Advia. Aligarh: AMU. p-108–109.

Rahman, M. 2011. A review: pharmacognostics & pharmacological property of *N. jatamansi* DC. *Elixir Pharmacy* (39): 5017–5020.

Rahman, M. 2014. Phytochemical, cytotoxic and antibacterial activity of two medicinal plants of Bangladesh. *Pharmacology Online* 4: 3–10.

Ram, S. 1997. Immunomodulatory effects of NIM-76, a volatile fraction from Neem oil. *Journal of Ethnopharmacology* 55(2):133–9. doi: 10.1016/s0378-8741(96)01487-0.

Ramer, R., and B. Hinz. 2015. New insights into antimetastatic and antiangiogenic effects of cannabinoids. *International Review of Cell and Molecular Biology*. (314): 43–116.

Rao V.S., and A. Rao. 2005. Anticonvulsant and neurotoxicity profile of *Nardostachys jatamansi* in rat. *Journal of Ethnopharmacology* 102:351–6

Rashid, B. 2015. *Areca Catechu:* Enfolding of historical and therapeutic traditional knowledge with modern update. *Indian Journal of Pharmacology* 2(5): 221–228.

Razi, Z. 1991. Kitab ul Mansoori, 1st edition, (Urdu Translation by CCRUM, New Delhi). p-25–29.

Rehman, R., and M. Akram. 2010. *Zingiber officinale* Roscoe (pharmacological activity) *Journal of Medicinal Plants Research* 5(3):344–348.

Ribeiro, R.D.A., M. de Melo, and F. de Barros. 1986. Acute antihypertensive effect in conscious rats produced by some medicinal plants used in the state of São Paulo. *Journal of Ethnopharmacology* 15(3): 261–269.

Rizwan, K. 2010. Shareh Asbab. Urdu Translation. Central Council for Research in Unani Medicine New Delhi. Ministry of Health & Family Welfare, Govt. of India. 3: 61–77.

Ross, G., R.S. Selvasubramnium, and S. Jayasunder. 2001. Immunomodulatory activity of *Punica granatum* in rabbits. A preliminary study. *Journal of Ethanopharmacology* 78(1):85–7.

Rubnov, S. 2001. Suppressors of cancer cell proliferation from fig (*Ficus carica*) resin: isolation and structure elucidation. *Journal of Natural Products* 64(7): 993–996.

Rushd, I. 1997. Kitab ul kulliyat (Urdu Translation). New Delhi: CCRUM. p-165–172.

Ryu, H.S., and H., Kim 2004. Effect of *Zingiber officinale* Roscoe extracts on mice immune cell activation. Korean Journal of Nutrition 37(1): 23–30.

Saada, H.N. 2009. Grape seed extract *Vitis vinifera* protects against radiation-induced oxidative damage and metabolic disorders in rats. *Phytotherapy Research* 23:434–438.

Saha, J., T. Mitra, K. Gupta, et al. 2012. Phytoconstituents and HPTLC analysis in *Saraca asoca* (Roxb.) Wilde. *International Journal of Pharmacy and Pharmaceutical Sciences.* 4(1): 96–99.

Sakshima, S. 2014. Antioxidant Activity of Essential Oil and Extracts of Valeriana jatamansi Roots. *BioMedical Research International.* Article ID 614187.

Salim, M.N. 2003. Protective effect of *Nardostachys jatamansi* in rat cerebral ischemia. *Pharmacology and Biochemical Behaviour* (74): 481–486.

Samarqandi, N. 1906. Risala Al Asbab wal Alamat. Matba Nami, 1st edition. Munshi Nawal Kishore, Lucknow. PP. 236–240.

Sampath, K.P., D. Bhowmik, S. Duraivel, and M. Umadevi. 2012. Traditional and Medicinal uses of Banana. *Journal of Pharmacognosy and Phytochemistry.* 1(3): 52–53.

Sari, L.M., R.F. Hakim, Z. Mubarak, and A. Andriyanto. 2020. Analysis of phenolic compounds and immunomodulatory activity of areca nut extract from Aceh, Indonesia, against *Staphylococcus aureus* infection in Sprague-Dawley rats. *Veterinary World* 13(1): 134–140.

Sari, L.M. 2021. Antioxidant activity of areca nut to human health: Effect on oral cancer cell lines and immunomodulatory activity. *Bioactive Compounds in Nutraceutical and Functional Food for Good Human Health.*

Satyal, P. 2013. Bioactivities and compositional analyses of Cinnamomum essential oils from Nepal: C. camphora, C. tamala, and C. glaucescens. *Natural Product Communications* 8(12):1777–1784.

Schubert, S.Y., E.P. Lansky, and I. Neeman. 1999. Antioxidant and eicosanoid enzyme inhibition properties of pomegranate seed oil and fermented juice flavonoids. *Journal of Ethnopharmacology* (66): 11–17.

Shamsi, T.N., R. Parveen, S. Afreen, et al. 2014. *In vitro* Antibacterial and Antioxidant Activities of Sandalwood (*Santalum album*). *Austin Journal of Biotechnology & Bioengineering* 1(2): 3.

Sharma, M.K., M. Kumar, and A. Kumar, 2002. *Ocimum sanctum* aqueous leaf extract provides protection against mercury induced toxicity in Swiss albino mice. *Indian Journal of Experimental Biology* 40(9): 1079–82.

Shi, C., C. Jianyun, Y. Xiaofei, et al. 2014. Grape seed and clove bud extracts as natural antioxidants in silver carp (Hypophthalmichthys molitrix) fillets during chilled storage: Effect on lipid and protein oxidation. *Food Control* 40(1): 134–139.

Silva, R.M., V.M. Campanholo, and A.P. Paiotti. 2015. Chemopreventive activity of grape juice concentrate (G8000TM) on rat colon carcinogenesis induced by azoxymethane. *Environment Toxicological Pharmacology* 40: 870–875.

Sina, I. 2010. Al qanoon Fit Tib (Urdu Translation). New Delhi: Idara kitabul shifa. p-16, 17, 18, 28, 35, 83, 89, 203, 204.

Singanan, V., M. Singanan, and H. Begum. 2007. The hepatoprotective effect of bael leaves (Aegle marmelos) in alcohol induced liver injury in albino rats. *International Journal of Science & Technology* 2(2): 83–92.

Singh, P., D. Singh, and R.K. Goel. 2014. *Ficus religiosa* L. figs - a potential herbal adjuvant to phenytoin for improved management of epilepsy and associated behavioural comorbidities. *Epilepsy Behaviour* 41:171–178.

Singh, S.K., A.N. Kesari, and P.K. Rai. 2007. Assessment of glycemic potential of *Musa paradisiaca* Stem Juice. *Indian Journal of Clinical Biochemistry* 22(2): 48–52.

Sogut, B., I. Celik, and Y. Tuluce. 2008. The effects of diet supplemented with the black Cumin (*Nigella sativa* L.) upon immune potential and antioxidant marker enzymes and lipid peroxidation in broiler chicks. *Journal of Animal and Veterinary Advances* 7(10): 1196–1199.

Soni, N., S. Mehta, G. Satpathy, and R.K. Gupta. 2014. Estimation of nutritional, phytochemical, antioxidant and antibacterial activity of dried fig (*Ficus carica*). *Journal of Pharmacognosy and Phytochemistry* 3(2):158–165.

Sumner, M.D. 2005. Effects of pomegranate juice consumption on myocardial perfusion in patients with coronary heart disease. *American Journal of Cardiology* 96:810–4.

Sydney, S., N.C. Sanford, J. Freeman, M. HillReba, M.K. Benjamin, and K. Ralph. 1978. Camphor: Who Needs It? American Academy of Pediatrics 62(3): 404–06.

Tabri, A.R. 2003. Firdous al Hikmat. Faisal Publications. Deoband. P-28.

Talhaoui, N., A. Taamalli, A. María Gómez-Caravaca, A. Fernández-Gutiérrez, and A. Segura-Carretero. 2015. Phenolic compounds in olive leaves: Analytical determination, biotic and abiotic influence, and health benefits. *Food Research International* 77: 92–108.

Tan, B.K., and J. Vanitha. 2004. Immunomodulatory and antimicrobial effects of some traditional Chinese medicinal herbs: a review. *Current Medicinal Chemistry* 11(11):1423–30. Doi: 10.2174/0929867043365161. PMID: 15180575.

Tariq, N.A. 2010. Taju-ul Mufradaat, Khawas-ul Advia. Published by Idara-e-Kitabus shifa, New Delhi, 63–65.

Teunisdie, M.S. 1983. Evaluation of Asoka Aristha, an indigenous medicine in Sri Lanka. *Journal of Ethnopharmacology* 8(3): 313–320.

Thippeswamy, D. 2011. Anxiolytic activity of *Nymphaea alba* Linn.in mice as experimental models of anxiety, *Indian Journal of Pharmacology* 43(1): 50–55.

Tong, H., X. Song, X. Sun., G. Sun., and F. Du.2011. Immunomodulatory and antitumor activities of grape seed proanthocyanidins. *Journal of Agricultural and Food Chemistry* 59(21):11543–7.

Tresina, P.S., K. Paulpriya, V. Sornalakshmi, and V.R. Mohan. 2018. Antioxidant activity of *Saraca asoca* (Roxb.) wilde flower: an *in vitro* evaluation. *International Journal of Pharmacognosy and Phytochemical Research* 10(4): 139–145.

Umar, S., J. Zargan, and K. Umar., et al. 2012. Modulation of the oxidative stress and inflammatory cytokine response by thymoquinone in the collagen induce arthritis in Wistar rats. *Chemico-Biological Interactions* 197(1): 40–46.

Upadhyay, S. 1992. Immuno-modulatory effects of neem (*Azadirachta indica*) oil. *International Journal of Immunopharmacology* 14(7):1187–93. doi: 10.1016/0192-0561(92)90054-o.

USDA.gov: https://plants.usda.gov/core/profile.

Van D.N. 1987. Immunomodulatory activity of an aqueous extract of *Azadirachta indica* stem bark. *Journal of Ethnopharmacology* 19(2): 125–13.

Vardanian, S.A. 1978. Phytotherapy of bronchial asthma in medieval Armenian medicine. *Terapevticheskiĭ Arkhiv* 50(4): 133–136.

Venkatachalam, V.V., and B. Rajinikanth. 2013. Immuno-modulatory Activity of Aqueous Leaf Extract of *Ocimum sanctum*. *Recent Advancements in System Modelling Applications*. 188: 425–432. https://doi.org/10.1007/978-81-322-1035-1_37

Verma, S.N. 2010. Analgesic activity of various leaf extracts of *Saraca indica* Linn. *Der pharmacia Lettre*. (2): 352–57.

Viollon, C., and J.P. Chaumont. 1994. Antifungal properties of essential oils and their main components upon Cryptococcus neoformans. *Mycopathologia* 128(3): 151–153.

Viswanathan, S.1990. Antiinflammatory and mast cell protective effect of *Ficus religiosa*. *Ancient Science Life* 10(2): 122–125.

Vlase, M.N. 2014. Evaluation of antioxidant and antimicrobial activities and phenolic profile for *Hyssopus officinalis*, *Ocimum basilicum* and *Teucrium chamaedrys*. *Molecules*. 19(1): 5490–5507.

Vogel, H.G. 2002. Analgesic, anti-inflammatory and antipyretic activity. Drug discovery & evaluation Pharmacological Assays, 2nd edition: 759–767.

Wilasrusmee, D. 2002. In vitro immunomodulatory effects of herbal products. *American Surgeon* 68:860–864.

Xu, K.Z., C. Zhu, and M.S. Kim, et al. 2009. Pomegranate flower ameliorates fatty liver in an animal model of type 2 diabetes and obesity. *Journal of Ethnopharmacology* 123:280–7.

Yadav, Y.C. 2015. Hepatoprotective effect of *Ficus religiosa* latex on cisplatin induced liver injury in Wistar rats. *Revista Brasileira de Farmacognosia* 25: 278–283.

Yancheva, S.D. 2005. Efficient agrobacterium-mediated transformation and recovery of transgenic fig (*Ficus carica* L.) plants. *Plant Science* 6(168):1433–1441.

Yanni, A.E., V. Efthymiou, and P. Lelovas, et al. 2015. Effects of dietary Corinthian currants (Vitis vinifera L., var. Apyrena) on atherosclerosis and plasma phenolic compounds during prolonged hypercholesterolemia in New Zealand White rabbits. *Food Function* 6: 963–971.

Yin, X., J. Quan, and T. Kanazawa. 2008. Banana prevents plasma oxidative stress in healthy individuals. Plant Foods Hum. Nutrition 63: 71–76.

You, T. and B.J. Nicklas. 2006. Chronic inflammation: role of adipose tissue and modulation by weight loss. *Current Diabetes Reviews* 2(2): 29–37.

Zaidi, I. and A. Hasan. 2011. Textbook on Kulliyat e Umoor e tabi'yah. Aligarh. p-1, 15, 81, 96.

Zhao, S. 2020. Immunomodulatory effects of fermented fig (*Ficus carica* L.) fruit extracts on cyclophosphamide-treated mice. *Journal of Functional Foods* 75: 104219.

Zuccarini, P. 2009. Camphor: risks and benefits of a widely used natural product. *Journal of Applied Science and Environvenmental Management* 13(2):69–74.

11 Molecular Features of Potential Herbal Products in Enhancing Human Immune System

Chandrabose Selvaraj, Chandrabose Yogeswari, and Sanjeev Kumar Singh

CONTENTS

11.1 INTRODUCTION

The survival of human beings is greatly influenced by the defensive mechanism of the immune system against various types of harmful pathogens and some of the elements. The immune system potentially helps the host cells to prevent the entry of microorganisms and the development of major health issues like cancer

(Mak et al. 2014). The occurrence of defects in the immune system leads to response impairment against various infectious agents and cancer. Both extrinsic and intrinsic pathways heavily influence the impairment of the immune system. Some of the pathogens, including human immunodeficiency virus or the advanced stage of some of the chronic diseases, may cause impairments (Chinen and Shearer 2010; Abbas et al. 2016). Several medical systems, like Chinese traditional medicine, traditional Thai medicine, African traditional medicine, along with Indian traditional medicine, are currently practiced all around the world by using potential medicinal plants for treating the diseases. In particular, microbial infections, insect, and reptile bites are well treated through the use of available medicinal plants. Due to the range and diversity of the various secondary plant metabolites, herbal remedies are also strongly involved in the development of conventional drugs. Most secondary metabolites are significantly active as potent immunomodulators and improve cell- and humoral-mediated immunity. Secondary metabolites with immunomodulatory properties induce immune modulation in organisms and trigger immune system stimulation against a variety of harmful pathogenic microbial infections. Similarly, they also cause the activation of specialized cells, such as macrophages, natural killer (NK) cells, and granulocytes, subsequently activating the production of cytokines. These cytokines are of core importance for the enhancement of immune response (Lesourd 2006; Vigila and Baskaran 2008). For example, the plant extract of *Mentha longifolia* (mint) has been extensively used in the pharmaceutical industry and in the food and chemical industries. It has potent activities, including antimicrobial, antioxidant, and immunomodulatory effects, with no side effects (Mikaili et al. 2013).

Many plant-derived compounds have been identified from their source plant and their structure elucidated and subsequently used as potential lead molecules for the development of commercial, single-chemical drugs to treat a number of diseases. For example, the widely used drug aspirin was purified from the willow tree bark extract and used as an important painkiller and antipyretic activity (Dias et al. 2012). The major bioactive components of traditionally used plants, including quinine and opium, are commonly used as powerful drug molecules for the treatment of several diseases (Wadood et al. 2013). As a consequence of the successful use of medicinal plants for an extended period into the current day has resulted in a number of researchers focusing on plant-derived lead molecules that have immunomodulating effects to find and develop novel and effective drug molecules to reduce the usage of toxic synthetic chemicals and to reduce the high risk of many chronic diseases. A wide variety of secondary plant metabolites, including flavonoids, terpenoids, phenolics, and curcumins, have potent effects in inhibiting DNA synthesis and stimulating the action of several protective enzymes, such as phase II enzymes. Many medicinal plants are rich in antioxidant molecules that provide efficient protection against chronic disease, maintain low-density lipoprotein (LDL)-cholesterol, and also inhibit both lipoxygenase and cyclooxygenase enzymes to prevent lipid peroxidation (Kyo et al. 2001; Gebreyohannes and Gebreyohannes 2013). This support from the scientific literature provides support for herbal medicines and their effective action against a variety of infectious diseases as an effective alternative approach to current chemotherapy (Dutt 2013). Moreover, it is well known that plant compounds with immunomodulatory effects may also act as highly effective adjuvants to vaccines (Wilson and Warise 2008). Hence, this present book chapter describes the various plant-derived immunomodulatory compounds and their source, mode of action, and their crucial role in immune response to stimulate the immune system.

11.2 ROLES OF MEDICINAL PLANTS

11.2.1 Role in Modern Medicine

In recent years, medicinal plants are often used as the alternative healthcare system in both developing and developed countries. The mixture of natural compounds primarily derived from plants has great potential to treat a wide range of diseases. However, owing to poor absorption, herbal medicines have less effectiveness than other modern, synthetic medicines (Gauttam et al. 2003; Sagar et al. 2005). WHO (the World Health Organization) states that about 80% of the world population have been using medicinal plants in the traditional herbal medicine herbal medicine system for primary health care. The evaluation of modern drugs since the beginning of the 19th century led to the isolation of the first active compound, morphine, purified from the opium poppy by a German pharmacist, followed by the isolation and characterization of a number of plant-based compounds as effective molecules (Hamilton et al. 2000; Joo et al. 2014). Among them, a number are still used in traditional medicine. After the invention of advanced chemical technologies, the development of synthetic compounds has significantly reduced the usage and importance of natural products, although natural products are still used to find potent novel lead molecules in the treatment of cancer, hypertension, and other diseases (Newman et al. 2003). The identification of novel lead molecules in most of the pharmaceutical companies is well developed, with high-throughput synthesis and combinatorial chemistry-based approaches since the 1980s. Some of the pharma industries are facing challenges to develop novel drugs, and, over recent decades, they have focused their attention on natural products for the development of novel drugs with help of modern technology, including high-throughput screening (Zhu et al. 2012; Ngo et al. 2013).

11.2.2 Role in Traditional Chinese Medicine

In addition to Ayurveda and Siddha, Chinese medicine plays a significant role in boosting the immune system and its activity and function. Traditional Chinese medicine was considered to be the most advanced medical science in the late 17th century, and around 12,000 medical classics were distributed through China. In the Chinese medicinal system, several surgeries were practised, like Ayurveda, though, in recent years, only acupuncture and herbal-based therapy are used as major branches of the Chinese medicine system. Basically, two important therapeutic approaches have attracted particular attention in the field of complementary and alternative medicine.

The combination of one or more herbs in a single formulation was one of the most prominent steps in Chinese medicine. The 'Theory of the Five Elements' is widely used in Chinese medicine to describe the relationship between the human body and the five elemental qualities, namely earth, metal, water, wood, and fire. Before the 20th century, Chinese medicine was intensively used for the treatment of various pathological diseases (Xue 1991; Zhang et al. 1996).

Several studies demonstrated that Chinese medicines are highly effective at stimulation of the immune system. Wang et al. (2015) reported that the polysaccharides isolated from the medicinal plant ginseng (*Panax ginseng*) exhibited anticancer properties and also had the ability to improve the size of the organs associated with the immune system; for instance, PGFP1 is a polysaccharide from *Panax ginseng* with potent inhibitory activity in cancer-bearing mice, which reduced the size of the spleen and thymus, also suppressing lipopolysaccharide (LPS) or Concanavalin-A (ConA) -mediated T cell proliferation. The interactions between several compounds in Chinese herbal medicine result in good therapeutic effects, so that the isolation and purification of major active compounds from herbal plant preparations are carefully studied both in preclinical and clinical trials to develop potent novel anti-cancer natural compounds (Zhou et al. 2014). Polysaccharides are among the most important active molecules used in Chinese medicine, with significant anticancer and immune-enhancing properties with fewer side effects, hence the significance of polysaccharides in the widely used Chinese medicine system.

11.2.3 ROLE IN AYURVEDA

Ayurveda is one of the oldest traditional medicinal systems in India, which has been applied and organized since around 1500 BC. The system of Ayurveda is literally defined as the 'Science of Life' and contains 114 hymns and their associated formulations for the management of a number of diseases. Two major schools, Dhanvantari Sampradaya and Atreya Sampradaya, have been nurtured and have gathered the knowledge of Ayurveda over the centuries. The school Atreya Sampradaya represents the compilation of Charaka Samhita with another school of medicine and surgery (Sushruta Samhita). More than one thousand five hundred plant-derived molecules and potent molecules from animal and mineral sources have been described in this medical system. Since the medieval period, only the Ayurveda medicine system existed in the Indian sub-continent for healthcare requirements, and that period is considered to be the golden period of Ayurveda. In the 20th century, the system of Ayurveda received official recognition and a national healthcare network, based on Ayurveda was set up to treat various diseases. After independence, the Indian Government initiated several procedures to enhance the position of Ayurveda as a major health system. Recently, several colleges and hospitals for Ayurveda have been established, regulating the education and registration of Ayurveda, Siddha, and Unani systems of medicine. The use of medicinal plants in the Ayurvedic system has a strong effect on the body and activates the immune system. The classical preparations of Ayurvedic medicines are 90% made from plants with combinations of several plant products for optimal effect. Studies have demonstrated that, compared with a single herbal formulation, the polyherbal preparation shows a longer-lasting effect. Approximately thirty plant species are used in a polyherbal combination in the Ayurveda system of medicine and the major active components are accurately combined in such a way as to make an effective formulation. In the polyherbal formulation, one or more constituents plays the main role and others will support and show different properties, or, in some cases, act as a catalyst for the proper absorption and transportation of major active molecules, to reduce the toxic effects. Generally, the Ayurvedic formulations are safer and show fewer side effects (Kurup 2004; Ravishankar and Shukla 2007).

For instance, the widely used plants, such as pippali, tulsi, and guduchi, show strong and potent activity against infectious diseases. All the plant parts, including leaves, flowers, bark, roots, and seed are selected, with the selection of a specific part of the plant also being important for the development of a good formulation. A particular combination of the plant parts results in the formulation achieving the greatest effect (Jagetia 2004). Polyherbal formulations have the potential to enhance their therapeutic effects compared to single plant products, with this interactive phenomenon being called synergy. Most of the active components of medicinal plants and some in the herb extract have potent pharmacological actions. There are two basic mechanisms of synergistic action, namely pharmacokinetic synergy and pharmacodynamic synergy, which have been employed to facilitate the ADME (absorption, distribution, metabolism, and elimination) properties of the active plant molecules (Parasuraman et al. 2014). Later, this synergistic effect of molecules can be exploited to target similar receptors. Several factors are involved in most of the disease-oriented pathways, the polyherbal formulation targetting the multiple receptors at the same time, thus providing lasting relief (Chorgade 2007). Most of the conventional medicines are preferably administered after food, but, in Ayurveda, medications are directed to be taken on an empty stomach, with the absorption of drugs occurring as part of normal metabolism. The most advanced scientific techniques are used for the identification and characterization of major active compounds from the polyherbal formulation. A combination of three herbs, like long pepper, black pepper, and ginger, significantly improves their mucus-reducing effects, whereas another combination, of neem and ginger, positively offsets any extreme effects (Ponnusankar et al. 2011).

11.2.4 Role in Siddha

The medicinal practice belonging to the Siddha system is considered to be a great achievement of Tamil culture, which is derived from Dravidian culture and practiced in the time of the civilization of the Indus Valley, Chinese culture, and Taoism. Since ancient times, the Siddha system of medicine combines proper diet and health measures (Ajmal et al. 2017). In Tamil culture, Siddha categorized human diseases into 4448 different types, and used medicinal plants as the main source by which to treat different types of diseases. Medicinal plants greatly influence the characteristic features of physiology and have been used to alleviate the effect on the number of pathophysiological states of immunity and immunomodulatory for more than several centuries in the history of medicine. The potent immunomodulator can significantly influence the immune system components and its associated function in either specific or non-specific ways, including both immune responses (innate and adaptive) (Figure 11.1). Hence, the immunomodulators are referred to as substances that can modify and improve the defence mechanism of host cells against pathogenic organisms, to reduce the impact of diseases. The major active components of the medicinal plants regulate the immune system by interacting with different types of immune cells and effector mechanisms. For example, the basic functions involved in the immune systems destroy the non-self cells to induce the mechanisms to detect and eliminate the harmful pathogens (Hubbard et al. 2006). Siddha medicine in India is still used to treat various diseases, including respiratory disease (asthma and chronic obstructive pulmonary disease (COPD)), which are the most important causes of human mortality (Viegi et al. 2006).

Three main sources of natural products are used in the Siddha medicinal system: products from plants (mulavargam), from an animal source (jivavargam), and inorganic materials (thathuvargam), based on the five characteristic features like the taste, quality, potency, post-digestive taste, and action (Zysk 2008). Of the three sources, plant products are dominantly used in the Siddha system and the plant sources predominantly use 108 herbs (karpa mooligai) to treat human ailments. The traditionally used medicinal plants include *Withania somnifera, Solanum trilobatum, Cuminum cyminum, Aloe barbadensis, Azadirachta indica, Zingber officinale, Phyllanthus emblica,* and *Phyllanthus amarus*, which represent a few of those dominantly used in the Siddha system (Ram et al. 2009). These plants greatly influence the immune response and prevent chronic diseases. The medicinal plant formulations are also used in the Siddha system. In recent years in India, more plant

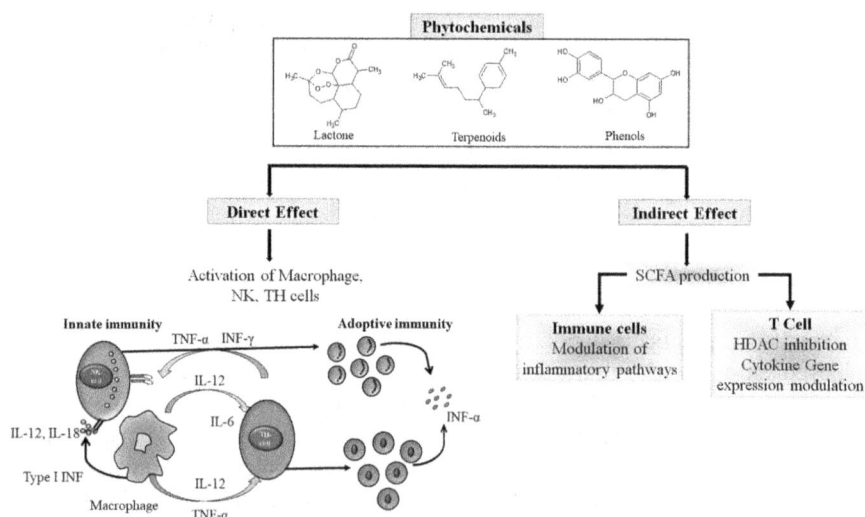

FIGURE 11.1 Schematic representation of phytochemical effects in terms of direct and indirect benefits towards the immune cells.

formulations are used and manufactured commercially by various pharmaceutical companies, including TAMPCOL, IMCOPS, and SKM SIDDHA, and prescribed by Siddha physicians (Ram et al. 2009).

11.2.5 ROLE IN OTHER REGIONAL MEDICINAL SYSTEMS

The growing popularity of traditional remedies, along with its massive commercial potential, has attracted the attention of the pharmaceutical industry, which are eyeing each medicinal system operating around the world. As stated above, the WHO reports that about 65% to 80% of the world's population uses traditional medicines. Apart from above-discussed medicinal systems, African traditional medicine is also a notable holistic discipline that uses ethnic herbalism, combined with spirituality aspects. Much research suggests that modern medicine rooted in this ancient medicine, and exploiting the traditional medicinal practice based on African biodiversity will provide new remedies to the world in the future. This policy is not limited to African traditional medicine but is also appropriate to all the regional traditional medicinal systems.

11.3 MEDICINAL PLANTS AND IMMUNOLOGICAL REGULATION

The body's immune system plays a key role in defence mechanisms and is composed of central immune organs where unique immune cells can develop and exert the effects that subsequently impact host immunity. The major immune system is composed of immune organs like bone marrow and peripheral immune organs, producing numerous immune cells like lymphocytes and a number of phagocytes that monitor cancerogenesis and influence the expression of cytokines to exert anticancer activity, becoming the principal target for cancer treatment. Hence, the status of immune organs is more important for developing novel drug molecules against cancer and other chronic diseases (Wu et al. 2016). The common assembly of the immune system is depicted as being multilayered, achieving a high level of defence. For example, the skin is recognized as a primary immune system, acting as a potent barrier against various infectious diseases as well as being involved in maintaining the temperature and pH of the body, providing an inappropriate environment for harmful organisms. Once the pathogenic microorganism has entered the host body, it is addressed by either an innate and/or an acquired immune system, which has a multitude of cells and molecules which interact with each other to form a complex to detect and attack the pathogen (Hofmeyr, 2001). Several *in-vitro* and *in-vivo* reports have demonstrated the effects of herbal medicines on cytokines, showing that they significantly influence many cytokines. Cytokines are a group of proteins present in the form of interleukins, interferons, and chemokines, which are essential for maintaining physiological stability and their secretion in cells *via* intermolecular crosstalk (Mogensen 2009). Numbers of novel molecules are needed as antagonists, agonists, and initiators. Interferons act as an agonist for hairy cell leukaemia, and tumour necrosis factor has been proposed as an agonist for rheumatoid arthritis (Gomes et al. 2016). Cytokines have diverse pleiotropic characters and play a crucial role in some disorders which are not related to the immune system. In some cases, interferon leads to depression and fatigue due to this adverse effect on patients; recently, phytotherapy has been used as an alternative to modifying the expression of cytokines. The medicinal plant *Astragalus membranaceus* is often used in the Chinese medicinal system to cure several diseases. The extract obtained from root of this plant significantly reduced the level of interleukin IL-6 in an *in-vitro* assay (Suzuki et al. 2008; Denzler et al. 2010). Another plant widely and commonly used in Indian herbal medicine is garlic (*Allium sativum*), which reduces the levels of IL-1 and IL-6 and acts as a potent anti-inflammatory, antioxidant, and angiotensin-converting enzyme inhibitor (Singh et al. 2001). Both innate and adaptive immune systems work together functionally, where the innate immune system distinguishes the signals from the infection, the adaptive system is involved in antigen production and is responsible for major histocompatibility complex proteins. The innate cells secrete the chemical signals, including cytokines and chemokines, to stimulate the adaptive immune system. Specifically, the B and T lymphocytes are well-known regulatory cells that maintain the immune response (Josefowicz et al. 2012; Mauri and Bosma, 2012).

11.3.1 IMMUNOMODULATOR AGENTS

Any biological or synthetic substance which can modulate the expression and aspect of the immune response is known as an immunomodulator, having the capability to stimulate or suppress both the innate and acquired immune systems. Clinically, immunomodulators are classified into three major categories, namely immunostimulants, immunosuppressants, and immunoadjuvants. Immunostimulants are non-specific agents that significantly improve the body's resistance to infection *via* an innate and adaptive immune response. In some cases, immunostimulants act as prophylactic and promoting agents to enhance the basic level of the immune response (Casa et al. 2014). Immunoadjuvants are effectively used for the enhancement of vaccine efficacy and can result in promising effects on the immune response. It has been reported that the immunoadjuvants may be active as selectors among the cellular and humoral helper cells 1 and 2 (Th1 and Th2). Another type of immunosuppressant is a heterogeneous group often concomitantly administered to cure several forms of organ transplant rejection and autoimmune disorders (Casa et al. 2014). A number of medicinal plants have been used as potent immunomodulators in the traditional medicine system of Rasayana to enhance the body's resistance. The medicinal plants also have various pharmacological activities, including antioxidant, anti-inflammatory, cardiotonic, hepatoprotective and antifungal properties. Various major active constituents from medicinal plants and their immunomodulatory role are listed in Table 11.1. Glycosides are one of the classes of plant-derived immunomodulators involved in enzymatic and acid hydrolysis to yield sugar molecules; structurally, they are sugar ethers which can interact with hydroxyl groups of both sugar and non-sugar molecules. A number of glycosides are known to influence immunomodulatory action, such as iridoid glycosides from *Picrorhiza scrophulariiflora*, anthraquinone glycosides, from *Andrographis paniculata*, and sesquiterpene glycosides

TABLE 11.1

Various Types of Immunomodulators and Their Action and Source

Plant name	Active Compound(s)	2-D Structure of the Compound	Mode of Action	Reference
Nigella sativa	Thymoquinone		Modulates pro- and anti-inflammatory cytokines	Majdalawieh and Fayyad 2015
Cuminum cyminum	Cumin oil, *p*-cymene		Activate cytotoxic CD8+ and CD4+ cells	Chauhan et al. 2010
Piper longum	Piperine		Increases total WBC count, bone marrow cellularity, total antibody production	Sunila et al. 2004

(Continued)

TABLE 11.1 (CONTINUED)
Various Types of Immunomodulators and Their Action and Source

Plant name	Active Compound(s)	2-D Structure of the Compound	Mode of Action	Reference
Hydrastis canadensis	Berberine		Significant reduction of plasma TNF-α, IFN-γ, and NO levels	Li et al. 2006
Stephania tetrandra	Tetrandrine		Suppresses cytokine production. Inhibits NF-κB- mediated release of inflammatory factors	Xue et al. 2008

(Continued)

TABLE 11.1 (CONTINUED)
Various Types of Immunomodulators and Their Action and Source

Plant name	Active Compound(s)	2-D Structure of the Compound	Mode of Action	Reference
Sinomenium acutum	Sinomenine		Graft survival	Mark et al.2003
Urtica dioica	Isorhamnetin-3-O-glucoside		*In-vitro* immunomodulatory potential	Akbay et al. 2003

(Continued)

TABLE 11.1 (CONTINUED)
Various Types of Immunomodulators and Their Action and Source

Plant name	Active Compound(s)	2-D Structure of the Compound	Mode of Action	Reference
Boerhavia diffusa	Betuletrin		Inhibits PHA-stimulated proliferation of peripheral blood mononuclear cells, IL-2 and TNF-α	Pandey et al., 2005
Plantago major	Aucubin		Enhances lymphocyte proliferation and secretion of IFN-γ	Chiang et al., 2003
Mangifera indica	Mangiferin		Enhances the production of IgG1 and IgG2b	Garcia et al. 2003

(Continued)

TABLE 11.1 (CONTINUED)
Various Types of Immunomodulators and Their Action and Source

Plant name	Active Compound(s)	2-D Structure of the Compound	Mode of Action	Reference
Phyllanthus embelica	Gallic acid		B cell proliferation, inhibition of mast cell degranulation	Serrano et al. 1998
Punica granatum	Ellagic acid		Antiproliferative and antioxidant activities	Seeram et al. 2005
Plantago major	Chlorogenic acid		Enhances lymphocyte proliferation and secretion of IFN	Chiang et al., 2003

(Continued)

TABLE 11.1 (CONTINUED)
Various Types of Immunomodulators and Their Action and Source

Plant name	Active Compound(s)	2-D Structure of the Compound	Mode of Action	Reference
Plantago major	Ferulic acid		Enhances lymphocyte proliferation and secretion of IFN	Chiang et al., 2003
Plantago major	*p*-Coumaric acid		Enhances lymphocyte proliferation and secretion of IFN	Chiang et al., 2003
Plantago major	Vanillic acid		Enhances lymphocyte proliferation and secretion of IFN	Chiang et al., 2003
Curcuma longa	Curcumin		Enhances bone marrow cellularity.	Yadav et al. 2005

(Continued)

TABLE 11.1 (CONTINUED)
Various Types of Immunomodulators and Their Action and Source

Plant name	Active Compound(s)	2-D Structure of the Compound	Mode of Action	Reference
Bidens pilosa	Centaurein		Augmentation of IFN-γ promoter activity	Chang et al. 2007
Jatropha curcas	Apigenin		Stimulation of humoral- and cell- mediated immune response	Abd-Alla et al. 2009
Jatropha curcas	Apigenin 7-*O*-β-D-galactoside		Stimulation of humoral- and cell-mediated immune response	Abd-Alla et al. 2009

(Continued)

TABLE 11.1 (CONTINUED)
Various Types of Immunomodulators and Their Action and Source

Plant name	Active Compound(s)	2-D Structure of the Compound	Mode of Action	Reference
Jatropha curcas	Orientin		Stimulation of humoral- and cell-mediated immune response	Abd-Alla et al. 2009
Jatropha curcas	Vitexin		Stimulation of humoral and cell-mediated immune response	Abd-Alla et al. 2009
Plantago major	Luteolin		Enhances lymphocyte proliferation and secretion of IFN	Chiang et al., 2003

(Continued)

TABLE 11.1 (CONTINUED)
Various Types of Immunomodulators and Their Action and Source

Plant name	Active Compound(s)	2-D Structure of the Compound	Mode of Action	Reference
Plantago major	Baicalein		Enhances lymphocyte proliferation and secretion of IFN	Chiang et al., 2003
Urtica dioica	Quercetin-3-O-rutinoside		Immunomodulation	Akbay et al. 2003
Urtica dioica	Kaempherol-3-O-rutinoside		Immunomodulation	Akbay et al. 2003

(Continued)

TABLE 11.1 (CONTINUED)
Various Types of Immunomodulators and Their Action and Source

Plant name	Active Compound(s)	2-D Structure of the Compound	Mode of Action	Reference
Cleome gynandra	Kaempferol		Anti-inflammatory mechanism	van der Meijden, 2001
Rubus fruticosus	Peonidin		Antioxidant and anti-inflammatory mechanism	Rechner et al. 2005; Wang et al. 2008
Terminalia chebula	Chebulagic acid		Down regulation of TNF-α and IL-6	Reddy et al. 2009

(Continued)

TABLE 11.1 (CONTINUED)
Various Types of Immunomodulators and Their Action and Source

Plant name	Active Compound(s)	2-D Structure of the Compound	Mode of Action	Reference
Terminalia chebula	Corilagin		Neuroprotection	Chang et al. 2012
Punica granatum	Punicalagin		Free radical scavenging and immunosuppressive action	Lee et al. 2008

(Continued)

TABLE 11.1 (CONTINUED)
Various Types of Immunomodulators and Their Action and Source

Plant name	Active Compound(s)	2-D Structure of the Compound	Mode of Action	Reference
Centella asiatica	Asiaticoside		Enhances phagocytic index and total WBC count	Punturee et al. 2005
Glycyrrhiza glabra	Glycyrrhizin		Inhibits classical complement pathway	Ablise et al. 2004
Andrographis paniculata	Andrographolide		Enhances the expression of IL-2. Inhibition of NO in endotoxin -stimulated macrophages	Chiou et al. 2000

(Continued)

TABLE 11.1 (CONTINUED)
Various Types of Immunomodulators and Their Action and Source

Plant name	Active Compound(s)	2-D Structure of the Compound	Mode of Action	Reference
Bowella serrata	Boswellic acid		Significant inhibition of mast cell degranulation	Singh et al. 2008
Rosmarinus officinalis	Ursolic acid		Activates intracellular killing effect of macrophages	Podder et al. 2015
Withania somnifera	Withanolide		Activates murine macrophages, phagocytosis and lysosomal enzyme activity	Ghosal et al. 1989
Corchorus fascicularis	β-Sitosterol		Activates human peripheral lymphocyte proliferation	Bouic et al. 1996

(Continued)

TABLE 11.1 (CONTINUED)
Various Types of Immunomodulators and Their Action and Source

Plant name	Active Compound(s)	2-D Structure of the Compound	Mode of Action	Reference
Artemisia annua	Artemisinin		Inhibit iNOS transcription,	(Aldieri et al. 2003
Lithospermum erythrorhizon	Shikonin		Inhibits the promoter/ transcriptional activity of the pro-inflammatory cytokine TNF-α	(Staniforth et al. 2004
Polygonum cuspidatum	Resveratrol		Regulates various transcription factors	(Harikumar and Aggarwal 2008
Zingiber officinale	6-Gingerol		Regulates the expression of NF-κB, AP-1, PKCα, cyclin D	Kim et al. 2004

(Continued)

TABLE 11.1 (CONTINUED)

Various Types of Immunomodulators and Their Action and Source

Plant name	Active Compound(s)	2-D Structure of the Compound	Mode of Action	Reference
Camellia sinensis	Epigallocatechin gallate		Activates EGFR, AKT, NF-κB, AP-	Babu and Liu (2008)
Copits chinensis	Berberine		Regulates T-helper cells	Lin and Lin 2011
Chelidonium majus	Chelerythrine		Regulates Cox-2 activity	Yun et al. 2021

(Continued)

TABLE 11.1 (CONTINUED)
Various Types of Immunomodulators and Their Action and Source

Plant name	Active Compound(s)	2-D Structure of the Compound	Mode of Action	Reference
Gelsemium elegans	Gelselegine		Inhibits NF-kB	Xu et al. 2012
Corydalis turtschaninovii	Pseudo-coptisine		Inhibits NF-kB	Yun et al. 2009
Boerhavia diffussa	β-D-galactopyranoside H		Activates NK cells	Pandeya et al. 2005

(Continued)

TABLE 11.1 (CONTINUED)
Various Types of Immunomodulators and Their Action and Source

Plant name	Active Compound(s)	2-D Structure of the Compound	Mode of Action	Reference
Rhododendron spiciferum	Proanthocyanidin		Enhances the expression of NK cells	Liu et al. 2010
Nardostachys jatamansi	Spirojatamol,		Plays a role in central nervous system (CNS)	Chatterjee et al. 2012

(Continued)

TABLE 11.1 (CONTINUED)
Various Types of Immunomodulators and Their Action and Source

Plant name	Active Compound(s)	2-D Structure of the Compound	Mode of Action	Reference
Nardostachys jatamansi	Nardostachysin,		Plays a role in CNS	Chatterjee et al. 2012
Nardostachys jatamansi	Jatamols A		Plays a role in CNS	Bagchi et al. 1991
Nardostachys jatamansi	Jatamols B		Plays a role in CNS	Bagchi et al. 1991

(Continued)

TABLE 11.1 (CONTINUED)
Various Types of Immunomodulators and Their Action and Source

Plant name	Active Compound(s)	2-D Structure of the Compound	Mode of Action	Reference
Centella asiatica	Asiatic acid		Modulates oxidative stress response	Cervenka and Jahodar 2006
Centella asiatica	Asiaticoside		Modulates oxidative stress response	Cervenka and Jahodar 2006
Bacopa monnieri	Bacoside A		Modulates intracellular oxidative stress	Limpeanchob et al. 2008

(Continued)

TABLE 11.1 (CONTINUED)
Various Types of Immunomodulators and Their Action and Source

Plant name	Active Compound(s)	2-D Structure of the Compound	Mode of Action	Reference
Bacopa monnieri	Jujubogenin		Modulates intracellular oxidative stress	Limpeanchob et al. 2008
Andrographis paniculata	Andrographolide		Regulates proliferation of lymphocytes and production of interleukin	Varma et al. 2011
Tinospora cordifolia	Cordifolioside A		Immunomodulation, anticancer	Sharma et al. 2019

(Continued)

TABLE 11.1 (CONTINUED)
Various Types of Immunomodulators and Their Action and Source

Plant name	Active Compound(s)	2-D Structure of the Compound	Mode of Action	Reference
Tinospora cordifolia	Syringin		Immunomodulation, anticancer	Sharma et al. 2019
Syzygium guineense	Arabinogalactan		Activates the cytokines	Ghildyal et al. 2010

(Continued)

TABLE 11.1 (CONTINUED)

Various Types of Immunomodulators and Their Action and Source

Plant name	Active Compound(s)	2-D Structure of the Compound	Mode of Action	Reference
Bergenia crassifolia	Bergenin		Exhibits immuno-modulatory and wound healing properties	Patel et al. 2012
Stellera chamaejasme	Eudesmin		Exhibits immunomodulatory activity	Xu et al. 2001
Hydrangea dulcis folium	Concanavalin-A		Regulates splenocyte proliferation	Matsuda et al. 1998

(Continued)

TABLE 11.1 (CONTINUED)
Various Types of Immunomodulators and Their Action and Source

Plant name	Active Compound(s)	2-D Structure of the Compound	Mode of Action	Reference
Hydrangea dulcis folium	Thunberginol A		Regulates splenocyte proliferation	Matsuda et al. 1998
Hydrangea dulcis folium	Hydrangenol		Regulates splenocyte proliferation	Matsuda et al. 1998
Phlomis younghusbandii	Barlerin		Exhibits immunomodulatory activity	Fan et al. 2010

(Continued)

TABLE 11.1 (CONTINUED)
Various Types of Immunomodulators and Their Action and Source

Plant name	Active Compound(s)	2-D Structure of the Compound	Mode of Action	Reference
Imperata cylindrica	5-Methoxy-flavone		Exhibits immunomodulatory activity	Fu et al. 2010
Polygonum aviculare	Rosmarinic acid		Exhibits immunomodulatory activity	Hu et al. 2006

(Continued)

TABLE 11.1 (CONTINUED)
Various Types of Immunomodulators and Their Action and Source

Plant name	Active Compound(s)	2-D Structure of the Compound	Mode of Action	Reference
Prunus mume	Isorhamnetin		Exhibits immunomodulatory activity	Zhang et al. 2008
Euphorbia hirta	Quercitol		Anti-inflammatory activity	Kumar et al. 2010
Euphorbia hirta	Myricitrin		Sedative and anxiolytic activity	Kumar et al. 2010

(Continued)

TABLE 11.1 (CONTINUED)
Various Types of Immunomodulators and Their Action and Source

Plant name	Active Compound(s)	2-D Structure of the Compound	Mode of Action	Reference
Aristolochia spp	Aristolochic acid		Antiangiogenic activity	Wei et al. 2007
Cordia superba	Alpha-amyrin		Anti-inflammatory, antimicrobial activity	Jamkhande et al. 2013
Lagenaria siceraria	Cucurbitacin		Purgative, emetic activity	Ramalingam et al. 2010

(Continued)

TABLE 11.1 (CONTINUED)
Various Types of Immunomodulators and Their Action and Source

Plant name	Active Compound(s)	2-D Structure of the Compound	Mode of Action	Reference
Panax ginseng	Ginsenosides		Adaptogenic properties, Anti-arrhythmic	Lee et al. 2010
Panax ginseng	Panaxtriol		Adaptogenic properties, Anti-arrhythmic	Lee et al. 2010
Panax ginseng	Oleanolic acid		Adaptogenic properties, antiarrhythmic	Raphael et al. 2003

(Continued)

TABLE 11.1 (CONTINUED)
Various Types of Immunomodulators and Their Action and Source

Plant name	Active Compound(s)	2-D Structure of the Compound	Mode of Action	Reference
Murraya koenigii	Coumarin		Antifungal	Igor et al. 2008
Ocimum sanctum	Eugenol		Antispasmodic,	Vaghasiya et al. 2010
Panax ginseng	Panaxdiol		Adaptogenic properties	Lee et al. 2010
Tinospora cordifolia	Berberine		Hypoglycemic agent	Sinha et al. 2004
Cleome gynandra	Kaempferol		Anti-inflammatory	Gaur et al. 2009

(Continued)

TABLE 11.1 (CONTINUED)
Various Types of Immunomodulators and Their Action and Source

Plant name	Active Compound(s)	2-D Structure of the Compound	Mode of Action	Reference
Hyptis suaveolens	Lupeol		Antispasmodic	Jain et al. 2005
Chelidomium majus	Chelerythrine		Enhances the production of IL-6, TNF-α	Li et al. 2012
Chelidomium majus	Sanguinarine		Inhibits degranulation	Agarwal et al. 1999

(Continued)

TABLE 11.1 (CONTINUED)

Various Types of Immunomodulators and Their Action and Source

Plant name	Active Compound(s)	2-D Structure of the Compound	Mode of Action	Reference
Bidens pilosa	Centaurcin		Induces nuclear factor activation	Chang et al. 2007
Jatropha curcas	Orientin		Stimulates humoral- and cell-mediated immune response	Abd-Alla et al. 2009

(Continued)

TABLE 11.1 (CONTINUED)
Various Types of Immunomodulators and Their Action and Source

Plant name	Active Compound(s)	2-D Structure of the Compound	Mode of Action	Reference
Jatropha curcas	Vitexin		Stimulates humoral- and cell-mediated immune response	Abd-Alla et al. 2009
Cedrus deodara	Dihydroquercetin		Exhibits immunomodulatory effects	Arreola et al. 2012

(Continued)

TABLE 11.1 (CONTINUED)
Various Types of Immunomodulators and Their Action and Source

Plant name	Active Compound(s)	2-D Structure of the Compound	Mode of Action	Reference
Opuntia polyacanth	Galactose		Used as potent immunotherapeutic adjuvant	Igor et al. 2008
Opuntia polyacanth	Galactourcinic Acid		Used as potent immunotherapeutic adjuvant	Igor et al. 2008
Vaccinium spp.	Peonidins		Inflammatory response	DeFuria et al. 2009

(Continued)

TABLE 11.1 (CONTINUED)
Various Types of Immunomodulators and Their Action and Source

Plant name	Active Compound(s)	2-D Structure of the Compound	Mode of Action	Reference
Vaccinium spp.	Malvidins		Inflammatory response	DeFuria et al. 2009
Vaccinium spp.	Delphinidins		Inflammatory response	DeFuria et al. 2009
Tinospora cordifolia	14-Deoxy-11, 12-didehydroandro grapholide		Immunostimulatory effect	Sinha et al. 2004

(Continued)

TABLE 11.1 (CONTINUED)
Various Types of Immunomodulators and Their Action and Source

Plant name	Active Compound(s)	2-D Structure of the Compound	Mode of Action	Reference
Boswellia serrata	Boswellic acid		Inhibits pro-inflammatory mediators	Singh et al. 2008
Ilex hainanensis	Ilexgenin A		Lipid disorders	Li et al. 2015
Ilex pubescens	Ilexolide A		Anti-inflammatory effect	Zhou et al. 2017

from *Dendrobium nobile*, a widely used plant in Chinese medicine. Dendrosides A and B from *D. nobile* caused significant stimulation of the proliferation of murine T and B lymphocytes (Dinesh Kumar et al. 2012).

11.3.2 Mechanism of Action of Immunomodulators

Immunomodulators are nutritional supplements that exert strong activity against various diseases owing to the presence of high concentrations of antioxidants. They also have antagonistic action and are involved in the formation of different free radicals. Hence, immunomodulators are mainly used to fight the effects of ageing factors, cancer, diabetes, and autoimmune diseases. The medicinal effect of this Rasayana herb is effectively mediated *via* activities of immunostimulants and immunosuppressants or is mediated through disturbing the effector arm of the immune response (Chulet and Pradhan, 2010). The mechanism of action of these immunomodulatory activities mainly occurs through the basic cellular process, including phagocytosis and macrophage activation. In addition, lymphoid cell stimulation, increase in cellular immune function, increased antigen-specific immunoglobulin production, and increases in the number of natural killer cells and white cells also play a key role in Rasayana-mediated cell response and its effect on immune systems (Singh et al. 2007; Anonymous, 2009; Vaghasiya et al. 2010). The modulatory activity of medicinal plant extracts on the immune response operates *via* stimulatory and suppressive effects and plays a crucial role in maintaining the disease-free state in normal and unhealthy persons. Phytochemicals show significant activity towards host defence mechanisms, even in an impaired immune response, and can provide supportive therapy to chemotherapy (Wagner et al. 1984). The increased level of cell proliferation in bone marrow cells is considered a potentially sensitive target for the various cytotoxic drugs because the bone marrow is one of the organs most affected during immunosuppression therapy. The plant-derived saponins play a significant role in various pharmacological activities, including antitumour, antiviral, immunomodulating, antihepatotoxic, and antifungal activity. Recently, the saponins isolated from *Paris polyphylla* showed active immunostimulant properties. Several studies have demonstrated that the saponins are considered to be important immunomodulating agents (Bafna et al. 2006; Xiu-feng et al. 2007).

11.3.3 Immunosuppressive Agents

Medicinal plants having strong immunosuppressive activity can be used as an alternative to conventional chemotherapy. The currently used chemotherapeutic agents shows various adverse effects. Several plant species have the ability to inhibit both the innate and the humoral immune response by activating the B and T lymphocytes. For example, *Cannabis sativa* significantly suppresses the hyperactivity of the immune system *via* activating the cannabinoid receptors such as CB1 and CB2 (Cannabinoid receptor 1 and 2). CB1 receptors are abundantly present in brain cells and CB2 are present in immune cells, which are used for the management of cancer and inflammatory disorders (Bettini and Vignali 2009). The phytochemical brasilicardin-A, purified from *Nocardia brasiliensis* IFM0406, shows effective immunosuppressive activity; it contains amino acids and perhydro-phenanthrene as important chemical moieties, which may influence the immunosuppressive effect of the molecule. Another compound isolated from green tea (*Camellia sinensis*) acts as a potent immunosuppressive agent and is used for the treatment of autoimmune arthritis. The major active constituent of green tea is catechin, a phenolic compound possessing significant anti-inflammatory action (Kunz and Ibrahim, 2009). The extract of *Artemisia annua* has been extensively used in the treatment of autoimmune diseases, including rheumatoid arthritis and lupus erythematodes, due to the existence of major bioactive compounds artemisinins; the derivatives of artemisinin, such as artesunate and artemether, also have a significant immunomodulatory effect (Perretti et al. 2009). The steroids of the sarsaparilla plant, such as smilagenin, saponins, stigmasterol, and sarsasapogenin, are the major beneficial components extensively used in the treatment of arthritis owing to their inhibitory effect on TNF-α (De Bosscher et al. 2008). The Zingiberaceae family member turmeric (*Curcuma longa*) is one of the most widely and often used medicinal plants in Indian traditional medicine, as well as in the Indian diet. It possesses strong antimicrobial activity and significant anti-inflammatory effect. Curcumin is the major bioactive compound present in *C. longa*; it is a yellow pigment that effectively regulates the immune response *via* cell- and humoral-mediated immunity (Kunz et al. 2009). Ashwagandha is another widely used medicinal plant that has diverse inhibitory activities. The alkaloids derived from Ashwagandha, such as iso-pelletierine anaferine, lactones (withanolides, withaferin), saponins (sitoindoside VII and VIII), and withanolides are main constituents of *Withania somnifera*, which greatly influence the activation of B and T cells and produce immunosuppressive action. Another important medicinal plant used both as medicine and in the diet is ginger (*Zingiber officinale*), mainly used for the reduction of pain in arthritis (Dooley and Nair, 2008). The major bioactive component zingiberene is effectively involved the anti-inflammation effect *via* inhibiting the major pathways such as cyclooxygenase (COX) and lipoxygenase. Figure 11.2 shows that the major active compound has an immunosuppressive effect.

11.4   MEDICINAL PLANTS AS IMMUNE BOOSTERS

Several studies have reported that medicinal plants can strongly boost up the immune system, by which they can cure several pathological diseases. *Abrus precatorius* is a member of the Fabaceae, with seed and root being the key parts of the plants, with major constituents like gallic acid, hypaphorine, glycyrrhizin, squalene, and 5-beta cholanic acid. The plant extract is widely used for the treatment of helminthiasis, vomiting, cancer, malaria, and jaundice. In addition, the seed and root extract of this plant exhibits the immunosuppression effect by inhibiting the expression of antibodies and delaying the hypersensitivity response. The reports stated that the extract of *A. precatorius* significantly increased the serum immunoglobulin levels and the activity of phagocytosis, stimulating the cell-mediated immunity (Tripathi et al. 2005). Another medicinal plant, *Acacia concinna*, exhibits an immunostimulatory effect by increasing the numbers of Th1 and Th2 helper cells. Pods and leaves are mainly used in this plant, containing lupeol, nicotine, spinasterol, ascorbic acid, rhamnose, and

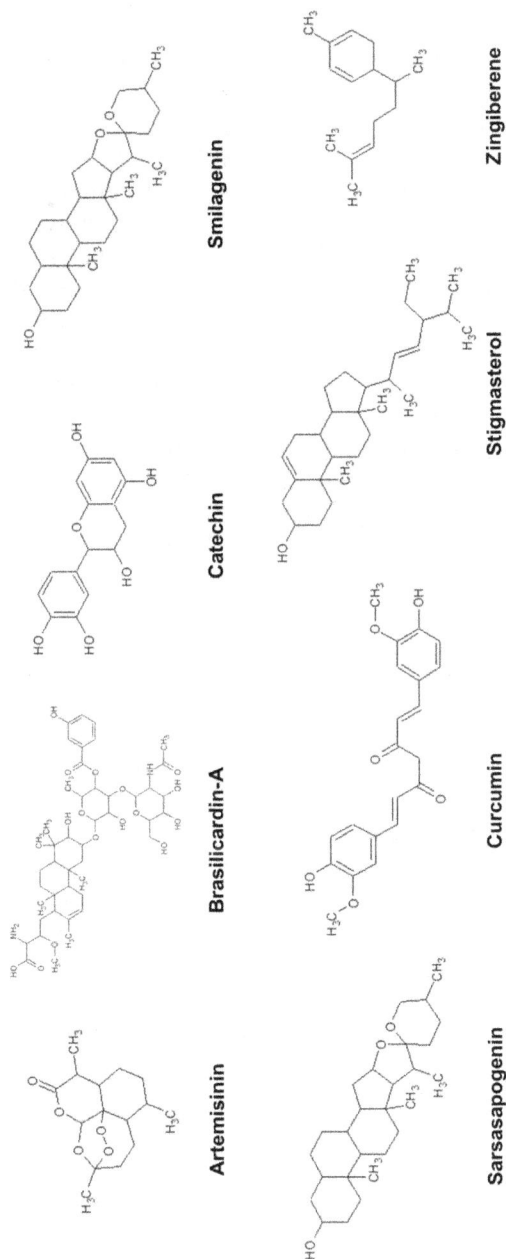

FIGURE 11.2 Major bioactive compounds with an immunosuppressive effect.

spinasterone as major active components that may be responsible for the antimalarial and anti-dandruff activity. The saponin extract from pods of *A. concinna* reported significant immunological adjuvant activity (Kukhetpitakwong et al. 2006; Ismail and Asad, 2009). The bulb extract of *Allium sativum* has major active components like allin, phytocidin, scordinin, and diallyl-disulphide, and is mainly used for treating various pathological conditions, including hyperlipidaemia, diabetes, bacterial infection, hypertension, cancer, and tuberculosis. It also exhibits antiviral, antirheumatic and antispasmodic activity. Garlic extract shows immunostimulatory activity by increasing the mitogenic activity of human peripheral blood lymphocytes, murine splenocytes, and thymocytes (Clement et al. 2010). It effectively promotes the Th2 cells like interleukin-4, -10, and -13 subsequently induce the expression of Th1 cells, such as INF-γ. The activation of IL-10 significantly suppressed pro-inflammatory cytokines like IL1, IL12, which are essential to produce antigen-presenting cells. The up-regulation of INF-γ can induce nitric oxide synthase and mRNA expression, which produce the NO and destroy *Leishmania*. Hence, the extract of *A. sativum* generates a potent immunomodulatory effect (Hodge et al. 2002; Liu and Uzonna, 2012). *Andrographis paniculata* is another widely used medicinal plant used for the management of helminthiasis, cholera, jaundice, and dyspepsia. Extracts of leaf, bark, and root of *A. paniculata* has chemical constituents like apigenin, kalmeghin, and andrographolide. Owing to the presence of these active molecules, *A. paniculata* exhibits an immunostimulatory effect and is also used for its hepatoprotective, alterative, and anthelmintic properties. It greatly influences the activation of antibody secretion and delayed-type hypersensitivity. The brown seaweed *Ascophyllum nodosum* contains tetraphlorethol C, tetrafucol A, and phlorotannins as major active compounds, hence showing a good anti-inflammatory effect, as well as acting as an immunostimulant, enhancing the production of natural killer cells. The medicinal plant *Boerhavia diffusa* is used to treat diabetes mellitus, cancer, leukaemia, and several bacterial infections. The chemical constituents include sitosterol, tetracosanoic acid, triacontanol, ursolic acid, and punarnavine. The pharmacological activities of *B. diffusa* include antioxidant, antiestrogenic, and immunomodulant properties. It effectively inhibits the natural killer cells, which prompt the production of NO, interleukin IL-2 and TNF-α (Nakano et al. 2012; Mehrotra et al. 2002). The widely used medicinal plant *Camellia sinensis* contains several essential and potent active molecules like catechin, saponins, epicatechin gallate, adenine, gallic acid, tannic acid, quercetin, and xanthine which are used to treat asthma, cancer, and bacterial infections, while also exhibiting an antioxidant effect. The essential chemical constituents of *C. sinensis*, the catechin-polysaccharide complexes, showed significant immunomodulatory activity in an animal model and in human peripheral mononuclear cells.

11.5 MOLECULAR CHEMISTRY OF PLANT-DERIVED IMMUNITY BOOSTERS

Several avenues of scientific research have reported that most of the plant-derived active molecules act as an essential source of clinical therapeutics by providing diverse chemical molecules with effective pharmacological activity. For many years, medicinal plants have been used in the traditional way to cure various diseases (Chattopadhyay et al. 2012). Most of the natural molecules have the appropriate pharmacological activity and are used in drug discovery strategies. Polyphenols derived from medicinal plants have potent antioxidant activity, hence these molecules are often used in the human diet. A number of studies have supported the concept of the beneficial and pharmacological activity of medicinal plants (Annuzzi et al. 2014; Estrela et al. 2017). In addition, some plants also have the capacity to control the immune system response, especially those plants which are rich in polyphenols, polysaccharides, flavonoids and alkaloids, which are often studied for their immunomodulatory activities (Farzaei et al. 2015; Ferreira et al. 2015; Andreicut et al. 2018). The plant-derived immunomodulators are inexpensive and more effective molecules, so have great potential value in medicine, though, due to the lack of standardization and characterization of most active components, evaluation of both qualitative and quantitative changes and the lack of a suitable test for efficacy are limitations to reported results on immunomodulatory effects of traditional medicinal systems. The preparation of *Echinacea* is an effective flower formulation used as an herbal remedy and reduces the symptoms of a severe cold, though there are reports of both high and low therapeutic efficacy, based on formula preparation. The efficacy of this formulation was noted only in certain preparations, mainly from *Echinacea purpurea* (Karsch-Völk et al. 2015). Balan et al. (2016) compared the effects of three different formulations, namely IMMUNAL drops prepared from a succus (concentrated liquid extract) of *E. purpurea*, IMMUNAL FORTE tablets prepared from *E. purpurea* herbae succus siccum, and ECHINACEA FORTE drops prepared from the juice of fresh flowers of *E. purpurea*, and the results revealed that the three formulations showed significant differences in immunomodulatory effect in the female Balb/c mice model. The formulation IMMUNAL drops and ECHINACEA FORTE shows effective immunostimulatory activity, whereas the IMMUNAL tablet showed immunoinhibitory activity and ECHINACEA FORTE had no effect on antibody production. This study highlights that the type of preparation greatly influenced the modulatory effects. However, a lot of studies have supported the concept that *Echinacea* be used as an immunostimulant which effectively enhances both innate and specific immunity (Sultan et al. 2014). In addition, *Echinacea* also exhibits antiviral and anti-inflammatory activity and plays a crucial role in traditional medicine. This wide range of actions of *Echinacea* depends on the plant parts extracted in particular, leaves, flowers, and roots having several active constituents. The different solvents used to create the preparation, like water, alcohol, or oil, also influenced the activity due to the different components that are extracted by the different solvents formed. The standardization of preparation and testing methods is also crucial before administration for evaluation of effect on the different immune systems. The phytochemical profile of each *Echinacea* product is highly dependent on the choice of plant material and extraction methods. The traditional use of *Echinacea* is mainly shown to be effective as a therapeutic agent; Rondanelli et al. (2018) reported that the prophylactic use of an *Echinacea* extract, containing specific bioactive molecules (polysaccharides and phenylethanoid), as a source was effective at preventing colds and enhancing the immune response. These reports suggested that *Echinacea* significantly stimulates the immune response in healthy as well in immune-suppressed animals (Di Pierro et al. 2012). It enhances the immune system *via* activation of phagocytosis, production of macrophages, and cytokine production, subsequently increasing the expression of TNF-α, interleukins, and interferons. Treatment with the *Echinacea* preparation activates the leukocyte mobility and induces the natural killer cells, which are responsible for the immunomodulatory effect on animals and humans (Vetvicka et al. 2014). The polysaccharide-rich *Echinacea* can stimulate the phenotype and maturation of dendritic cells *via* modulating pathways like JNK, MAPK and NF-kB, which favour the polarization of macrophages (Fu et al. 2017). The study was carried out by Wang et al. (2006) comparing four different extracts of *Echinacea* (whole plant, root, aerial parts, and flower) on dendritic cells over a 24-h period. The results revealed that there was a reduced level of CD32 and HLA-DR expression following treatment. Among the four preparations, the cells treated with extracts of the whole plant or the aerial parts showed the greatest inhibitory activity on CD32 expression, suggesting that, compared with the other extracts, the whole plant and aerial parts extracts had greater ability to inhibit dendritic cell maturation. Fu et al. (2017) demonstrated that an extract of *Echinacea* with a concentration of 100 μg/ml effectively activated the macrophages of murine bone marrow by stimulating the expression of essential markers like CD80, MHCII and CD86, and upregulating the macrophages, and was also involved in the production of interleukins, interferons and NO and in enhancing phagocytosis.

11.6 MOLECULAR CHEMISTRY OF PHYTOCONSTITUENTS

Phytochemicals are chemical compounds that are present in plants. Most of the chemical molecules have diverse pharmacology activity and biological significance. For instance, the main molecules present, flavonoids, carotenoids, and coumarins are considered essential. Approximately 4,000 different phytochemicals have been reported, all having potential biological activity. In the early period of the sixteenth century, most of the traditional medicinal systems used wild plants as their mainstream medical system (Venketeshwer Rao, 2015). In garlic extract, more than 200 chemicals have been reported with diverse properties (Fallah-Rostami et al. 2013), being particularly rich in sulphur compounds, which play the key role in the flavour of garlic and its various beneficial effects. The main constituents of garlic extract are carbohydrate and water, with organosulphur compounds, amino acids, proteins, and fibres in smaller but still significant amounts. The active molecules of garlic extracts are classified into two major categories, based on their chemical composition. The first are the nonvolatile sulphur-containing compounds and organosulphur compounds. Allin, allyl-L-cysteine sulphoxides, and γ-glutamyl-allyl-L-cysteines are the main precursors of nonvolatile sulphur-containing compounds; this category contains around 33 sulphur-containing molecules, enzymes, and amino acids, as well as lectins and glycosides (Kaku et al. 1992). The organosulphur-containing compounds are synthesized during production of the garlic preparation. Allicin is the most biologically active molecule that is not present in the normal condition, but is generated when the garlic is damaged, crushed, pulverized or boiled, which activates the production of the enzyme alliinase, which activates metabolism of the alliin to allicin (Londhe et al. 2011). The allicin immediately decomposes into the other essential compounds, such as diallyl disulphide, ajoene, and the formation of allyl-cysteines from γ-glutamyl cysteine (Rana et al. 2011). The organosulphur-containing compounds are further classified into three subgroups based on their chemical nature, such as thiosulphinates, organosulphur volatiles, and water-soluble compounds. The thiosulphinates are formed *via* the conversion of sulphoxides in the enzymatic reaction. For example, the allicin is considered as a transient compound that decomposes into sulphur- containing compounds which are not found in an active form in undamaged garlic (Amagase et al. 2006). The second group of compounds are the organosulphur volatiles, which includes a large variety of molecules in the processed garlic form, with methyl allyl trisulphide, diallyl trisulphide, 3-dithiin, 2-dithiin, and (E,Z)-ajones being the major and typical volatiles present in the processed garlic. Around twenty sulphides have been reported in the steam-boiled garlic oil and extract; all have allyl groups and are responsible for the flavor and taste of garlic (Amagase et al. 2006). The water-soluble sulphur compounds are extracted with water and contain S-allyl-L-cysteine as the major compound formed from γ-glutamyl-S-allyl-L-cysteines (Amagase et al. 2006). Other compounds, like lectins, pectin, fructan, vitamins, and glycolipids also have important biological activities and contribute to the inhibitory effect on cancer and pathogenic microbes (Suleria et al. 2013).

Ginger is another widely used spice which is also used in traditional herbal medicine. It has a significant health-promoting effect due to its high concentration of bioactive molecules (Shukla and Singh 2007). The origin and the form of ginger (fresh or dry) greatly influence the number and concentration of the chemical constituents. The rhizome contains many phytocompounds, including minerals, carbohydrates, and phytochemicals. The proteolytic enzyme zingibain is a potent enzyme present in the rhizomes, and there are also a moderate number of vitamins, while oleoresins are basic components and are responsible for some pharmacological effects of ginger. The extraction of ginger essential oils by gas chromatography techniques shows that sesquiterpenes are the major bioactive compounds, followed by carbonyl compounds, alcohols, and terpenes. In another study, Jolad et al. (2004) reported around sixty compounds in fresh ginger, which were categorized as volatile and non-volatile compounds, contributing specifically to the spiciness, whereas the sesquiterpene and hydrocarbons provide the aroma and taste of the ginger. Gong et al. (2004) reported 140 and 136 compounds from fresh and dry ginger, respectively, using gas chromatography–mass spectrometric (GC–MS) analysis. Compounds such as α-zingiberene and β-sesquiphellandrene are the main volatile components, while other bioactive molecules, curcumene, [6]-gingerol and [6]-shogaol, are mainly responsible for the spiciness. Gingerols are phenolics present in the ginger to which are mainly attributed the spiciness, with the concentration of [6]-gingerol acting as a key component of spiciness in the fresh rhizome being converted into shogaol during drying, with hydration and this conversion being heavily influenced by temperature and pH (Wohlmuth et al. 2005).

11.7   PHARMACOLOGY AND TOXICITY OF MEDICINAL PLANTS

The development of a drug from traditional plants is valuable and is a potent alternative to the modern drug development process, but also has a wide context for use in non-Western medical approaches and their activities. A single herb or a polyherb formulation usually have several bioactive molecules that have the potential for various pharmacological activities. Most of the medicinal plants extensively used, for example, have potent inhibitory activity against pathogenic bacteria. For a long period of time, medicinal plants were extensively used for maintaining human health. The methanol extracts of *Acacia nilotica*, *Withania somnifera*, and *Sida cordifolia* also show significant antimicrobial activity against *Pseudomonas* spp., *Staphylococcus* spp., and *Xanthomonas* spp. The leaf extracts of *T. cordifolia*, *Z. mauritiana* and *A. flavus* show effective antifungal activity (Gupta et al. 1993). Some medicinal plants possess anthelmintic activity, with the alcoholic extract of *Wedelia biflora* showing effective anthelmintic activity against the Indian earthworm. The aqueous extract of *Thespesia lampas* showed inhibitory activity against tapeworms and roundworms (Satish and Ravindra, 2009). Most importantly, medicinal plants also have potent anticancer properties. The currently employed approaches like chemotherapy, surgery, and radiotherapy cause several adverse effects in normal tissues while treating cancerous tissues. Hence, there is a need for alternative medicines (Veerakumar et al. 2016). A number of studies has supported the anticancer activity of several medicinal plants in attempts to find novel therapeutic agents without toxic effects. In recent decades, herbal medicines and plants have effectively proven their anticancer properties with limited side effects. In India, only a few plants have attracted enough attention to identify the active biomolecules and assess their role in the control/prevention of cancer proliferation (Shaikh et al. 2014). The plant-based secondary metabolites such as camptothecin, flavopiridol, resveratrol, vinblastine, and vincristine are plant-based compounds used as potent anticancer agents worldwide (Ghasemzadeh et al. 2011).

11.8   CURRENT DEVELOPMENTS IN IMMUNOMODULATOR RESEARCH

Schisandra chinensis is a Chinese herb used in clinical practice owing to its effective enzyme-inhibiting and hepatoprotective activity. In the 1960s, Chinese scientists started to isolate the potent bioactive molecules from *S. chinensis* and reported that schisandrin C was the major constituent with strong pharmacological activity. It was also used to decrease enzyme levels in the treatment of the hepatitis B virus (Yang et al. 2009). The structure–activity relationship of bifendate and its analogues was studied and a series of novel derivatives were synthesized then subjected to screening with respect to a number of chemical and pharmaceutical injury modes. It was noticed that the derivatives having hepatoprotective activity showed closely related dimethylenedioxy functional group in two benzene rings with long carboxyl side chains. Finally, a new compound, bicyclol, was synthesized. Due to the presence of the carbomethoxy side chain and the hydroxymethyl group, bicyclol has great bioavailability and biological activity (Liu et al. 2010). It also significantly inhibited the replication of the hepatitis B virus though it exhibited a more effective and it was discontinued due to fewer side effects (Bao et al. 2008; Li et al. 2011). Another plant-derived compound, paclitaxel, a potent anticancer compound extracted from *Taxus brevifolia*. Paclitaxel has a unique chemical structure and a radically distinct mechanism of action against cancer and has been tested successfully in treatment of several cancer types and has been involved in clinical trials. It received US Food and Drug Administration (FDA) approval for the treatment of ovarian cancer in the year 1992–93. (Wani and Horwitz, 2014). Owing to its low solubility in an aqueous medium, however, yields from the natural plant source were low.

11.9   LIMITATIONS

Several challenges and limitations exist to accurately assess the toxicological and epidemiological effects and other activities in the verification of herbal material use. The management of risk factors within ranges, pharmacological and clinical documentation, and an understanding of harmful additives need to be evaluated. The limits with clinical trials, standardization, and safety and efficacy assessments need to be overcome. The identification of novel herbal products has the following six essential steps: identification and characterization of potent molecules, activity of the molecule, identification of any side effects or adverse reaction, its pharmacological activity, and assessment of the toxicity and carcinogenicity in clinical trials. Low yields of the active molecules, lack of adequate research on the development of domestication of the plant source, insufficient techniques to yield product of consistently high quality, lack of good manufacturing practice, poor quality control measures, limited marketing, and lack of proper equipment are the major constraints associated with handling the medicinal plants in alternative approaches to current therapeutic strategies (Rukangira 2000). Another major constraint when dealing with herbal medicine is that the extract contains a mixture of organic substances and it is often difficult to find which molecules have good biological activity. In addition, owing to the complex nature of bioactive molecules, it is difficult to determine the structural and functional features. When determining the concentration of major components, temperature, dissolution, and atmospheric humidity may alter the concentration and sometimes the functions of active ingredients of herbal medicines. Other environmental factors affecting the yield of active ingredients from herbal plants, like pests/diseases, planting density, seeding time, and generic factors may also play an essential role; hence, the collection of plants and the time of harvest are important. Several ways are commonly used for adulteration of herbal plant material by substituting the target plant with inexpensive but readily available local plant relatives (Thillaivanan and Samraj, 2014).

11.10   CONCLUSION

Plant-based immunomodulators are naturally available substances that represent an interesting tool for the handling the immune system within a clinical setting, owing to their wide range of bioactivities. Medicinal plant products and active compounds are effectively studied and characterized to understand the basic phytochemical constituents with valid analytical methods and extraction protocols. The bioactive components are specifically analyzed and used as active markers to ensure the pharmacological efficacy of the molecule for comparative studies. The purified molecule can then be characterized to understand the beneficial effect of specific components of the molecule. For example, polyphenols are highly involved in the immunomodulatory activity due to polyunsaturated fatty acids (PUFA) -enriched fatty acids. Hence, the identification of major bioactive molecules with clinical evidence for their efficacy and safety is a major task for medicinal plant-induced immunomodulation due to limited studies. Hence, the selection of concentration, experimental protocols, and comparative standard compounds are reported in the preclinical studies (Heinrich et al. 2020; Izzo et al. 2020). Traditional medicinal systems in India provide the major bioactive molecules with multiple pleiotropic activities. Most of the medicinal plants have immunomodulatory effects achieved by an immune booster of the immune system to eradicate the pathogenic microorganisms and exogenous injuries. To control the impaired immune response due to autoimmune disorders, it is influenced by non-immune targets. In this chapter, we emphasize the immunomodulating effect of the traditional medicinal system and its pharmacological effect. In addition, molecular chemistry and the mechanism of action are also discussed. Traditional medicinal plants and their phytoconstituents are used as promising molecules for identification of plant-based drugs, and these molecules act as potential lead compounds for the development of effective, inexpensive immunomodulatory agents.

ACKNOWLEDGEMENT

The authors Chandrabose Selvaraj and Sanjeev Kumar Singh gratefully acknowledge RUSA-Phase 2.0 Policy (TNmulti-Gen), Department of Education, Government of India (Grant No: F.24-51/2014-U). The author Chandrabose Yogeswari gratefully acknowledges Vetri Siddha Medical College Hospital & Research Institute, Thanichayam, Madurai, for providing necessary information on this topic, along with facilities.

REFERENCES

Abbas, A.K., Lichtman, A.H.H., and S. Pillai. 2016. *Basic Immunology: Functions and Disorders of the Immune System*. 5th ed. Philadelphia, PA: Saunders Elsevier Science, pp. 239–43.

Abd-Alla, H.I., Moharram, F.A., Gaara, A.H., and M.M. El-Safty. 2009. Phytoconstituents of *Jatropha curcas* L. leaves and their immunomodulatory activity on humoral and cell-mediated immune response in chicks. *A Journal of Biosciences*. 64:495–501.

Ablise, M., Leininger-Muller, B., Wong, C.D., Siest, G., Loppinet, V., and S. Visvikis. 2004. Synthesis and *in vitro* antioxidant activity of glycyrrhetinic acid derivatives tested with the cytochrome P450/NADPH system. *Chemical and Pharmaceutical Bulletin (Tokyo)*. 52:1436–9.

Agarwal, S.S., and V.K. Singh. 1999. Immunomodulators: a review of studies on Indian medicinal plants and synthetic peptides. Part I: medicinal plants. *Proceedings of the Indian National Science Academy.* 65:179e204.

Ajmal, S.M., Naga Lakshmi, M., Nandhini, M., Meenadharshini, G., Kowshika shree, P.J. and T. Keerthiga et al. 2017. Standard operative procedure on external therapies in siddha system of medicine. *International Journal of Research in Medical Sciences.* 3:112–127.

Akbay, P., Basaran, A.A., Undeger, U., and N. Basaran. 2003. *In vitro* immunomodulatory activity of flavonoid glycosides from *Urtica dioica* L. *Phototherapy Research.*17:34–7.

Aldieri, E., Atragene, D., Bergandi, L., Riganti, C., Costamagna, C., Bosia, A. and D. Ghigo. 2003. Artemisinin inhibits inducible nitric oxide synthase and nuclear factor NF-kB activation, *FEBS Letters.* 552.

Amagase, H. 2006. Clarifying the real bioactive constituents of garlic. *Journal of Nutrition.* 136 Supplement:S716–S725.

Andreicut, A.D., Pârvu, A.E., Mot, A.C., Pârvu, M., Fischer Fodor, E., Cătoi, A.F., Feldrihan, V., Cecan, M., and A. Irimie. 2018. Phytochemical analysis of anti-inflammatory and antioxidant effects of Mahonia aquifolium flower and fruit extracts. *Oxidative Medicine and Cellular Longevity.* 2018:1–12.

Annuzzi, G., Bozzetto, L., Costabile, G., Giacco, R., Mangione, A., Anniballi, G., Vitale, M., Vetrani, C., Cipriano, P., and G. Della Corte, et al. 2014. Diets naturally rich in polyphenols improve fasting and postprandial dyslipidemia and reduce oxidative stress: a randomized controlled trial. *American Journal of Clinical Nutrition.* 99:463–471.

Anonymous 2009. *Panax ginseng.* Monograph. *Alternative Medicinal Reviews.*14:172e6.

Arreola, R., Becerril-Villanueva, E., Cruz-Fuentes, C., Velasco- Velázquez, M.A., Garcés-Alvarez, M.E., Hurtado-Alvarado, G., Quintero-Fabian, S., and Pavón, L. 2015. Immunomodulatory effects mediated by serotonin. *Journal of Immunology Research.* 2015:354957.

Babu, P.V, and D. Liu. 2008. Green tea catechins and cardiovascular health: an update. *Current Medicinal Chemistry.* 15(18):1840–50.

Bafna, A.R., and S.H. Mishra. 2006. Immunostimulatory effect of methanol extract of Curculigo orchioides on immunosuppressed mice. *Journal of Ethnopharmacology.* 104:1e4.

Bagchi, A., Oshima, Y., and H. Hikino. 1991. Jatamols A and B: sesquiterpenoids of Nardostachys jatamansi roots. *Planta Medica.* 57:282–3.

Bałan, B.J., Sokolnicka, I., Skopińska-Różewska, E., and P. Skopiński. 2016. The modulatory influence of some *Echinacea*-based remedies on antibody production and cellular immunity in mice. *Central-European Journal of Immunology.* 1:12–18.

Bao, X.Q., and G.T. Liu. 2008. Bicyclol: a novel antihepatitis drug with hepatic heat shock protein 27/70-inducing activity and cytoprotective effects in mice. *Cell Stress Chaperones.* 13:347–355.

Bettini, M., and D.A. Vignali. 2009. Regulatory T cells and inhibitory cytokines in autoimmunity. *Current Opinion in Immunology.* 21(6):612–8.

Bouic, P.J., Etsebeth, S., Liebenberg, R.W., Albrecht, C.F., Pegel, K., and P.P. Van Jaarsveld. 1996. Beta-Sitosterol and beta-sitosterol glucoside stimulate human peripheral blood lymphocyte proliferation: Implications for their use as an immunomodulatory vitamin combination. *International Journal of Immunopharmacology.* 18:693–700.

Casa, R., Sacanella, E., and R. Estruch. 2014. The immune protective effect of the Mediterranean diet against chronic low-grade inflammatory disease. *Endocrine, Metabolic & Immune Disorders Drug Targets.* 14:245–54.

Cervenka, F., and L. Jahodar. 2006. Plant metabolites as nootropics and cognitives. *Ceska a Slovenska Farmacie.* 55:219–229.

Chang, C.L., and C.S. Lin. 2012. Phytochemical composition, antioxidant activity, and neuroprotective effect of *Terminalia chebula* retzius extracts. *Evidence-based Complementary and Alternative Medicine.* 2012:125247.

Chang, S.L., Chiang, Y.M., Chang, C.L., Yeh, H.H., Shyur, L.F., and Y.H. Kuo, et al. 2007. Flavonoids, centaurein and centaureidin, from *Bidens pilosa*, stimulate IFN-gamma expression. *Journal of Ethnopharmacology*. 112:232–6.

Chatterjee, A., Basak, B., Datta, U., Banerji, J., Neuman, A., and T. Prange. 2005. Studies on the chemical constituents of N. jatamansi DC (Valerianaceae). *Indain Journal of Chemistry B*. 44:430–3.

Chattopadhyay, C., Chakrabarti, N., and M. Chatterjee. 2012. Black tea (Camellia sinensis) decoction shows immunomodulatory properties on an experimental animal model and in human peripheral mononuclear cells. *Pharmacognosy Research*. 4:15–21.

Chauhan, P.S., Satti, N.K., Suri, K.A., Amina, M., Bani, S. 2010. Stimulatory effects of Cuminum cyminum and flavonoid glycoside on cyclosporine-A and restraint stress induced immune-suppression in swiss albino mice. *Chemico-Biological Interactions.185*: 66–72.

Chiang, L.C., Ng, L.T., Chiang, W., Chang, M.Y., and C.C. Lin. 2003. Immunomodulatory activities of flavonoids, monoterpenoids, triterpenoids, iridoid glycosides and phenolic compounds of Plantago species. *Planta Medica*. 69:600–4.

Chinen, J., and W.T. Shearer. 2010. Secondary immunodeficiencies, including HIV infection. *Journal of Allergy and Clinical Immunology*. 125(2) Supplement 2:S195–203.

Chiou, W.F., Chen, C.F., and J.J. Lin. 2000. Mechanisms of suppression of inducible nitric oxide synthase (iNOS) expression in RAW 264.7 cells by andrographolide. *British Journal of Pharmacology*. 129:1553–60.

Chorgade, M.S. 2007. *Drug Discovery and Development*. Vol. 2. Hoboken, NJ: John Wiley.

Chulet, R., and P. Pradhan. 2010. A review on rasayana. *Pharmacognosy Reviews*. 3(6):229e34.

Clement, F., Pramod, S.N., and Y.P. Venkatesh. 2010. Identity of the immunomodulatory proteins from *Allium sativum* with the major garlic lectins or agglutinins. *International Journal of Immunopharmacology*. 10:316–24.

De Bosscher, K., Van Craenenbroeck, K., Meijer, O.C., and G. Haegeman. 2008. Selective transrepression versus transactivation mechanisms by glucocorticoid receptor modulators in stress and immune systems. *European Journal of Pharmacology*. 583:290–302.

DeFuria, J., Bennett, G., K.J. Strissel, et al. 2009. Dietary blueberry attenuates whole-body insulin resistance in high fat-fed mice by reducing adipocyte death and its inflammatory sequelae. *Journal of Nutrition*.139:1510–1516.

Denzler, K.L., Waters, R., Jacobs, B.L., Rochon, Y., and J.O. Langland. 2010. Regulation of inflammatory gene expression in PBMCs by immunostimulatory botanicals. *PLoS One*. 5:e12561.

Di Pierro, F., Rapacioli, G., Ferrara, T., and S. Togni. 2012. Use of a standardized extract from Echinacea angustifolia (Polinacea) for the prevention of respiratory tract infections. *Alternative Medicine Review: A Journal of Clinical Therapeutic*. 17:36–41.

Dias, D.A., and S.U. Roessner. 2012. A historical overview of natural products in drug discovery. *Metabolites*. 2:303–36.

Kumar, D., Arya, V., Kaur, R., Ali Bhat, Z., Gupta, V.K., and V. Kumar. 2012. A review of immunomodulators in the Indian traditional health care system. *Journal of Microbiology, Immunology and Infection*, 45:165e184

Dooley, M.A., and R. Nair. 2008. Therapy insight: preserving fertility in cyclophosphamide-treated patients with rheumatic disease. *Nature Clinical Practice Rheumatology*. 4:250–7.

Dutt, S.B. 2013. A review on immunomodulator activity of some indiginious medical plants. *Ancient Science of Life*. 32:S55.

Estrela, J.M., Mena, S., Obrador, E., Benlloch, M., Castellano, G., Salvador, R., and R.W. Dellinger. 2017. Polyphenolic phytochemicals in cancer prevention and therapy: Bioavailability versus bioefficacy. *Jouranl of Medicinal Chemistry*. 60:9413–9436.

Fallah-Rostami, F., Tabari, M.A., Esfandiari, B., Aghajanzadeh, H., and M.Y. Behzadi. 2013. Immunomodulatory activity of aged garlic extract against implanted fibrosarcoma tumor in mice. *North American Journal of Medicine & Science*. 5:207–212.

Fan, K., Wang, P., Zhang, X.L., Hao, S.H., Huang, S., J.Q. Wang. 2010. Study on the chemical constituents of Phlomisyoung husbandii. *Zhongyaocai (Journal of Chinese Medicinal Materials)*.33:1884–1886.

Farzaei, M., Rahimi, R., and M. Abdollahi. 2015. The role of dietary polyphenols in the management of inflammatory bowel disease. *Current Pharmaceutical Biotechnology*.16:196–210.

Ferreira, S.S., Passos, C.P., Madureira, P., Vilanova, M., and M.A. Coimbra. 2015. Structure–function relationships of immunostimulatory polysaccharides: a review. *Carbohydrate Polymers*. 132:378–396.

Fu, A., Wang, Y., Wu, Y., Chen, H., Zheng, S., Li, Y., Xu, X., and W. Li. 2017. *Echinacea purpurea* extract polarizes M1 macrophages in murine bone marrow-derived macrophages through the activation of JNK: *E CHINACEA P URPUREA E XTRACT P OLARIZES M1 M ACROPHAGES*. *Journal of Cellular Biochemistry*. 118:2664–2671.

Fu, L.N., Chen, L.Y., Liu, R.H., and D.F. Chen. 2010. Chemical constituents of Rhizoma imperatae and their anti-complementary activity. *Zhongyaocai (Journal of Chinese Medicinal Materials)*. 33:1871–1874.

Garcia, D., Leiro, J., Delgado, R., Sanmartín, M.L., and F.M. Ubeira. 2003. *Mangifera indica* L. extract (Vimang) and mangiferin modulate mouse humoral immune responses. *Phytotherapy Research*.17:1182–7.

Gaur, K., Kori, M.L., and R.K. Nema. 2009. Comparative screening of immunomodulatory activity of hydro-alcoholic extract of Hibiscus rosa sinensis Linn. and ethanolic extract of Cleome gynandra Linn. *GJP*. 3:85e9.

Gautam, V., Raman, R.M.V., and K. Ashish. 2003. Exporting indian healthcare (Export potential of Ayurveda and Siddha products and services) Road beyond boundaries (the case of selected Indian healthcare system). Export-Import Bank of India, Mumbai, pp4–54.

Gebreyohannes, G., and M. Gebreyohannes. 2013. Medicinal values of garlic: a review. *International Journal of Medical Sciences*. 5:401–8.

Ghasemzadeh, A. and N. Ghasemzadeh. 2011. Flavonoids and phenolic acids: role and biochemical activity in plants and human. *Journal of Medicinal Plants Research*. 5: 6697–6703.

Ghildyal, P., Grønhaug, T.E. and A. Rusten, et al. 2010. Chemical composition and immunological activities of polysaccharides isolated from the malian medicinal plant syzygium guineense. *Journal of Pharmacognosy and Phytotherapy*. 2:76–85.

Ghosal, S., Srivastava, R.S., Bhattacharya, S.K., Upadhyay, S.N., Jaiswal, A.K., and U. Chattopadhyay. 1989. Immunomodulatory and CNS effects of sitoindosides IX and X, two new glycowithanolides form *Withania somnifera*. *Phytotherapy Research*. 2:201–6.

Gomes, F.I., Aragão, M.G., Barbosa, F.C., Bezerra, M.M., de Paulo, Teixeira Pinto, V., and H.V. Chaves. 2016. Inflammatory cytokines interleukin-1ß and tumour necrosis factor-a - Novel biomarkers for the detection of periodontal diseases: a literature review. *Journal of Oral & Maxillofacial Research*. 7:e2.

Gong, F., Fung, Y.S., and Y.Z. Liang. 2004. Determination of volatile components in ginger using gas chromatography-mass spectrometry with resolution improved by data processing techniques. *Journal of Agricultural and Food Chemistry*. 52: 6378–6383.

Gupta, S., Yadava, J.N.S., and J.S. Tandon. 1993. Antisecretory (antidiarrhoeal) activity of Indian medicinal plants against Escherichia Coli enterotoxin-induced secretion in rabbit and guinea pig ileal loop models. *Pharmaceutical Biology*. 31:198–204.

Hamilton, G.R., and T.F. Baskett. 2000. In the arms of Morpheus the development of morphine for postoperative pain relief. *Canadian Journal of Anaesthesia*. 47:367–374.

Harikumar, K., Aggarwal, B., Harikumar, K.B., and B.B. Aggarwal. 2008. Resveratrol: a multitargeted agent for age-associated chronic diseases. *Cell Cycle*.7: 1020–1035.

Heinrich, M., Appendino, G., Eerth, T., Fürst, R., Izzo, A.A., Kayser, O., Pezzuto, J.M., and A. Viljoen. 2020. Best practice in research—Overcoming common challenges in phytopharmacological research. *Journal of Ethnopharmacology*. 246:112230.

Hodge, G., Hodge, S., and P. Han. 2002. *Allium sativum* (garlic) suppresses leukocyte inflammatory cytokine production in vitro: potential therapeutic use in the treatment of inflammatory bowel disease. *Cytometry*. 48:209–215.

Hofmeyr, S.A. 2001. An interpretative introduction to the immune system. In: Cohen I, Segel L, editors. *Design Principles for the Immune System and Other Distributed Autonomous Systems*. NY, USA: Oxford University Press, Inc; p. 3e24.

Hu, H.B., Wang, G.W., Liu, J.X., Cao, H., and X.D. Zheng. 2006. Studies on phenolic compounds from Polygonum aviculane. *Zhongguo Zhong Yao ZaZhi*. 31:740–742.

Hubbard, R., Tattersfield, A., Smith, C., West, J., Smeeth, L. and A. Fletcher. 2006. Use of inhaled corticosteroids and the risk of fracture. *Chest*. 130:1082–8

Igor, A., Schepetkina, Gang Xiea, Liliya, N., Kirpotinaa, Robyn, A., Kleinb, Mark, A., and T. Jutilaa, Mark. 2008. Quinna. Macrophage immunomodulatory activity of polysaccharides isolated from Opuntia polyacantha. *International Immunopharmacology*. 8:1455–1466.

Ismail, S., and M. Asad. 2009. Immunomodulatory activity of Acacia catechu. *Indian Journal of Physiology and Pharmacology*. 53:25–3.

Izzo, A.A., Teixeira, M., Alexander, S., Cirino, G., Docherty, J.R., George, C.H., Insel, P.A., Ji, Y., Kendall, D.A., R.A. Panattieri, et al. 2020. A practical guide for transparent reporting of research on natural products in the British Journal of Pharmacology: reproducibility of natural product research. *British Journal Pharmacology*. 177:2169–2178.

Jagetia, G.C., Malagi, K.J., Baliga, M.S., Venkatesh, P., Veruva, and R.R., Triphala. 2004. An ayurvedic rasayana drug, protects mice against radiation-induced lethality by freeradical scavenging. *Journal of Alternative and Complementary Medicine*. 10:971–978.

Jain, V., Bhagwat, D., Jat, R.C., and S. Bhardwaj. 2005. The immunomodulation potential of Hyptis suaveolens. *IJPRD*. 1:1e6.

Jamkhande, P.G., Barde, S.R., Patwekar, S.L., and P.S. Tidke. 2013. Plant profile, phytochemistry and pharmacology of Cordia dichotoma (Indian cherry): a review. *Asian Journal of Pacific Journal of Tropical Biomedicine*. 3:1009–1016.

Jolad, S.D., Lantz, R.C., Solyom, A.M., Chen, G.J., Bates, R.B. and B.N. Timmermann. 2004. Fresh organically grown ginger (Zingiber officinale): composition and effects on LPS-induced PGE2 production. *Phytochemistry*. 65: 1937–1954.

Joo, Y.E. 2014. Natural product-derived drugs for the treatment of inflammatory bowel diseases. *Intestinal Research*. 12:103–109.

Josefowicz, S.Z., Lu, L.F., and A.Y. Rudensky. 2012. Regulatory T cells: Mechanisms of differentiation and function. *Annual Review of Immunology*. 30:531–564.

Kaku, H., Goldstein, I.J., VanDamme, E.J.M., and W.J. Peumans. New mannose-specific lectins from garlic (Allium sativum) and ramsons (Allium ursinum) bulbs. *Carbohydrate Research*. 229: 347–353.

Karsch-Völk, M., Barrett B., and K. Linde. 2015. *Echinacea* for preventing and treating the common cold. *JAMA*. 313:618.

Kim, S., Chun, K., Kundu, J., and Y.-J. Surh. 2004. Inhibitory effects of [6]-gingerol on PMA-induced COX-2 expression and activation of NF-kappaB and p38 MAPK in mouse skin. *BioFactors (Oxford, England)*. 21. 27–31.

Kukhetpitakwong, R., Hahnvajanawong, C., and P. Homchampa. 2006. Immunological adjuvant activities of saponin extracts from the pods of Acacia concinna. *International Journal Immunopharmacology*. 6:1729–35.

Kumar, S., Malhotra, R., and D. Kumar. 2010. Euphorbia hirta: Its chemistry, traditional and medicinal uses, and pharmacological activities. *Pharmacognocy Reviews*. 4:58–61.

Kunz, M., and S.M. Ibrahim. 2009. Cytokines and cytokine profiles in human autoimmune diseases and animal models of autoimmunity. *Mediators Inflammation*. 2009: 979258.

Kurup, P.N.V., 2004. Ayurveda- a potential global medical system. In *Scientific Basis for Ayurvedic Therapies*. (Mishra, L.C. Ed.). CRC Press- New York. pp 1–15.

Kyo, E., Uda, N., Kasuga, S., Y. Itakura. 2001. Immuno modulatory effects of aged garlic extract. *Journal of Nutrition*. 131:1075S–9S.

Lee, S.I., Kim, B.S., Kim, K.S., Lee, S., Shin, K.S., and J.S. Lim. 2008. Immune-suppressive activity of punicalagin via inhibition of NFAT activation. *Biochemical and Biophysical Research Communications*. 371:799–803.

LeSourd, B. 2006. Nutritional factors and immunological ageing. *Proceedings of the Nutrition Society*. 65:319–325.

Li, F., Wang, H.D., Lu, D.X., Wang, Y.P., Qi, R.B., and Y.M. Fu. et al. 2006. Neutral sulfate berberine modulates cytokine secretion and increases survival in endotoxemic mice. *Acta Pharmaceutica Sinica B*. 27:1199–205.

Li, S., Wang, N., and Brodt, P. 2012. Metastatic cells can escape the proapoptotic effects of TNF-α through increased autocrine IL-6/STAT3 signaling. *Cancer Research*. 72(4):865–75.

Li, Y., Yang, J., Chen, M.H., Wang, Q., Qin, M.J., Zhang, T., Chen, X.Q., Liu, B.L., and Wen, X.D. 2015. Ilexgenin A inhibits endoplasmic reticulum stress and ameliorates endothelial dysfunction via suppression of TXNIP/NLRP3 inflammasome activation in an AMPK dependent manner. *Pharmacological Research*. 99:101–115.

Li, Y.T., Du, L.P., and D. Mei. 2011. Progress in the study on the pharmacokinetics of Bicyclol. *Medical Research Journal*. 40:18–20.

Limpeanchob, N., Jaipan, S., Rattanakaruna, S., Phrompittayarat, W., and K. Ingkaninan. 2008. Neuroprotective effect of Bacopa monnieri on beta-amyloid-induced cell death in primary cortical culture. *Journal of Ethnopharmacology*. 120:112–117.

Lin, W., and J. Lin. 2011. Berberine down-regulates the Th1/Th2 cytokine gene expression ratio in mouse primary splenocytes in the absence or presence of lipopolysaccharide in a preventive manner. *International Journal of Immunopharmacology*. 11:1984–90.

Liu, D., and J.E. Uzonna. 2012. The early interaction of *Leishmania* with macrophages and dendritic cells and its influence on the host immune response. *Frontiers in Cellular and Infection Microbiology*. 2:83.

Liu, G.T., Zhang, C.Z., and Y. Li. 2010. Study of the anti-hepatitis new drug bicyclol. *Medical Research Journal*. 39.

Liu, Y., Cao, Y., Ye, J., Wang, W., Song, K., Wang, X., Wang, C., Li, R., and X. Deng. 2009. Immunomodulatory effects of proanthocyanidin A-1 derived in vitro from Rhododendron spiciferum. *Fitoterapia*. 81:108–14.

Londhe, V.P., Gavasane, A.T., Nipate, S.S., Bandawane, D.D., and P.D. Chaudhari. 2011. Role of garlic (Allium sativum) in various diseases: an overview. *Journal of Pharmaceutical Research and Opinion*. 4:129–134.

Mak, T.W., Saunders, M.E., B.D. Jett. 2014. Innate Immunity. In *Primer to the Immune Response*, 2nd ed.; Elsevier Science Publishing Co. Inc.: New York, NY, USA, pp. 55–83.

Majdalawieh, A.F., and M.W. Fayyad. 2015. Immunomodulatory and anti-inflammatory action of Nigella sativa and thymoquinone: a comprehensive review. *International Immunopharmacology*. 28:295–304,

Mark, W., Schneeberger, S., Seiler, R., Stroka, D.M., Amberger, A., and F. Offner, et al. 2003. Sinomenine blocks tissue remodeling in a rat model of chronic cardiac allograft rejection. *Transplantation*. 75:940–5.

Matsuda, H., Shimoda, H., Yamahara, J., and M. Yoshikawa. 1998. Immunomodulatory activity of thunberginol A and related compounds isolated from Hydrangeae dulcis Folium on splenocyte proliferation activated by mitogens. *Bioorganic and Medicinal Chemistry Letters.* 8: 215–220.

Mauri, C., and A. Bosma. 2012. Immune regulatory function of B cells. *The Annual Review of Immunology.* 30:221–241.

Mehrotra, S., Mishra, K., and R. Maurya. 2002. Immunomodulation by ethanolic extract of Boerhaavia diffusa roots. *International Journal Immunopharmacology.* 2:987–96.

Mikaili, P., Mojaverrostami, S., Moloudizargari, M., and S. Aghajanshakeri. 2013. Pharmacological and therapeutic effects of Mentha Longifolia L. and its main constituent, menthol. *Ancient Science of Life.* 33:131–8.

Mogensen, T.H. 2009. Pathogen recognition and inflammatory signaling in innate immune defenses. *Clinical Microbiology Reviews.* 22:240–73.

Nakano, K., Kim, D., and Z. Jiang. Immunostimulatory activities of the sulfated polysaccharide ascophyllan from Ascophyllum nodosum in vivo and in vitro systems. *Bioscience, Biotechnology and Biochemistry.* 76: 157376.

Newman, D.J., Cragg, G.M., and K.M. Snader. 2003. Natural products as sources of new drugs over the period 1981–2002. *Journal of Natural Products.* 66:1022–1037.

Ngo, L.T., Okogun, J.I., and W.R., Folk. 2013. 21st Century natural product research and drug development and traditional medicines. *Journal of Natural Products.* 30:584–592.

Pandey, R., Maurya, R., Singh, G., Sathiamoorthy, B., and S. Naik. 2005. Immunosuppressive properties of flavonoids isolated from *Boerhaavia diffusa* Linn. *International Immunopharmacology.* 5:541–53.

Parasuraman, S., Thing, G.S., and S.A. Dhanaraj. 2014. Polyherbal formulation: concept of ayurveda. *Pharmacognocy Reviews.* 8:73–80.

Patel, D.K., Patel, K., Kumar, R., Gadewar, M., and V. Tahilyani. 2012. Pharmacological and Analytical aspects of bergenin a concise report. *Asian Pacific Journal of Tropical Biomedicine.* 2012:163–167.

Perretti, M., and F. D'Acquisto. 2009. Annexin A1 and glucocorticoids as effectors of the resolution of inflammation. *Nature Reviews Immunology.* 9:62–70.

Podder, B., Jang, W.S., Nam, K.W., Lee, B.E., and H.Y. Song. 2015. Ursolic acid activates intracellular killing effect of macrophages during *Mycobacterium tuberculosis* infection. *Journal of Microbiology and Biotechnology.* 25:738–44.

Ponnusankar, S., Pandit, S., Babu, R., Bandyopadhyay, A., and P.K. Mukherjee. 2011. Cytochrome P450 inhibitory potential of triphala—a rasayana from ayurveda. *Journal of Ethnopharmacology.* 133:120–125.

Punturee, K., Wild, C.P., Kasinrerk, W., and U. Vinitketkumnuen. 2005. Immunomodulatory activities of *Centella asiatica* and *Rhinacanthus nasutus* extracts. *Asian Pacific Journal of Cancer Prevention.* 6:396–400.

Ram, A., Arul Joseph, D., Balachandar, S., and V. Pal Singh. 2009. Medicinal plants from Siddha system of medicine useful for treating respiratory diseases. *International Journal of Pharmaceuticals Analysis*, ISSN: 0975-3079, 1:20–30.

Ramalingam, B., and C.N. Patel. 2010. Studies on anthelmintic and antimicrobial activity of the leaf extracts of Lagenaria siceraria. *Molecular Journal of Global Pharma Technology.* 2: 66–70.

Rana, S.V., Pal, S.V.R., Vaiphei, K., Sharma, S.K., and R.P. Ola. 2011. Garlic in health and disease. *Nutrition Research Reviews.* 24:60–71.

Raphael, T., and J.G. Kuttan. 2003. Effect of naturally occurring triterpenoids glycyrrhizic acid, ursolic acid, oleanolic acid and nomilin on the immune system. *Phytomedicine.* 10:483e9

Ravishankar, B., V.J. Shukla. 2007. Indian systems of medicine: a brief profile. *African Journal of Traditional, Complementary and Alternative Medicines.* 4: 319–337.

Rechner, A.R., and C. Kroner. 2005. Anthocyanins and colonic metabolites of dietary polyphenols inhibit platelet function. *Thrombosis Research.* 116:327–34.

Reddy, D.B., and P. Reddanna. 2009. Chebulagic acid (CA) attenuates LPS-induced inflammation by suppressing NF-kappaB and MAPK activation in RAW 264.7 macrophages. *Biochemistry Biophysics Research Communication.* 381:112–7.

Rondanelli, M., Miccono, A., Lamburghini, S., Avanzato, I., Riva, A., Allegrini, P., Faliva, M.A., Peroni, G., Nichetti, M., and S. Perna. 2018. Self-care for common colds: The pivotal role of vitamin D, vitamin C, zinc and *Echinacea* in three main immune interactive clusters (physical barriers, innate and adaptive immunity) involved during an episode of common colds—Practical advice on dosages and on the time to take these nutrients/botanicals in order to prevent or treat common colds. *Evidence Based Complementary and Alternative Medicine.* 2018:1–36.

Rukangira, E. 2000. The African Herbal Industry: constraints and challenges, Proc: "The natural Products and Cosmeceutcals 2001conference". Africa. 2000: 1–20.

Sagar, B.P.S., Zafar, R., and R. Panwar. 2005. Herbal drug standardization. *The Indian Pharmacist.* 4:19–22.

Satish, B.K., Ravindra, A.F. (2009). Investigation of In vitro anthelmintic activity of Thespesia lampas (Cav.). *Asian Journal of Pharmaceutical and Clinical Research.* 2(2): 69–71.

Seeram, N.P, Adams, L.S., Henning, S.M., Niu, Y., Zhang, Y., and M.G. Nair, et al. 2005. *In vitro* anti-proliferative, apoptotic and antioxidant activities of punicalagin, ellagic acid and a total pomegranate tannin extract are enhanced in combination with other polyphenols as found in pomegranate juice. *Journal of Nutritional Biochemistry.* 16:360–7.

Serrano, A., Papacios, C., Roy, G., Cespon, C., Villar, M.L., and M. Nocito et al. 1998. Derivatives of gallic acid induces apoptosis in tumoral cell lines and inhibit lymphocyte proliferation. *Archives of Biochemistry and Biophysics.* 350:49–54.

Shaikh, R., Pund, M., Dawane, A., and S. Iliyas. 2014. Evaluation of anticancer, antioxidant, and possible anti-inflammatory properties of selected medicinal plants used in indian traditional medication. *Journal of Traditional and Complementary Medicine.* 4: 253–257.

Sharma, P., Dwivedee, B.P., Bisht, D., Dash, A.K., and D. Kumar. 2019. The chemical constituents and diverse pharmacological importance of Tinospora cordifolia. *Heliyon.* 5:e02437.

Shukla, Y. and M. Singh. 2007. Cancer preventive properties of ginger: a brief review. *Food and Chemical Toxicology.* 45: 683–690.

Singh, S., Khajuria, A., Taneja, S.C., Johri, R.K., Singh, J., and G.N. Qazi. 2008. Boswellic acids: a leukotriene inhibitor also effective through topical application in inflammatory disorders. *Phytomedicine.* 15:400–7.

Singh, S., Taneja, M., and D.K. Majumdar. 2007. Biological activities of Ocimum sanctum Linn. fixed oil e an overview. *Indian Journal of Experimental Biology.* 45:403e12.

Singh, U.P., Prithiviraj, B., Sarma, B.K., Singh, M., and A.B. Ray. 2001. Role of garlic (Allium sativum L.) in human and plant diseases. *Indian Journal of Experimental Biology.* 39:310–22.

Sinha, K., Mishra, N.P., Singh, J., and S.P.S. Khanuja. 2004. Tinospora cordifolia, a reservoir plant for therapeutic applications. *Indian Journal of Traditional Knowledge.* 3: 257–270.

Sinha, S., Perdomo, G., Brown, N.F., and O'Doherty, R.M. 2004. Fatty acid-induced insulin resistance in L6 myotubes is prevented by inhibition of activation and nuclear localization of nuclear factor kappa B. *Journal of Biological Chemistry.* 279(40):41294–301.

Sook Young Lee, Yong Kyoung Kim, Nam Park, Chun Sung Kim, Chung Yeol Le, and Sang Un Park. 2010. Chemical constituents and biological activities of the berry of *Panax ginseng*. *Journal of Medicinal Plants Research*. 4: 349–353.

Vanisree, S., Sheng-Yang, W., Lie-Fen, S., and Y. Ning-Sun. 2004. Shikonins, Phytocompounds from Lithospermum erythrorhizon, Inhibit the Transcriptional Activation of Human Tumor Necrosis Factor Promoter in Vivo. *The Journal of Biological Chemistry*. 279:5877–85.

Rao, V. (Ed.), Matos, M.J., Santana, L., Uriarte, E., Abreu, O.A., Molina, E., and E.G. Yordi. 2015. Chapter 5 Coumarins - An Important Class of Phytochemicals; Phytochemicals - Isolation, Characterisation and Role in Human Health. ISBN: 978-953-51-2170-1.

Staniforth, V., Wang, S.Y., Shyur, L.F., and Yang, N.S. 2004. Shikonins, phytocompounds from *Lithospermum erythrorhizon*, inhibit the transcriptional activation of human tumor necrosis factor alpha promoter in vivo. *Journal of Biological Chemistry*. 279(7):5877–85.

Suleria, H.A.R., Butt, M.S., Anjum, F.M., Sultan, S., and N. Khalid. 2013. Aqueous garlic extract; natural remedy to improve haematological, renal and liver status. *Journal of Nutrition and Food Sciences*. 4:252.

Sultan, M.T., Buttxs, M.S., Qayyum M.M.N., and H.A.R. Suleria. 2014. Immunity: Plants as effective mediators. *Critical Reviews in Food Science*. 54:1298–1308.

Sunila, E.S., and G. Kuttan. 2004. Immunomodulatory and antitumor activity of *Piper longum* Linn. And piperine. *Journal of Ethnopharmacology*. 90:339–46.

Suzuki, T., Chow, C.W., and G.P. Downey. 2008. Role of innate immune cells and their products in lung immunopathology. *International Journal of Biochemistry and Cell Biology*. 40:1348–61.

Thillaivanan, S., and K. Samraj. 2014. Challenges constraints and opportunities in herbal medicines – a review. *International Journal of Herbal Medicine*. 2: 21–24.

Tripathi, S., and T. Maiti. 2005. Imrnunomodulatory role of native and heat denatured agglutinin from Abrus precatorius. *International Journal of Biochemistry and Cell Biology*. 37:45162.

Vaghasiya, J., Datani, M., Nandkumar, K., Malaviya, S., and N. Jivani. 2010. Comparative evaluation of alcoholic and aqueous extracts of Ocimum sanctum for immunomodulatory activity. *International Journal of Biological & Pharmaceutical Research*. 1:25e9.

van der Meijden, A.P. 2001. Non-specific immunotherapy with Bacille Calmette-Guérin (BCG). *Clinical and Experimental Immunology*. 123:179–80.

Varma, A., Padh, H., and N. Shrivastava. 2011. Andrographolide: a new plant-derived antineoplastic entity on horizon. *Evidence Based Complementary and Alternative Medicine*. 2011:815390.

Veerakumar, S., Amanulla, S.D, and K. Ramanthan. 2016. Anti-cancer efficacy of ethanolic extracts from various parts of Annona squamosa on MCF-7 cell line. *Journals of Pharmacognosy and Phytotherapy*. 8: 147–154.

Vetvicka, V., and J. Vetvickova. 2014. Natural immunomodulators and their stimulation of immune reaction: true or false? *Anticancer Research*. 34:2275–2282.

Viegi, G., Maio, S., Pistelli, F., Baldacci, S. and L. Carrozzi. 2006. Definition, epidemiology and natural history of COPD. *Respirology*. 11:523–532.

Vigila, A.G., and X. Baskaran. 2008. Immunomodulatory effect of coconut protein on cyclophosphamide induced immune suppressed Swiss Albino mice. *Ethnobotanical Leaflets*. 12:1206–12.

Wadood, A, Ghufran, M., Jamal, S.B., Naeem, M., Khan, A., and R. Ghaffar, et al. 2013. Phytochemical analysis of medicinal plants occurring in local area of Mardan. *Biochemistry and Analytical Biochemistry*. 2(4):1–4.

Wagner, H. In., Hikino, H., and N.R. Farnsworth. 1984. *Economic and Medicinal Plant Research*, vol. 1. London: Academic Press;. p. 113e53.

Wang, C.Y., Chiao, M.T., Yen, P.J., Huang, W.C., Hou, C.C., Chien, S.C., Yeh, K.C., Yang, W.C., Shyur, L.F., and N.S. Yang. 2006. Modulatory effects of Echinacea purpurea extracts on human dendritic cells: a cell- and gene-based study. *Genomics*. 88:801–808.

Wang, L.S., and G.D. Stoner. 2008. Anthocyanins and their role in cancer prevention. *Cancer Letters*. 269:281–90.

Wang, Y., Huang, M., Sun, R., and L. Pan. 2015. Extraction, characterization of a Ginseng fruits polysaccharide and its immune modulating activities in rats with Lewis lung carcinoma. *Carbohydrate Polymer*.127: 215–221.

Wani, M.C., and S.B. Horwitz. 2014. Nature as a remarkable chemist: a personal story of the discovery and development of Taxol. *Anticancer Drugs*. 25: 482–487.

Wei J., Mo Y., and S. Liang. 2007. Limit detection of aristolochic acid in Ganteling Capsules. *Chinese Traditional Patent Medicine*. 29:1266–1267.

Wilson, D.R., and L. Warise. 2008. Cytokines and their role in depression. *Perspectives in Psychiatric Care*. 44:285–9.

Wohlmuth, H., Leach, D.N., Smith, M.K., and S.P. Myers. 2005. Gingerol content of diploid and tetraploid clones of ginger (Zingiber officinale Roscoe). *Journal of Agriculture Food Chemistry*. 53: 5772–5778.

Wu, S., Powers, S., Zhu, W., and Y.A. Hannun. 2016. Substantial contribution of extrinsic risk factors to cancer development. *Nature*. 529:43–7.

Xiu-feng, Z., Yan, C., Jia-jun, H., Ya-zhou, Z., Zhou, N., Lan-fen, W., Bao-zhen, Y., Ya-lin, T., and L. Yang. 2007. Immuno-stimulating properties of diosgenyl saponins isolated from Paris polyphylla. *Bioorganic Medicinal Chemistry Letters*. 17:2408e13.

Xu, Z.H., Qin, G.W., Li, X.Y., and R.S. Xu. 2001. New biflavanones and bioactive compounds from Stellera chamaejasme. *Yao Xue Xue Bao*. 36:669–671.

Xu, Y, Liao, S, Na, Z, Huabin L, Yan L, and Huai-Rong. 2012. Gelsemium alkaloids, immunosuppressive agents from Gelsemium elegans. *Fitoterapia*. 83:1120–4.

Xue, Q.L. 1991. *Union Catalog of Chinese Medical Literature*. Beijing.

Xue, Y., Wang, Y., Feng, D.C., Xiao, B.G., and L.Y. Xu. 2008. Tetrandrine suppresses lipopolysaccharide-induced microglial activation by inhibiting NF-kappaB pathway. *Acta Pharmacologica Sinica*. 29:245–51.

Yadav, V.S., Mishra, K.P., Singh, D.P., Mehrotra, S., and V.K. Singh. 2005. Immunomodulatory effects of curcumin. *Immunopharmacology and Immunotoxicology*. 27:485–97.

Yang, Y.F., Yang, B.C., and L.L. Jin, 2009. Retrospection, strategy, and practice on innovative drug research and development of Chinese materia medica. *Chinese Traditional and Herbs Drugs*. 40:1513–1519.

Yun, D., Yoon, S.Y., Park, S.J., and Park, Y.J. 2021. The anticancer effect of natural plant alkaloid isoquinolines. *International Journal of Molecular Sciences*. 22(4):1653.

Yun, K., Shin, J.-S., Choi, J., Back, N., Chung, H., and K. Lee. 2009. Quaternary alkaloid, pseudocoptisine isolated from tubers of Corydalis turtschaninovi inhibits LPS-induced nitric oxide, PGE2, and pro-inflammatory cytokines production via the down-regulation of NF-??B in RAW 264.7 murine macrophage cells. *International Journal of Immunopharmacology*. 9:1323–31.

Zhang, M.Q. 1996. A treatise on the standardization of prescription's name. In: Chang I.M., editor. *Experts Meeting for the Standardization of Titles of Chinese Prescriptions*. Seoul: Natural Products Research Institute, Seoul National University, WHO Collaborating Center for Traditional Medicine. 33–9.

Zhang, Q.H., Zhang, L., Shang, L.X., Shao, C.L., and Y.X. Wu. 2008. Studies on the chemical constituents of flowers of Prunusmume. *Journal of Chinese Medicinal Materials*. 31: 1666–1668.

Zhou, B., Yang, Z., Feng, Q., Liang, X., Li, J., Zanin, M., and Zhong, N. 2017. Aurantiamide acetate from baphicacanthus cusia root exhibits anti-inflammatory and anti-viral effects via inhibition of the NF-κB signaling pathway in Influenza A virus-infected cells. *Journal of Ethnopharmacology.* 199:60–7.

Zhou, J, Zhou, T., Jiang, M., Wang, X., and Q. Liu, et al. 2014. Research progress on synergistic anti-cancer mechanisms of compounds in traditional Chinese medicine. *Journal of Traditional Chinese Medicine.* 34: 100–105.

Zhu, F., Ma, X.H., Qin, C., Tao, L., Liu, X., Shi, Z., Zhang, C.L., Tan, C.Y., Chen, Y.Z., and Y.Y. Jiang. 2012. Drug discovery prospect from untapped species: Indications from approved natural product drugs. *PLoS ONE.* 7:e39782.

Zysk, K.G. 2008. Siddha Medicine in Tamil Nadu. © Nationalmuseet og Kenneth G. Zysk, Tranquebar Initiativets Skriftserie, ISBN: 978-87-7602-102-3.

12 Specific Plant Nutrients and Vitamins that Fortify Human Immune System

Kirubel Teshome Tadele and
Gebeyanesh Worku Zerssa

CONTENTS

12.1 INTRODUCTION

From the instant of birth in the process of joining this world, a living organism's body is bombarded by pathogenic microorganisms, the solitary goal of which is living and replicating under favorable conditions based on their natural behaviour and a nutrient-rich environment. Harmful microorganisms reproduce and infect a body by very specialized mechanisms which may even lead to mortality unless managed properly. These microorganisms also use infected bodies as a route for spreading to new hosts (Gombart et al. 2020). Nowadays, the challenging global problems, such as environmental and water pollution, provide extra opportunities for infection by microorganisms, which is facilitated by the technology-aided high mobility of people and commodities around the world. There is no better example than COVID-19 for this, which spread throughout the world within a couple of months after its

DOI: 10.1201/9781003137955-12

outbreak in December 2019 and may be considered to be the most detrimental event of the 21st century.

Nature is not passive, allowing microorganisms to attack and damage living organisms at will. There is an immune system whose main functions are to protect the host's body against infection and damage from the pathogens, removing unwanted damaged tissues, and providing persistent reconnaissance of harmful cells that grow in the body of the host (Wu et al. 2019). The system consists of innate (non-specific) and adaptive (specific) immune systems (Li et al. 2007) as functional branches. Although the immune system has a complicated defensive strategy, orchestrated by specialized tissues, organs, cells, and chemicals (Rondanelli et al. 2018), their organization can be described into three core cooperative clusters, including physical barriers, and innate and adaptive immunity (Calder and Kew 2002; Maggini et al. 2007). The first barrier contains physical barriers with an acidic medium due to the availability of different fatty acids and enzymes, which are able to limit the growth of nearly all bacteria, secreting pathogen-destroying mucus, and enhancing the acidity of the stomach. The second barrier is innate immunity, which contains cells such as natural killer (NK) cells, cytokines, macrophages, and neutrophil granulocytes as elements for its functions (Rondanelli et al. 2018). The innate immune system takes immediate action to distinguish and destroy foreign threats through inflammatory processes, resolving the inflammation, and repairing the damage caused (Murphy and Weaver 2017). Hence, the innate immune system provides the first line of defence against invading pathogens in vertebrates (Narnaware et al. 1994). The problem of the innate immune system is its inability to increase the responding efficacy when there is a repeated pathogenic attack. Then, the additional help needed opens the door for the adaptive (specific) immune system to act subsequently. Antigen-specific cells like T lymphocytes, which play a key role in killing virally-infected cells, as well as B lymphocytes, that are responsible for secretion of antibodies specific to the infecting pathogen after being activated, operate under the adaptive immune system (van Gorkom et al. 2018). Although the adaptive immune system responds more slowly than the innate immune system, it is more efficient in eliminating infections because of the exquisite specificity of antigen recognition by its lymphocytes. But the adaptive immune system is not independent of the innate immune since it interacts with, and relies upon, cells of the innate immune system for many of its functions (Murphy and Weaver 2017).

Innate immunity is strongly influenced by nutrition and the interconnection between nutrition and immunity is considered to be absolute (Mainous and Deitch 1994). Nutrition, taking into account the content and nature of the nutrients as well as the duration of the intake, has a profound impact on human health (Nobs et al. 2020). However, for the immune system to generate an efficient immune response, adequate and balanced nutrition is required to supply it with the necessary components (Marcos et al. 2003). In general, nutrition determines the development of the immune system in infants and their efficiency in adult life (Sima et al. 2016). The enormous influence of nutrition on immune function was confirmed after being studied for several decades and transformed research in the field to a specific discipline called nutritional immunology (Wu et al. 2019). The research findings in this area greatly emphasize the use of immunity-boosting plant nutrients asone of the most promising methods of controlling diseases (Harikrishnan et al. 2011). Nutrition provides certain micronutrients upon which every stage of an immune response depends (Gombart et al. 2020). Considering the risk of premature death as a result of the persistent infectious diseases globally, the plants containing immune system-boosting nutrients and vitamins are in great demand. The main aim of this chapter is to explore the specific immune system-boosting plant nutrients and vitamins to our current understanding of the field. It also describes some suggested mechanisms by which the nutrients enhance the efficacy of the immune system, although the mechanism is still not fully understood.

12.2 SPECIFIC PLANT NUTRIENTS AND THEIR IMMUNE SYSTEM STIMULATING EFFECT

The great health benefits of functional and nutraceutical foods are making them popular around the world (Suleria et al. 2015). The strong interaction between nutrients and the immune system has been proved and has attracted particular attention to nutrition. Currently, some plants with immune system-boosting specific nutrients, such as garlic, ginger, green tea, echinacea, broccoli, and black pepper are on target to manage the morbidity and mortality due to pathogens causing infectious diseases (Table 12.1).

12.2.1 GARLIC

Garlic (*Allium sativum*) is a bulb-forming annual plant belonging to the genus *Allium* of the Amaryllidaceae family (Lee et al. 2012), native to Central and South Asia (Rouf et al. 2020). The numerous health benefits of garlic make it one of the most used plants in herbal medicine. Garlic has been used to treat as well as to prevent diseases by the Chinese, Greeks, and Romans for centuries. The efficacy of the plant in treating and preventing diseases like cancer, cardiovascular, and obesity is indicated in the literature (Miguel 2011; ia-Ul-Haq et al. 2011; Zia-Ul-Haq et al. 2013; Khanra et al. 2015). Presently, garlic is cultivated throughout the world, with countries like China, India, South Korea, Egypt, and the USA being among the leaders in garlic production (Medina and Garcia 2007; Rehman et al. 2019). Garlic is an edible crop that has been used as medicine (Gruhlke et al. 2019), a functional food, spice, and seasoning herb (Rehman et al. 2019; Rouf et al. 2020) since ancient times. The plant is among one of those most widely used for its health-giving benefits and it is also used as a flavouring agent, enhancing physical and mental health (Shin and Kim 2004). Garlic is used to treat common viral diseases, such as the common cold, fever, coughs, asthma, and wounds in Asia and Europe (Rehman et al. 2019; Rouf et al. 2020). The oil extracted from garlic has also been used to mitigate the pain of ear infections (Al Abbasi, 2008). In African countries, like Ethiopia and Nigeria, garlic has been used as a traditional remedy for the treatment of several infections, such as sexually transmitted infections, tuberculosis (TB), respiratory system diseases, and wounds due to injuries and damage of different tissues (Gebreyohannes and Mebrahtu 2013; Abiy and Asefaw 2016).

TABLE 12.1

Summary of Major Findings of Immune System Boosting Activity of Some Medicinal Plant Nutrients

Medicinal Plant	Bioactive Compounds	Immune System Stimulating Compounds	Activity	References
Garlic	Organosulphur compounds (G-SAC, alliin, allicin)	Allicin	Activated the release of Zn^{2+} from proteins S-thioallylated 332 proteins of human Jurkat cell proteome	(Gruhlke et al. 2019)
Ginger	Gingerol, shogoal, zingiberol, zingiberene	Gingerol	Inhibited the gene expression of Th2 cytokines and IFN-γ Stimulated both innate and adaptive immune response mechanisms	(Kawamotoa et al. 2016; Bauer et al. 2014)
Green tea	Catechin flavonoids (EGCG, EGC, EC, ECG, phenolic acid, theobromine, theanine, theophylline, and caffeine)	EGCG	Sustained the levels of CD4+ and CD8+ lymphocytes at the required level and increased the secretion of sIgA in BALF mice Prevented skin erythema formation in mice Supported the restoration of T cell activity by mediating PD-L1 inhibition	(Tang et al. 2020; Jung et al. 2019; Rawangkan et al. 2018)
Echinacea (the most potent immuno stimulating)	Polysaccharides, alkaloids, glycoproteins, caffeic acid derivatives, alkylamides, and volatile oils	Polysaccharides Alkamides Glycoproteins	Activated the synthesis of pro-inflammatory cytokine TNF-α in RAW 264.7 macrophage-like cells Enhanced the production and secretion of macrophages	(Balciunaite et al. 2015; Rininger et al. 2000; Todd et al. 2015; Luettig et al.1989; Roesler et al. 1991)
Broccoli	Glucosinolates, dithiolthiones, indoles, glucoraphanin, S-methyl cysteine sulfoxide, isothiocyanates	Sulphoraphane	Decreased the oozing of pro- inflammatory cytokines	(Aguado et al. 2014: Ruiz-Jiménez et al. 2003; Bessler and Djaldetti, 2018; Busato et al. 2020; Geisel et al. 2014)
Red Pepper	Capsaicin, capsisin, capsantine polyphenol, flavonoids, and flavonols	Capsaicin	Augmented activated macrophages in number as well as phagocytic activity Inhibited IL-12 and IL-23 expression Augmented the immunoglobulin (IgM) levels Elevated the leucocytes cells	(Zaki et al. 2017: Puvaca, 2018; Abdelnour *et al.* 2018; Abdelnour et al. 2018: Afolabi et al. 2017)

The enormous health benefits of garlic are mainly associated with its organo-sulphur compounds (Suleria et al. 2015). The organosulphur compound content (1.1–3.5%) content of garlic is much higher than that in other plants, which is the main reason behind its superior health- benefits relative to other plants. Glutamyl-S-allyl-L-cysteines (G-SAC) are the principal organosulphur compounds of intact garlic. These compounds hydrolyze and oxidize, forming S-allyl-l-cysteine sulphoxides (alliin) when stored (Matsuura and Lachance 1997).

Alliin is highly unstable, being converted to the chief bioactive components, allicin and other thiosulphates, by an enzyme, alliinase, released by crushing, chopping, or chewing of garlic (Amagase 2006).

Allicin is mainly responsible for the medicinal role of garlic (Larry et al. 2018). This bioactive organosulphur compound provides the necessary components for the immune system to defend the host against pathological microorganisms, making garlic the source of numerous health benefits (Gardner et al. 2007). Fresh garlic has a distinctive pleasant flavour, which is also associated with volatile compounds released from the unstable alliin by the help of the enzyme allinase (Krest et al. 2000). About 10 g of edible garlic (one single clove) produces up to 5 mg of allicin (Gruhlke et al. 2019). A diet containing garlic, either raw or crushed, is proved to act as an immune modulator, influencing the expression of immunity in humans (Abdullah 2000; Charron et al. 2015).

Daily consumption of food containing aged garlic extract (AGE) modulates the immune system response of healthy but obese adults by stimulating the immune cells and inflammatory mediators (Xu et al. 2018). Although the mechanism by which the extract plays the role is still in doubt, a hydrogen sulphide (H_2S) -based mechanism is considered to be a potential one. This mechanism deactivates the pathway of NF-kappa-beta signaling, facilitating the production of pro-inflammatory cytokines (Ha et al. 2015; Rios et al. 2015). The bioactive organosulphur compounds in AGE, like S-allyl-L-cysteine (SAC), increase the endogenous production of H_2S and act as its mediators (Gu and Zhu 2011; Chulah et al. 2007), driving the suppression of obesity induced-inflammation (Xu et al. 2018). Aging makes garlic nearly odorless by converting its strong organosulphur compounds into hydrophilic compounds, like SAC and S-allylmercaptocysteine (SAMC). There are compounds such as lectins and fructooligosaccharides in aged garlic with proven immunomodulating activity (Chandrashekar and Venkatesh 2009; Chandrashekar et al. 2011). Allicin, the main organosulphur compound in garlic, stimulates the immune response by activating the release of Zn^{2+} from proteins to enhance the production of IL-2 in murine EL-4 T cells. It inhibits the activity of enolase, a targeted enzyme in cancer therapy. Allicin also inhibits some selected S-thioallylated proteins, which are one of the components of the garlic action mechanism, causing the actin cytoskeleton disruption.

These activities of allicin and other organosulfur compounds of garlic are respon-sible for modulating the immune system in humans. The strong immunostimulating activity of allicin on mammalian cells at its higher doses is manifested by its abil-ity to achieve S-thioallylation of 332 proteins in the human Jurkat cell proteome (Gruhlke et al. 2019).

Identification of garlic or lemon aqueous extracts, as well as their combination, as antiproliferative in mice indicated the good activity of the two, especially when combined. Thus, the garlic and lemon extract combination is a promising option for anticancer food and therapy development, although the molecular mechanisms need to be further studied. The combination of garlic and lemon extracts activated the immune system by inhibiting angiogenesis and inducing apoptosis. The combination enhanced the immunity-boosting ability of garlic due to the acidic environment provided by the lemon extract which activates organosulphur compound production (Talib 2017).

It was reported in a randomized crossover garlic-containing meal feeding study that garlic intake up-regulated the nuclear factor of activated T cells (NFAT) activating protein with the immune receptor tyrosine-based activation motif 1 (NFAM1) gene, modulating the immune system (Charron et al. 2015). A study carried out to determine the influence of aged garlic dietary augmentation on the immune system function, targeting the innate immune NK cell and adaptive immune $\gamma\delta$-T cell functions, revealed a lowering of inflammatory cytokine secretion by the garlic-treated cells. The significantly lower secretion of IFN-γ suggests that the immune system easily destroys the pathogens with a smaller amount of the inflammatory cytokine. The supplementation also reduced cold and flu symptoms, which might be related to lowering in inflammatory cytokine secretion, $\gamma\delta$-T and NK cell function, and thiol status improvement (Nantz et al. 2012). The modification of the innate immune cells by dietary compounds has been reported (Meadows et al. 1992; Percival et al. 2005; Hanson et al. 2007; Schink et al. 2007). Garlic powder supplemented as natural feed additives for broiler chickens improved their red blood cells (RBC) and haemoglobin content (Hb). It also improved the weight of the liver and immune-related organs, which was due to the bioactive molecules in garlic powder, enhancing the immune system (Ismail et al. 2020).

Garlic, onion lemon, and juice supplementation as natural additives to the diet of buffalo calves increased the digestibility of all nutrients. It also significantly increased blood components GPT and GOT; erythrocytes and leukocytes numbers also increased. Glutamate-pyruvate transaminase (GPT) is highly active glutamate degrading enzyme found in the liver and other tissues, while glutamateoxaloacetic transaminase (GOT) is found in mitochondrial and cytosolic forms, catalyzing amino acid metabolism as well as urea and tricarboxylic acid cycles. Furthermore, the increasing immunity (globulin fractions) was manifested by the elimination of harmful bacteria, avoiding early infections (Ahmed et al. 2009). Post dietary supplementation of garlic and ginger to Sasso broiler chicks modulated their immune system response. The most likely mechanism for this activity included amplification of phagocytosis, increased antifungal activity, and minimization of nitric oxide (NO) synthesis. Phagocytic cells increased, showing 90% engulfing capacity of *Candida albicans* in broiler chicks treated with the two medicinal plant extracts. The antimicrobial activity of garlic which might be associated with its bioactive compounds is reported. The suggested mechanism of the action is *via* hindering the functions of the microbial membrane and the associated membrane proteins (Hafidh et al. 2011). The antibacterial potential of garlic might be attributed to its increased production of TNF-α cytokines and lymphocyte-triggering abilities (Mojani et al. 2016). The extracts have bioactive compounds which interact with innate lymphocytes and natural killer cells (Percival 2016). It is also reported that the bioactive compounds activate macrophages and B cells, enhance immunoglobulin production, and regulate cytokine secretion (Li et al. 2015). The downregulation of NO production after treatment of the birds with garlic and ginger additives might reduce the pathological damage occurring as a result of excess NO production (Amirghofran et al. 2011).

12.2.2 GINGER

Ginger (*Zingiber officinale*) is a well-known spice and medicinal plant, which has been used throughout the world and is readily accessible in many Asian countries (Bauer et al. 2014; Sheikhi et al. 2015). Tropical Asians, especially in southern China or India, are believed to have been the first to use ginger (Semwal et al. 2015). Ginger rhizome (the actual botanical term for what is referred to as 'ginger root') is used as a spice globally (Kikuzaki and Nakatani 1996). The typical components of a dry ginger root powder are carbohydrates (60–70%), protein (9%), lipid (3–6%), fibre (3–8%), proteases (2–6%), volatile bioactive compounds (1–3%), and vitamins (Murray 1995). Ginger possesses numerous biological activities, such as antidiabetic, anti-inflammatory, and antitumour properties, due to the bioactive compounds such as gingerol, gingerdiol, and gingerdione (Kikuzaki and Nakatani 1996). The bioactive compounds of ginger increase host resistance to infectious diseases by stimulating the immune system response mechanisms of the host (Bauer et al. 2014). It is also reported that cell-mediated immune response, as well as the non-specific proliferation of T lymphocytes, are influenced by ginger oil (Wilasrusmee et al. 2002).

Compounds of phenolic ketone derivatives make ginger a good antioxidant. Gingerol is one of the typical volatile compounds of ginger, which is responsible for the pungent odour and taste of the plant. This compound also increases the palatability of food as well as increasing the secretion of digestive enzymes (Mansour et al. 2012; Jesudoss et al. 2017; Ahmadifar et al. 2019). Ginger has been used to treat gastrointestinal disorders for many centuries (Sheikhi et al. 2015). Ginger is also used as a treatment option for nausea and vomiting (Sharifi-Rad et al. 2017; Tóth et al. 2018). However, it is not recommended for pregnant women since it has mutagenic effects *in vitro* (Nakamura and Yamamoto 1983; Nagabhushan et al. 1987; Srinivasan 2017; Tóth et al. 2018).

Supplementation with ginger powder for patients with active rheumatoid arthritis (RA) decreased the manifestation of the disease by enhancing the expression of FoxP3 genes and declining the expression of RORγt and T-bet genes to improve RA symptoms. The anti-inflammatory activity of ginger is indicated by its ability to reduce T-bet. The immunomodulatory effects of ginger were verified by increases in FoxP3 expression in patients who consumed ginger (Aryaeian et al. 2019). The increase in FoxP3 expression activated Tregs function, modulating the immune system (Nazari et al. 2013). The improvement of RA showed the potential of ginger to boost the immune system to prevent the damage caused by autoimmune diseases (Aryaeian et al. 2019).

A range of concentrations of feed supplementation with ginger and organic selenium improved the growth and immune system function of broiler chickens. The improvement was directly related to the increase in secretion of gastrointestinal enzymes such as disaccharidases, lipase and maltase, which improve digestion and food intake (Zhang et al. 2009). The combined feeding of ginger and selenium improved immune response with no synergistic effect on the performance of broiler chickens (Safiullah et al. 2019).

It was recently reported for the first time that ginger rhizome extract has benefits even for smokers. Ginger consumption increased the concentration of haemoglobin to compensate for its reduction as a result of smoking, a finding which benefits smokers with anaemia. Ginger consumption enhances the thyroid gland activity in smokers as well as in non-smokers. It also enhanced IgM levels of non-smokers for better humoral immunity, antibody response, and defence against infections (Mahassni et al. 2019).

Nanoparticles prepared from compounds isolated from ginger protected mice from alcohol-induced liver damage. It is suggested that the nanoparticles activated nuclear factor erythroid 2-related factor 2 (Nrf2), which plays a key role in the expression of liver detoxifying genes. This also inhibits the production of oxygen free radicals to support the safety of the liver (Zhuang et al. 2015).

An antiallergic effect of ginger is reported, with the major bioactive phenolic compound 6-gingerol suggested to play the role. The potential of 6-gingerol to inhibit the expression of genes encoding Th2 cytokines and IFN-γ was indicated clearly (Kawamotoa et al. 2016). In addition, feeding with ginger prohibited Th2-mediated immune responses and 6-gingerol suppressed eosinophilia in a mouse model (Ahui et al. 2008), so it could be a good option for the prevention of IgE-mediated allergic disorders. 6-Gingerol is a proven immunosuppressing agent (Kawamotoa et al. 2016).

12.2.3 GREEN TEA

After water, tea is the leading beverage to be consumed globally today (Costa et al. 2002; Rietveld and Wiseman 2003). A leaf of *Camellia sinensis* plant is used for the preparation of tea. The plant belongs to the Theaceae family and all types of tea are prepared from its leaf. The beginning of tea usage goes back 5,000 years in Southwest China. In preparing black tea, the basic processes include oxidation, a curing process of maceration and exposure to atmospheric oxygen, and black tea is the preferred form in Western countries (Graham 1992; Langley-Evans 2002). The majority of tea consumed in the USA is black ice tea (Il'yasova et al. 2003). The complex chemical composition of dried green tea contains carbohydrates (7–25%), proteins (15–20%), minerals (5%), flavonoids (25–35%), xanthic bases (3.5%), pigments (0.5–2%) and aromatic organic acids (Graham 1992; Cabrera et al. 2006). Both tea leaves and the tea beverage obtained by processing the leaves are rich in polyphenols (flavonoids), particularly the most biologically active flavanols, the catechins (Crespy and Williamson 2004), and several vitamins (Sato and Miyata 2000; Higdon and Frei 2003). Green tea is rich in catechins and also includes phenolic acid, theobromine, theophylline, theanine, and caffeine (Barbalho et al. 2019).

In the catechins in green tea, epigallocatechin-3-gallate (EGCG) is the most abundant (32–50%), followed by epigallocatechin (EGC) (18–28%), then others like epicatechin (EC) (6%) and epicatechin-3-gallate (ECG) (8–12%). These bioactive compounds are responsible for the biological activities of the plant, such as its antioxidant and anti-inflammatory properties. These biological activities are very important for the prevention and treatment of numerous diseases such as diabetes, cancer, obesity and cardiovascular diseases (Inoue-Choi et al. 2010; Geetha and Santhy 2013; Najeeb et al. 2016; Cazzola et al. 2018). The immune system stimulating potential of green tea polyphenols has been reported (Shimizu et al. 2010; Kim et al. 2016; Sharma et al. 2017).

It has been reported that tea drinkers showed better immune system stimulation than coffee drinkers through greater γδ-T-T cell proliferation *in vivo*, which is associated with the presence of the unique amino acid, L-theanine, in tea. L-theanine is converted to glutamic acid, alkylamine and ethylamine *via* hydrolyzation (Kamath et al. 2003). The most abundant bioactive compound, catechin, increased levels of immunoglobulin in the rat model, which demonstrated its potential for stimulating the immune system (Ganeshpurkar and Saluja 2018). The immunomodulating activity of catechins is associated with increasing the level of phagocytic cell production in animals (Banacerraf 1978). Supplementation of feed with green tea by-products showed a positive impact on immune cell proliferation in goats by increasing the proliferation of T and B cells (Ahmed et al. 2015). Anticancer activity of green tea catechins has been reported. EGCG showed immune checkpoint inhibition activity and supported the restoration of T cell activity by mediating PD-L1 inhibition, making T cells kill cancer cells more effectively (Rawangkan et al. 2018). The main polyphenol in green tea, EGCG, restored the immune system disturbed by overdose supplementation of the toxic food contaminant, Perfluorodecanoic acid (PFDA) in mice and significantly reduced their mortality (Wang et al. 2020).

Supplementation with green tea for one week stimulated the function of the skin barrier by modulating skin metabolites and inhibiting metabolome changes in response to UV stress in mice exposed to external UV radiation. It is suggested that this effect prevents the formation of skin erythema (Jung et al. 2019). The components of green tea, such as epigallocatechin gallate, caffeine, and theanine, defend the skin against UV stress by repairing the disturbed immune system caused by UV exposure and by enhancing its functions. (–)-Epigallocatechin-3-gallate (EGCG) enhanced the immune system in mice through maintaining the normal levels of CD4+ and CD8+ lymphocytes and increasing the secretion of sIgA in BALB/c mice and blocked infection by microorganisms in the respiratory tract. However, the activity of the compound was dose-dependent and the risk of immune suppression was reported at overdose levels. In addition, EGCG inhibited the release of the main stress hormones in normal mice, preventing the restraint stress to minimize the liver injury (Tang et al. 2020).

12.2.4 ECHINACEA

Echinacea, commonly known as the purple coneflower, is an herbal medicine that was first recognized by Native Americans in the eighteenth century. Today, the plant is well distributed all over the world and widely found in the USA and Europe.

Echinacea is rich in bioactive metabolites, such as glycoproteins, caffeic acid derivatives, alkaloids, flavonoids, polysaccharides, glycoproteins, and volatile oils (Mirjalili et al. 2006; Göllner et al. 2013; Balciunaite et al. 2015; Moazami et al. 2015). Echinacea and its pharmaceutics have been used for the treatment of breathing-system-related illnesses like influenza, cough and sore throat, of immunity-related cases like sepsis, and animal-related injuries, such as rabies and snake bites in the developing as well as in the developed world (Hu and Kitts 2000; Binns et al. 2002; Jawad et al. 2012; Rauš et al. 2015; Li et al. 2017). The *Echinacea* genus is in the Asteraceae family and has various species, such as *Echinacea purpurea*, *Echinacea angustifolia*, and *Echinacea pallida* (O'Hara et al. 1998). *E. purpurea* is the most used species and among the most popular medicinal plants worldwide today (Hudson 2012). These species possess several biological activities, such as bactericidal, free radical scavenging, anti-inflammatory, antiproliferative, antihypertensive, and immunomodulation properties (LaLone et al. 2007; Aarland et al. 2017; Chiou et al. 2017). *E. purpurea* is considered to be an efficient medicinal plant due to its low toxicity and few adverse effects.

E. purpurea is rich in numerous bioactive compounds, such as polysaccharides, alkaloids, glycoproteins, caffeic acid derivatives, and alkylamides. The immunomodulatory activities of this plant are also associated with the abundant presence of alkylamides, glycoproteins, and polysaccharides in its roots (Balciunaite et al. 2015). The immunostimulatory activity of *Echinacea* has been reported to be associated with its polysaccharide bioactive compounds (Luettig et al. 1989; Roesler et al. 1991). Although the immunomodulation mechanisms involving plant metabolites are not well understood, it is reported that the immunomodulatory effect of *E. purpurea* is associated with the biochemical changes its phytochemicals cause in immune cells (Todd et al. 2015). The potential of certain standardized *E. purpurea* preparations to treat viral and microbial respiratory infections has been reported (Sharma et al. 2009, 2010).

It has also been reported that ethanolic extracts of *E. purpurea* showed a dual effect on immune system function: activation of production of the pro-inflammatory cytokine TNF-α in RAW 264.7 macrophage-like cells to fortify the immune system response in one way and it suppresses the generation of TNF-α in response to LPS exposure (Todd et al. 2015). Both of the activities are vital for regulation of the host immune response.

Children treated with combined Echinacea and Azithromycin showed a low frequency of tonsillitis recurrence, with reduced symptoms (Awad 2020). Echinacea has immunostimulating properties, for which alkamides are thought to be responsible among the bioactive constituents of the plant (Rininger et al. 2000). The plant can also reduce the severity of symptoms in early infections of the common cold and flu, which is believed to be one of the outcomes of its stimulatory effect on the immune system (Barrett 2003). *Echinacea purpurea* supplementations decreased the death rates of chickens infected with *Escherichia coli* bacteria, which might be due to the enhancement of immune response by the medicinal plant (Hashem et al. 2020). The immunostimulatory potential of *Echinacea purpurea* is believed to increase the resistance of the birds against infection (Gharieb and Youssef 2014).

The addition of 2% *E. purpurea* extracts in the drinking water for broiler chickens increased their immune response (Hassan and Sobhan 2017). *E. purpurea* is the most potent immune system stimulator because it has a high potential to increasing the non-specific immune system.

The immune system stimulating effect of tetraploid (CPE4) wolfberry fruit and diploid (CPE2) *Echinacea purpurea* polysaccharide was compared and reported. The immunoregulatory effect of tetraploid (CPE4) polysaccharide is found to be double that of the diploid (CPE2) polysaccharide, a finding which is clearly related to chromosome doubling (Yang et al. 2018). Polyploidization oF this bioactive component (polysaccharide) of the plant enhanced their biological activities (Shi and Liu, 1998). Several studies indicated a direct influence of *E. purpurea* on the immune system function (Cech et al. 2010; King et al. 2014). Cellular immunity was promoted in young Wistar rats treated with E. *purpurea* extract, a finding which was confirmed by a level of immunoregulatory cytokines and immunoglobulins comparable with those in adult rats (Wang et al. 2017).

12.2.5 Broccoli

Broccoli (*Brassica oleracea* var. *italica*) is an edible vegetable plant belonging to the family Brassicaceae (Vallejo et al. 2004; Eberhardt et al. 2005). It is indigenous to the eastern Mediterranean and Asia Minor, and was distributed to England and the USA in the eighteenth century. This fast-growing leafy vegetable has attracted much interest recently due to its high value in terms of nutrition and health care (Axelsson et al. 2017). Broccoli has been one of the top research targets (Jones et al. 2010) due to health benefits attributed to phytochemicals such as glucosinolates, glucoraphanin, dithiolthiones, isothiocyanates, indoles and its derivatives, and *S*-methyl cysteine sulphoxide (Ruiz-Jiménez et al. 2003; Aguado et al. 2014).

A common and bioactive compound in cruciferous vegetables, including broccoli, sulphoraphane is an isothiocyanate formed by glucoraphanin hydrolysis (Fahey et al. 2002; Ares et al. 2014; Bricker et al. 2014; Baenas et al. 2015). Sulphoraphane is an important bioactive compound which possesses various biological activities including immunomodulatory activity (Thejass and Kuttan 2007).

Pectin FB extracted from broccoli modulated the immune system of mice *in vivo* in a concentration-dependent way *via* increasing the number of activated macrophages and phagocytic activity. The reported ability of this polysaccharide to modulate the immune system makes it a potential contributor to immunomodulating drug development (Busato et al. 2020).

Sulphoraphane decreased the secretion of pro-inflammatory cytokines in a dose-dependent manner. This compound is reported to have the potential of enhancing the response of the immune system (Bessler and Djaldetti 2018).

Sulphoraphane is a successful therapy in mice against a T cell-mediated autoimmune disease through a suggested inhibition of IL-12 and IL-23 expression (Geisel et al. 2014). ESAT-6 protein, obtained from genetically modified broccoli, enhanced the humoral immune response in mice against *Mycobacterium tuberculosis* (Saba et al. 2020). The concentration of the ESAT-6 antigen derived from this plant is higher than that obtained from other edible plants (Uvarova et al. 2013; Permyakova et al. 2015), showing its potential for the development of an edible plant-based vaccine against tuberculosis.

Dietary supplementation of broccoli in lower concentrations improved response in ligand-sensitive Ahrb/b mice and improved the resistance of the intestine to the chemical through host-microbiome alteration. This effect of broccoli consumption is partly associated with heightened AHR activity. It also significantly modulated the expression of numerous genes, like the up-regulation of the expression of cyclin and cell cycle regulatory genes. The potential of broccoli to play a therapeutic role in intestinal homoeostasis is also suggested (Hubbard et al. 2017).

The water-soluble polysaccharides of broccoli, whose structure has been elucidated for the first time, showed good anticancer activity against HepG2 liver, MDA-MB-231 cell line, and Sihacervical carcinoma cells. One of the three mechanisms by which natural polysaccharides act as an anticancer agent is by regulating the immune system to increase resistance against the cancer (Zong et al. 2012), which might be the mechanism by which the polysaccharides acted here. However, confirmation of the mechanism requires further investigation (Xu et al. 2015).

Dietary supplementation of young broccoli sprout homogenates for smokers decreased viral infection and a similar effect was manifested in a cohort of healthy nonsmokers. The observed effect was related to viral replication minimization due to oxidative stress reduction in nasal cells. This further emphasizes how much the immune system function is influenced by nutritional factors and the broccoli sprout homogenates supplied might alter specific host defense responses (Noah et al. 2014).

12.2.6 RED PEPPER

Red chilli pepper (*Capsicum annuum*) is a plant species from the Solanaceae family which is indigenous to central America. The plant is edible and grown for its fruit which can be consumed either fresh or cooked. The fruit can also be processed to be used as spices (Jancso et al. 1997). At present, hot red peppers are the most important spices in human nutrition globally. However, strong care is needed especially regarding its dose since it is recognized to cause pain to the mucous membranes when consumed in surplus (Nwaopara et al. 2004, 2007). They are well known medicinal plants with several biological activities (Johann et al. 2010; Freires et al. 2013) which are related to their main bioactive component capsaicin (Abdelnour et al. 2018; Puvaca 2018). There are also other bioactive phytochemicals in this herbal plant such as capsisin and capsantine. The plant has chemopreventive and chemotherapeutic effects, which are due to these bioactive compounds (Al-Kassie et al. 2012). Jancso et al. (1997) reported that red pepper exclusively produces the alkaloids known as the capsaicinoids, about 50% of which is represented by capsaicin. The pungent and irritating effect of hot red pepper is due to capsaicin. The spicy feature of hot pepper is also associated with capsaicin (Govindarajan and Sathyanarayana 1991). The capsaicinoids and capsaicin of hot red pepper increases metabolism in terms of body temperature, oxygen consumption, and energy promotion in humans (Ohnuki et al. 2001). There are subclass compounds of capsaicin, such as dihydrocapsaicin, nordihydrocapsaicin, homodihydrocapsaicin, and homocapsaicin (Fattori et al. 2016), which also contribute to the medicinal role of the plant. Vitamin C is also abundantly found in hot red pepper as well as pro-vitamin A, which contributes to the antioxidant and anti-stressor activities of the plant (Lee et al. 2005; Puvaca 2018; Puvaca et al. 2019). Hot red pepper has potential to decrease cholesterol and fat deposition which helps the vascular system through participating in the lowering of triglyceride levels (Al-Kassie et al. 2012). Hot red pepper powder supplementation as a feed additive for broiler chicks increased their bacterial inhibitory potential and villi length, improving their performance. The improved bacterial defense might be due to morphological modification of the small intestine *via* a reduction in the growth of pathogenic or nonpathogenic microorganisms in the intestine. This may cause a reduction in the inflammatory reactions at the intestinal mucosa, which directs the increasing villus area to improve secretion, digestion, and nutrient absorption functions. However, it did not affect the weight of the immune organ, the spleen (Soliman and Al-Afifi 2020).

The improvement of immunity parameters, like immunoglobulin G (IgG), by feeding hot red pepper to rabbits has been reported. The improvement of immune system function is linked with increase in the immunoglobulin (IgM) levels (Abdelnour et al. 2018). Moradi et al. (2016) also reported that supplementation with red pepper as a feed additive stimulated the immune system function of broiler chicks, suggesting that the bioactive components of the plant controls microbial growth *via* influencing biological processes of the key microflora like protein synthesis. The bioactive compounds in red pepper further inhibited the multiplication of *Methanobacterium* and *Escherichia coli* (Ghaedi et al. 2014). Afolabi et al. (2017) reported that addition of dried hot red pepper as feed additives for broilers enhanced their performance by stimulating their immune system, elevating the leucocyte cell numbers.

12.3 SELECTED VITAMINS FORTIFYING THE IMMUNE SYSTEM

Vitamins are micronutrients with various roles in the biological system. Several vitamins, including vitamins A, C, D, and E, are essential for effective immune system functioning (Maggini et al. 2007) (Table 12.2).

12.3.1 VITAMIN C

Vitamin C (ascorbic acid) is the most crucial vitamin which humans and other primates must obtain from fruits and vegetables since they cannot synthesize it (Kumar et al. 2013). Any compound carrying out the biological property of L-ascorbic acid is categorized under vitamin C (Kumar et al. 2013). The vitamin is also added widely to food as a scurvy-preventing food factor (Tee et al. 1988; Rasanu et al. 2005). The chemical composition of ascorbic acid is rich in hydroxyl groups which makes it polar and water soluble. The most important reaction of vitamin C is its oxidation that converts the diol group to a diketo group (Tee et al. 1988). Various critical functions of ascorbic acid in the human body make it an essential micronutrient for humans. Scurvy is a potentially fatal disease caused by a severe deficiency of

TABLE 12.2

Summary of Major Findings of Immune System Boosting Activity of Some Vitamins

Vitamins	Dietary sources for human	Bioactive form	Activity	References
Vitamin C	Fruits and vegetables	Ascorbic acid	Enhanced chemotaxis and phagocytosis of phagocytes Contributes to the maturation of T cells Decreased the heterophil count and heterophil: lymphocyte ratio Reduced antibody levels in viral infections Decreased the inflammatory markers and FiO_2 requirements in high-risk COVID-19 patients Augmented the levels of immunoglobulin A and the stimulation index of T lymphocytes	(van Gorkom et al. 2018; Nosrati et al. 2017; Mikirova and Hunninghake, 2014; Hiedra et al. 2020; Gan et al. 2020)
Vitamin D	Skin exposure to sunlight	1, 25(OH)2D	Decreased the inflammatory cytokines IFNx, TNF-α, and IL12p70 levels Decreased pro-inflammatory cytokines and high secretion of interleukin-10 (IL-10) Modulated the percentages and functions of peripheral blood lymphocyte subsets Suppressed the increased production of B cells and TNF-α	(Sharifi et al. 2019; Giraldo et al. 2018; Chen et al. 2016)
Vitamin E	Vegetable oils and nut oils	α-tocopherol	Enhanced humoral immune responses in several animal species Decreased IFN-γ expression Increased the levels of CD55 and CD47 of pneumonia patients	(Lee and Han, 2018; Awadin et al. 2019; Shen and Zhan, 2020)

vitamin C (Sauberlich 1997), leading to several metabolic disorders, such as collagenous structure weakening, delayed recovery from injury recovery, and weakened immunity. People suffering from scurvy are easily exposed to dangerous and potentially lethal diseases like pneumonia. The level of vitamin C in the host determines the degree of infection since deficiency causes inflammation in the biological system (Hemila 2017).

A small amount (~10 mg/day) of vitamin C is enough to combat scurvy (Krebs 1953), but higher dietary intakes (100–200 mg/day) are recommended since storage of vitamin C in the body is low because of its water solubility (Levine et al. 1995; Carr and Frei 1999). The essential nature of the vitamin is apparent in high dietary intakes of vitamin C, which are much higher than those of other vitamins. Vitamin C is a very strong free radical scavenger (antioxidant) and is involved as a cofactor in fifteen mammalian enzyme-catalyzed metabolic reactions *via* iron-, copper- and 2-oxoglutarate-dependent oxidoreductase enzymes. Most mammals synthesize ascorbic acid in their liver using gulono-gamma-lactone oxidase, a vital ascorbate biosynthesizing enzyme. But many primates and humans depend on dietary sources to fulfill their need for ascorbic acid.

Vitamin C has proved to play an extensive role in the immune system (Carr and Maggini 2017). Ascorbic acid promotes microbial killing by enhancing chemotaxis and phagocytosis of phagocytes, although its role in a diverse subclass of lymphocytes is less evident (van Gorkom et al. 2018). However, it is suggested that vitamin C has a crucial function in lymphocytic cells since these cells obtain vitamin C through either its sodium-dependent or -independent transporter (Wilson 2005), having intracellular ascorbic acid concentrations higher than plasma levels (Evans et al. 1982; Omaye et al. 1987). van Gorkom et al. (2018) reported that ascorbic acid contributes to the maturation of T cells. Furthermore, ascorbic acid stimulates Th2 to Th1 shifting of immune responses, which is confirmed by increasing the interferon (IFN)-γ/interleukin (IL)-5 cytokines secretion ratio percentage in bronchoalveolar lavage fluid after ascorbic acid supplementation in mice (Chang et al. 2009). Although the mechanism of the effect is still in doubt, dendritic cell mediation has been suggested. The secretion of more IL-12 and production of more IFN- and less IL-5 dendritic cells (DCs) after treatment of dendritic cells with ascorbic acid is an indication of this (Jeong et al. 2011).

Supplementation of vitamin C in drinking water for broiler chicks significantly augmented the level of lymphocytes and decreased the number of heterophils as well as increasing the lymphocyte/heterophil ratio, which indicated the improvement in their immune response (Nosrati et al. 2017).

It is reported that even an elevated dose of this vitamin has an encouraging outcome on Epstein-Barr Virus (EBV)-caused infectious disease as long-term intravenous (IV) infusions of vitamin C reduced EBV EA IgG and EBV VCA IgM antibody levels (Mikirova and Hunninghake 2014). The mechanism suggested for this is higher cellular glucose uptake rates due to viral infection, leading to increased oxidative stress (Yongjun et al. 2011), which enhances the assimilation rate of ascorbic acid as the vitamin enters cells in the form of dehydroascorbate through the same glucose transporters (Rose 1988; Vera et al. 1993; Vera et al. 1995).

Rondanelli et al. (2018) reported that both the duration and severity of the common cold is reduced by regular supplementation of vitamin C with about a two-fold higher positive effect in children than in adults. The level of vitamin C in SARS-CoV-2 patients was analyzed and the level was found to be undetectable in most of the patients. The reduced level of the vitamin might be associated to its higher metabolic consumption due to the virus (Chiscano-Camón et al. 2020). Therefore, increasing the dose of vitamin C consumption may compensate for the reduced level and help the immune system to efficiently fight the virus, minimizing the severity of the disease and the need for hospitalization of the patients.

It has been reported that treating high-risk COVID-19 patients of advanced age and with multiple comorbidities with IV vitamin C showed a positive effect. The treatment significantly decreased the inflammatory markers and FiO_2 requirements (Hiedra et al. 2020). This emphasizes that regular consumption of vitamin C might be a potential preventive route for viral infection and a higher dose might be required for patients.

Dietary supplementation of vitamin C for broilers challenged with the bacterium *Salmonella enteritidis* improved the microbial population structure and intestinal morphology of the birds. The crucial outcome of the vitamin supplementation was the improvement of the immune response. The effect enhanced the intestinal health of the birds and increased their productivity, while minimizing their death rate (Gan et al. 2020).

12.3.2 VITAMIN D

Vitamin D refers to a cluster of fat-soluble secosteroids that play a key role in boosting assimilation of micronutrients such as zinc, calcium, iron, magnesium, and phosphate (Holick 2007). Humans obtain vitamin D either from skin exposure to sunlight (80–100%) and/or from the food they eat, either as a daily diet or from supplements. The two most important compounds from fat-soluble secosteroid groups in humans are vitamin D3 and vitamin D2. Particularly, the body can synthesize the former one in the skin from a cholesterol-inadequate sunlight UVB-supplying environment, unlike other fat- or water-soluble vitamins. Although it is suggested that sunlight UVB exposure for vitamin D synthesis is regulated by a negative feedback loop to avoid toxicity, the doubt over cancer development due to prolonged sunlight exposure has remained a problem when setting the quantity of sunlight exposure needed to fulfill vitamin D requirements by national bodies. The adequate synthesis of vitamin D by many mammals including humans *via* sunlight exposure means that it should not be considered strictly as a vitamin. Rather, it is a vital nutrient required in limited amounts and may be considered a hormone after hydroxylation in the body to 1, 25(OH)2D since its production and application take place in different sites (He et al. 2016). Vitamin D was discovered and its chemical structure elucidated by Adolf Windaus, who was awarded the Nobel Prize for Chemistry in 1928 for his key contributions (Wolf 2004). The biologically active form, 1, 25(OH)2D, is obtained by two-time hydroxylation of the inert vitamin D by the 25-hydroxylase enzyme. The main storage form, as well as the chief circulating metabolite of the vitamin, is 25(OH)D, and muscles and adipose tissue are its storage sites (Baeke et al. 2010).

The important effect of the vitamin on the functioning of both innate and adaptive immune systems (He et al. 2016) was confirmed after the discovery of its receptor in almost all immune cells (Baeke et al. 2010), which have the potential to change 25(OH)D to 1, 25(OH)2D by expressing the mitochondrial vitamin D-activating enzyme. The conversion is regulated by the major circulating metabolite of vitamin D, 25(OH)D (Bikle 2009). It is interesting that vitamin D often prominently upregulates immune system-related genes although genes involved in cellular metabolism are less sensitive to the nuclear hormone (Neme et al. 2017). Thus, vitamin D deficiency affects the immune system function (Holick 2007) in addition to the bone disorders ('rickets') it causes (Carlberg 2014).

The occurrence of the initial COVID-19 outbreak in winter and the declining of cases in the southern Hemisphere about the end of the summer, when there is the highest quantity of 25-hydroxyvitamin D (25(OH)D) in the cell showed that higher vitamin D3 doses might be useful to treat COVID-19-infected people. It has also been suggested that raising the concentration of 25(OH)D *via* vitamin D supplementation in winter might help in influenza prevention (Grant et al. 2020). Supplementation of magnesium is recommended along with vitamin D supplementation since it activates the vitamin for better regulation of calcium and phosphate homoeostasis. Magnesium is required by all vitamin D-metabolizing enzymes, acting as a cofactor for enzymatic reactions in the liver and kidneys (Uwitonze and Razzaque 2018).

A long-term high-dose supplementation of vitamin D resulted in hypercalcaemia, rendering T cells more prone to pro-inflammatory activation which can promote the worsening of CNS demyelinating disease. It also stimulated the activation as well as the division of both myeloid antigen-presenting cells (APC) and T cells in mice (Häusler et al. 2019). This novel finding is not in agreement with the previous reports suggesting that the moderate dose of the vitamin is safe in short-term supplementation (Sotirchos et al. 2016). However, the longer-term supplementation of high-dose vitamin D in the novel finding might make it more efficient and recommended as it broadly activated the immune system cells. It is finally suggested that the moderate level may cause an immediate regulatory influence, whereas the continuous high-dosage supplementation might activate multiple sclerosis disease activity by enhancing mean levels of T cell excitatory calcium (Häusler et al. 2019).

Treatment of ulcerative colitis patients with vitamin D3 decreased the inflammatory cytokines (TNF-α, IFN-γ, and IL12p70) levels without affecting the circulatory amount of IL-4 and IL-10. This highlighted the inhibition potential of vitamin D toward Th1 immune responses but not Th2 responses, suggesting the therapeutic immunomodulatory potential of vitamin D (Sharifi et al. 2019).

Addition of vitamin D as a food supplement significantly decreased the level of pro-inflammatory cytokines and the elevated production of interleukin-10 (IL-10), enhancing the resistance of healthy individuals to DENV-2 infection. The dose-dependent inhibitory effect of the vitamin against DENV infection indicated its influence on the immune response and its ability to act as an immunity modulator (Giraldo et al. 2018). Chen et al. (2016) reported that 1,25(OH)2D supplementation might regulate the cellular immune response abnormalities caused due to deficiency of vitamin D in patients with recurrent miscarriage (RM). The deficiency of vitamin D observed in most of the patients indicated the key role of the vitamin in the modulation of blood lymphocyte subsets.

12.3.3 VITAMIN E

Vitamin E comprises eight fat-soluble compounds divided into tocopherols (α-, β-, γ-, and δ-tocopherol) and tocotrienols (α-, β-, γ-, and δ-tocotrienol) (Traber 2006). Although all members of vitamin E are bioactive, α-tocopherol (α-TOH) is the most biologically active in mammals (Hosomi et al. 1997; Traber 2006), which is related to the absence of interconversion between these forms. As a result, the only vitamin E form meeting the human requirement is α-tocopherol (Traber, 2007). The tocopherols and tocotrienols have a common chromanol ring and their differences lie in their tails: a phytyl tail for tocopherols, but an unsaturated tail for tocotrienols. The α -, β-, γ-, and δ- forms differ in the quantity and attachments of methyl groups on the ring. There is also a difference in stereochemistry between natural and synthetic tocopherols: natural tocopherols have a single (RRR) stereochemistry, while the synthetic groups are a mixture of eight stereoisomers (Lee and Han 2018).

Vegetable oils and oils from sources such as cottonseed, soybean, wheat germ, corn, walnut, sunflower, palm (Sheppard et al. 1980; Lee and Han, 2018), avocados (Dreher and Davenport 2013), olives (Piroddi et al. 2017), and legumes (Soba et al. 2020) are well-known dietary sources of vitamin E. There is no toxic accumulation level of vitamin E in the liver unlike other fat-soluble vitamins since its metabolism increases with its intake, resulting in the removal of its catabolic products from biological system *via* urine and faeces. The most likely three compartments in the liver for the metabolism of the vitamin E (mainly α-TOH) are the endoplasmic reticulum, peroxisomes, and mitochondria (Sontag and Parker 2002).

The molecular structure of vitamin E has three functionally distinct units: the first (I) is a functional unit, the second (II) is a signalling unit, and the third (III) is a hydrophobic domain which determines the properties of the vitamin (Wallert et al. 2020).

The biological activity, especially the free radical scavenging potential, of vitamin E is reported (Olcott and Mattill 1931). The most potent form of vitamin E, in terms of the above-mentioned activity and ensuring fertility, α-tocopherol has a biological activity as a result of units I and II (Neuzil et al. 2002). These units possess phenolic groups which are good free radical scavengers and the antioxidant potential of the vitamin is directly related to this group. The third unit is responsible for the hydrophobicity of the vitamin which facilitates the integration into lipoproteins and membranes (Neuzil et al. 2002).

The immunomodulating property of vitamin E in animals, including humans, is reported in which dendritic cells are suggested to play the role in initiating adaptive immune responses by connecting innate and specific immune systems. It is also well reported that dietary supplementation with the vitamin enhances humoral immune responses in several types of animals *via* increasing lymphocytic proliferation, the level of immunoglobulins, the degree of antibody responses, the activity of NK cells, and interleukin IL-2 production. The increased lymphocytic proliferation in humans due to high-dose (above the recommended levels) supplementation of vitamin E enhanced delayed-type hypersensitivity (DTH) response, increased IL-2 production, and decreased IL-6 production (Lee and Han 2018). Vitamin E greatly supports defence against pathogens due to its immunostimulatory activity with a reported mechanisms of increased macrophage activity and antibody (Ab) production for *Streptococcus pneumoniae* type 1 (Heinzerling 1974), and higher NK activity and Th1 response to the influenza virus (Hayek et al. 1997; Han et al. 2000). Thus, the deficiency of vitamin E vastly contributes to the oxidation of unsaturated fatty acids to increase oxidative stress which could also happen in the elderly, potentially reducing the immune system function (Fukui et al. 2001; Muller 2010; Wu and Meydani 2014; Lee and Ulatowski 2019; Lewis et al. 2019). Furthermore, vitamin E deficiency causes abnormal functioning of the central nervous system and the reproductive system (Saito et al. 2020).

The immune-system-stimulating potential of vitamin E in chickens has been reported. Supplementation of the vitamin with Fetomune Plus® for experimentally AIV H9N2-infected chickens improved their immunological and pathological effects through decreasing IFN-gamma expression. The improvement of immune system response was further indicated by a significantly reduced mortality rate of the chickens (Awadin et al. 2019). Supplementation of vitamin E as a feed additive stimulated the immune system function of goats and increased their resistance to epsilon toxin D of *Clostridium perfringens* (Khan et al. 2019).

Treatment of patients with stroke-associated pneumonia with vitamin E increased resistance to the disease due to an auxiliary therapeutic effect of the vitamin which increased the levels of CD55 and CD47. The effect was dose dependent in which the high-dose vitamin E group showed better resistance and shorter duration of hospitalization (Shen and Zhan 2020). The potential of vitamin E in inhibiting PMN apoptosis was reported in which the enhancement of CD55 and GPI binding stability is suggested as a potential mechanism (Witt et al. 2000). Polymorphonuclear neutrophil (PMN) are the most abundant circulating immune cells.

Dietary supplementation with vitamin E improved the immune response by increasing the total antioxidant capacity in pigs. However, the effect was insignificant in pigs fed with peroxidized lipids since the concentration of vitamin E was not adequately increased as the vitamin was consumed by peroxidized lipids to save cells from oxidative damage caused as a result of oxidative stress by the oxidants. However, addition of peroxidized lipids canceled the immune system stimulation by the vitamin and no improvement in immune response was recorded (Silva-Guillen et al. 2020).

Dietary supplementation of 30 IU vitamin E/kg for *Salmonella enteritidis*-challenged laying hens improved their immunity response by alleviating the oxidative and immune stress due to the challenge, decreasing the mortality rate of the birds (Liu et al. 2019). Dalia et al. (2018) reported that the combination of vitamin E with bacterial organic selenium as a feed additive (ADS18-Se) improved the immune system in broiler chickens by regulating some cytokine expression levels and immunoglobulin levels. The immune system-stimulating activity of the two combined was better than that of the bacterial organic selenium alone.

12.4　CONCLUSION

The immune system is one of the critical parts of a biological system, with its key roles including protection against infection and the removal of damaged tissues. However, the system greatly depends on nutrients and vitamins to efficiently perform its activities. Although specific bioactive compounds of some medicinal plants show immune system strengthening activities, there is still a need to identify the mechanism by which they operate in order to improve the use of plants as immune system enhancers to cope with the problems caused by infectious diseases and drug resistance of pathogenic microorganisms.

REFERENCES

Aarland, R.C., A.E. Bañuelos-Hernández, M. Fragoso-Serrano, E.D. Sierra-Palacios, F.D. de León-Sánchez, L.J. Pérez-Flores, F. Rivera-Cabrera, and J.A. Mendoza-Espinoza. 2017. Studies on phytochemical, antioxidant, anti-inflammatory, hypoglycaemic and antiproliferative activities of *Echinacea purpurea* and *Echinacea angustifolia* extracts. *Pharmaceutical Biology* 55(1):649–656.

Abdelnour S., M. Alagawany, M.E. Abd El-Hack, A.M. Sheiha, I.M. Saadeldin, and A.A. Swelum. 2018. Growth, carcass traits, blood hematology, serum metabolites, immunity, and oxidative indices of growing rabbits fed diets supplemented with red or black pepper oils. *Animals* 8(10):168.

Abdullah, T. 2000. A strategic call to utilize Echinacea-garlic in flu-cold seasons. *Journal of the National Medical Association* 92(1):48–51.

Abiy, E., and B. Asefaw, 2016. Anti-bacterial effect of garlic (*Allium sativum*) against clinical isolates of *Staphylococcus aureus* and *Escherichia coli* from patients attending Hawassa Referral Hospital, Ethiopia. *Journal of Infectious Diseases and Treatment* 2(2):1–5.

Afolabi, K.D., N.E. Kelechi, A.O. Mobolaji, and O. Rotimi. 2017. Hot Red Pepper (*Capsicum annum* L.) Meal Enhanced the Immunity, Performance and Economy of Broilers Fed in Phases. *Journal of Biology, Agriculture and Healthcare* 7(8):1–7.

Ahmadifar, E., N. Sheikhzadeh, K. Roshanaei, N. Dargahi, C. Faggio. 2019. Can dietary ginger (*Zingiber officinale*) alter biochemical and immunological parameters and gene expression related to growth, immunity and antioxidant system in zebrafish (*Danio rerio*)? *Aquaculture* 507:341–348.

Ahmed A.A., N.I. Bassuony, S.E.S. Awad, A.M. Aiad and S.A. Mohamed. 2009. Adding natural juice of vegetables and fruitage to ruminant diets (b) nutrients utilization, microbial safety and immunity, effect of diets suplemented with lemon, onion and garlic juice fed to growing buffalo calves. *World Journal of Agricultural Sciences* 5(4):456–465.

Ahmed, S.T., J.W. Lee, H.S. Mun, and C.J. Yang. 2015. Effects of supplementation with green tea by-products on growth performance, meat quality, blood metabolites and immune cell proliferation in goats. *Journal of Animal Physiology and Animal Nutrition* 99(6):1127–1137.

Ahui, M.L., P. Champy, A. Ramadan, L.P. Van, L. Araujo, K.B. Andre, S. Diem, D. Damotte, S. Kati-Coulibaly, M.A. Offoumou, M. Dy, N. Thieblemont, and A. Herbelin. 2008. Ginger prevents Th2-mediated immune responses in a mouse model of airway inflammation. *International Immunopharmacology* 8(12):1626–1632.

Aguado, S., J. Quirós, J. Canivet, D. Farrusseng, K. Boltes, and R. Rosal. 2014. Antimicrobial activity of cobalt imidazolate metal–organic frameworks. *Chemosphere* 113:188–192.

Al Abbasi, A. 2008. Efficacy of garlic oil in treatment of active chronic suppurative otitis media. *Kufa Medical Journal* 11(1):495–500.

Al-Kassie, G.A.M., G.Y. Butris, and S.J. Ajeena. 2012. The potency of feed supplemented mixture of hot red pepper and black pepper on the performance and some hematological blood traits in broiler diet. *International Journal of Advanced Biological of Research* 2:53–57.

Amagase H. 2006. Clarifying the real bioactive constituents of garlic. *The Journal of Nutrition* 136(3) Supplement:716–725.

Amirghofran Z., S. Malek-Hosseini, H. Golmoghaddam, F. Kalantar, M. Shabani. 2011. Inhibition of nitric oxide production and proinflammatory cytokines by several medicinal plants. *Iranian Journal of Immunology* 8(3):159–169.

Ares, A.M., J. Bernal, M.T. Martín, J.L. Bernal, and M.J. Nozal. 2014. Optimized formation, extraction, and determination of sulforaphane in broccoli by liquid chromatography with diode array detection. *Food Analytical Methods* 7(3):730–740.

Aryaeian, N., F. Shahram, M. Mahmoudi, H. Tavakoli, B. Yousefi, T. Arablou, and S.J. Karegar. 2019. The effect of ginger supplementation on some immunity and inflammation intermediate genes expression in patients with active Rheumatoid Arthritis. *Gene* 698:179–185.

Awad, O.G.A. 2020. Echinacea can help with Azithromycin in prevention of recurrent tonsillitis in children. *American Journal of Otolaryngology* 41:102344.

Awadin, W.F., A.H. Eladl, R.A. El-Shafei, M.A. El-Adl, and H.S. Ali. 2019. Immunological and pathological effects of vitamin E with Fetomune Plus® on chickens experimentally infected with avian influenza virus H9N2. *Veterinary Microbiology* 231: 24–32.

Axelsson, A.S., E. Tubbs, B. Mecham, S. Chacko, H.A. Nenonen, Y. Tang, J.W. Fahey, J.M.J. Derry, C.B. Wollheim, N. Wierup, M.W. Haymond, S.H. Friend, H. Mulder, and A.H. Rosengren. 2017. Sulforaphane reduces hepatic glucose production and improves glucose control in patients with type 2 diabetes. *Science Translational Medicine* 9(394):4477.

Baeke, F., T. Takiishi, H. Korf, C. Gysemans and C. Mathieu. 2010.Vitamin D: modulator of the immune system. *Current Opinion in Pharmacology* 10(4):482–496.

Baenas, N., J.M. Silván, S. Medina, S. de Pascual-Teresa, C. García- Viguera, D.A. Moreno. 2015. Metabolism and antiproliferative effects of sulforaphane and broccoli sprouts in human intestinal(Caco-2) and hepatic (HepG2) cells. *Phytochemistry Reviews* 14(6):1035–1044.

Balciunaite G., J. Juodsnukyte, A. Savickas, O. Ragazinskiene, L. Siatkute, G. Zvirblyte, E. Mistiniene, and N. Savickiene. 2015. Fractionation and evaluation of proteins in roots of *Echinacea purpurea* (L.) Moench, *Acta Pharmaceutica* 65(4):473–479.

Banacerraf, B. 1978. A hypothesis to relate the specificity of T lymphocytes. *Journal of Immunology* 120(6):1809–1812.

Barbalho, S.M., H. Bosso, L.M.S. Pescinini, and R.A. Goulart. 2019.Green tea: a possibility in the therapeutic approach of inflammatory bowel diseases?: Green tea and inflammatory bowel diseases. *Complementary Therapies in Medicine* 43:148–153.

Barrett, B. 2003. Medicinal properties of Echinacea: a critical review. *Phytomedicine* 10(1):66–86.

Bauer D., E. Mazzio, K.F. Soliman, E. Taka, E. Oriaku, T. Womble, and S. Darling-Reed. 2014. Diallyl disulfide inhibits TNFá-induced CCL2 release by MDA-MB-231 cells. *Anticancer Research.* 34(6):2763–2770.

Bessler H., and M. Djaldetti. 2018. Broccoli and human health: immunomodulatory effect of sulforaphane in a model of colon cancer. *International Journal of Food Sciences and Nutrition* 69(8):946–953.

Bikle, D. 2009. Nonclassic actions of vitamin D. *The Journal of Clinical Endocrinology and Metabolism* 94(1):26–34.

Binns, S.E., J. Hudson, S. Merali, and J.T. Arnason. 2002. Antiviral activity of characterized extracts from echinacea spp. (Heliantheae: Asteraceae) against herpes simplex virus (HSV-I), *Planta Medica* 68 (9):780–783.

Bricker, G.V., K.M. Riedl, R.A. Ralston, K.L. Tober, T.M. Oberyszyn, and S.J. Schwartz. 2014. Isothiocyanate metabolism, distribution, and interconversion in mice following consumption of thermally processed broccoli sprouts or purified sulforaphane. Molecular Nutrition and Food Research 58(10):1991–2000.

Busato, B., E.C.A. Abreu, C.L.O. Petkowicz, G.R. Martinez, and G.R. Noleto. 2020. Pectin from *Brassica oleracea var. italica* triggers immunomodulating effects in vivo. *International Journal of Biological Macromolecules* 161:431–440.

Cabrera, C., R. Artacho, and R. Giménez. 2006. Beneficial effects of green tea—a review. *The Journal of the American College of Nutrition.* 25(2):79–99.

Carlberg, C. 2014. The physiology of vitamin D-far more than calcium and bone. *Frontiers in Physiology* 5:335.

Calder, P.C., and S. Kew. 2002. The immune system: a target for functional foods? *British Journal of Nutrition* 88(2) Supplement 2:165–176.

Carr, A.C., and B. Frei. 1999. Toward a new recommended dietary allowance for vitamin C based on antioxidant and health effects in humans. *The American Journal of Clinical Nutrition* 69(6):1086–1087.

Carr, A.C., and S. Maggini. 2017. Maggini Vitamin C and immune function. *Nutrients* 9(11):1211.

Cazzola, M., S. Ferraris, F. Boschetto, A. Rondinella, E. Marin, W. Zhu, G. Pezzotti, E. Vernè, and S. Spriano. 2018. Green tea polyphenols coupled with a bioactive titanium alloy surface: in vitro characterization of osteoinductive behavior through a KUSA A1 cell study. *International Journal of Molecular Sciences* 19(8):2255.

Cech, N.B., V. Kandhi, J.M. Davis, A. Hamilton, D. Eads, and S.M. Laster. 2010. Echinacea and its alkylamides: effects on the influenza A-induced secretion of cytokines, chemokines, and PGE(2) from RAW 264.7 macrophage-like cells. *International Immunopharmacology* 10(10):1268–1278.

Chandrashekar, P.M., and Y.P. Venkatesh. 2009. Identification of the protein components displaying immunomodulatory activity in aged garlic extract. *Journal of Ethnopharmacology* 124:384–390.

Chandrashekar, P.M., K.V.H. Prashanth, Y.P. Venkatesh. 2011. Isolation, structural elucidation and immunomodulatory activity of fructans from aged garlic extract. *Phytochemistry* 72:255–264.

Chang, H. H., C. Chen, and J. Y Lin. 2009. High dose vitamin C supplementation increases the Th1/Th2 cytokine secretion ratio, but decreases eosinophilic infiltration in bronchoalveolar lavage fluid of ovalbumin-sensitized and challenged mice. *Journal of Agricultural and Food Chemistry* 57(21):10471–10476.

Charron, C.S., H.D. Dawson, G.P. Albaugh, P.M. Solverson, B.T. Vinyard, G.I. Solano-Aguilar, and J.A. Novotny. 2015. A single meal containing raw, crushed garlic influences expression of immunity and cancer related genes in whole blood of humans. The Journal of Nutrition 145(11):2448–2455.

Chen, X., B. Yin, R.C. Lian, T. Zhang, H.Z. Zhang, L.H. Diao, Y.Y. Li, C.Y. Huang, D.S. Liang, and Y. Zeng. 2016. Modulatory effects of vitamin d on peripheral cellular immunity in patients with recurrent miscarriage. *American Journal of Reproductive Immunology* 76:432–438.

Chiou, S.Y., J.M. Sung, P.W. Huang, and S.D. Lin. 2017. Antioxidant, antidiabetic, and antihypertensive properties of *echinacea purpurea* flower extract and caffeic acid derivatives using in vitro models. *Journal of Medicinal Food*, 20(2):171–179.

Chiscano-Camón, L., J.C. Ruiz-Rodriguez, A. Ruiz-Sanmartin, O. Roca and R. Ferrer. 2020. Vitamin C levels in patients with SARS-CoV-2-associated acute respiratory distress Syndrome. *Research Letter* 24:522.

Chuah, S.C., P.K. Moore, and Y.Z. Zhu. 2007. S-allylcysteine mediates cardioprotection in an acute myocardial infarction rat model via a hydrogen sulfide-mediated pathway. *American Journal of Physiology- Heart and Circulatory Physiology* 293(5):2693–2701.

Costa, L.M., S.T. Gouveia, and J.A. Nobrega.2002. Comparison of heating extraction procedures for Al, Ca, Mg, and Mn in tea samples. *Analytical Sciences* 18(3):313–318.

Crespy, V., and G. Williamson. 2004. A review of the health effects of green tea catechins in In vivo animal models. *The Journal of Nutrition* 134(12) Supplement:3431–3440.

Dalia, A.M., T.C. Loh, A.Q. Sazili, M.F. Jahromi and A.A. Samsudin. 2018. Effects of vitamin E, inorganic selenium, bacterial organic selenium, and their combinations on immunity response in broiler chickens. *BMC Veterinary Research* 14:249.

Dreher, M.L., and A.J. Davenport. 2013. Hass avocado composition and potential health effects. *Critical Reviews in Food Science and Nutrition* 53(7):738–50.

Eberhardt, M.V., K. Kobira, A. Keck, J.A. Juvik, and E.H. Jeffery. 2005. Correlation analyses of phytochemical composition, chemical, and cellular measures of antioxidant activity of broccoli (Brassica oleracea L.var. italica), *Journal of Agricultural and Food Chemistry* 53(19): 7421–7431.

Evans, R.M., L. Currie, and A. Campbell. 1982. The distribution of ascorbic acid between various cellular components of blood, in normal individuals, and its relation to the plasma concentration. *British Journal of Nutrition* 47(3):473–482.

Fahey, J.W., X. Haristoy, P.M. Dolan, T.W. Kensler, I. Scholtus, K.K. Stephenson, P. Talalay, and A. Lozniewsk. 2002. Sulforaphane inhibits extracellular, intracellular, and antibiotic-resistant strains of *Helicobacter pylori* and prevents benzo[a] pyrene-induced stomach tumors. *Proceedings of the National Academy of Sciences of the United States of America* 99(11):7610–7615.

Fattori, V., M.S.N. Hohmann, C.R. Ana, F.A. Pinho-Ribeiro and A.V. Waldiceu. 2016. Capsaicin: current understanding of its mechanisms and therapy of pain and other preclinical and clinical uses. *Molecules* 21(7):844.

Freires, I.A., L.A. Alves, G.L. Ferreira, V.C. Jovito, R.D. Castro, and A.L. Cavalcanti. 2013. A randomized clinical trial of Schinus terebinthifolius mouthwash to treat biofilm-induced gingivitis. *Evidence-Based Complementary and Alternative Medicine* 1–8.

Fukui, K., K. Onodera, T. Shinkai, S. Suzuki, and S. Urano. 2001. Impairment of learning and memory in rats caused by oxidative stress and aging, and changes in antioxidative defense systems. *Annals of the New York Academy of Sciences* 928:168–175.

Gan L., H. Fan, T. Mahmood, and Y. Guo. 2020. Dietary supplementation with vitamin C ameliorates the adverse effects of Salmonella Enteritidis-challenge in broilers by shaping intestinal microbiota. *Poultry Science* 99(7):3663–3674.

Ganeshpurkar, A., and A.K. Saluja. 2018. Protective effect of catechin on humoral and cell mediated immunity in rat model. *International Immunopharmacology* 54:261–266.

Gardner, C.D., L.D. Lawson, E. Block, L.M. Chatterjee, A. Kiazand, R.R. Balise, H.C. Kraemer. 2007. Effect of raw garlic vs. commercial garlic supplements on plasma lipid concentrations in adults with moderate hypercholesterolemia: A randomized clinical trial. *Archives of Internal Medicine* 167(4):346–353.

Gebreyohannes, G., and G. Mebrahtu. 2013. Medicinal values of garlic: a review. *International Journal of Medicine and Medical Sciences* 5(9):401–408.

Geetha, B., and K.S. Santhy, 2013. Anti-proliferative activity of green tea extract in human cervical cancer cells (HeLa). *International Journal of Current Microbiology and Applied Sciences* 2(9):341–346.

Geisel, J., J. Bruck, I. Glocova, K. Dengler, T. Sinnberg, O. Rothfuss, M. Walter, K. Schulze-Osthoff, M. R€ocken, and K. Ghoreschi. 2014. Sulforaphane protects from T cellmediated autoimmune disease by inhibition of IL-23 and IL-12 in dendritic cells. *The Journal of Immunology* 192(8):3530–3539.

Ghaedi, H., J. Nasr, F. Kheiri, Y. Rahimian, and Y. Miri. 2014. The effect of virginiamycin and black pepper (*Piper nigrum* L.) extract on performance of broiler chicks. *Research Opinions in Animal and Veterinary Sciences* 4(2):91–95.

Gharieb, M., and F. Youssef. 2014. Effect of *Echinacea purpurea* and garlic on growth performance, immune response, biochemichal and hematological parameters in broiler chicks. *Assiut Veterinary Medical Journal* 60(140):218–228.

Giraldo, D.M., A. Cardona, S. Urcuqui-Inchima. 2018. High-dose of vitamin D supplement is associated with reduced susceptibility of monocyte-derived macrophages to dengue virus infection and proinflammatory cytokine production: an exploratory study. *Clinica Chimica Acta*, 478:140–151.

Göllner, E.M., J.C. Gramann, and B. Classen. 2013. Antibodies against Yariv's reagent for immunolocalization of arabinogalactan-proteins in aerial parts of Echinacea purpurea. *Planta Medica* 79(2):175–180.

Gombart, A.F., A. Pierre, and S. Maggini. 2020. A review of micronutrients and the immune system–working in harmony to reduce the risk of infection. *Nutrients* 12(1):236.

Govindarajan, V.S., and M.N. Sathyanarayana. 1991. Capsicum production, echnology, chemistry and quality. PartV. Impact on physiology, pharmacology, nutrition and metabolism: Structure, pungency, pain and desensitization sequences. *Critical Reviews in Food Science and Nutrition* 29(6):435–474.

Graham, H.N. 1992. Green tea composition, consumption, and polyphenol chemistry. *Preventive Medicine* 21(3): 334–350.

Grant, W.B., H. Lahore, S.L. McDonnell, C.A. Baggerly, C.B. French, J.L. Aliano and H.P. Bhattoa. 2020. Evidence that vitamin D supplementation could reduce risk of influenza and COVID-19 infections and deaths. *Nutrients* 12(4):988.

Gruhlke, M.C.H., H. Antelmannb, J. Bernhardtc, V. Kloubertd, L. Rinkd, A.J. Slusarenkoa. 2019. The human allicin-proteome: S-thioallylation of proteins by the garlic defence substance allicin and its biological effects. *Free Radical Biology and Medicine* 131:144–153.

Gu, X., and Y.Z. Zhu. 2011. Therapeutic applications of organosulfur compounds as novel hydrogen sulfide donors and/or mediators. *Expert Review of Clinical Pharmacology* 4(1):123–133.

Ha, C., S. Tian, K. Sun, D. Wang, J. Lv, and Y. Wang. 2015. Hydrogen sulfide attenuates IL-1binduced inflammatory signaling and dysfunction of osteoarthritic chondrocytes. *International Journal of Molecular Medicine* 35(6):1657–1666.

Hafidh, R.R., A.S. Abdulamir, L.S. Vern, F.A. Bakar, F. Abas, F. Jahanshiri, and Z. Sekawi. 2011. Inhibition of growth of highly resistant bacterial and fungal pathogens by a natural product. *Open Microbiology Journal* 5:96–106.

Han, S.N., D. Wu, W.K. Ha, A. Beharka, D.E. Smith, B.S. Bender, and S.N. Meydani. 2000. Vitamin E supplementation increases T helper 1 cytokine production in old mice infected with influenza virus. *Immunology* 100(4):487–493.

Hanson, M.G., V. Ozenci, M.C. Carlsten, B.L. Glimelius, J.E. Frodin, G. Masucci, K. Malmberg, and R.V.R. Kiessling. 2007. A short-term dietary supplementation with high doses of vitamin E increases NK cell cytolytic activity in advanced colorectal cancer patients. *Cancer Immunol Immunother* 56(7):973–984.

Harikrishnan, R., C. Balasundaram, and M.S. Heo. 2011. Impact of plant products on innate and adaptive immune system of cultured finfish and shellfish. *Aquaculture* 317(1–4):1–15.

Hashem, M.A., A.N.F. Neamat-Allah, H.E.E. Hammza, and H. M Abou-Elnaga. 2020. Impact of dietary supplementation with Echinacea purpurea on growth performance, immunological, biochemical, and pathological findings in broiler chickens infected by pathogenic E. coli. *Tropical Animal Health and Production* 52:1599–1607.

Hassan H., and F. Sobhan. 2017. Performance, serum biochemical parameters and immunity in broiler chicks fed dietary *Echinacea purpurea* and *Thymus vulgaris* extracts. *Journal of Worlds's Poultry Research* 7(3):123–128.

Häusler, D., S. Torke, E. Peelen, T. Bertsch, M. Djukic, R. Nau, C. Larochelle, S.S. Zamvil, W. Brück, and M.S. Weber. 2019. High dose vitamin D exacerbates central nervous system autoimmunity by raising T-cell excitatory calcium. *Brain* 142(9):2737–2755.

Hayek, M.G., S.F. Taylor, B.S. Bender, S.N. Han, M. Meydani, D.E. Smith, S. Eghtesada, and S.N. Meydani. 1997. Vitamin E supplementation decreases lung virus titers in mice infected with influenza. *Journal of Infectious Disease* 176(1):273–276.

He, C.S., X.H. Aw Yong, N.P. Walsh, and M. Gleeson. 2016. Is there an optimal vitamin D status for immunity in athletes and military personnel? *Exercise Immunology Review* 22:42–64.

Heinzerling, R.H., R.P. Tengerdy, L.L. Wick, and D.C. Lueker. 1974. Vitamin E protects mice against *Diplococcus pneumoniae* type I infection. *Infection and Immunity* 10(6):1292–1295.

Hemila, H. 2017. Vitamin C and Infections. *Nutrients* 9(4):339.

Hiedra, R., K.B. Lo, M. Elbashabsheh, F. Gul, R.M. Wright, J. Albano, Z. Azmaiparashvili, and G.P. Aponte. 2020. The use of IV vitamin C for patients with COVID-19: a case series. *Expert Review of Anti-infective Therapy*. DOI: 10.1080/14787210.2020.1794819

Higdon, J.V., and B. Frei. 2003. Tea catechins and polyphenols: health effects, metabolism, and antioxidant functions. *Critical Reviews in Food Science and Nutrition* 43:89–143.

Holick, M.F. 2007. Vitamin D deficiency. *The New England Journal of Medicine* 357:266–281.

Hosomi, A., M. Arita, Y. Sato, C. Kiyose, T. Ueda, O. Igarashi, H. Arai, and K. Inoue. 1997. Affinity for alpha-tocopherol transfer protein as a determinant of the biological activities of vitamin E analogs. *FEBS Letters* 409(1):105–108.

Hu, C., and D.D. Kitts. 2000. Studies on the antioxidant activity of Echinacea root extract. *Journal of Agriculture and Food Chemistry*. 48(5):1466–1472.

Hubbard, T.D., I.A. Murray, R.G. Nichols, K. Cassel, M. Podolsky, G. Kuzu, Y. Tian, P. Smith, M.J. Kennett, A.D. Patterson, and G.H. Perdew. 2017. Dietary broccoli impacts microbial community structure and attenuates chemically induced colitis in mice in an Ah receptor dependent manner. *Journal of Functional Foods* 37:685–698.

Hudson, J.B. 2012. Applications of the phytomedicine *Echinacea purpurea* (Purple Coneflower) in infectious diseases. *Journal of Biomedicine and Biotechnology* 769896.

Il'yasova, D., C. Martín, and R.S. Sandler. 2003. Tea intake and risk of colon cancer in African-Americans and Whites: North Carolina colon cancer study cancer causes control. 14:767–772.

Inoue-Choi, M., J.M. Yuan, C.S. Yang, D.J. Van Den Berg, M. Lee, Y. Gao, and M.C. Yu. 2010. Genetic association between the COMT genotype and urinary levels of tea polyphenols and their metabolites among daily green tea drinkers. *International Journal of Molecular Epidemiology and Genetics* 1(2):114–123.

Ismail, I.E., M. Alagawany, A.E. Taha, N. Puvaca, V. Laudadio, and V. Tufarelli. 2020. Effect of dietary supplementation of garlicpowder and phenyl acetic acid on productive performance, bloodhaematology, immunity and antioxidant status of broiler chickens. *Asian-Australasian Journal of Animal Sciences*. https://doi.org/10.5713/ajas.20.0140

Jancso, G., E. Kiraly, and A. Jansco-Gabor. 1997. Pharmacologically induced selective degeneration of chemosensitive primary sensory neurons. *Nature* 270:741–743.

Jawad, M., R. Schoop, A. Suter, P. Klein, and R. Eccles. 2012. Safety and efficacy profile of Echinacea purpurea to prevent common cold episodes: a randomized, double-blind,placebo-controlled trial, *Evidence-Based Complementary and Alternative Medicine*. 841315.

Jeong, Y.J., S.W. Hong, J.H. Kim, D.H. Jin, J.S. Kang, W.J. Lee, and Y.I. Hwang. 2011. Vitamin C-treated murine bone marrow-derived dendritic cells preferentially drive naive T cells into Th1 cells by increased IL-12 secretions. *Cellular Immunology* 266(2):192–199.

Jesudoss, V.A.S., S.V.A. Santiago, K. Venkatachalam, and P. Subramanian. 2017. Zingerone (ginger extract): antioxidant potential for efficacy in gastrointestinal and liver disease, *Gastrointestinal Tissue* 289–297.

Johann, S., N.P. Sá, L.A. Lima, P.S. Cisalpino, B.B. Cota, T.M. Alves, E.P. Siqueira, and C.L. Zani. 2010. Antifungal activity of schinol and a new biphenyl compound isolated from Schinus terebinthifolius against the pathogenic fungus Paracoccidioides brasiliensis. *Annals of Clinical Microbiology and Antimicrobials* 9(30):1–6.

Jones, R.B., C.L. Frisina, S. Winkler, M. Imsic and R.B. Tomkins. 2010. Cooking method significantly effects glucosinolate content and sulforaphane production in broccoli florets. *Food Chemistry* 123(2):237–242.

Jung, E.S., J. Park, H. Park, W. Holzapfel, J.S. Hwang, and C.H. Lee. 2019. Seven-day Green Tea Supplementation Revamps Gut Microbiome and Caecum/Skin Metabolome in Mice from Stress. *Scientific Report* 9:18418.

Kamath, A.B., L. Wang, H. Das, L. Li, V.N. Reinhold, and J.F. Bukowski. 2003. Antigens in teabeverage prime human Vgamma 2Vdelta 2 T cells in vitro and in vivo formemory and nonmemory antibacterial cytokine responses. *Proceedings of the National Academy of Sciences of the United States of America* 100(10):6009–6014.

Kawamotoa, Y., Y. Uenob, E. Nakahashia, M. Obayashia, K. Sugiharaa, S. Qiaoa, M. Iidac, M.Y. Kumasakac, I. Yajimac, Y. Gotod, N. Ohgamic, M. Katoc, and K. Takedaa. 2016. Prevention of allergic rhinitis by ginger and the molecular basis of immunosuppression by 6-gingerol through T cell inactivation. *The Journal of Nutritional Biochemistry* 27:112–122.

Khan, M.A., S.B. Khan, S. Ahmad, I. Ahmad, I. Haq, K. Prince, A. Ullah, M. Shoaib, S. Zaman, A.I. Aqib, G. Rashid, M. Ali, I.U. Khan, I. Khan, N. Ullah, and M. Shahid. 2019. Effect of vitamin E supplementation on humoral immunity following the administration of enterotoxaemia vaccine in goats. *Pakistan Journal of Zoology* 51(6):1–3.

Khanra, R., S. Dewanjee, T.K. Dua, R. Sahu, M. Gangopadhyay, V. De Feo, and M. Zia-Ul-Haq. 2015. *Abroma augusta* L. (Malvaceae) leaf extract attenuates diabetes induced nephropathy and cardiomyopathy via inhibition of oxidative stress and inflammatory response. *Journal of Translational Medicine* 13(1):1–14.

Kikuzaki, H., and N. Nakatani, 1996. Cyclic diaryl heptanoids from rhizomes of *Zingiber officinale*. *Phytochemistry* 43(1):273–277.

Kim, Y.H., Y.S. Won, X. Yang, M. Kumazoe, S. Yamashita, A. Hara, A. Takagaki, K. Goto, F. Nanjo, and H. Tachibana. 2016. Green tea catechin metabolites exert immunoregulatory effects on $CD_4(+)$ T cell and natural killer cell activities. *Journal of Agricultural and Food Chemistry* 64:3591–3597.

King, S., J. Glanville, M.E. Sanders, A. Fitzgerald, and D. Varley, 2014. Effectiveness of probiotics on the duration of illness in healthy children and adults who develop common acute respiratory infectious conditions: a systematic review and meta-analysis. *British Journal of Nutrition* 112(1):41–54.

Krebs, H.A. 1953. The sheffield experiment on the vitamin C requirement of human adults. *Proceedings of the Nutrition Society* 12(3):237–246.

Krest, I., J. Glodek, M. Keusgen. 2000. Cysteine sulfoxides and alliinase activity of some allium species. *Journal of Agricultural and Food Chemistry* 48(8):3753–3760.

Kumar V.G., A. Kumar, K. Raghu, G.R. Patel and S. Manjappa. 2013. Determination of vitamin C in some fruits and vegetables in Davanagere City, (Karanataka) – India. *International Journal of Pharmacy and Life Sciences* 4(3):2489–2491.

LaLone, C.A., K.D. Hammer, L. Wu, J. Bae, N. Leyva, Y. Liu, A.K.S. Solco, G.A. Kraus, P.A. Murphy, E.S. Wurtele, O.K. Kim, M.P. Widrlechner, and D.F. Birt. 2007. Echinacea species and alkamides inhibit prostaglandin E₂ production in RAW264.7 mouse macrophage cells. *Journal of Agriculture and Food Chemistry* 55(18):7314–7322.

Langley-Evans, S.C. 2002. The role of tea in human health: an update. *Journal of the American College of Nutrition* 51:181–188.

Larry, D., S. Lawson, and M. Hunsaker. 2018. Allicin bioavailability and bioequivalence from garlic supplements and garlic foods. *Nutrients* 10(7):812.

Lee, D.H., C.S. Ra, Y.H. Song, K. Sung, and J.D. Kim. 2012. Effects of dietary garlic extract on growth, feed utilization and whole body composition of juvenile sterlet sturgeon *(Acipenser ruthenus)*. *Asian-Australasian Journal of Animal Sciences* 25(4): 577–583.

Lee G.Y., and S.N. Han. 2018. The role of vitamin E in immunity. *Nutrients* 10(11):1614.

Lee, J.J., K.M. Crosby, K.S. Yoo, and D.I. Lescobar. 2005. Impact of genetic and environmental variation of development of flavonoids and carotenoids in pepper (*Capsicum* spp.). *Scientia Horticulturae* 106:341–352.

Lee, P. and L.M. Ulatowski. 2019. Vitamin E: Mechanism of transport and regulation in the CNS. *IUBMB Life* 71(4):424–429.

Levine, M., K.R. Dhariwal, R.W. Welch, Y. Wang, and J.B. Park. 1995. Determination of optimal vitamin C requirements in humans. *The American Journal of Clinical Nutrition* 62(6) Supplement:1347–1356.

Lewis, E.D., S.N. Meydani, and D. Wu. 2019. Regulatory role of vitamin E in the immune system and inflammation. *IUBMB Life* 71(4):487–494.

Li, G., X. Ma, L. Deng, X. Zhao, Y. Wei, Z. Gao, J. Jia, J. Xu, and C. Sun. 2015. Fresh garlic extract enhances the antimicrobial activities of antibiotics on resistant strains in vitro. *Jundishapur Journal of Microbiology* 8(5):14814.

Li, P., Y.L. Yin, D. Li, S.W. Kim, and G. Wu. 2007. Amino acids and immune function. *British Journal of Nutrition* 98(2):237–252.

Li, Y., Y. Wang, Y. Wu, B. Wang, X. Chen, X. Xu, H. Chen, W. Li, and X. Xu. 2017. Echinacea pupurea extracts promote murine dendritic cell maturation by activation of JNK, p3⁸ MAPK and NF-κB pathways. *Developmental and Comparative Immunology* 73:21–26.

Liu, Y.J., L.H. Zhao, R. Mosenthin, J.Y. Zhang, C. Ji, and Q.G. Ma. 2019. Protective Effect of Vitamin E on laying performance, antioxidant capacity, and immunity in laying hens challenged with *Salmonella Enteritidis*. *Poultry Science* 98(11):5847–5854.

Luettig B., C. Steinm̈uller, G.E. Gifford, H. Wagner, and M.- L. Lohmann-matthes. 1989. Macrophage activation by the polysaccharide arabinogalactan isolated from plant cell cultures of *Echinacea purpurea*. *Journal of the National Cancer Institute* 81(9):669–675.

Mahassni, S.H., and O.A. Bukhari. 2019. Beneficial effects of an aqueous ginger extract on the immune system cells and antibodies, hematology, and thyroid hormones in male smokers and non-smokers. *Journal of Nutrition & Intermediary Metabolism* 15:10–17.

Mainous, M.R., and E.A. Deitch. 1994. Nutrition and infection. *Surgical Clinics of North America* 74(3):659–676.

Mikirova, N.A. and R. Hunninghake. 2014. Effect of high dose vitamin C on Epstein-Barr viral infection. *Medical Science Monitor* 20:725–732.

Maggini, S., E.S. Wintergerst, S. Beveridge, and D.H. Hornig. 2007. Selected vitamins and trace elements support immune function by strengthening epithelial barriers and cellular and humoral immune responses. *British Journal of Nutrition* 98(1) Supplement 1:29–35.

Mansour, M.S., Y.M. Ni, A.L. Roberts, M. Kelleman, A. Roychoudhury, and M.P. St-Onge. 2012. Ginger consumption enhances the thermic effect of food and promotes feelings of satiety without affecting metabolic and hormonal parameters in overweight men: a pilot study, Metabolism. 61(10):1347–1352.

Marcos, A., E. Nova, and A. Montero. 2003. Changes in the immune system are conditioned by nutrition. *European Journal of Clinical Nutrition* 57(1) Supplement 1:66 – 69.

Matsuura, H. and Lachance, P.A. 1997. *Phytochemistry of Garlic Horticultural and Processing Procedures*, Food and Nutrition Press: Trumbull, CT.

Meadows, G.G., M. Wallendal, A. Kosugi, J. Wunderlich, and D.S. Singer. 1992. Ethanol induces marked changes in lymphocyte populations and natural killer cell activity in mice. *Alcoholism Clinical and Experimental Research* 16:474–479.

Medina, J.D.L.C., and H.S. Garcia. 2007. Garlic: Post hervest operations. In D. Mejia (Ed.), *INPho- Post herbest compendium*. Mexico: Food and Agricultural Organization of the United States. 1–43.

Murray, M.T. 1995. *The Healing Power of Herbis: the Enlightened Person's Guide to the Worders of Medicinal Plants*, USA Prima Publ., Rocklin, CA.

Miguel, M. 2011. *Anthocyanins*: Antioxidant and/or anti-infl ammatory activities. *Journal of Applied Pharmaceutical Science*, 1(6):7–15.

Mirjalili, M.H., P. Salehi, H.N. Badi, and A. Sonboli. 2006. Volatile constituents of the flowerheads of threeEchinacea species cultivated in Iran. *Flavour and Fragrance Journal* 21 (2):355–358.

Moazami, Y., T.V. Gulledge, S.M. Laster, and J.G. Pierce. 2015. Synthesis and biological evaluation of a series of fatty acid amides from Echinacea. *Bioorganic and Medicinal Chemistry Letters* 25(16):3091–3094.

Mojani, M.S., A. Rahmat, R. Ramasamy, V.H. Sarmadi, P. Sandrasaigaran, S. Vellasamy, and S.M.A. Hejazi. 2016. Metabolic and immunologic alterations of ginger rhizome among streptozotocin-nicotinamide induced diabetic rats. *Malaysian Journal of Nutrition* 22(3):421–432.

Moradi, S., M. Mousavinia and B.A. Galeh. 2016. Effect of use black and red pepper powder as feed additive on performance and some immune parameters of Cobb 500 broiler chicks. *CIBTech Journal of ZoologyB* 5(2):45–50.

Muller, D.P. 2010. Vitamin E and neurological function. *Molecular Nutrition Food Research* 54(5):710–718.

Murphy, K. and C. Weaver. 2017. *Janeway's Immunobiology*. Philadelphia: Taylor & Francis.

Nagabhushan, M., A.J. Amonkar, and S.V. Bhide.1987. Mutagenicity of gingerol and shogaol and antimutagenicity of zingerone in Salmonella/microsome assay. *Cancer Letters* 36(2): 221–233.

Najeeb U, A. Mahboob, A. Hasnain, M.A. Tahir, M. Aftab, N. Bibi, and S. Ahmad. 2016. Green tea phytocompounds as anticancer: a review. *Asian Pacific Journal of Tropical Disease* 6(4):330–336.

Nakamura, H., and T. Yamamoto. 1983. The active part of the [6]-gingerol molecule in mutagenesis. *Mutation Research Letters* 122(2):87–94.

Nantz, M.P., C.A. Rowe, C.E. Muller, R.A. Creasy, J.M. Stanilka, and S.S. Percival 2012. Supplementation with aged garlic extract improves both NK and γδ-T cell function and reduces the severity of cold and flu symptoms: a randomized, double-blind, placebo-controlled nutrition intervention. *Clinical Nutrition* 31:337–344.

Narnaware, Y.K., B.I. Baker, and M.G. Tomlinson. 1994. The effects of various stresses, corticosteroids and adrenergic agents on phagocytosis in the rainbow trout *Oncorhynchus mykiss. Fish Physiology and Biochemistry* 13:31–40.

Nazari, B., A. Amirzargar, B. Nikbin, M. Nafar, P. Ahmadpour, B. Einollahi, M.L. Pezeshki, S.M.R. Khatami, B. Ansaripour, H. Nikuinejad, F. Mohamadi, M. Mahmoudi, S. Soltani, and M.H. Nicknam. 2013. Comparison of the Th1, IFN-γ secreting cells and FoxP3 expression between patients with stable graft function and acute rejection post kidney transplantation, 12(3):262–268.

Neme, A., S. Seuter, and C. Carlberg. 2017. Selective regulation of biological processes by vitamin D based on the spatio-temporal cistrome of its receptor. *Biochimica et Biophysica Acta-Gene Regulatory Mechanisms* 1860(9):952–61.

Neuzil, J., K. Kagedal, L. Andera, C. Weber, and U.T. Brunk. 2002. Vitamin E analogs: a new class of multiple action agents with anti-neoplastic and anti-atherogenic activity, *Apoptosis* 7(2):179–187.

Noah, T.L., H. Zhang, H. Zhou, E. Glista-Baker, L. Muller, R.N. Bauer, M. Meyer, P.C. Murphy, S. Jones, B. Letang, C. Robinette, and I. Jaspers. 2014. Effect of broccoli sprouts on nasal response to live attenuated influenza virus in smokers: a randomized, double-blind study. *PLoS One* 9(6):98671.

Nobs, S.P., N. Zmora, and E. Elinav. 2020. Nutrition regulates innate immunity in health and disease. *Annual Review of Nutrition* 40:189–219.

Nosrati, M., F. Javandel, L.M. Camacho, A. Khusro, M. Cipriano, A. Seidavi, and A.Z.M. Salem. 2017. The effects of antibiotic, probiotic, organic acid, vitamin C, and *Echinacea purpurea* extract on performance, carcass characteristics, blood chemistry, microbiota, and immunity of broiler chickens. *Journal of Applied Poultry Research* 26(2):295–306.

Nwaopara, A.O., L.C. Anyanwu, C.A. Oyinbo, and I.C. Anaikot. 2004. The histological changes in pancreas of Wister rats fed with diets containing Yaji (Local meat sauce). *Journal of Experimental and Clinical Anatomy* 3:44–47.

Nwaopara, A.O., M.A.C. Odike, U. Inegbenebor, and M.I. Adoye, 2007. The combined effects of excessive consumption of ginger, clove, red pepper and black pepper on the histology of the liver. *Pakistan Journal of Nutrition* 6(6):524–527.

O'Hara, M.A., D. Kiefer, K. Farrell, K. Kemper. 1998. A review of the 12 commonly used medicinal herbs. *Archives of Family Medicine* 7(6):523–536.

Ohnuki, K., S. Niwa, S. Maeda, N. Inoue, S. Yazawa and T. Fushiki. 2001. CH-19 sweet, a non-pungent cultivar of red pepper, increased body temperature and oxygen consumption in *humans. Bioscience, Biotechnology, and Biochemistry* 65(9):2033–2036.

Olcott, H., and H. Mattill. 1931. The unsaponifiable lipids of lettuce. 3. Antioxidant. *The Journal of Biological Chemistry* 93(1):65–70.

Omaye, S.T., E.E. Schaus, M.A. Kutnink, and W.C. Hawkes. 1987. Measurement of vitamin C in blood components by high-performance liquid chromatography. Implication in assessing vitamin C status. *Annals of the New York Academy of Sciences* 498:389–401.

Percival, S.S. 2016. Aged garlic extract modifies human immunity. *The Journal of Nutrition* 146(2):433–436.

Percival S.S., S.A. Nelson, and J.A. Milner. 2005. Workshop executive summary report. *The Journal of Nutrition* 135:2898–2907.

Permyakova, N.V., A.A. Zagorskaya, P.A. Belavin, E.A. Uvarova, O.V. Nosareva, A.E. Nesterov, A.A. Novikovskaya, E.L. Zav'Yalov, M.P. Moshkin, and E.V. Deineko. 2015. Transgenic carrot expressing fusion protein comprising M. tuberculosis antigens induces immune response in mice. *BioMed Research International*, 417565.

Piroddi, M., A. Albini, R. Fabiani, L. Giovannelli, C. Luceri, F. Natella, P. Rosignoli, T. Rossi, A. Taticchi, M. Servili, and F. Galli. 2017. Nutrigenomics of extra-virgin olive oil: a review. *BioFactors*, 43(1):17–41.

Puvača, N. 2018. Bioactive compounds in selected hot spices and medicinal plants. *Journal of Agronomy, Technology and Engineering Management* 1(1):8–17.

Puvača, N., D.L. Pelić, S. Popović, P. Ikonić, O. Đuragić, T. Peulić, and L. Lević. 2019. Evaluation of Broiler Chickens Lipid Profile Influenced by Dietary Chili Pepper Addition *Journal of Agronomy, Technology and Engineering Management* 2(5):318–324.

Rasanu N., V. Magearu, N. Matei, and A. Soceanu. 2005. Determination of Vitamin C in different stages of fruits growing. *Analele Universităńii Din Bucuresti* 2–3:167–172.

Rauš, K., S. Pleschka, P. Klein, R. Schoop, P. Fisher. 2015. Effect of an Echinacea-based hot drink versus Oseltamivir in influenza treatment: a randomized, double-blind, double-dummy, multicenter, noninferiority clinical trial. *Current Therapeutic Research, Clinical and Experimental* 77:66–72.

Rawangkan A., P. Wongsirisin, K. Namiki, K. Iida, Y. Kobayashi, Y. Shimizu, H. Fujiki and M. Suganuma. 2018. Green tea catechin is an alternative immune checkpoint inhibitor that inhibits pd-11 expression and lung tumor growth. *Molecules* 23(8):2071.

Rehman, R., S. Saif, M.A. Hanif, and M. Riaz. 2019. *Medicinal plants of South Asia*: Garlic. Amsterdam: Elsevier.

Rietveld, A., and S. Wiseman. 2003. Antioxidant Effects of Tea: Evidence from Human Clinical Trials. *The Journal of Nutrition* 133(10): 3275–3284.

Rininger, J.A., S. Kickner, P. Chigurupati, A. Mclean, Z. Franck. 2000. Immunopharmacological activity of Echinacea preparations following simulated digestion on murine macrophages and human peripheral blood mononuclear cells. *Journal of Leukocyte Biology* 68(4):503–510.

Rios, E., B. Szczesny, F.G. Soriano, G. Olah, and C. Szabo. 2015. Hydrogen sulfide attenuates cytokine production through the modulation of chromatin remodeling. *International Journal of Molecular Medicine* 35(6):1741–1746.

Roesler J., A. Emmend¨orffer, C. Steinm¨uller, B. Luettig, H. Wagner, and M.-L. Lohmann-Matthes. 1991. Application of purified polysaccharides from cell cultures of the plant Echinacea purpurea to test subjects mediates activation of the phagocyte system. *International Journal of Immunopharmacology* 13(7):27–37.

Rondanelli, M., A. Miccono, S. Lamburghini, I. Avanzato, A. Riva, P. Allegrini, M.A. Faliva, G. Peroni, M. Nichetti, and S. Perna. 2018. Self-care for common colds: the pivotal role of vitamin D, vitamin C, zinc, and *echinacea* in three main immune interactive clusters (physical barriers, innate and adaptive immunity) involved during an episode of common colds—practical advice on dosages and on the time to take these nutrients/botanicals in order to prevent or treat common colds. *Evidence-Based Complementary and Alternative Medicine* 5813095.

Rose, R.C. 1988. Transport of ascorbic acid and other water-soluble vitamins. *Biochimica et Biophysica Acta - General Subjects* 947(2): 335–366.

Rouf, R., S.J. Uddin, D.K. Sarker, M.T. Islam, E.S. Ali, J.A. Shilpi, L. Nahar, E. Tiralongo, S.D. Sarker. 2020. Antiviral potential of garlic (*Allium sativum*) and its organosulfur compounds: a systematic update of pre-clinical and clinical data. *Trends in Food Science and Technology* 104:219–234.

Ruiz-Jiménez, J., J. Luque-Garcıa, and M.L. de Castro. 2003. Dynamic ultrasound-assisted extraction of cadmium and lead from plants prior to electrothermal atomic absorption spectrometry. *Analytica Chimica Acta* 480(2):231–237.

Saba, K., M. Sameeullah, A. Asghar, J. Gottschamel, S. Latif, A.G. Lossl, B. Mirza, O. Mirza, and M.T. Waheed. 2020. Expression of ESAT-6 antigen from *Mycobacterium tuberculosis* in broccoli: An edible plant. *Biotechnology and Applied Biochemistry* 67(1):148–157.

Safiullah, N. Chand, R.U. Khan, S. Naz, M. Ahmad, and S. Gul. 2019. Effect of ginger (*Zingiber officinale Roscoe*) and organic selenium on growth dynamics, blood melanodialdehyde and paraoxonase in broilers exposed to heat stress. *Journal of Applied Animal Research* 47(1):212–216.

Saito H, K. Hara, S. Kitajima, and K. Tanemura. 2020. Effect of Vitamin E deficiency on spermatogenesis in mice and its similarity to aging, *Reproductive Toxicology*. https://doi.org/10.1016/j.reprotox.2020.10.003

Sato T, and G. Miyata. 2000. The nutraceutical benefit, part I: green tea. *The Journal of Nutrition* 16(14):315–17.

Sauberlich, H.E. 1997. A history of scurvy and vitamin C: In Vitamin C in Health and Disease; Packer, L., Fuchs, J., Eds.; Marcel Dekker, 1–24. New York, NY.

Schink, M., W. Troger, A. Dabidian, A. Goyert, H. Scheuerecker, J. Meyer, I.U. Fischer, and F. Glaser. 2007. Mistletoe extract reduces the surgical suppression of natural killer cell activity in cancer patients. a randomized phase III trial. *Forsch Komplementarmed* 14(1): 9–17.

Semwal, R.B., D.K. Semwal, S. Combrinck, and A.M. Viljoen. 2015. Gingerols and shogaols: Important nutraceutical principles from ginger. *Phytochemistry* 117:554–568.

Sharifi, A., H. Vahedi, S. Nedjat, H. Rafiei, and M.J. Hosseinzadeh-Attar. 2019. Effect of single-dose injection of vitamin D on immune cytokines in ulcerative colitis patients: a randomized placebo-controlled trial. *Journal of Pathology, Microbiology and Immunology* 127:681–687.

Sharifi-Rad, M., E.M. Varoni, B. Salehi, J. Sharifi-Rad, K.R. Matthews, S.A. Ayatollahi, F. Kobarfard, S.A. Ibrahim, D. Mnayer, Z.A. Zakaria, M. Sharifi-Rad, Z. Yousaf, M. Iriti, A. Basile, D. Rigano. 2017. Plants of the genus zingiber as a source of bioactive phytochemicals: from tradition to pharmacy. *Molecules* 22(12):2145.

Sharma, M., S.A. Anderson, R. Schoop, and J.B. Hudson. 2009. Induction of multiple proinflammatory cytokines by respiratory viruses and reversal by standardized Echinacea, a potent antiviral herbal extract. *Antiviral Research* 83(2):165–170.

Sharma, R.A. Sharma, A. Kumari, P.M. Kulurkar, R. Raj, A. Gulati, and Y.S. Padwad, Consumption of green tea epigallocatechin-3-gallate enhances systemic immune response, antioxidative capacity and HPA axis functions in aged male Swiss albino mice. *Biogerontology* 2017, 18, 367–382.

Sharma, S.M., M. Anderson, S.R. Schoop, and J.B. Hudson. 2010. Bactericidal and anti-inflammatory properties of a standardized Echinacea extract (Echinaforce): dual actions against respiratory bacteria. *Phytomedicine* 17:563–568.

Sheikhi, M.A., A. Ebadi, A. Talaeizadeh, and H. Rahmani. 2015. Alternative methods to treat nausea and vomiting from cancer chemotherapy. Chemotherapy Research and Practice 818759.

Shen H., and B. Zhan 2020. Effect of vitamin E on strokeassociated Pneumonia. *Journal of International Medical Research* 48(9):1–12.

Sheppard, A.J., J.A.T. Pennington, J. L. Weihrauch. 1980. Analysis and distribution of vitamin E in vegetable oils and foods: In Vitamin E in Health and Disease; Packer, L., Fuchs, J., Eds.; Marcel Dekker, 7–65. New York, NY.

Shi, W.J. and Y.Q. Liu, 1998. Acomparison of nutritional components of fruit of tetraploid and diploid Lycium barbarum. *Journal of Ningxia Medical University* 20:17–18.

Shimizu, K., N.K. Shimizu, W. Hakamata, K. Unno, T. Asai, N. Oku. 2010. Preventive effect of green tea catechins on experimental tumor metastasis in senescence-accelerated mice. *Biological and Pharmaceutical Bulletin* 33:117–121.

Shin, S.H., and M.K. Kim. 2004. Effect of dired powders or ethanol extracts of garlic flesh and peel on lipid metabolism and antithrombogenic capacity in 16-month-old rats. *The Korean Journal of Nutrition.* 37(7):515–524.

Silva-Guillen Y.V., C. Arellano, R.D. Boyd, G. Martinez, and E. van Heugten. 2020. Growth performance, oxidative stress and immune status of newly weaned pigs fed peroxidized lipids with or without supplemental vitamin E or polyphenols. *Journal of Animal Science and Biotechnology* 11(22).

Sima, P., V. Vetvicka, and L. Vannucci. 2016. Co-evolution of nutrition and immunity. *Journal of Food Science & Nutrition* 2:1–3.

Soba, D., M. Muller, I. Aranjuelo, and S. Munne-Bosch. 2020. Vitamin E in legume nodules: Occurrence and antioxidant function. *Phytochemistry* 172:112261.

Soliman N.K., and S.F. AlAfifi. 2020. The productive performance, intestinal bacteria and histomorphology of broiler chicks fed diets containing hot red pepper. *Egyptian Poultry Science Journal* 40:345–357.

Sontag, T.J., and R.S. Parker. 2002. Cytochrome P450 omega-hydroxylase pathway of tocopherol catabolism. Novel mechanism of regulation of vitamin E status. *Journal of Biological Chemistry* (28) 25290–25296.

Sotirchos, E.S., P. Bhargava, C. Eckstein, K. Van Haren, M. Baynes, A. Ntranos, A. Gocke, L. Steinman, E.M. Mowry, and P.A. Calabresi. 2016. Safety and immunologic effects of high- vs lowdose cholecalciferol in multiple sclerosis. *Neurology* 86:382–390.

Srinivasan, K. 2017. Ginger rhizomes (Zingiber officinale): a spice with multiple health beneficial potentials. *Pharma Nutrition* 5(1):18–28.

Suleria, H.A., M.S. Butt, N. Khalid, S. Sultan, A. Raza, M. Aleem, M. Abbas. 2015. Garlic (Allium sativum): diet based therapy of 21st century–a review. *Asian Pacific Journal of Tropical Disease* 5(4):271–278.

Talib, W.H. 2017. Consumption of garlic and lemon aqueous extracts combination reduces tumor burden by angiogenesis inhibition, apoptosis induction, and immune system modulation. *Nutrition* 43–44:89–97.

Tang, H., S. Hao, X. Chen, Y. Li, Z. Yin, Y. Zou, X. Song, L. Lixia, G. Ye, L. Zhao, H. Guo, R. He, C. Lv, J. Lin, and F. Shi. 2020. Epigallocatechin-3-gallate protects immunity and liver drug-metabolism function in mice loaded with restraint stress. *Biomedicine and Pharmacotherapy* 129:110418.

Tee E.S., S.I. Young, S.K. Ho and S.S. Mizura. 1988. Determination of vitamin c in fresh fruits and vegetables using the dye-titration and microfluorometric methods. *Pertanika* 11(1):39–44.

Thejass, P., and G. Kuttan. 2007. Immunomodulatory activity of sulforaphane, a naturally occurring isothiocyanate from broccoli (*Brassica oleracea*). *Phytomedicine* 14:538–545.

Todd, D.A., T.V. Gulledge, E.R. Britton, M. Oberhofer, M. Leyte-Lugo, A.N. Moody, T. Shymanovich, L.F. Grubbs, M. Juzumaite, T.N. Graf, N.H. Oberlies, S.H. Faeth, S.M. Laster, and N.B. Cech. 2015. Ethanolic Echinacea purpurea extracts contain a mixture of cytokine-suppressive and cytokine-inducing compounds, including some that originate from endophytic bacteria. *PLoS One* 10:0124276.

Tóth, B., T. Lantos, P. Hegyi, R.Viola, A. Vasas, R. Benkő, Z. Gyöngyi, Á. Vincze, P. Csécsei, A. Mikó, D. Hegyi, A. Szentesi, Mária Matuz, and D. Csupor. 2018. Ginger (Zingiber officinale): An alternative for the prevention of postoperativenausea and vomiting. A meta-analysis. Phytomedicine 50:8–18.

Traber, M.G. 2007. Vitamin E regulatory mechanisms. *Annual Review of Nutrition* 27:347–362.

Traber, M.G. 2006. Vitamin E: modern nutrition in health and disease. In: M.E. Shils, A.C. Ross, B Caballero, R Cousins, 396–411. Lippincott Williams & Wilkins, Baltimore.

Uvarova, E.A., P.A. Belavin, N.V. Permyakova, A.A. Zagorskaya, O.V. Nosareva, A.A. Kakimzhanova, and E.V. Deineko. 2013. Oral Immunogenicity of Plant-Made *Mycobacterium tuberculosis* ESAT6 and CFP10, *BioMed Research International* 316304.

Uwitonze, A.M., and M.S. Razzaque. 2018. Role of magnesium in vitamin D activation and function. *The Journal of the American Osteopathic Association* 118:181–189.

Vallejo, F., F. Tomás-Barberán, and F. Ferreres. 2004. Characterisation of flavonols in broccoli (Brassica oleracea L. var. italica) by liquid chromatography–UV diode-array detection– electrospray ionisation mass spectrometry. *Journal of Chromatography A* 1054(1):181–193.

van Gorkom, G.N.Y., R.G.J.K. Wolterink, C.H.M.J. Van Elssen, L. Wieten, W.T.V. Germeraad, and G.M.J. Bos. 2018. Influence of vitamin C on lymphocytes: an overview. *Antioxidants* 7(3):41.

Vera, J.C., C.I. Rivas, F.V. Velasquez, R.H. Zhang, I.I. Concha, and D.W. Golde. 1995. Resolution of the facilitated transport of dehydroascorbic acid from its intracellular accumulation as ascorbic acid. Journal of Biological Chemistry 270(40):23706–12.

Vera, J.C., C.I. Rivas, J. Fischbarg, D.W. Golde. 1993. Mammalian facilitative hexose transporters mediate the transport of dehydroascorbic acid. *Nature* 364(6432):79–82.

Wallert, M., L. Börmel, and S. Lorkowski. 2020. Inflammatory Diseases and Vitamin E—What Do We Know and Where Do We Go? *Molecular Nutrition Food Research* 2000097.

Wang, C., Y. Hou, Y. Lv, S. Chen, X. Zhou, R. Zhu, J. Wang, W. Jia, and X. Wang. 2017. *Echinacea purpurea* Extract Affects the Immune System, Global Metabolome, and Gut Microbiome in Wistar Rats. *Journal of Agricultural Science* 9(4):1–14.

Wang, D., Q. Gao, T. Wang, Z. Kan, X. Li, L. Hu, C. Peng, F. Qian, Y. Wanga, and D. Granato. 2020. Green tea polyphenols and epigallocatechin-3-gallate protect against perfluorodecanoic acid induced liver damage and inflammation in mice by inhibiting NLRP3 inflammasome activation. *Food Research International* 127:108628.

Wilasrusmee, C., S. Kittur, J. Siddiqui, D. Bruch, S.Wilasrusmee, and D.S. Kittur. 2002. *In vitro* immunomodulatory effects of ten commonly used herbs on murine lymphocytes. *The Journal Alternative and Complementary Medicine* 8(4):467–475.

Wilson, J.X. 2005. Regulation of vitamin C transport. *Annual Review of Nutrition* 25:105–125.

Witt, W., I. Kolleck, and B. Rustow. 2000. Identification of high density lipo protein binding proteins, including a glycosyl phosphatidylinositol-anchored membrane dipeptidase, in rat lung and type II pneumocytes. *American Journal of Respiratory Cell and Molecular Biology* 22:739 –746.

Wolf, G. 2004. The discovery of vitamin D: the contribution of Adolf Windaus. *The Journal of Nutrition* 134(6):1299–1302.

Wu, D., and S.N. Meydani. 2014. Age-associated changes in immune function: impact of vitamin E intervention and the underlying mechanisms. *Endocrine, Metabolic and Immune Disorders-Drug Targets* 14(4):283–289.

Wu, D., E.D. Lewis, M. Pae and S.N. Meydani. 2019. Nutritional modulation of immune function: analysis of evidence, mechanisms, and clinical relevance. *Frontiers in Immunology Function* 9:3160.

Xu, C., A.E. Mathews, C. Rodrigues, B.J. Eudy, C.A. Rowe, A. O'Donoughue, and S.S. Percival. 2018. Aged garlic extract supplementation modifies inflammation and immunity of adults with obesity: a randomized, double-blind, placebo-controlled clinical trial. *Clinical Nutrition ESPEN* 24:148–155.

Xu, L., J. Cao, and W. Chen. Structural characterization of a broccoli polysaccharide andevaluation of anti-cancer cell proliferation effects. *Carbohydrate Polymers* 126 (2015):179–184.

Yang, G., K. Li, C. Liu, P. Peng, M. Bai, J. Sun, Q. Li, Z. Yang, Y. Yang, and H. Wu. 2018. A comparison of the immunostimulatory effects of polysaccharides from tetraploid and diploid *Echinacea purpurea*. *BioMed Research International* 8628531.

Yongjun, Y., T.G. Maguire, and J.C. Alwine. 2011. Human cytomegalovirus activates glucose transporter 4 expression to increase glucose update during infection. *Journal of Virology* 85(4):1573–80.

Zaki, N., A. Hasib, K.C. Eddine, F. Dehbi, H.E. Batal, and A. Ouatmane. 2017. Comparative Evaluation of the Phytochemical Constituents and the Antioxidant Activities of Five Moroccan Pepper Varieties (*Capsicum annuum* L.). *Journal of Chemical, Biological and Physical Sciences* 7(4):1294–1306.

Zhang, G.F., Z.B. Yang, Y. Wang, W.R. Yang, S.Z. Jiang, G.S. Gai. 2009. Effects of ginger root (*Zingiber officinale*) processed to different particle sizes on growth performance, antioxidant status, and serum metabolites of broiler chickens. *Poultry Science* 88(10):2159–2166.

Zhuang, X., D. Zhong-Bin, J. Mu, L. Zhang, J. Yan, D. Miller, W. Feng, C.J. McClain and H. Zhang. 2015. Ginger-derived nanoparticles protect against alcohol-induced liver damage. *Journal of Extracellular Vesicles*, 4(1): 28713.

Zia-Ul-Haq, M., B.A. Khan, P. Landa, Z. Kutil, S. Ahmed, M. Qayum, S. Ahmad. 2011. Platelet aggregation and anti-infl ammatory effects of garden pea, Desi chickpea and Kabuli chickpea. *Acta Poloniae Pharmaceutica* 69 (4):707–711.

Zia-Ul-Haq, M., P. Landa, Z. Kutil, S. Ahmed, M. Qayum, S. Ahmad. 2013. Evaluation of antiinflammatory activity of selected legumes from Pakistan: In vitro inhibition of Cyclooxygenase-2. *Pakistan Journal of Pharmaceutical Sciences*, 26 (1):185–187.

Zong, A.Z., H.Z. Cao, and F.S. Wang. 2012. Anticancer polysaccharides from natural resources: A review of recent research. *Carbohydrate Polymers* 90(4):1395–1410.

13 Role of Specific Spices in Fortifying the Human Immune System

Yashdeep Srivastava, Swati Upadhyay,
Mohd Ahmad, Deepak Kumar Verma,
and Vinod Kumar Mishra

CONTENTS

13.1 INTRODUCTION

Since ancient times, spices have been known for their medicinal properties and health benefits, as well as their culinary impact. In the wake of the COVID-19 outbreak, there is a growing concern in strengthening our immune system in order to protect our bodies from infectious diseases. The immune system is a network of biological processes that protects an organism against disease. It involves many types

DOI: 10.1201/9781003137955-13

of cells, tissues, and organs. Immunity is the key mechanism for the protection of the host against infectious agents. A very important role in the immune system is played by the cytokines, which are a broad group of low-molecular-weight glycoproteins, secreted by specific immune system cells and categorized as signalling messengers that mediate and regulate immunity, inflammation, and haematopoiesis. Basically, immunity is of two types, namely innate immunity, which is the first line of protection, in which phagocytic cells and macrophages play an important role, and adaptive immunity, which is capable of specifically recognizing and selectively removing various foreign microorganisms and molecules. In addition, the processing and presentation of antigens is also a complex process mediated by the Major Histocompatibility Complex (MHC), which is categorized as either Class-I or Class-II MHC. An endogenous antigen can be processed and presented by class-I MHC to antigen-presenting cells (APCs), where it can be recognized by $CD8^+$ cells. An exogenous antigen can be processed and presented by class-II MHC to APCs, where it can be recognized by $CD4^{+/}$ T cells. Although the immune system does a remarkable job of defending our body against disease-causing microorganisms, if it is weakened, pathogens will invade successfully and may lead to disease. Is it possible to intervene in this process and boost our immune system?

Recently, many studies have shown the conclusive role of food-derived substances in modulation of immune function, such as nutrients (Field et al. 2002; Amati et al. 2003), amino acids (Takegoshi et al. 1998), fatty acids (Kaminogawa and Nanno 2004), vitamins (Meydani et al. 1990; Coutsoudis et al. 1992), minerals (Sempertegui et al. 1996), nucleotides (Nagafuchi et al. 2000), and probiotics (Arak et al. 1999; Hatakka et al. 2001).

Correlation study data from 163 countries between COVID-19 incidence and spice consumption has revealed the potential of spices to fight COVID-19 (Elsayed and Khan 2020). Recently, there has been growing interest in inexpensive natural immunomodulatory molecules, derived from spices, for strengthening and boosting immune response. It has been reported that coumarins and flavonoids from some spices exhibited immunomodulatory activity, i.e., directly enhancing lymphocyte activation and/or secretion of the multipotent cytokine, interferon gamma (IFN-γ) (Cherng et al. 2008). Curcumin, a polyphenol derived from the spice turmeric, is reported to activate the host innate immunity (Catanzaro et al. 2018). Given the proven immunomodulatory properties of some spices, the aim of this chapter was to research the immune booster properties of spices, such as Turmeric (*Curcuma longa*), Cinnamon (*Cinnamomum zeylanicum* and *Cinnamomum cassia)*, Black pepper (*Piper nigrum*), Star Anise (*Illicium verum*), Clove (*Syzygium aromaticum*), Fenugreek (*Trigonella foenum-graecum*), Black Cumin (*Nigella sativa*), Garlic (*Allium sativum*), Ginger (*Zingiber officinale*), *Capsicum* sp. and Omum (*Trachyspermum ammi*).

13.2   SPECIFIC SPICES FOR A STRONG IMMUNE SYSTEM

13.2.1   TURMERIC (*CURCUMA LONGA* L., FAMILY ZINGIBERACEAE)

The use of turmeric has been known in India since the Vedic period, for almost 4,000 years. In food, it is used as a colouring agent and is often referred to as "Indian saffron" and also "the golden spice". In the traditional system of medicine, it has been widely used for treatment of various ailments, such as respiratory illness (e.g., asthma, bronchial hyperactivity, and allergy), liver disorders, anorexia, rheumatism, diabetic wounds, sprain, and swelling. Modern interest in turmeric started in the 1970s when researchers found that the spice may possess biological anti-inflammatory and antioxidant properties and may prove effective in hepatobiliary diseases (Hu et al. 2017). Health benefits of turmeric are attributed to curcumin, obtained from the rhizome (Nelson et al. 2017).

13.2.1.1 Curcumin

The transcription factor, nuclear factor-kappa B (NF-κB) has been reported to be constitutively active in many types of cancer (Giuliani et al. 2018). Curcumin down-regulates the constitutive activity of NF-κB and induces apoptosis in novel mouse melanoma cells (Marín et al. 2007). Tumour necrosis factor-α (TNF-α) is an inflammatory cytokine produced by macrophages/monocytes during acute inflammation and the reduction of its concentration is a therapeutic target in several inflammatory diseases. The results of several preclinical studies on the effect of curcumin on TNF-α have shown that it effectively blocked TNF-α (Sahebkar et al. 2016). Studies showed that inhibition of the JAK/STAT pathway by curcumin is involved in reduced migration and invasion of cancer cells (Ashrafizadeh et al. 2020). Curcumin exerts anti-diabetic, renoprotective, and neuroprotective impacts by normalizing the expression of the JAK/STAT signalling pathway (Ashrafizadeh et al. 2020). Several studies have demonstrated immunomodulatory properties of curcumin on immune cells and mediators, such as various T lymphocytes, dendritic cells, NK cells, monocytes and macrophages, B cells, neutrophils, eosinophils, mast cells, and different inflammatory cytokines (Srivastava et al., 2011; Momtazi-Borojeni et al. 2018).

13.2.2 Cinnamon (*Cinnamomum zeylanicum* and *Cinnamomum cassia*)

The bark of various cinnamon species is used worldwide for cooking and also in traditional and modern medicines. Cinnamaldehyde is one of the major constituents of cinnamon essential oil, which is known to possess anti-inflammatory properties. It was found that cinnamaldehyde inhibits TNF-α-induced inflammation through suppression of NF-κB activation (Liao et al. 2008) and TLR4, and NLRP3 signalling pathways (Lee et al. 2015).

13.2.3 Black Pepper (*Piper nigrum*)

Black pepper has long been used in many cuisines and it holds a very valuable place among herbal medicinal plants. Piperine exhibits a strong anti-inflammatory function. Clinical studies have demonstrated remarkable immunomodulatory potential of piperine, together with antioxidant, antitumour, and drug availability-enhancing properties. It possesses the potential to treat lipopolysaccharide (LPS)-induced inflammation. Results indicated that piperine inhibited LPS-induced expression of IRF-1 and IRF-7 mRNAs, inhibited phosphorylation of IRF-3, type1 IFN mRNA, and down-regulation of STAT-1 activity (Bae et al. 2010). Similarly, Wang-Sheng et al. (2016) reported that piperine inhibited LPS-induced TNF-α, IL-6, IL-1β, and prostaglandin E2 (PGE-2) production in BV2 microglial cells. It found to inhibit the production of IL-2, and IFN-γ in activated human peripheral blood mononuclear cells (PBMCs) (Chuchawankul et al. 2012). Also, piperine reduced the level of proinflammatory cytokines IL-1β, IL-6, and TNF-α, and lowered the expression of COX-2, NOS-2, and NF-κB in cerebral ischaemia in rats (Vaibhav et al. 2012).

13.2.4   STAR ANISE (*ILLICIUM VERUM*)

Star anise (*Illicium verum*) is an important medicinal plant in traditional Chinese medicine and is widely known for its antiviral properties. It is source of shikimic acid, which is used in the manufacture of oseltamivir (Tamiflu®), an antiviral medication for influenza A and influenza B (Patra et al. 2020). *Staphylococcus aureus* cultures treated with *trans*-anethole (a terpenoid from anise or from star anise essential oils) have shown human neutrophil phagocytic activity as well as IL-8 production, suggesting an innate immune response (Kwiatkowski et al. 2020). An extract from this plant was found to reduce expression of IL-4, IL-6, TNF-α, TARC, RANTES, ICAM-1, and VCAM-1, but not IFN-γ in atopic dermatitis in a mouse model (Sung et al. 2012a). The extract inhibited TNF-α/IFN-γ-induced chemokines, pro-inflammatory cytokines, and adhesion molecules *via* blockade of NF-κB, STAT1, MAPK, and Akt activation (Sung et al. 2012b), indicating therapeutic properties of *Illicium verum* extract against inflammatory skin diseases like atopic dermatitis.

13.2.5   CLOVE (*SYZYGIUM AROMATICUM*)

Clove (*Syzygium aromaticum*, from the plant family Myrtaceae) is an aromatic flower bud which is native to the small islands of Maluku in Indonesia, also known as the "Spice Islands". Recently, the application of natural spices as immunomodulators has attracted increasing attention. Clove shows great potential as an immunostimulant (Halder et al. 2011). Eugenol is the major constituent of *Syzygium aromaticum*. The immunomodulatory effect of *S. aromaticum* essential oil has been attributed to an augmentation of humoral and cell-mediated immune responses (Halder et al. 2011). Islamuddin et al. (2016) demonstrated antileishmanial activity of a eugenol emulsion through potentiating Th1 immunostimulation without adverse side effects, and may help to alleviate the depressed cell-mediated immunity and hence complement the antileishmanial activity. Inflammation is known as adaptive immunity response of the body. Eugenol possesses anti-inflammatory potential, with *in-vitro* studies revealing that clove oil polyphenol inhibits nuclear factor-kB (NF-kB) activation in lipopolysaccharide-initiated macrophages induced by inactivated cyclooxygenase activity (COX-2) and tumour necrosis factor (TNF-α) (Kim et al. 2003). Thus, eugenol may serve as a plausible lead candidate for developing the COX-2 inhibitor as an anti-inflammatory or anticancer chemopreventive agent. Eugenol reduced levels of TNF-α and neutrophils in the mouse during pulmonary inflammation. It also protected against nicotine-induced dysfunction of murine macrophages through down-regulating the Th1 cytokines (TNF-α, IL-12) with concurrent activation of

Th2 responses (IL-10, TGF-β) (Kim et al. 2003). Studies on collagen-induced arthritis in the murine model showed the anti-arthritic property of eugenol. It inhibits mononuclear cell infiltration into the knee joints of arthritic mice and also decreases the levels of cytokines, such as tumour necrosis factor (TNF-α), interferon (IFNγ), and tumour growth factor (TGF-β) within the ankle joints (Grespan et al., 2012). The eugenol shows significant potential against dermatitis as an anti-inflammatory molecule which inhibited the release of myeloperoxidase (MPO) in degranulation of PMA-stimulated neutrophils (Lopes et al. 2018). It is reported that MPO displays cytokine-like properties that can activate leukocytes in an inflammatory response (Lau et al. 2005). It prevents neutrophil degranulation and can be used as an anti-inflammatory compound against dermatitis disease (Sheppard et al. 2005). Han et al. (2017) reported significant inhibitory effects of eugenol in human dermal fibroblasts that exhibited antiproliferative activity and also significantly decreased the levels of inflammatory biomarkers, such as vascular cell adhesion molecule-1 (VCAM-1), interferon gamma-induced protein 10 (IP-10), interferon-inducible T-cell α chemoattractant (I-TAC), and monokine induced by gamma interferon (MIG).

13.2.6 FENUGREEK (*TRIGONELLA FOENUM-GRAECUM*)

Fenugreek (*T. foenum-graecum*) is an important species of the Fabaceae family. It is an annual herb that has been used widely in the Indian (Ayurvedic) system of medicine. Medicinal properties of this herb are due to the presence of alkaloids, saponins, and flavonoids (Yadav et al. 2011). Apart from its traditional medicinal uses, fenugreek is found to have many pharmacological properties, such as antidiabetic, antinociceptive, anticarcinogenic, antioxidant, anti-inflammatory, and hypocholesterolaemic activities (Goyal et al. 2016). Several studies have shown that seeds of fenugreek possess significant immunomodulatory functions. The dietary administration of fenugreek enhances the humoral immune response and the expression of immune-associated genes, particularly IgM gene expression in fish (Bahi et al. 2017). An extract of this plant elicited a significant increase in phagocytic index and phagocytic capacity of macrophages and showed a stimulatory effect on immune functions in mice (Bin-Hafeez et al. 2003). Fenugreek extract cured Th2-induced allergic skin inflammation by enhancing Th1 differentiation and may prove to be a useful therapeutic agent for treatment of allergic inflammatory diseases according to traditional use, as well as Th2-mediated allergic response (Bae et al. 2012). The seeds of this plant also exhibit anti-inflammatory activity by suppressing the production of pro-inflammatory cytokines and IgE-mediated immune response. It also regulates the balance between helper T (T_h) cells (Piao et al. 2017). The administration of *T. foenum-graecum* extract improved metabolic features, and corrected inflammatory alterations associated with ovariectomy and helped in reducing the metabolic and inflammatory alternations associated with menopause (Abedinzade et al. 2015a). Fenugreek seed has been shown to affect immunological responses in piglets after weaning. The addition of fenugreek increased the relative concentration of the γδ T cell population (TCR1+CD8α−) in the blood with a simultaneous reduction of antigen-presenting cells (MHCII+CD5−) (Zentek et al. 2013).

13.2.7   Black Cumin (*Nigella sativa*)

Nigella sativa (black cumin) is a medicinal belonging to the Ranunculaceae family and is native to Southwest Asia, southern Europe, and North Africa, but it is cultivated and used in different parts of the world (Gholamnezhad et al. 2015). Mainly, the seeds of this plant are found to possess immunomodulatory functions along with other medicinal properties, such as antidiabetic, anticancer, analgesic, antimicrobial, anti-inflammatory, gastroprotective, hepatoprotective, and antioxidant properties (Abel-Salam, 2012). Phytochemical analyses of *N. sativa* displayed the presence of alkaloids, saponins, sterols, and essential oil (Ghahramanloo et al. 2017).

Thymoquinone (TQ) is one of the main active components of the volatile oil of *N. sativa* seeds and most effects and actions of *N. sativa* are mainly related to TQ concentration (Samarghandian et al. 2018). The oil and extracts of this plant were found to suppress humoral immune response while alleviating the cell-mediated response (Majdalawieh and Fayyad, 2015). The oil of *N. sativa*, combined with artemether (ART) and praziquantel (PZQ), was used to check the immune and inflammatory response of mice infected with *Schistosoma mansoni*. Immunity of host was improved after administration of *N. sativa* oil, and levels of cytokines and IgG in the blood significantly increased (Sheir et al. 2015). Due to its ability to suppress the inflammatory mediators, *N. sativa* oil was also reported to enhance cell-mediated immunity in immuno-suppressed male rabbits (Salem, 2005). Another study revealed the immunostimulatory effect of *N. sativa* seeds on non-phytohaemagglutinin (PHA) -stimulated proliferation of human peripheral blood mononuclear cells (PBMCs). PHA was used to trigger B and T lymphocyte proliferation by interaction between active components of extracts and cell surface molecules or growth factors involved in non-PHA activation. *N. sativa* was reported to have chemopreventive or anticancer activities as a result of immunostimulatory activity (Alshatwi, 2014). Elmowalid et al. (2013) reported that an extract of this plant showed prominent increases in the microbicidal activity of monocyte-derived macrophages against yeast or bacteria, enhancing the activity of macrophages (innate immunity) and also regulating adaptive immunity to infectious diseases (Elmowalid et al. 2013). Recently, it was also observed that *N. sativa* has potential antiviral activity against COVID-19. The seeds and oil of *N. sativa* can be considered to be a first aid kit as a preventive measure against COVID-19. The bioactive compounds, thymoquinone, α-hederin, or nigellidine, could be promising alternative herbal drugs with which to combat COVID-19 (Islam et al. 2021). *In-silico* studies proved that the bioactive constituents of this plant can bind with the ACE2 receptors, while the bioactive phytoconstituents are involved in molecular pathways like HIF1, VEGF, IL-17, AGE-RAGE, chemokine and calcium signalling pathways, which can be particularly helpful in combating hypoxia and inflammation caused by a compromised immune system and oxidative stress (Jakhmola et al. 2020).

13.2.8   Garlic (*Allium sativum*)

Garlic (*A. sativum*; Amaryllidaceae) originates from Central Asia and has been used as a medicinal plant for thousands of years. It contains organosulphur compounds, such as ajoene, allicin, alliin, allixin, γ glutamyl-S-2-propenyl cysteine, diallyl disul-phide, methyl allyl disulphide, S-allyl-cysteine, and 1,2-vinyldiithin (Martin et al. 2016). Allicin inhibited TNF-α-induced secretion of IL-1β, IL-8, IP-10, and IFN-γ and also achieved suppression of the degradation of the NF-κB inhibitory protein IκB in intestinal epithelial cells (Lang et al. 2004). Thus, allicin may have the poten-tial to attenuate intestinal inflammation. Garlic appears to enhance the functioning of the immune system by stimulating certain cell types, such as macrophages, lym-phocytes, natural killer (NK) cells, dendritic cells, and eosinophils *via* modulation of cytokine secretion, immunoglobulin production, phagocytosis, and macrophage activation (Arreola et al. 2015). Several garlic associated compounds, such as ajoene, allicin, allyl, methyl thiosulphinate, and methyl allyl thiosulphinate, have been found to possess high viricidal activity (Mikaili et al. 2013).

13.2.9 Ginger (*Zingiber officinale*)

Ginger (*Z. officinale*; family Zingiberaceae) is widely used in folk medicine and as a spice. The bioactive molecules present in ginger include α-zingiberene, α-farnesene, β-bisabolene, α-curcumene, [6]-gingerol and [6]-shogaol, paradol, zingerones, and allied derivatives (Zhan et al., 2008). Ginger is consumed in many cultures as an immune booster (Kannappan et al., 2011). Ginger extracts have been reported to have anti-inflammatory, anti-oxidant, and anti-cancer effects. 6-Shogaol is one of the most bioactive components of ginger rhizomes and possesses neuroprotective, neurotrphic, and anti-inflammatory properties. It was shown to suppress the release of pro-inflammatory cytokines and decreased the level of inducible nitric oxide synthase (iNOS), cyclooxygenase-2 (COX-2), and phospho-NF-kB in LPS-treated astrocytes, as well as up-regulated histone H3 acetylation and suppressed histone deacetylase (HDAC)1 expression (Shim et al. 2011). [6]-Gingerol inhibits COX-2 expression by blocking the activation of p38 MAP kinase and NF-κB in phorbol ester-stimulated mouse skin (Kim et al. 2005). Ginger ameliorated allergic asthma by reducing inflammation of the allergic airway and suppressed Th2-mediated immune responses in mice with ovalbumin-induced allergic asthma (Khan et al. 2015). An *in-vitro* study indicated that 6-gingerol could alleviate allergic rhinitis by reducing cytokine production for T cell activation and inhibiting the activation of B cells and mast cells (Kawamoto et al. 2016).

13.2.10 Capsicum

Capsaicin (*trans*-8-methyl-*N*-vanillyl-6-nonenamide) is the principal component of hot peppers, in the genus *Capsicum*. It has been employed in pain relief, weight loss, and cancer prevention (Luo et al. 2011). Capsaicin from juice of *Capsicum baccatum* exhibited an anti-inflammatory effect by inhibition of the production of pro-inflammatory cytokines (TNF-alpha and IL-1-beta) at the inflammatory site in mouse inflammatory immune peritonitis. Furthermore, capsaicin was able to inhibit the neutrophil migration towards the inflammatory site (Spiller et al. 2008). Capsaicin has been shown to suppress cell proliferation and to trigger apoptosis of Multiple Myeloma (MM) cells, by reducing STAT3 phosphorylation and activation

(Bhutani et al. 2007). Cytotoxic anticancer therapeutics induce immunogenic cell death (ICD), inducing tumour cells to undergo apoptosis while eliciting the emission of a spatiotemporally defined combination of damage-associated molecular patterns (DAMPs) which is decoded by the immune system to activate antitumour immunity for long-term therapeutic success. The neurotoxin capsaicin (CPS) can induce both cancer cell apoptosis and immune-mediated tumour regression (D'Eliseo et al., 2013). It has been reported that capsaicin reduced the Mcl-1 expression level, leading to the capsaicin-mediated cell death and autophagy induction (Granato et al. 2015).

13.2.11   OMUM (*TRACHYSPERMUM AMMI*)

Omum (*T. ammi*), commonly known as ajwain, ajowan, caraway, Bishop's weed, or carom, is an annual herb of the family Apiaceae (previously, the Umbelliferae). It has been used in food preparation and also as a traditional medicine in Ayurveda. Although a number of pharmacological activities have been attributed to ajowan, its role in immunomodulation is not known. Ajowan glycoprotein (Agp) showed effective mitogenic activity towards splenocytes, induced proliferation of B cell-enriched murine splenocytes and activated macrophages to release NO, promoted phagocytosis, and produced pro-inflammatory cytokines (IL-12, TNF-α and IFN-γ) (Shruthi et al. 2017). Seed extracts of *T. ammi* exhibited an immunomodulatory effect on cell-mediated immunity through the delayed-type hypersensitivity assay skin thickness method (Siddiqui et al. 2019). The carvacrol present in ajwain oil showed an inhibitory effect on TNF-α, IL-1β, and TGF-β (Liu et al. 2012). Carvacrol also inhibited secretion of TNF-α and IL-1β in porcine alveolar macrophages (Liu 2011).

13.2.12   ASAFOETIDA (*FERULA ASSAFOETIDA*)

Asafoetida (known as Heeng in India), an oleo-gum-resin obtained from the roots of *Ferula assafoetida*, is used in different countries for various purposes. This oleo-gum-resin has been known to possess antifungal, antidiabetic, anti-inflammatory, antimutagenic, and antiviral activities (Iranshahi and Iranshahi 2010). The oleogum-resin, ferulic acid, and the essential oil of *F. assafoetida* has shown cytotoxic effect on 4T1 breast cancer cells (Bagheri et al. 2017).

13.2.13   SAFFRON (*CROCUS SATIVUS*)

The dark red stigma of *C. sativus* has a very long history as a food colouring and flavouring agent. The main bioactive metabolites of the saffron spice are the carotenoids (Poma et al. 2012; Hosseini et al. 2018). Saffron has an inhibitory effect on production of the inflammatory cytokines, IL-1β, IL-4, IL-5, IL-6, IL-8, IL-13, tumour necrosis factor alpha (TNF-α), interferon gamma (IFN-γ), TGF-β, and VEGF (Umigai et al. 2012; Zeinali et al. 2019). Saffron down-regulates the key pro-inflammatory enzymes such as myeloperoxidase (MPO), cyclooxygenase-2 (COX-2), inducible nitric oxide synthase (iNOS), phospholipase A2, and prostanoids (Zeinali et al. 2019).

13.3 CONCLUSION AND FUTURE PERSPECTIVES

An ancient Indian text says, 'aushadham ucchyathe sarvam', which implies that food is the absolute cure and healer. Ayurveda promotes a number of herbs and spices for boosting immunity. However, scientific exploration of diet–health linkages is a significant area of research. Spices and their active ingredients possess immunomodulatory properties acting through activation/or suppression of immune systems *via* interfering with several pathways, culminating in improved immune responses. In addition, some of these spices possess antioxidant properties which are important for their anti-inflammatory and anticancer activities. Evidence from *in-vitro* and *in-vivo* studies into the active constituents of spices indicate that many of the active phytochemicals from various spices may reduce the risk or severity of disease by boosting immunity. However, before the therapeutic use of spices as immune booster, this must be thoroughly investigated and information must be disseminated to the various stakeholders with respect to the efficacies and health benefit claims associated with the respective spices.

REFERENCES

Abedinzade, M., S. Nasri, M.J. Omodi, E. Ghasemi, and A. Ghorbani. 2015a. Efficacy of *Trigonella foenum-graecum* seed extract in reducing metabolic and inflammatory alterations associated with menopause. *Iranian Red Crescent Medical Journal* 17: 362–365.

Abedinzade, M., S.Nasri, M. Jamal Omodi, E. Ghasemi, and A. Ghorbani. 2015b. Efficacy of *Trigonella foenum-graecum* seed extract in reducing metabolic and inflammatory alterations associated with menopause. *Iranian Red Crescent Medical Journal* 17: e26685.

Abel-Salam, B.K. 2012. Immunomodulatory effects of black seeds and garlic on alloxan-induced diabetes in albino rat. *Allergologia et Immunopathologia (Madr)* 40: 336–40.

Alshatwi, A.A.,2014. Bioactivity-guided identification to delineate the immunomodulatory effects of methanolic extract of *Nigella sativa* seed on human peripheral blood mononuclear cells. *Chinese Journal of Integrative Medicine* 2: 1–6.

Amati, L., D. Cirimele, V. Pugliese, V. Covelli, F. Resta, and E. Jirillo. 2003. Nutrition and immunity: laboratory and clinical aspects. *Current Pharmaceutical Design* 9: 1924–1931.

Araki K., T. Shinozaki, Y. Irie, and Y. Miyazawa. 1999. Trial of oral administration of *Bifidobacterium breve* for the prevention of rotavirus infections. *Kansenshogaku Zasshi* 73: 305–310.

Arreola, R., S. Quintero-Fabián, R.I. López-Roa, E.O. Flores-Gutiérrez, J.P. Reyes-Grajeda, L. Carrera-Quintanar, and D. Ortuño-Sahagún. 2015. Immunomodulation and anti-inflammatory effects of garlic compounds. *Journal of Immunology Research* 2015: 401630.

Ashrafizadeh, M., H. Rafiei, R. Mohammadinejad, E.G. Afshar, T. Farkhondeh, and S. Samarghandian. 2020. Potential therapeutic effects of curcumin mediated by JAK/STAT signaling pathway: a review. *Phytotherapy Research* https://doi.org/10.1002/ptr.6642

Bae, G.S., M.S. Kim, W.S. Jung, S.W. Seo, S.W. Yun, S.G. Kim, R.K Park, E.C Kim, H.J. Song, and S.J. Park. 2010. Inhibition of lipopolysaccharide-induced inflammatory responses by piperine. *European Journal of Pharmacology* 642: 154–162.

Bae, M.J., H.S. Shin, D.W. Choi, and D.H. Shon. 2012. Antiallergic effect of *Trigonella foenum-graecum* L. extracts on allergic skin inflammation induced by trimellitic anhydride in BALB/c mice. *Journal of Ethnopharmacology* 144: 514–22.

Bagheri, S.M., A.A. Asl, A. Shams, S.A. Mirghanizadeh-Bafghi, and Z. Hafizibarjin. 2017. Evaluation of cytotoxicity effects of oleo-Gum-Resin and its essential oil of *Ferula assa-foetida* and ferulic acid on 4T1 breast cancer cells. *Indian Journal of Medical and Paediatric Oncology: Official Journal of Indian Society of Medical and Paediatric Oncology* 38: 116.

Bahi, A., F.A. Guardiola, C.M. Messina, A. Mahdhi, R. Cerezuela, A. Santulli, ... & M.A. Esteban. 2017. Effects of dietary administration of fenugreek seeds, alone or in combination with probiotics, on growth performance parameters, humoral immune response and gene expression of gilthead seabream (*Sparus aurata* L.). *Fish and Shellfish Immunology* 60: 50–58.

Bhutani, M., A.K. Pathak, A.S. Nair, A.B. Kunnumakkara, S. Guha, G. Sethi, and B.B. Aggarwal. 2007. Capsaicin is a novel blocker of constitutive and interleukin-6-inducible STAT3 activation. *Clinical Cancer Research* 13: 3024–3032.

Bin-Hafeez, B., Haque, R., and S. Parvez. 2003. Immunomodulatory effects of fenugreek (*Trigonella foenum-graecum* L.) extract in mice. *International Immunopharmacology* 3: 257–65.

Catanzaro, M., E. Corsini, M. Rosini, M. Racchi, and C. Lanni. 2018. Immunomodulators inspired by nature: a review on Curcumin and Echinacea. *Molecules (Basel, Switzerland)*, 23: 2778.

Cherng, J.M., W. Chiang, and L.C. Chiang. 2008. Immunomodulatory activities of common vegetables and spices of umbelliferae and its related coumarins and flavonoids. *Food Chemistry* 106: 944–950.

Coutsoudis, A., P. Kiepiela, H.M. Coovadia, and M. Broughton. 1992. Vitamin A supplementation enhances specific IgG antibody levels and total lymphocyte numbers while improving morbidity in measles. *Pediatric Infectious Disease Journal* 11: 203–209.

Chuchawankul, S., N. Khorana, and Y. Poovorawan. 2012. Piperine inhibits cytokine production by human peripheral blood mononuclear cells. *Genetics and Molecular Research* 11: 617–27.

de Lopes, A., F.N. da Fonseca, T.M. Rocha, L.B. de Freitas, E.V.O. Araújo, D.V.T. Wong, R.C.P.L. Júnior, and L.K.A.M. Leal. 2018. Eugenol as a promising molecule for the treatment of dermatitis: antioxidant and anti-inflammatory activities and its nanoformulation. *Oxidative Medicine and Cellular Longevity.* https://doi.org/10.1155/2018/8194849

D'Eliseo, D., L. Manzi, and F. Velotti. 2013. Capsaicin as an inducer of damage-associated molecular patterns (DAMPs) of immunogenic cell death (ICD) in human bladder cancer cells. *Cell Stress & Chaperones*, 18: 801–808.

Elsayed, Y., and N.A. Khan. 2020. Immunity-boosting spices and the novel Coronavirus. *ACS Chemical Neuroscience* 11(12).

Elmowalid, G., A.M. Amar, and A.A. Ahmad. 2013. *Nigella sativa* seed extract: 1. Enhancement of sheep macrophage immune functions *in vitro*. *Research in Veterinary Science* 95: 437–443.

Field, C.J., I.R. Johnson, and P.D. Schley. 2002. Nutrients and their role in host resistance to infection. *Journal of Leukocyte Biology* 71: 16–32.

Ghahramanloo, K.H., B. Kamalidehghan, H.A. Javar, R.T. Widodo, K. Majidzadeh, and M.I. Noordin. 2017. Comparative analysis of essential oil composition of Iranian and Indian *Nigella sativa* L. Extracted using supercritical fluid extraction and solvent extraction. *Drug Design Development and Therapy* 11: 2221–2226.

Gholamnezhad, Z., R. Keyhanmanesh, and M.H. Boskabady. 2015. Anti-inflammatory, antioxidant, and immunomodulatory aspects of *Nigella sativa* for its preventive and bronchodilatory effects on obstructive respiratory diseases: a review of basic and clinical evidence. *Journal of Functional Foods* 17: 910–927.

Giuliani, C., I. Bucci, and G. Napolitano. 2018. The role of the transcription factor nuclear factor-kappa b in thyroid autoimmunity and cancer. *Frontiers in Endocrinology* 9: 471.

Goyal, S., N. Gupta, and S. Chatterjee. 2016. Investigating therapeutic potential of *Trigonella foenum-graecum* L. as our defense mechanism against several human diseases. *Journal of Toxicology* 2016: Article ID 1250387.

Granato, M., M.S.G. Montani, M. Filardi, A. Faggioni, and M. Cirone. 2015. Capsaicin triggers immunogenic PEL cell death, stimulates DCs and reverts PEL-induced immune suppression. *Oncotarget* 6: 29543–29554.

Grespan, R., M. Paludo, L.H. de Paula, C.P. Barbosa, C.A. Bersani-Amado, M.M. Dalalio, and R.K.N. Cuman. 2012. Anti-arthritic effect of eugenol on collagen-induced arthritis experimental model. *Biological and Pharmaceutical Bulletin* 35: 1818–1820.

Halder, S, A.K. Mehta, P.K. Mediratta, and K.K. Sharma. 2011. Essential oil of clove (*Eugenia caryophyllata*) augments the humoral immune response but decreases cell mediated immunity. *Phytotherapy Research* 25: 1254–1256.

Han, X. and T.L. Parker. 2017. Anti-inflammatory activity of clove (*Eugenia caryophyllata*) essential oil in human dermal fibroblasts. *Pharmaceutical Biology* 55: 1619–1622.

Hatakka, K., E. Savilahti, A. Pönkä, J.H. Meurman, T. Poussa, L. Näse M. Saxelin, and R. Korpela. 2001. Effect of long term consumption of probiotic milk on infections in children attending day care centers: Double blind, randomized trial. *British Medical Journal* 322: 1–5.

Hosseini, A., B.M. Razavi, and H. Hosseinzadeh. 2018. Pharmacokinetic properties of Saffron and its active components. *European Journal of Drug Metabolism and Pharmacokinetics* 43: 383–390.

Hu, R.W., E.J. Carey, K.D. Lindor, and J.H.Tabibian. 2017. Curcumin in hepatobiliary disease: Pharmacotherapeutic properties and emerging potential clinical applications. *Annals of Hepatology* 16: 835–841.

Iranshahi, M., and M. Iranshahi. 2010. Traditional uses, phytochemistry and pharmacology of Asafoetida (*Ferula assa-foetida* oleo-gum-resin)—a review. *Journal of Ethnopharmacology* 134: 1–10.

Islam, M.N., K.S. Hossain, P.P. Sarker, J. Ferdous, M.A Hannan, M.M. Rahman, D.T. Chu, and M.J. Uddin. 2021. Revisiting pharmacological potentials of *Nigella sativa* seed: A promising option for COVID-19 prevention and cure. *Phytotherapy Research* 35: 1329–1344.

Islamuddin, M., G. Chouhan, M.Y. Want, H.A. Ozbak, H.A. Hemeg, and F. Afrin. 2016. Immunotherapeutic potential of eugenol emulsion in experimental visceral Leishmaniasis. *PLOS Neglected Tropical Disease* 10: e0005011.

Jakhmola, M.R., N. Sehgal, N. Dogra, S. Saxena, and D.P. Katare, 2020. Deciphering underlying mechanism of Sars-CoV-2 infection in humans and revealing the therapeutic potential of bioactive constituents from *Nigella sativa* to combat COVID19: *in-silico* study. *Journal of Biomolecular Structure and Dynamics* 28: 1–13.

Kaminogawa, S., and M. Nanno. 2004. Modulation of immune functions by foods. *Evidence-Based Complementary and Alternative Medicine 1*: Article ID 928435, 10 pages.

Kannappan, R., S.C. Gupta, J.H. Kim, S. Reuter, and B.B. Aggarwal. 2011. Neuroprotection by spice-derived nutraceuticals: You are what you eat. *Molecular Neurobiology* 44: 142–159.

Kawamoto, Y., Y. Ueno, E. Nakahashi, M. Obayashi, K. Sugihara, S. Qiao, M. Iida, M.Y. Kumasaka, I. Yajima, Y. Goto, N. Ohgami, M. Kato, and K. Takeda. 2016. Prevention of allergic rhinitis by ginger and the molecular basis of immunosuppression by 6-gingerol through T cell inactivation. *Journal of Nutritional Biochemistry* 27: 112–122.

Khan, A.M., M. Shahzad, M.B.R. Asim, M. Imran, and A. Shabbir. 2015. *Zingiber officinale* ameliorates allergic asthma via suppression of Th2-mediated immune response. *Pharmaceutical Biology* 53: 359–367.

Kim, S.S., O.J. Oh, H.Y. Min, E.J. Park, Y. Kim, H.J. Park, Y.N. Han, and S.K. Lee 2003. Eugenol suppresses cyclooxygenase-2 expression in lipopolysaccharide-stimulated mouse macrophage RAW264.7 cells. *Life Science* 73: 337–348.

Kim, S.O., J.K. Kundu, Y.K. Shin, J.H. Park, M.H. Cho, T.Y. Kim, and Y.J. Surh. 2005. [6]-Gingerol inhibits COX-2 expression by blocking the activation of p38 MAP kinase and NF-κ B in phorbol ester-stimulated mouse skin. *Oncogene* 24: 2558–2567.

Kwiatkowski, P., B.Wojciuk, I. Wojciechowska-Koszko, Ł. Łopusiewicz, B. Grygorcewicz, A. Pruss, M. Sienkiewicz, K. Fijałkowski, E. Kowalczyk, and B. Dołęgowska, 2020. Innate immune response against *Staphylococcus aureus* preincubated with subinhibitory concentration of *trans*-Anethole. *International Journal of Molecular Sciences* 21: 4178.

Lang A, M. Lahav, E. Sakhnini, I. Barshack, H.H. Fidder, B. Avidan, E. Bardan, R. Hershkoviz, S. Bar-Meir, and Y. Chowers. 2004. Allicin inhibits spontaneous and TNF-alpha induced secretion of proinflammatory cytokines and chemokines from intestinal epithelial cells. *Clinical Nutrition (Edinburg Scotland)* 23: 1199–1208.

Lau, D., H. Mollnau, J.P. Eiserich, B.A. Freeman, A. Daiber, U.M. Gehling, J. Brümmer, V. Rudolph, T. Münzel, T. Heitzer, T. Meinertz, and S. Baldus. 2005. Myeloperoxidase mediates neutrophil activation by association with CD11b/CD18 integrins, *Proceedings of the National Academy of Sciences of the United States of America* 102: 431–436.

Lee, S.C, J.S. Hsu, C.C. Li, K.M. Chen, and C.T. Liu. 2015. Protective effect of leaf essential Oil from *Cinnamomum osmophloeum* Kanehira on endotoxin-induced intestinal injury in mice associated with suppressed local expression of molecules in the signaling pathways of TLR4 and NLRP3. *PLoS ONE* 10: e0120700.

Liao, B.C., C.W. Hsieh, Y.C. Liu, T.T. Tzeng, Y.W. Sun, and B.S. Wung. 2008. Cinnamaldehyde inhibits the tumor necrosis factor-alpha-induced expression of cell adhesion molecules in endothelial cells by suppressing NF-kappaB activation: effects upon IkappaB and Nrf2. *Toxicology and Applied Pharmacology* 229: 161–171.

Liu, Y. 2011. *Effects of Plant Extracts on Immune Function and Disease Resistance in Pigs*, University of Illinois, Urbana, Ill, USA, 2011.

Liu, Y., M. Song, T.M. Che, D. Bravo, and J.E. Pettigrew. 2012. Anti-inflammatory effects of several plant extracts on porcine alveolar macrophages in vitro. *Journal of Animal Science* 90: 2774–2783.

Luo, X.J., J. Peng, and Y.J. Li. 2011. Recent advances in the study on capsaicinoids and capsinoids. *European Journal of Pharmacology* 650: 1–7.

Majdalawieh, A.F., and M.W. Fayyad. 2015. Immunomodulatory and anti-inflammatory action of *Nigella sativa* and thymoquinone: a comprehensive review. *International Immunopharmacology* 28: 295–304.

Marín, Y.E., B.A. Wall, S. Wang, J. Namkoong, J.J. Martino, J. Suh, H.J. Lee, A.B. Rabson, C.S. Yang, S. Chen, and J.H. Ryu. 2007. Curcumin down regulates the constitutive activity of NF-kappaB and induces apoptosis in novel mouse melanoma cells. *Melanoma Research* 17: 274–283.

Martins, N., S. Petropoulos, and I.C. Ferreira. 2016. Chemical composition and bioactive compounds of garlic (*Allium sativum* L.) as affected by pre-and post-harvest conditions: a review. *Food Chemistry* 211: 41–50.

Meydani, S.N., M.P. Barklund, Liu S, M. Meydani, R.A. Miller, J.G. Cannon, F.D. Morrow, R. Rocklin, and J.B. Blumberg. 1990. Vitamin E supplementation enhances cell-mediated immunity in healthy elderly subjects. *American Journal of Clinical Nutrition* 52: 557–563.

Mikaili, P., S. Maadirad, M. Moloudizargari, S. Aghajanshakeri, and S. Sarahroodi 2013. Therapeutic uses and pharmacological properties of garlic, shallot, and their biologically active compounds. *Iranian Journal of Basic Medical Sciences*, 16: 1031.

Momtazi-Borojeni, A.A., S.M. Haftcheshmeh, S.A. Esmaeili, T.P. Johnston, E. Abdollahi, and A. Sahebkar. 2018. Curcumin: a natural modulator of immune cells in systemic lupus erythematosus. *Autoimmunity Review* 17: 125–135.

Nagafuchi, S., M. Totsuka, S. Hachimura, M. Goto, T. Takahashi, T. Yajima, T. Kuwata, and S. 2000. Dietary nucleotides increase the proportion of a TCR gammadelta+ subset of intraepithelial lymphocytes (IEL) and IL-7 production by intestinal epithelial cells (IEC); implications for modification of cellular and molecular cross-talk between IEL and IEC by dietary nucleotides. *Bioscience, Biotechnology, and Biochemistry* 64: 1459.

Nelson, K.M., J.L. Dahlin, J. Bisson, J. Graham, G.F. Pauli, and M.A. Walters. 2017. The essential medicinal chemistry of Curcumin. *Journal of Medicinal Chemistry* 60: 1620–1637.

Patra, J.K., G. Das, S. Bose, S. Banerjee, C.N. Vishnuprasad, M.D.P. Rodriguez-Torres, and H.S. Shin. 2020. Star anise (*Illicium verum*): chemical compounds, antiviral properties, and clinical relevance. *Phytotherapy Research* 34: 1248–1267.

Piao, C.H., T.T. Bui, C.H.Song, H.S Shin, D.H Shon, and O.H. Chai. 2017. *Trigonella foenum-graecum* alleviates airway inflammation of allergic asthma in ovalbumin-induced mouse model. *Biochemical and Biophysical Research Communications* 482: 1284–88.

Poma, A., Fontecchio, G., Carlucci, G., and G. Chichiricco. 2012. Anti-inflammatory properties of drugs from saffron crocus. anti-Inflammatory and anti-allergy agents in medicinal chemistry. *Anti-Inflammatory & Anti-Allergy Agents in Medicinal Chemistry (Formerly Current Medicinal Chemistry-Anti-Inflammatory and Anti-Allergy Agents)* 11: 37–51.

Sahebkar, A., A.F.G. Cicero, L.E. Simental-Mendía, B.B. Aggarwal, and S.C. Gupta. 2016. Curcumin downregulates human tumor necrosis factor-α levels: a systematic review and meta-analysis of randomized controlled trials. *Pharmacology Research* 107: 234–242.

Salem, M. 2005. Immunomodulatory and therapeutic properties of the *Nigella sativa* L. seed. *Journal of International Immunopharmacology* 5: 1749–1770.

Samarghandian, S., T. Farkhondeh, and F. Samini. 2018. A review on possible therapeutic effect of Nigella sativa and Thymoquinone in neurodegenerative diseases. *CNS and Neurological Disorders Drug Targets* 17: 412–420.

Sempertegui, F., B. Estrella, E. Correa, L. Aguirre, B. Saa, M. Torres, F. Navarrete, C. Alarcón, J. Carrión, Rodríguez, and J.K. Griffiths. 1996. Effects of short-term zinc supplementation on cellular immunity, respiratory symptoms, and growth of malnourished Equadorian children. *European Journal of Clinical Nutrition* 50: 42–46.

Sheir, S.K., A.M Maghraby, A.H. Mohamed, G.Y. Osman, and S.A. Al-Qormuti, 2015. Immunomodulatory and ameliorative role of *Nigella sativa* oil on *Schistosoma mansoni* infected mice. *Canadian Journal of Pure and Applied Sciences* 9: 3345–55.

Sheppard, F.R., M.R. Kelher, E.E. Moore, N.J. McLaughlin, A. Banerjee, and C.C. Silliman. 2005. Structural organization of the neutrophil NADPH oxidase: phosphorylation and translocation during priming and activation. *Journal of Leukocyte Biology* 78: 1025–1042.

Spiller, F., M.K. Alves, S.M. Vieira, T.A. Carvalho, C.E. Leite, A. Lunardelli, J.A. Poloni, F.Q. Cunha, and J.R. de Oliveira. 2008. Anti-inflammatory effects of red pepper (*Capsicum baccatum*) on carrageenan and antigen-induced inflammation. *Journal of Pharmacy and Pharmacology* 60: 473–478.

Shim S., S. Kim, D.S. Choi, Y.B. Kwon, and J. Kwon. 2011. Anti-inflammatory effects of [6]-shogaol: potential roles of HDAC inhibition and HSP70 induction. *Food and Chemical Toxicology* 49: 2734–2740.

Shruthi, R.R., Y.P. Venkatesh, and G. Muralikrishna. 2017. Structural and functional characterization of a novel immunomodulatory glycoprotein isolated from ajowan (*Trachyspermum ammi* L.). *Glycoconjugate Journal* 34: 499–514.

Siddiqui, M.J., A. Aslam, and T. Khan. 2019. Comparison and evaluation of different seed extracts of Trachyspermum ammi for immunomodulatory effect on cell-mediated immunity through delayed-type hypersensitivity assay skin thickness method. *Journal of Pharmacy and Bioallied Sciences* 11: 43.

Srivastava R.M., S. Singh S.K. Dubey, K. Misra, and A. Khar. 2011. Immunomodulatory and therapeutic activity of curcumin. *International Immunopharmacology* 11: 331–41.

Sung Y.Y., Y.S. Kim, and H.K. Kim. 2012. *Illicium verum* extract inhibits TNF-α- and IFN-γ-induced expression of chemokines and cytokines in human keratinocytes. *Journal of Ethnopharmacoly* 144: 182–189.

Takegoshi, K., H. Nanasawa, H. Itoh, T. Yasuyama, Y. Ohmoto, and K. Sugiyama. 1998. Effects of branched-chain amino acid-enriched nutrient mixture on natural killer cell activity in viral cirrhosis. *Arzneimittelforschung* 48: 701–706.

Umigai, N., Tanaka, J., Tsuruma, K., Shimazawa, M., and Hara, H. 2012. Crocetin, a Carotenoid derivative, inhibits VEGF-induced angiogenesis via suppression of p38 phosphorylation. *Current Neurovascular Research* 9: 102–109.

Vaibhav, K., P. Shrivastava, H. Javed, A. Khan, M.E. Ahmed, R. Tabassum, M.M. Khan, G. Khuwaja, F. Islam, M.S. Siddiqui, M.M. Safhi, and F. Islam. 2012. Piperine suppresses cerebral ischemia-reperfusion-induced inflammation through the repression of COX-2, NOS-2, and NF-κB in middle cerebral artery occlusion rat model. *Molecular and Cellular Biochemistry* 367: 73–84.

Wang-Sheng, C., A. Jie, L. Jian-Jun, H. Lan, X. Zeng-Bao, and L. Chang-Qing 2016. Piperine attenuates lipopolysaccharide (LPS)-induced inflammatory responses in BV2 microglia. *International Immunopharmacology* 42: 44–48.

Yadav, R., R. Kaushik, and D. Gupta. 2011. The health benefits of *Trigonella foenum-graecum*: a review. *International Journal of Engineering Research Applications* 1: 32–35.

Zeinali, M., M.R. Zirak, S.A. Rezaee, G. Karimi, and H. Hosseinzadeh. 2019. Immunoregulatory and anti-inflammatory properties of *Crocus sativus* (Saffron) and its main active constituents: a review. *Iranian Journal of Basic Medical Sciences* 22: 334.

Zentek, J., S. Gärtner, L. Tedin, K. Männer, A. Mader, and W. Vahjen. 2013. Fenugreek seed affects intestinal microbiota and immunological variables in piglets after weaning. *British Journal of Nutrition* 109: 859–866.

Zhan, K., C. Wang, K. Xu, and H. Yin. 2008. Analysis of volatile and non-volatile compositions in ginger oleoresin by gas chromatography-mass spectrometry. *Chinese Journal of Chromatography* 26: 692–696.

14 Specific Fruits and Berries for a Strong Human Immune System

Rakesh Kumar

CONTENTS

14.1 INTRODUCTION

The immune system consists of organs, tissues, cells, and some proteins which collaborate to defend the body against attacks by foreign agents. These agents can be infectious microbes, such as bacteria, viruses, fungi, and parasites. Many microbes and pathogens find our bodies very favourable for their growth, so, they try to enter into our body to achieve multiplication but our immune system tries to check their entry and destroy them. If the immune system fails to check the entry and multiplication of a pathogen, our body becomes infected. The immune system is able to kill each and every pathogen, by recognizing and remembering each different pathogen. Several cells and chemicals take part in this mechanism. These cells work in a collaborative manner to secrete and move powerful chemicals from one site to another. The system automatically upgrades its defences as it is attacked by a new enemy.

Immunity is a complex mechanism which achieves resistance against foreign agents by either inbuilt ('innate immunity') or acquired means ('adaptive immunity'), functioning in a collaborative manner. Nutrition plays an important role in developing natural resistance. Poor nutrition or, worse, malnutrition badly affects our immune system and suppress its function (Coico and Sunshine 2009). Our

DOI: 10.1201/9781003137955-14

immune system can be boosted by balanced nutrition, so diet can be very important for improving the efficiency of immune system. Immunity functions can be damaged by a low-nutrient diet deficient in either macronutrients or micronutrients. The strength of body defence can be enhanced or improved if a balanced diet or proper nutrition are provided. Reports indicate that a balanced diet is important to carry out the vital role supporting the immune system (Chandra 1997). Negative mental state, anxiety, or traumas lead to malfunctioning of the immune system and decrease body resistance by destruction of proteins. Malnutrition during childhood causes infections and its complications compromise immunity, leading to illness and premature mortality (Chandra 1997, 2003). This book chapter highlights the structure of the immune system and the role of nutrition on immune function. It also describes the effect of the intake of specific fruits and berries on immune function.

14.2   STRUCTURE OF THE IMMUNE SYSTEM

The defence system in our bodies that protects us against harmful substances or pathogens is called the immune system. It consists of many physical (e.g., skin) and biochemical barriers for self-defence (Karacabey 2012). Macrophages and neutrophils are non-specific cells that can enhance the defence competency of phagocytes and stimulate the immune system. The production of many substances, like interferons, interleukins, and other sophisticated compounds, is stimulated when these substances are added onto the surfaces of phagocytes and lymphocyte cells, so that the immune system is activated (Karacabey 2012).

A healthy immune system has the capability to identify and distinguish the body's own cells and foreign cells. The body's own cells and foreign cells are known as 'self' cells and 'non-self' cells, respectively. The defence system behaves in a friendly and peaceful manner with cells that are identified as self cells, but it quickly launches an attack against non-self or foreign cells. This type of response of immune system is called an autoimmune reaction (Basoglu and Turnagol 2004; Akalin and Unal 2005; Coskun 2005; Karacabey 2005; Saygin et al. 2006; Palmer 2011; Cantorna et al. 2012). Technically, an antigen is an element that can trigger the immune response. An antigen can be any foreign element, like a bacterium, virus, or any other microbe or even a part of it. Tissue or cells from of a different genotype also act as antigens. Such behaviour of the immune system explains how the body rejects transplanted tissues or organs. But, during abnormal behaviour, sometimes, the defence system can make a mistake in distinguishing self and non-self cells and can harm self cells; this type of behaviour of body is called an *autoimmune disorder* or disease. Sometimes, in special cases, the defence system reacts against comparatively harmless substances like pollen, identifying them as antigens, and this type of antigen may be termed an allergen.

Our defence or immune system consists of various parts like the lymphoid organs, thymus, spleen, lymphoid nodes, and several cell types located throughout the body. As soon as pathogenic substances enter into the body, the immune system starts working against invaders; this type of act of immune system is known as the *immune response* (Keith and Jeejeebhoy 1997; Coico and Sunshine 2009; Bistrian 2011).

14.3   IMMUNITY: TYPES AND MECHANISMS

The immunity has been conceptually divided into two types, namely innate and adaptive immunity. Innate immunity is inbuilt. Basically, it is the first line of defence in the form of physical and biochemical barriers and is represented by some specialized cells. It activates instantly when the body comes into contact with a foreign agent (Medzhitov and Janeway 2000). The mechanism of innate immunity is composed of various specialized cells, like macrophages, neutrophils, dendritic cells, and natural killer cells. Its mechanism depends upon the process of phagocytosis, the release of inflammatory mediators, activation of proteins of the complement system, and synthesis of acute phase proteins (Medzhitov et al. 1997). During the process of phagocytosis, the pathogen attaches to surface receptors on the phagocyte, which then starts internalizing into vesicles. These vesicles are called phagosomes, which later fuse to form a lysosome, and subsequently digestion of the pathogen starts (Abbas and Lichtman 2003).

The acquired or adaptive immune response is different from the innate response. The acquired immune response basically depends on lymphocyte activation and on the production of soluble molecules. The main features of the acquired response are specificity and diversity of recognition, memory, specialized response, self-restraint, and tolerance of self components of the organism. In the mechanism of acquired immune response, antigen-presenting cells play a key role in the activation of lymphocytes, and presenting antigens are associated with molecules of the major histocompatibility complex (MHC) to the T lymphocytes (Delves and Roitt 2000). The outline of immunity, the various types and its components is depicted in Figure 14.1.

14.4   EFFECTS OF NUTRITION ON THE IMMUNE SYSTEM

Malnutrition is a very serious problem in the world, especially in developing countries. According to estimates, approximately 6 million children of the world die due to infection because of breakdown of the immune system caused by malnutrition. Therefore, our diet must be balanced and rich in adequate proteins to keep our immune system strong (Chandra 2003). Vitamins, mineral nutrients, and beta-carotene are also very important components of our daily diet, which are thought to contribute to our first line of defence against free radicals. Our body requires free radicals for smooth metabolic functioning but, when present in excessive quantities, they become dangerous ('reactive oxygen species', ROS). Compounds which provide protection against free radicals, and the oxidation and subsequent damage of substances such as membrane fats are called antioxidants. Antioxidants trap or quench ROS and prevent the oxidation of substances like fats (Greiner 2011).

It has been very well reviewed and documented by various researchers and authors that micronutrients (vitamins and minerals) play a very important role in boosting

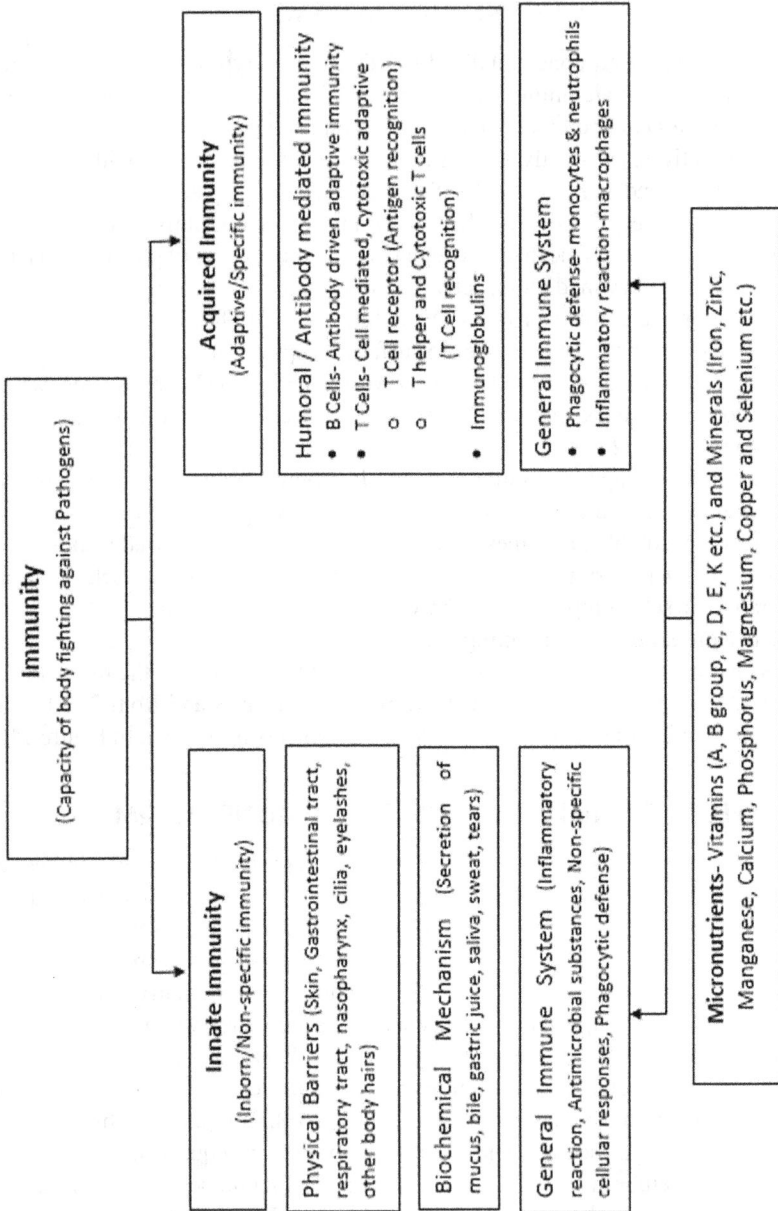

FIGURE 14.1 Outline of the immune system of our body and the role of micronutrients.

the immune system. Various vitamins and minerals has been reported to maintain the structural and functional integrity of physical barriers, such as the skin, digestive tract, and respiratory tract (Clairmont et al. 1996; Gniadecki et al. 1997; Palmer et al. 2001; Chew and Park 2004; Gombart 2009; Yin et al. 2011; Haryanto et al. 2015; Sirisinha 2015; Biesalski 2016; Clark and Mach 2016; Levy 2016; Carr and Maggini 2017; Lin et al. 2017; Mihajlovic et al. 2017; Yoshii et al. 2019); to allow differentiation, proliferation, movement, and functioning of innate immune cells (Tanaka et al. 1991; Sly et al. 2001; WHO 2006; Maggini et al. 2008, 2018; Sheikh et al. 2010; Wu and Meydani 2014; Haryanto et al. 2015; Saeed et al. 2016; Carr and Maggini 2017; Wishart 2017; Agoro et al. 2018; Gao et al. 2018; Bozonet and Carr 2019; Wu et al. 2019; MIC 2020); antimicrobial activity (Matsui et al. 1986; Reichel et al. 1987; Rigby et al. 1987; Inoue et al. 1998; Wang et al. 2004; Gombart et al. 2005; Weber and Heilborn 2005; Haryanto et al. 2015; Carr and Maggini 2017; Wu et al. 2019; MIC 2020); inflammation and antioxidant activity (Tanaka et al. 1991; Sly et al. 2001; Topilski et al. 2004; Wintergerst et al. 2006; Maggini et al. 2008; Sakakeeny et al. 2012; Zhang et al. 2012; Haryanto et al. 2015; Lin and Li 2016; Saeed et al. 2016; Carr and Maggini 2017; Jarosz et al. 2017; Ueland et al. 2017; Wishart 2017; Wu et al. 2019; MIC 2020); differentiation, proliferation, and normal functioning of T cells (Penna et al. 2000; Piemonti et al. 2000; Wintergerst et al. 2006; Maggini et al. 2008; Ross 2012; Haryanto et al. 2015; Bscheider and Butcher 2016; Saeed et al. 2016; Carr and Maggini 2017; Sassi et al. 2018; Wu et al. 2019; MIC 2020); antibody production and development (Maggini et al. 2008; Haryanto et al. 2015; Saeed et al. 2016; Carr and Maggini 2017; MIC 2020); and in antibody response to an antigen (Han et al. 2004; Maggini et al. 2008; Saeed et al. 2016; Wu et al. 2019).

Lack of micronutrients represses immune system by weakening individual immune functions. Malnutrition weakens the immunity functions by suppressing the immune system. Recently, increased cases of repressive immune systems have been reported (Palmer 2011). Basoglu and Turnagol (2004) reported that of the factors related to diet, particularly energy intake, macro- and micronutrients are the main effects of malfunction on the immune system.

14.5 ROLE OF FRUITS AND BERRIES ON HEALTH AND IMMUNITY

In botanical terminology, berries are fruits developed from a single flower containing a single ovary, which contain large numbers of seeds. Examples of berry fruits are tomatoes, banana, and grapes, but common 'berries' in the literature, like strawberries, blackberries, blueberries, cranberries, and raspberries, are not included as botanical berries (Figure 14.2). For the present chapter, both types of fruits, i.e., botanical berries and common (but non-botanical) berries are considered. Furthermore, the health effects of some common berry fruits, like grapes, have already been reviewed extensively by several authors (Yang and Xiao 2013; Georgiev et al. 2014; Singh et al. 2015a). Kolouchova-Hanzlikova et al. (2004) reported the presence of a key phytochemical, resveratrol, in grapes, which has been found to be beneficial with respect to improved health in terms of diseases like cancer and cardiovascular disease. Similar results have also been reported by various research groups (Pagliaro et al. 2015;

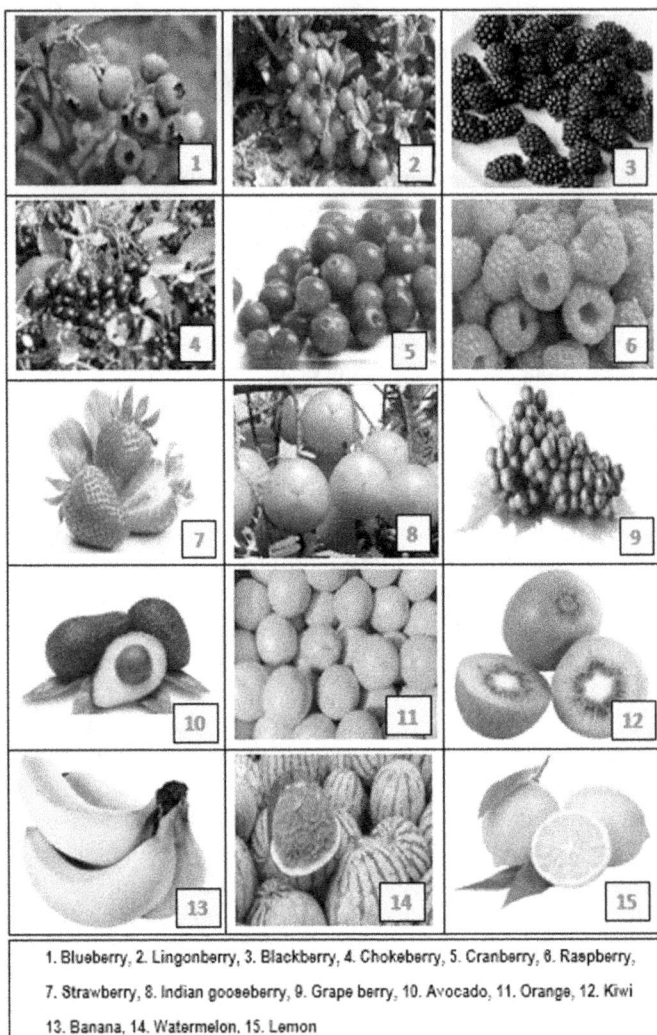

1. Blueberry, 2. Lingonberry, 3. Blackberry, 4. Chokeberry, 5. Cranberry, 6. Raspberry, 7. Strawberry, 8. Indian gooseberry, 9. Grape berry, 10. Avocado, 11. Orange, 12. Kiwi 13. Banana, 14. Watermelon, 15. Lemon

FIGURE 14.2 Immunomodulator fruits and berries.

Singh et al. 2015b; Zulueta et al. 2015; Kursvietiene et al. 2016). Due to the synergistic potential of various berry components, whole berry consumption has shown a clear advantage over consumption of phytochemical supplementation of the diet. Our digestive system also supports consumption of raw fruits in our diet because bioactive compounds (vitamins, minerals, and antioxidants) and beneficial phytochemicals are generally readily extracted by the enzymes, microbiota, and epithelium of the gut.

Several researchers have described and reviewed the beneficial effects of berry fruits due to their bioactive components in relation to various health conditions and diseases like diabetes and obesity (Tsuda 2016), cardiovascular diseases (Basu et al. 2010), cancer development (Kristo et al. 2016), and metabolic syndrome (Vendrame et al. 2016). Comparatively little research has been performed on the potential health benefits of berries on the digestive system but *in vivo* studies have demonstrated that intake of berry fruits had direct, positive effects on the health of the digestive tract, i.e., mouth, oesophagus, stomach, intestine, microbiota and, ultimately, on the immune system. As mentioned in the literature, berries support the function of the digestive system, immune cells, and cellular repair of damage due to cancer. It has been reported that immune cells educated in the gut migrated throughout the body and resulted in suppression of lung carcinoma (Hong et al. 2004). It is very well proved that specific illnesses can be cured by alterations of immune responses, with nutrition playing an important role in developing immunity. So, a comprehensive understanding of these alterations and applications of certain bioactive phytochemicals found in specific berries and fruits can help in improving the immunity of the body.

Fruits, especially berries, have been reported to contain phytochemicals and biochemicals showing antioxidant properties (Jia et al. 2012). The biochemical analysis of fruits shows that berries are excellent source of bioactive compounds like flavonoids, phenolics, and tannins, which, individually or in combination, may be helpful against chronic diseases such as cardiovascular disease, diabetes, cancer, and obesity (Wu et al. 2010). Slavin et al. (2012) and other workers have reviewed and described the relationship between fruit intake and the risk of disease development. Fruits, especially berries, have been reported for their high concentrations of phytochemicals, micronutrients, sugars, etc. (Table 14.1). Phytochemicals are bioactive substances, responsible for colour, aroma, defence, etc. of plants. More than 5,000 phytochemicals have been identified to date in plants. These may be classified into alkaloids, phenolics, nitrogen-containing components, organosulphur components, carotenoids, and phytosterols (Liu 2004). Research findings highlight the use of phytochemicals in the treatment of diseases, such as cancer metastases (Kim et al. 2016; Shankar et al. 2016), inflammatory bowel disease (Kaulmann and Bohn 2016), and obesity-induced insulin resistance (Younus and Anwar 2016), as well as their role in stimulating weight loss (Rupasinghe et al. 2016). Furthermore, studies are being conducted to determine the relationship between fruits and immunity and the mechanisms responsible for any such association.

The health effects of berries have been analysed in *in-vivo* and *in-vitro* studies conducted in animal and human systems. Both types of study have their own merits and demerits, with *in-vitro* studies being mostly conducted for screening and studying the mechanism of action, whereas *in-vivo* studies can be helpful to analyse the beneficial and harmful effects of berry fruit components. Research findings of *in-vivo* studies recommend consumption of whole berries for better results due to their high concentration of phytochemicals and their increased bioavailability and activity in the presence of other components. The phytochemical concentrations of various berries have been identified and listed by the United States Department of Agriculture (USDA) database. Several research groups (Wada and Ou, 2002; Rimando et al. 2004; Ehala et al. 2005; Mertz et al. 2007; Abe et al. 2012; Rodriguez-Mateos et al. 2012) have contributed to the USDA information regarding the consumption of berries.

TABLE 14.1
Various Fruits and Berries and Their Phytochemical and Micronutrient Components (adapted and modified from Giancarlo et al. (2011))

Common Name	Botanical Name	Phytochemicals and Micronutrients
Cornelian cherry	*Cornus mas*	Vitamin C, fructose, minerals and tannins
Red raspberry	*Rubus idaeus*	Phenols, flavonols, such as kaempferol, myricetin, and quercetin
Bilberry	*Vaccinium myrtillus*	Vitamin C, minerals (calcium and iron), fibre, and some antioxidant compounds such as anthocyanins and proanthocyanidins
Sea buckthorn	*Hippophaë rhamnoides*	Vitamins (A, C, E, F, K, and B group), flavonols, and mineral elements such as iron, calcium, magnesium, and copper.
Wild rose	*Rosa canina*	Vitamin C, flavonols, proanthocyanidins, polyphenols, and antioxidants
Elderberry	*Sambucus nigra*	Vitamins A, C, anthocyanins, cyanogenic glucosides
Barbados cherry	*Malpighia glabra*	Vitamins (C, A, B_1, B_6), flavonoids, and minerals (calcium, phosphorus, iron, potassium, and magnesium).
Guava	*Psidium guajava*	Vitamin C, tannins, polyphenols, terpenes, flavonoids, fibre, fatty acids, and minerals (calcium, phosphorus, iron, and manganese).
Pomegranate	*Punica granatum*	Polyphenols, particularly ellagitannins, and antioxidants
Tamarind	*Tamarindus indica*	Vitamin C, phenolics, and antioxidants
Grape	*Vitis vinifera*	Vitamins C, E, A, K, minerals (calcium, iron, phosphorus, zinc, manganese)
Indian gooseberry	*Phyllanthus emblica*	Vitamin C, tannins, and polyphenols
Blueberry	*Vaccinium corymbosum*	Vitamins C, K, micronutrients, and anthocyanins
Lingonberry	*Vaccinium vitis-idaea*	Vitamin C, A, B, minerals (potassium, calcium, magnesium, and phosphorus), and anthocyanins
Blackberry	*Rubus fruticosus*	Vitamins C, K, folic acid, minerals (e.g., manganese), and anthocyanins
Blackcurrant	*Ribes nigrum*	Vitamins C, E, fatty acids, polyphenols, and anthocyanins
Chokeberry	*Aronia* spp.	Vitamin C and polyphenols
Cranberry	*Vaccinium macrocarpon*	Vitamin C, manganese, and polyphenols
Raspberry	*Rubus* spp.	Vitamin A, thiamine, riboflavin, vitamin B_6, calcium, zinc, and anthocyanins
Strawberry	*Fragaria* × *ananassa*	Vitamin C, manganese, and polyphenols

14.6   ROLES OF FRUITS AND BERRIES IN DISEASE PREVENTION AND IMMUNITY

Various research reports have proved that our diet, with adequate fruits and vegetables, makes our immune system stronger and protects us against various chronic diseases, like cardiovascular disease, eye disease, and cancer of the digestive tract, pancreas, and urinary bladder (Crawford et al. 1994; Van Duyn and Pivonka 2000). It is also observed that the habit of mothers of regular fruit consumption has a positive impact on the health and food habits of their children. Studies show that requirement for consuming fruits and vegetables of males and females is different (Wardle et al. 2000; Wang et al. 2002).

Fruits and vegetables are rich source of micronutrients and provide various essential vitamins and elements, such as vitamin C, thiamine, niacin, riboflavin, folic acid, pyridoxine, calcium, potassium, zinc, phosphorus, and dietary fibre. The phytochemicals and bioactive substances present in fruits are powerful antioxidants, which activate metabolism and detoxify carcinogens from our body (Wargovich 2000). Several research groups have reported the value of fruits and berries in supporting and boosting the immune system (Kushi et al. 2012; Sinha et al. 2012; Calder 2013). The antioxidant capacity of various fruits and vegetables can vary greatly (Kalt 2002), so it is advisable to take a combination of various fruits and vegetables in our daily diet. Reports showed that the benefits of consumption of carotenoid-rich fruits has been found to be superior over carotenoid dietary supplements in increasing resistance to low-density lipoprotein (LDL) oxidation, and improving repair of our body cells and DNA (Southon 2000; Seifried et al. 2003). Normally, consumption of fruits like orange, mango, melon, pineapples, grapes, etc. is recommended for a better immune system.

The findings of several studies have shown that intake of fibre from fruit and vegetables is inversely proportional to the incidence of coronary heart disease. Meta-analyses of studies showed that cardiovascular events decreased, when intake of fruits was increased, meaning that consumption of fruits has a positive impact on cardiac health (Dauchet et al. 2005; He et al. 2006). Clinical and biological investigations also support the protective effect of fruit and vegetable intake against coronary heart disease (CHD), diabetes, dyslipidaemia, and hypertension (Appel et al. 1997; Ness and Powles 1997; Van Duyn et al. 2000; Ford and Mokdad 2001; Bazzano et al. 2003; Alonso et al. 2004; He et al. 2006). Similarly, different population studies have also observed a negative correlation between intake of adequate fruits and incidence rates of CHD. Lock et al. (2005), for example, noted a lower risk of cardiac arrest in persons who consumed adequate quantities of fruits.

Studies conducted by Block et al. (1992) and Steinmetz and Potter (1996) have indicated that a diet rich in fruits and vegetables can prevent different types of cancer, of the digestive tract (oropharynx, oesophagus, stomach, colon, and rectum); similarly, Galeone et al. (2007) reported that a high dietary intake of fruits and vegetables can reduce the risk of lung cancer in smokers as well as in non-smokers. Furthermore, adequate intake of fruits and vegetables was shown to reduce the risk of developing cancer by 19% (Van't Veer et al. 2000). It has been reported that dietary supplementation with berry fruits and vegetables is beneficial in arresting old-age-related problems in rats (Joseph et al. 1999). A diet rich in carotenoids, like lutein and zeaxanthin, can be beneficial in preventing damage to the retina caused by light or oxidants (Mares-Perlman et al. 2002). It has been found that these carotenoids are helpful to reduce the risk of age-related macular degeneration (Seddon et al. 1994; Snellen et al. 2002).

Romieu and Trenga (2001) reported that fruit and vegetable consumption is beneficial in reducing the risk of chronic obstructive pulmonary disease. The consumption of apple fruits has also been reported to be associated with better lung function by Tabak et al. (2001) and Butland et al. (2000). Although the actual reason for the beneficial effects of fruit intake in reducing the risk of chronic obstructive pulmonary disease is not known, it is suggested that antioxidants like vitamin C or flavonoids must be playing an important role in reducing the risk of the disease. Some other studies have also demonstrated that a diet rich in antioxidants is found to be beneficial in reducing the risk of developing Alzheimer's disease. This may be due to the fact that fresh fruit juice is rich in micronutrients (minerals and vitamins) which catalyze metabolic reactions occurring in the body. Fruits rich in vitamin C and antioxidants, like citrus fruits, pineapple, grapes, and tomatoes, are helpful in detoxifying the body (Cuthbertson 2002). According to the Department of Health, South Africa (2001), fruits are an important integral part of a healthy diet as they are rich source of vitamins, minerals and other substances that could be useful in boosting the immune function.

14.7   POSSIBLE MECHANISM OF ACTION OF FRUITS IN IMMUNITY AND DISEASE PREVENTION

According to biological concepts, cells are constantly exposed to a range of oxidizing agents. These oxidants may be produced by metabolic activities or food, air, or water may be sources of these agents. However, to sustain optimal physiological conditions, it is important to maintain the balance between oxidants and antioxidants. If the number of oxidants is large in comparison with antioxidants, it can lead to oxidative stress (Ames et al. 1993; Adom et al. 2003). This oxidative stress is responsible for oxidative damage to macromolecules such as lipids, proteins, and DNA, that consequently lead to increased risk of developing chronic diseases like cancer and cardiovascular disease (Ames et al. 1993; Liu et al. 1995). To reduce oxidative stress or improve the oxidant/antioxidant balance, a high concentration of antioxidants is needed. In order to fulfil the demand for sufficient quantities of antioxidants, adequate amounts of fruits rich in antioxidants, such as carotenoids and phenolics, need to be consumed. These antioxidant compounds may help to reduce the risk of developing chronic diseases by protecting cellular systems from oxidative damage (Wang et al. 1996; Vinson et al. 2001; Adom et al. 2003).

Phenolics are secondary plant metabolites of the utmost importance for both plants and humans. In plants, they provide support of reproductive functions and protection from enemies like pathogens, parasites, and predators, whereas, in humans, where they need to be supplied in our diet, phenolics are associated with reduced risk of chronic diseases (Sun et al. 2002). Different species of fruits and vegetables contain different phytochemicals in different quantities (Adom and Liu 2002; Adom et al. 2003). Fruits such as apple, orange, blueberry, and grapes contain diverse types of phytochemicals in various quantities, so, in combinations, different fruits show synergistic effects with respect to antioxidant activity.

Oxidative damage is linked to several mechanisms of tumour formation that lead to carcinogenesis (Ames et al. 1993; Liu et al. 1995). Oxidative stress induced by free radicals causes DNA damage, gene mutations, or chromosomal aberrations (Ames et al. 1993). Recent studies have demonstrated that phytochemicals in fruits and berries can have complementary and overlapping mechanisms of action. They have antioxidant activity and hence carry out the scavenging of free radicals, as well as the regulation of gene expression in determining cell functions. They protect cells from abnormal growth and development and boost the immune functions of cells (Ames et al. 1993; Liu et al. 1995; Adom and Liu 2002). Fruits and vegetables produce precursors to bicarbonate ions which form acidic buffers, which help to neutralize acids consumed in the diet and maintain the normal pH (New 2002).

14.8   CONCLUSION

The function of our immune system depends upon various factors like age, gender, food and dietary habits, genetics, and the physiology of the host. The nutrition level of the host plays an important role in boosting the immune system. Fruits, specifically berries, are generally considered to be beneficial in improving the health of our digestive tract and microbiome due to their phytochemical and micronutrient content. The studies show that efficiency of our immune system can be improved by consuming specific fruits and berries. But an extensive body of research is still needed to understand the functioning of our immune system in relation to the dietary intake of various fruits and berries. The studies have shown that phytochemicals supplied as whole fruits are relatively more beneficial than those in fruit juice or in the form of a dietary supplement. Fruits lose their nutrition level after prolonged storage, so it is advised to consume seasonal fresh fruits without any additives to strengthen the immune system.

BIBLIOGRAPHY

Abbas, A.K. and A.H. Lichtman. 2003. *Cellular and Molecular Immunology*. 6th ed. Saunders.
Abe, L.T., F.M. Lajolo and M.I. Genovese 2012. Potential dietary sources of ellagic acid and other antioxidants among fruits consumed in Brazil: jabuticaba (*Myrciaria jaboticaba* (Vell.) Berg). *Journal of the Science of Food and Agriculture* 92: 1679–1687.
Adom, K.K. and R.H. Liu. 2002. Antioxidant activity of grains. *Journal of Agricultural Food Chemistry* 50: 6182–6187.
Adom, K.K., M.E. Sorrells and R.H. Liu. 2003. Phytochemicals and antioxidant activity of wheat varieties. *Journal of Agricultural Food Chemistry* 51: 7825–7834.

Agoro, R., M. Taleb, V.F.J. Quesniaux and C. Mura. 2018. Cell iron status influences macrophage polarization. PLoS One 13(5), e0196921.

Akalin A.S. and G. Ünal. 2005. Probiyotikler ve Allerji Gida Dergisi 30(1): 43–48.

Alonso, A., C. de la Fuente, A.M. Martin-Arnau, J. de Irala, J.A. Martinez and M.A. Gonzalez. 2004. Fruit and vegetable consumption is inversely associated with blood pressure in a Mediterranean population with a high vegetable-fat intake. *British Journal of Nutrition* 92: 311–319.

Alpert, P. 2017. The role of vitamins and minerals on the immune system. *Home Health Care Management and Practice* 29: 199–202.

Ames, B.N., M.K. Shigenaga and L.S. Gold. 1993. DNA lesions, inducible DNA repair and cell division: the three key factors in mutagenesis and carcinogenesis. *Environmental Health Perspective* 101(S5): 35–44.

Appel, L.J., T.J. Moore and E. Obarzanek. 1997. A clinical trial of the effects of dietary patterns onblood pressure. DASH Collaborative Research Group. *The New England Journal of Medicine* 336(16): 117–1124.

Basoglu, S. and H. Turnagol. 2004. Egzersiz ve immün sistem: Karbonhidratlar ETKisi. Hacettepe *Journal of Sport Sciences* 15: 100–123.

Basu, A., M. Rhone and T.J. Lyons. 2010. Berries: emerging impact on cardiovascular health. *Nutrition Reviews* 68(3): 168–177.

Bazzano, L.A., M.K. Serdula and S. Liu. 2003. Dietary intake of fruits and vegetables and risks of cardiovascular disease. *Current Artherosclerosis Reports* 5: 492–499.

Beck, M.A. 1999. Trace minerals, immune function, and viral evolution. In *Military Strategies for Sustainment of Nutrition and Immune Function in the Field*; National Academy Press: Washington, DC, USA, p. 339.

Besold, A.N., E.M. Culbertson and V.C. Culotta. 2016. The Yin and Yang of copper during infection. *Journal of Biological Inorganic. Chemistry* 21: 137–144.

Biesalski, H.K. 2016. Nutrition meets the microbiome: Micronutrients and the microbiota. *Annals of the New York Academy of Sciences* 1372: 53–64.

Bistrian, B.R. 2011. Diet, lifestyle, and long-term weight gain. *The New England Journal of Medicine* 365: 1058–1059.

Block, G., B.H. Patterson and A.F. Subar. 1992. Fruit, vegetables and cancer prevention: a review of the epidemiological evidence. *Nutrition and Cancer* 18: 1–29.

Bozonet, S.M. and A.C. Carr. 2019. The role of physiological vitamin C concentrations on key functions of neutrophils isolated from healthy individuals. *Nutrients* 11(6): 1363.

Bscheider, M. and E.C. Butcher. 2016. Vitamin D immunoregulation through dendritic cells. *Immunology* 148(3): 227–236.

Bussiere, F.I., A. Mazur, J. L Fauquert, A. Labbe, Y. Rayssiguier and A. Tridon. 2002. High magnesium concentration in vitro decreases human leukocyte activation. *Magnesium Research* 15: 43–48.

Butland, B. K, A.M. Fehily and F.C. Elwood. 2000. Diet, lung function and lung decline in a cohort of 2512 middle aged men. Thorax 55(2): 102–108.

Calder, P.C. 2013. Feeding the immune system, *Proceedings of the Nutrition Society* 72(3): 299–309.

Cantorna, M.T., J. Zhao and L Yang. 2012. Vitamin D, invariant natural killer T-cells and experimental autoimmune disease. *Proceedings of the Nutrition Society* 71(1): 62–66.

Carr, A. and S. Maggini. 2017. Vitamin C and immune function. *Nutrients* 9(11): 1211.

Chandra, R.K. 1997. Nutrition and the immune system: an introduction. *The American Journal of Clinical Nutrition* 66(2): 460S–463S.

Chandra, R.K. 2003. Nutrient regulation of immune functions. *Forum of Nutrition* 56: 147–148.

Chew, B.P. and J.S. Park. 2004. Carotenoid action on the immune response. *Journal of Nutrition* 134: 257S–261S.

Clairmont, A., D. Tessman, A. Stock, S. Nicolai, W. Stahl and H. Sies. 1996. Induction of gap junctional intercellular communication by vitamin D in human skin fibroblasts is dependent on the nuclear Induction of gap junctional intercellular communication by vitamin D in human skin fibroblasts is dependent on the nuclear vitamin D receptor. *Carcinogenesis* 17: 1389–1391.

Clark, A. and N. Mach. 2016. Role of vitamin D in the hygiene hypothesis: the interplay between vitamin D, vitamin D receptors, gut microbiota, and immune response. *Frontiers in Immunology* 7: 627.

Coico, R. and G. Sunshine. 2009. *Immunology: A Short Course*. John Wiley and Sons.

Coskun, T. 2005. Fonksiyonel Besinlerin Sagligimiz Üzerine Etkileri. Çocuk Sagligi ve Hastaliklari Dergisi 48: 69–84.

Crawford, P.B., E. Obarzanek, J. Morrison and Z.I. Sabry. 1994. Comparative advantage of 3-dayfood records over 24 recall and 5-day food frequency validated by observation of 9-and10-year girls. *Journal of the American Dietetic Association* 94(6): 626–630.

Cuthbertson, W.F.J. 2002. Are the effects of dietary fruits and vegetables on human health related to those of chronic dietary restriction on animal longevity and disease?. *British Journal of Nutrition* 87(2): 187–188.

Dauchet L., P. Amouyel and J. Dallongeville. 2005. Fruit and vegetable consumption and risk of stroke: a meta-analysis of cohort studies. *Neurology* 65: 1193–1197.

Delves, P.J. and I.M. Roitt.2000. The immune system – first of two parts. *New England Journal of Medicine* 343(1): 37–49.

Department of Health, South Africa. 2001. South African national guidelines on nutrition for people living with TB, HIV/AIDS and other chronic debilitating conditions.

Ehala, S., M. Vaher and M. Kaljurand. 2005. Characterization of phenolic profiles of Northern European berries by capillary electrophoresis and determination of their antioxidant activity. *Journal of Agricultural and Food Chemistry* 53(16): 6484–6490.

Ford, E.S. and A.H. Mokdad. 2001. Fruit and vegetable consumption and diabetes mellitus incidence among USA adults. *Preventive Medicine* 32(1): 33–39.

Galeone, C., E. Negri, C. Pelucchi, C.L. Vecchia, C. Bosetti and J. Hu. 2007. Dietary intake of fruits and vegetables and lung cancer risk: a case-control study in Harbin, Northern China. *Annals of Oncology* 18(2): 388–392.

Gao, H., W. Dai, L. Zhao, J. Min and F. Wang. 2018. The role of zinc and zinc homeostasis in macrophage function. *Journal of Immunology Research* 2018, 6872621.

Georgiev, V., A. Ananga and V. Tsolova, 2014. Recent advances and uses of grape flavonoids as nutraceuticals. *Nutrients* 6(1): 391–415.

Giancarlo, B., G.L. Beccaro, M.G. Mellano and V. Novello. 2011. Nutraceutical content of berries and minor fruits. *Proceedings of ISMF and MP*, December 19–22, 2011, Kalyani, W.B., India

Gniadecki, R., B. Gajkowska and M. Hansen. 1997. 1,25-dihydroxyvitamin D3 stimulates the assembly of adherens junctions in keratinocytes: Involvement of protein kinase C. *Endocrinology* 138(6): 2241–2248.

Gombart, A.F. 2009. The vitamin D–antimicrobial peptide pathway and its role in protection against infection. *Future Microbiology* 4: 1151.

Gombart, A.F., A. Pierre and S. Maggini. 2020. A Review of Micronutrients and the Immune System–Working in Harmony to Reduce the Risk of Infection. *Nutrients* 12: 236.

Gombart, A.F., N. Borregaard, H.P. Koeffler. 2005. Human cathelicidin antimicrobial peptide (CAMP) gene is a direct target of the vitamin D receptor and is strongly up-regulated in myeloid cells by 1,25-dihydroxyvitamin D3. *FASEB Journal* 19(9): 1067–1077.

Greiner, T. 2011. Vitamins and minerals for women: recent programs and intervention trials. *Nutrition Research and Practice* 5(1): 3–10.

Han, S.N., O. Adolfsson, C. K Lee, T.A. Prolla, J. Ordovas and S.N. Meydani. 2004. Vitamin E and gene expression in immune cells. *Annals of the New York Academy of Science* 1031, 96–101.

Haryanto, B., T. Suksmasari, E. Wintergerst and S. Maggini. 2015. Multivitamin supplementation supports immune function and ameliorates conditions triggered by reduced air quality. *Vitamins and Minerals* 4(2), 1–15.

He, F.J., C.A. Nowson and G.A. MacGregor. 2006. Fruit and vegetable consumption and stroke: meta-analysis of cohort studies. *Lancet* 367: 320–326.

Heyworth, P.G., A.R. Cross and J.T. Curnutte. 2003. Chronic granulomatous disease. *Current Opinion in Immunology* 15(5): 578–584.

Hong, F., J. Yan, J.T. Baran, D.J. Allendorf, R.D. Hansen, G.R. Ostroff, P.X. Xing, N.K.V. Cheung, and G.D. Ross. 2004. Mechanism by which orally administered beta-1,3-glucans enhance the tumoricidal activity of antitumor monoclonal antibodies in murine tumor models. *Journal of Immunology* 173(2): 797–806.

Hurwitz, B.E., J.R. Klaus, M.M. Llabre, A. Gonzalez, P.J. Lawrence, K.J. Maher, J.M. Greeson, M.K. Baum, G. Shor-Posner, J.S. Skyler and N. Schneiderman. 2007. Suppression of human immunodeficiency virus type 1 viral load with selenium supplementation: A randomized controlled trial. *Archives of Internal Medicine* 167(2): 148–154.

Ibs, K.H. and, L. Rink. 2003. Zinc-Altered Immune function. *The Journal of Nutrition* 133 Supplement 1: 1452S–1456S.

Inoue, M., T. Matsui, A. Nishibu, Y. Nihei, K. Iwatsuki and F. Kaneko. 1998. Regulatory effects of 1alpha, 25-dihydroxyvitamin D3 on inflammatory responses in psoriasis. *European Journal of Dermatology* 8(1): 16–20.

Janeway, C.A. and R. Medzhitov. 2002. Innate immunity recognition. *Annual Review of Immunology* 20: 197–216.

Jarosz, M., M. Olbert, G. Wyszogrodzka, K. Młyniec and T. Librowski. 2017. Antioxidant and anti-inflammatory effects of zinc. Zinc-dependent NF-kB signaling. *Inflammopharmacology* 25(1): 11–24.

Jia, N., B. Kong, Q. Liu, X. Diao and X. Xia. 2012. Antioxidant activity of black currant (*Ribes nigrum* L.) extract and its inhibitory effect on lipid and protein oxidation of pork patties during chilled storage. *Meat Science* 91: 533–539.

Joseph, J.A., N.A. Denisova and G. Arendash. 1999. Blueberry supplementation enhances signaling and prevents behavioural deficits in an Alzheimer disease model. *Nutrtional Neuroscience* 6(3): 153–162.

Kalt, W. 2002. Health functional phytochemicals of fruits. *Horticulture Review* 27: 269–315.

Karacabey, K. 2005. Effect of regular exercise on health and disease. *Neuro Endocrinology Letters* 26(5): 617–623.

Karacabey, K. 2012. The Effect of nutritional elements on the immune system. *Journal of Obesity and Weight Loss Therapy* 2: 152, doi: 10.4172/2165-7904.1000152.

Kaulmann, A. and T. Bohn. 2016. Bioactivity of polyphenols: preventive and adjuvant strategies toward reducing inflammatory bowel diseases-promises, perspectives, and pitfalls. *Oxidative Medicine and Cellular Longevity* 2016: 9346470. doi: 10.1155/2016/9346470.

Keith, M.E. and K.N. Jeejeebhoy. 1997. Immunonutrition. *Bailliere's Clinical and Endocrinology Metabolism* 11(4): 709–738.

Kim, E.K., E.J. Choi and T. Debnath. 2016. Role of phytochemicals in the inhibition of epithelial-mesenchymal transition in cancer metastasis. *Food and Function* 7: 3677–3685.

Kitabayashi, C., T. Fukada, M. Kanamoto, W. Ohashi, S. Hojyo, T. Atsumi, N. Ueda, I. Azuma, H. Hirota, M. Murakami and T. Hirano. 2010. Zinc suppresses Th17 development via inhibition of STAT3 activation. *International Immunology* 22(5): 375–386.

Kolouchová-Hanzlíková, I., K. Melzoch, V. Filip, J. Šmidrkal, (2004). Rapid method for resveratrol determination by HPLC with electrochemical and UV detections in wines. *Food Chemistry* 87: 151–158.

Kristo, A.S., D. Klimis-Zacas and A.K. Sikalidis. 2016. Protective role of dietary berries in cancer. *Antioxidants (Basel)*. 5(4): 37. doi: 10.3390/antiox5040037.

Kursvietiene, L., I. Staneviciene, A. Mongirdiene and Jurga Bernatoniené. 2016. Multiplicity of effects and health benefits of resveratrol. *Medicina (Kaunas)* 52(3): 148–155.

Kushi, L.H., C. Doyle, M. McCullough, C.L. Rock, W. Demark-Wahnefried, E.V. Bandera, S. Gapstur, A. V Patel, K. Andrews, T. Gansler, American Cancer Society 2010 Nutrition and Physical Activity Guidelines Advisory Committee. 2012. American Cancer Society Guidelines on nutrition and physical activity for cancer prevention: reducing the risk of cancer with healthy food choices and physical activity. *CA: A Cancer Journal for Clinicians* 62(1), 30–67.

Laires, M.J. and C. Monteiro. 2008. Exercise, magnesium and immune function. *Magnesium Research* 21: 92–96.

Levy, M., C.A. Thaiss and E. Elinav. 2016. Metabolites: messengers between the microbiota and the immune system. *Genes and Development* 30(14): 1589–1597.

Lin, P.H., M. Sermersheim, H. Li, P.H.U. Lee, S.M. Steinberg and J. Ma. 2017. Zinc in wound healing modulation. *Nutrients* 10(1): 16.

Lin, Z. and W. Li. 2016. The roles of vitamin D and its analogs in inflammatory diseases. *Current Topics in Medicinal Chemistry* 16(11): 1242–1261.

Liu, R.H. 2004. Potential synergy of phytochemicals in cancer prevention: mechanism of action. *The Journal of Nutrition* 134(12 suppl) suppl: 3479S–3485S.

Liu, R.H. and J.H. Hotchkiss. 1995. Potential genotoxicity of chronically elevated nitric oxide: a review. *Mutation Research* 339(2): 73–89.

Lock, K, J. Pomerleau, L. Causer, D.R. Altmann and M. McKee. 2005. The global burden of disease attributable to low consumption of fruit and vegetables: implications for the global strategy on diet. *World Health Org* 83: 100–108.

Maggini, S.A. Pierre and P.C. Calder. 2018. Immune function and micronutrient requirements change over the life course. *Nutrients* 10(10): 1531.

Maggini, S., S. Beveridge, P.J.P. Sorbara and G. Senatore. 2008. Feeding the immune system: The role of micronutrients in restoring resistance to infections. *CAB Review* 3: 1–21.

Mares-Perlman J.A., A.E. Millen, T.L. Ficek and S.E. Hankinson. 2002. The body of evidence to support a protective role for lutein and zeaxanthin in decaying chronic disease. *Journal of Nutrition* 132 (3): 518S–524S.

Matsui, T., R. Takahashi, Y. Nakao, T. Koizumi, Y. Katakami, K. Mihara, T. Sugiyama and T. Fujita. 1986. 1,25-Dihydroxyvitamin D3-regulated expression of genes involved in human T-lymphocyte proliferation and differentiation. *Cancer Research* 46: 5827–5831.

Maywald, M., F. Wang and L. Rink. 2018. Zinc supplementation plays a crucial role in T helper 9 differentiation in allogeneic immune reactions and non-activated T cells. *Journal of Trace Elements in Medicine and Biology* 50: 482–488.

Medzhitov R. and C. Jr Janeway. 2000. Innate immunity. *New England Journal of Medicine* 343(5): 338–344.

Medzhitov, R., P. Preston-Hurlburt and C. Jr Janeway. 1997. A human homologue of the Drosophila Toll protein signals activation of adaptive immunity. *Nature* 388: 394–397.

Mertz, C., V. Cheynier, Z. Gunata and P. Brat. 2007. Analysis of phenolic compounds in two blackberry species (*Rubus glaucus* and *Rubus adenotrichus*) by high-performance liquid chromatography with diode array detection and electrospray ion trap mass spectrometry. *Journal of Agricultural and Food Chemistry* 55(21): 8616–8624.

Micronutrient Information Center (MIC). Immunity in Depth. Linus Pauling Institute. Available online: http://lpi.oregonstate.edu/mic/health-disease/immunity (accessed on 10 October 2020).

Mihajlovic, M., M. Fedecostante, M.J. Oost, S.K.P. Steenhuis, E. Lentjes, I. Maitimu-Smeele, M.J. Janssen, L.B. Hilbrands and R. Masereeuw. 2017. Role of Vitamin D in maintaining renal epithelial barrier function in uremic conditions. *International Journal Molecular Sciences* 18(12): 2531.

Ness, A.R. and J.W. Powles. 1997. Fruit and vegetables and cardiovascular disease: a review. *International Journal of Epidemiology* 26(1): 1–13.

New, S.A. 2002. Nutrition society medal lecture: the role of the skeleton in acid-base homeostasis. *The Proceedings of Nutrition Society* 61(2): 151–164.

Pagliaro, B., C. Santolamazza, F. Simonelli and S. Rubattu. 2015. Phytochemical compounds and protection from cardiovascular diseases: a state of the art. *Biomed Research International* 2015: 918069. doi: 10.1155/2015/918069.

Palmer, A.C. 2011. Nutritionally mediated programming of the developing immune system. *Advances in Nutrition* 2(5): 377–395.

Palmer, H.G., J.M. Gonzalez-Sancho, J. Espada, M.T. Berciano, I. Puig, J. Baulida, M. Quintanilla, A. Cano, A.G. de Herreros, M. Lafarga and A. Munoz. 2001. Vitamin D3 promotes the differentiation of colon carcinoma cells by the induction of E-cadherin and the inhibition of beta-catenin signaling. *Journal of Cell Biology* 154(2): 369–387.

Penna, G., L. Adorini. 2000. 1 Alpha, 25-dihydroxyvitamin D3 inhibits differentiation, maturation, activation, and survival of dendritic cells leading to impaired alloreactive T cell activation. *Journal of Immunology* 164(5): 2405–2411.

Petrovic, J., D. Stanic, G. Dmitrasinovic, B. Plecas-Solarovic, S. Ignjatovic, B. Batinic, D. Popovic and V. Pesic. 2016. Magnesium supplementation diminishes peripheral blood lymphocyte DNA oxidative damage in athletes and sedentary young man. *Oxidative Medicine and Cellular Longevity* 2016, 2019643. doi: 10.1155/2016/2019643.

Piemonti, L., P. Monti, M. Sironi, P. Fraticelli, B.E. Leone, E. Dal Cin, P. Allavena and V. Di Carlo. 2000. Vitamin D3 affects differentiation, maturation, and function of human monocyte-derived dendritic cells. *Journal of Immunology* 164(9): 4443–4451.

Reichel, H., H.P. Koeffler, A. Tobler and A.W. Norman. 1987. 1 alpha,25-Dihydroxyvitamin D3 inhibits gamma-interferon synthesis by normal human peripheral blood lymphocytes. *Proceedings of National Academy Science of United States of America* 84(10): 3385–3389.

Rigby, W.F., S. Denome and M.W. Fanger. 1987. Regulation of lymphokine production and human T lymphocyte activation by 1,25-dihydroxyvitamin D3. Specific inhibition at the level of messenger RNA. *Journal of Clinical Investigation* 79(6): 1659–1664.

Rimando, A.M., W. Kalt, J.B. Magee, J. Dewey and J.R. Ballington. 2004. Resveratrol, pterostilbene, and piceatannol in *Vaccinium* berries. *Journal of Agricultural and Food Chemistry* 52(15): 4713–4719.

Rodriguez-Mateos, A., T. Cifuentes-Gomez, S. Tabatabaee, C. Lecras and J.P.E. Spencer. 2012. Procyanidin, anthocyanin, and chlorogenic acid contents of highbush and lowbush blueberries. *Journal of Agricultural and Food Chemistry* 60(23): 5772–5778.

Romieu, I. and C. Trenga. 2001. Diet and obstructive lung diseases. *Epidemiologic Reviews* 23(2): 268–287.

Ross, A.C. 2012. Vitamin A and retinoic acid in T cell-related immunity. *American Journal of Clinical Nutrition* 96(5): 1166s–1172s.

Rupasinghe, H.P., S. Sekhon-Loodu, T. Mantso and M.I. Panayiotidis. 2016. Phytochemicals in regulating fatty acid beta-oxidation: potential underlying mechanisms and their involvement in obesity and weight loss. *Pharmacology and Therapeutics* 165: 153–163.

Saeed, F., M. Nadeem, R.S. Ahmed, M.T. Nadeem, M.S. Arshad and A. Ullah. 2016. Studying the impact of nutritional immunology underlying the modulation of immune responses by nutritional compounds—a review. *Food and Agricultural Immunology* 27(2): 205–229.

Sakakeeny, L., R. Roubeno, M. Obin, J.D. Fontes, E.J. Benjamin, Y. Bujanover, P.F. Jacques and J. Selhub. 2012. Plasma pyridoxal-5-phosphate is inversely associated with systemic markers of inflammation in a population of U.S. adults. *Journal of Nutrition* 142(7): 1280–1285.

Sassi, F., C. Tamone and P. D'Amelio. 2018. Vitamin D: nutrient, hormone, and immunomodulator. *Nutrients* 10(11): 1656.

Saygin, O., K. Karacabey, R. Ozmerdivenli, E. Zorba, F. Ilhan and V. Bulut. 2006. Effect of chronic exercise on immunoglobin, complement and leukocyte types in volleyball players and athletes. *Neuro Endocrinology Letters* 27(1): 271–276.

Seddon, J.M., U.A. Ajani, R.D. Sperduto, R Hiller, N Blair, T C Burton, M D Farber, E S Gragoudas, J Haller, and D T Miller (1994). Dietary carotenoids, vitamins A, C, and E, and advanced age-related macular degeneration. Eye disease case-control study group. *JAMA* 272(18): 1413–1420.

Seifried, H.E., S.S. McDonald, D.E. Anderson, P. Greenwald and J.A. Milner. 2003. The antioxidant conundrum in cancer. *Cancer Research* 63: 4295–4298.

Shankar, A.H. and A.S. Prasad. 1998. Zinc and immune function: the biological basis of altered resistance to infection. *American Journal of Clinical Nutrition* 68(2) Supplement: 447S–463S.

Shankar, E., R. Kanwal, M. Candamo and S. Gupta. 2016. Dietary phytochemicals as epigenetic modifiers in cancer: promise and challenges. *Seminar in Cancer Biology* 40–41: 82–89.

Sheikh, A., S. Shamsuzzaman, S.M. Ahmad, D. Nasrin, S. Nahar, M.M. Alam, A.A.l. Tarique, Y.A. Begum, S.S. Qadri, M.I. Chowdhury, A. Saha, C.P. Larson and F. Quadri. 2010. Zinc influences innate immune responses in children with enterotoxigenic Escherichia coli-induced diarrhea. *Journal of Nutrition* 140(5): 1049–1056.

Singh, C.K., M.A. Ndiaye and N. Ahmad. 2015. Resveratrol and cancer: challenges for clinical translation. *Biochimica et Biophysica Acta* 1852(6): 1178–1185.

Singh, C.K., X. Liu and N. Ahmad. 2015. Resveratrol, in its natural combination in whole grape, for health promotion and disease management. *Annals of New York Academy of Sciences* 1348: 150–160.

Sinha, N., J. Sidhu, J. Barta, J. Wu and M.P. Cano (Eds.). 2012. *Handbook of Fruits and Fruit Processing*, John Wiley and Sons.

Sirisinha, S. 2015. The pleiotropic role of vitamin A in regulating mucosal immunity. *Asian Pacific Journal of Allergy and Immunology* 33(2): 71–89.

Slavin, J.L. and B. Lloyd. 2012. Health benefits of fruits and vegetables. *Advances in Nutrition* 3(4): 506–516.

Sly, L.M., M. Lopez, W.M. Nauseef and N.E. Reiner. 2001. 1alpha,25-Dihydroxyvitamin D3-induced monocyte antimycobacterial activity is regulated by phosphatidylinositol 3-kinase and mediated by the NADPH-dependent phagocyte oxidase. *Journal of Biological Chemistry.* 276(38): 35482–35493.

Snellen, E.L.M., A.L.M. Verbeek, G.W.P. Van Den Hoogen, J.R.M. Cruysberg and C.B. Hoyng. 2002. Neovascular age-related macular degeneration and its relationship to antioxidant intake. *Acta Ophthalmologica Scandinavica* 80(4): 368–371.

Southon, S. 2000. Increased fruit and vegetable consumption within EU: potential health benefits. *Food Research International* 33(3–4): 211–217.

Steinmetz, K.A. and J.D. Potter. 1996. Vegetables, fruit and cancer prevention: a review. *Journal of the American Dietetic Association* 96(10): 1027–1039.

Sun, J., Y.F. Chu, X. Wu and R.H. Liu. 2002. Antioxidant and antiproliferative activities of common fruits. *Journal of Agricultural and Food Chemistry* 50: 7449–7454.

Tabak, C., I.C. Arts, H.A. Smit, D. Heederik and D. Kromhout. 2001. Chronic obstructive pulmonary disease and intake of catechins, flavonols and flavones: the MORGEN Study. *American Journal of Respiratory and Critical Care Medicine* 164(1): 61–64.

Tanaka, H., K.A. Hruska, Y. Seino, J.D. Malone, Y. Nishii and S.L. Teitelbaum. 1991. Disassociation of the macrophage-maturational effects of vitamin D from respiratory burst priming. *Journal of Biological Chemistry* 266(17): 10888–10892.

Topilski, I., L. Flaishon, Y. Naveh, A. Harmelin, Y. Levo and I. Shachar. 2004. The anti-inflammatory effects of 1, 25-dihydroxyvitamin D3 on Th2 cells in vivo are due in part to the control of integrin-mediated T lymphocyte homing. *European Journal of Immunology*. 34(4): 1068–1076.

Tsuda, T. 2016. Recent progress in anti-obesity and anti-diabetes effect of berries. Antioxidants (Basel) 5(2): 13. doi: 10.3390/antiox5020013.

Ueland, P.M., A. McCann, O. Midttun and A. Ulvik. 2017. Inflammation, vitamin B6 and related pathways. *Molecular Aspects of Medicine* 53, 10–27.

Van Duyn, M.A. and E. Pivonka. 2000. Overview of the health benefits of fruit and vegetable consumption for the dietetics professional: selected literature. *Journal of the American Dietetic Association* 100(12): 1511–1521.

Van't Veer, P., M.C. Jansen, M. Klerk and F.J. Kok. 2000. Fruits and vegetables in the prevention of cancer and cardiovascular disease. *Public Health Nutrition* 3(1): 103–107.

Vendrame S, C. Del Bo, S. Ciappellano, P. Riso and D. Klimis-Zacas. 2016. Berry fruit consumption and metabolic syndrome. Antioxidants (Basel) 5(4): 34. doi: 10.3390/antiox5040034.

Vinson, J., J. Proch and P. Bose. 2001. Determination of quantity of polyphenol antioxidants in foods and beverages. *Methods in enzymology* 335: 103–114.

Wada, L. and B. Ou. 2002. Antioxidant activity and phenolic content of Oregon caneberries. *Journal of Agricultural and Food Chemistry* 50(12): 3495–3500.

Wang, T.T., F.P. Nestel, V. Bourdeau, Y. Nagai, Q. Wang, J. Liao, L. Tavera-Mendoza, R. Lin, J.W. Hanrahan, S. Mader and J.H. White. 2004. Cutting edge: 1,25-dihydroxyvitamin D3 is a direct inducer of antimicrobial peptide gene expression. *Journal of Immunology* 173(5): 2909–2912.

Wang, Y., G.B. Douglas, G.C. Waghorn, T.N. Barry, A.G. Foote and R.W. Purchas. 1996. Effect of condensed tannins upon the performance of lambs grazing *Lotus corniculatus* and lucerne (*Medicago sativa*). *Journal of Agricultural Science* 126(1): 87–98.

Wang, Y., M.E. Bentley, F. Zhai and B.M. Popkin. 2002. Tracking dietary intake patterns of Chinese from childhood to adolescence over a six-year follow-up period. *Journal of Nutrition* 132(3): 430–438.

Wardle, J., K. Permenter and J. Waller. 2000. Nutrition knowledge and food intake. *Appetite* 34(3): 269–275.

Wargovich, M. 2000. Anticancer properties of fruits and vegetables. *HortScience* 35: 573–575.

Weber, G., J.D. Heilborn, C.I. Chamorro Jimenez, A. Hammarsjo, H. Törmä and M. Stahle. 2005. Vitamin D induces the antimicrobial protein hCAP18 in human skin. *Journal of Investigative Dermatology* 124(5): 1080–1082.

Wintergerst, E.S., S. Maggini and Hornig, D. 2007. Contribution of selected vitamins and trace elements to immune function. *Annals of Nutrition and Metabolism* 51(4): 301–323.

Wintergerst, E.; S. Maggini and D. Hornig. 2006. Immune-enhancing role of vitamin C and zinc and effect on clinical conditions. *Annals of Nutrition and Metabolism* 50(2): 85–94.

Wishart, K. 2017. Increased micronutrient requirements during physiologically demanding situations: Review of the current evidence. *Vitamins and Minerals* 6(3): 1–16.

World Health Organization (WHO). 2006. Food and Agricultural Organization of the United Nations. Part 2. Evaluating the public health significance of micronutrient malnutrition. In *Guidelines on Food Fortification with Micronutrients*, WHO: Geneva, Switzerland.

Wu, D. and S.N. Meydani. 2014. Age-associated changes in immune function: impact of vitamin E intervention and the underlying mechanisms. *Endocrine, Metabolic and Immune Disorders Drug Targets* 14(4): 283–289.

Wu, D., E.D. Lewis, M. Pae and S.N. Meydani. 2019. Nutritional modulation of immune function: Analysis of evidence, mechanisms, and clinical relevance. *Frontiers in Immunology* 9: 3160, doi: 10.3389/fimmu.2018.03160.

Wu, R., B. Frei, J.A. Kennedy and Y. Zhao. 2010. Effects of refrigerated storage and processing technologies on the bioactive compounds and antioxidant capacities of 'Marion' and 'Evergreen' blackberries. *LWT – Food Science and Technology*, 43(8): 1253–1264.

Yang, J., and Y.Y. Xiao. 2013. Grape phytochemicals and associated health benefits. *Critical Reviews in Food Science and Nutrition* 53(11): 1202–1225.

Yin, Z., V. Pintea, Y. Lin, B.D. Hammock and M.A. Watsky. 2011. Vitamin D enhances corneal epithelial barrier function. *Investigative Ophthalmology and Visual Science* 52(10): 7359–7364.

Yoshii, K., K. Hosomi, K. Sawane and J. Kunisawa. 2019. Metabolism of dietary and microbial vitamin B family in the regulation of host immunity. *Frontiers in Nutrition* 6: 48. doi: 10.3389/fnut.2019.00048

Younus, H. and S. Anwar. 2016. Prevention of non-enzymatic glycosylation (glycation): implication in the treatment of diabetic complication. *International Journal of Health Science (Qassim)* 10(2): 261–277.

Zhang, Y., D.Y.M. Leung, B.N. Richers, Y. Liu, L.K. Remigio, D.W. Riches and E. Goleva. 2012. Vitamin D inhibits monocyte/macrophage proinflammatory cytokine production by targeting MAPK phosphatase-1. *Journal of Immunology* 188(5): 2127–2135.

Zulueta, A., A. Caretti, P. Signorelli and G. Riccardo. 2015. Resveratrol: a potential challenger against gastric cancer. *World Journal of Gastroenterology* 21(37): 10636–10643.

15 Natural Immunity Boosters and Anticancer Medicinal Plants

Swati Agarwal, Sonu Kumari,
and Amrendra Kumar

CONTENTS

DOI: 10.1201/9781003137955-15

15.1 INTRODUCTION

Cancer is a disease which leads to uncontrolled cell growth and division, with the potential to spread and invade other parts of the body. It is one of the foremost causes of death worldwide. It mainly occurs because of genomic alterations in the DNA and it starts with a natural cell change, leading to abnormal growth (Krishnamurthi 2007). The number of cases of cancer is continuously rising and expected to reach 21 million by 2030 (Siegel et al. 2019). Almost 1,762,450 new cancer sufferers and 606,880 deaths were estimated in the United States alone in the year 2019. In 2014, the world cancer report released the data for year 2003, where around 4.7 million women and 5.3 million men were reported to develop a malignant growth annually, with 6.2 million people dying of cancer (McGuire 2016).

Nowadays, several methods are used to treat cancers. Some methods are conventional, like surgery, chemotherapy, radiotherapy, stem cell transplants, etc., but they all have one major side effect, which is non selectivity between the healthy and diseased cells (Sersa et al. 2003). On the other hand, some modern techniques are more specific for small populations of abnormal cells, such as proton therapy, robot-assisted surgery, stereotactic radiosurgery, etc. To avoid the harm to healthy cells during these treatments, research is now shifting towards more natural therapies and the use of phytochemicals. Phytochemicals are plant-derived chemicals. This process requires screening raw extracts of plants for potential anticancer phytochemicals, and then carrying out their purification, identification, characterization, and activity towards different cancerous cells.

The immune system can easily be improved through the use of medicinal plants as these have high concentrations and diversity of flavonoids, as well as vitamin C. These phytochemicals can behave as agents with anti-inflammatory and immunostimulant properties. Therefore, it can increase the action of lymphocytes, enhance phagocytosis, and stimulate interferon development. For instance, *Allium sativum* (garlic) acts mainly as an immune system booster. Several other plant species act as immune system stimulators, which achieve an immune-potentiating outcome by exciting usual killer cell action (Khodadadi 2015).

Medicinal plants are significant for cancer management because of the various chemical complexes present in the preparations (Ji et al. 2009). These compounds are known as secondary plant metabolites which are useful but not essential to the plant. Some important secondary plant metabolite classes are alkaloids, polyphenols, terpenoids, pigments, tannins, flavonoids, etc. These compounds have several curative properties on the human body, like anti-inflammatory, contraceptive, anticancer, antiseptic etc. Several secondary plant metabolites have been reported for the management of cancer. The method for treating cancer is by suppressing the cancer stimulating enzymes, inducing the production of anticancer enzymes, repairing the DNA, increasing the immunity of the body, and inducing antioxidant activity, etc. (Efferth 2010).

In this chapter, we will attempt to describe some of the more effective anticancer medicinal plants including their phytochemicals, herbal preparation, and their mechanism of action in cancer treatment.

15.2 MEDICINAL PLANTS: IMMUNE BOOSTERS

During the infection period, viruses, bacteria, and fungi are attacked by the body's immune system. It identifies the foreign body in the system through the action of particular receptors to generate an instant reaction through immune cell activation, and the production of cytokines and chemokines (Kumar et al. 2011). Plants with medicinal properties play important roles in the prevention of infection from a range of disease-causing microorganisms. Globally, several medicinal plants have been reported to act as immune boosters. Some medicinal plants are suggested to improve the patient's physical condition and to sustain natural resistance against illness through re-establishing body stability (Das et al. 2014). It is appealing to consider that the curative and tonic influences of these herbal medications may be because of their direct effect on the human immune system. There are number of medicinal plants which have been proposed to improve the natural resistance to various infections.

Certain therapeutic plants are particularly effective immune system boosters. Immunomodulator plants are considered to be most effective for the nervous and hormonal systems of the body, whereas other medicinal plants have antioxidant, antiviral, or anticancer properties, which decrease the ageing effects as well as improving immunity. In plant-based medications, preparation of single plant species as well as compound formulations of different species have been approved to treat illness (Saklani and Kutty 2008).

15.3 ANTICANCER MEDICINAL PLANTS

Medicinal plants are exploited by extracting their phytochemicals and other compounds, which are in addition to the conventional drugs synthesized to treat tumours and other cancerous growths (Desai et al. 2008). Approximately 35,000 plant species were selected by the National Cancer Institute (NCI) for their possible anticancer actions. Of them, about 3,000 plant species showed activity against cancer cell lines (Douros and Suffness 1980).

Some medicinal plants (Figure 15.1) and bioactive compounds derived from them have curative properties against cancers and immunity boosting abilities and are reported in detail in the next sections of this chapter, with others being presented in Table 15.1.

15.3.1 *ALLIUM SATIVUM*

Allium sativum (garlic) is a member of the Amaryllidaceae family. *A. sativum* is a native of northern Iran and central Asia. It has been used for several centuries for

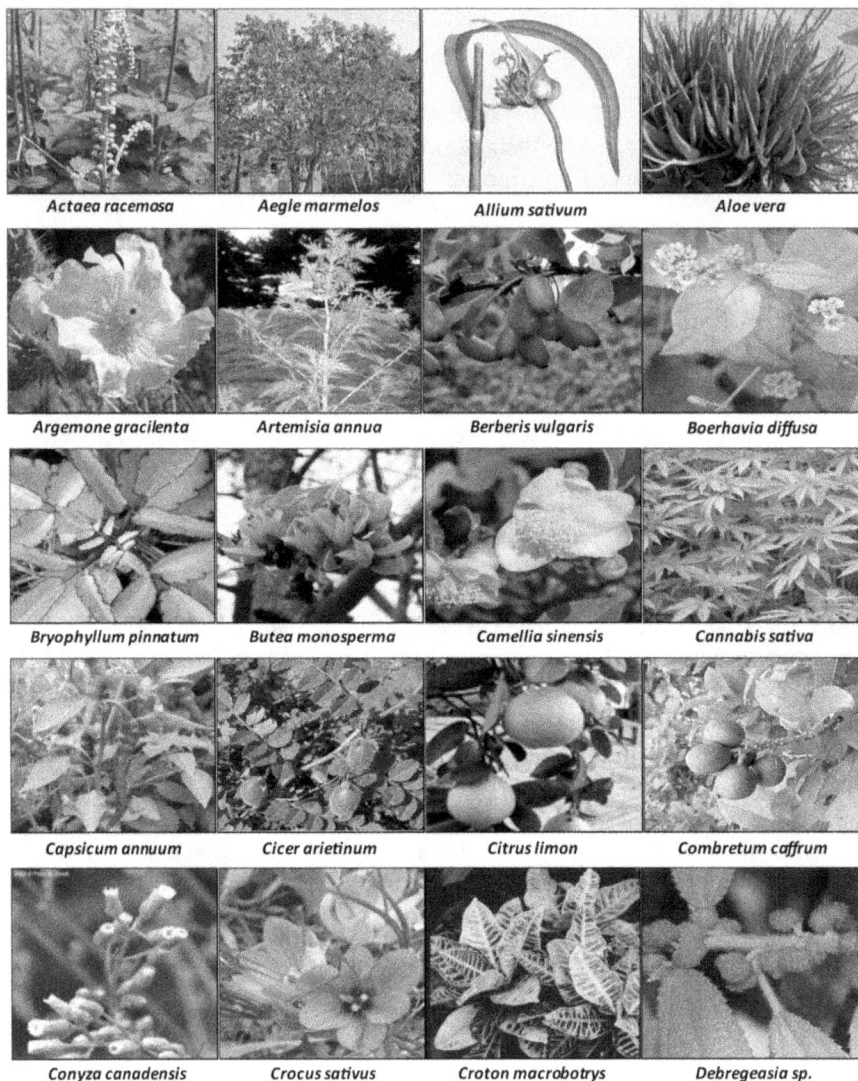

Actaea racemosa	Aegle marmelos	Allium sativum	Aloe vera
Argemone gracilenta	Artemisia annua	Berberis vulgaris	Boerhavia diffusa
Bryophyllum pinnatum	Butea monosperma	Camellia sinensis	Cannabis sativa
Capsicum annuum	Cicer arietinum	Citrus limon	Combretum caffrum
Conyza canadensis	Crocus sativus	Croton macrobotrys	Debregeasia sp.

FIGURE 15.1 Some important medicinal plants used in the treatment of cancer.

food flavouring and medicinal purposes. Traditionally, garlic is recognized as a noteworthy immune booster. Matured garlic extract shows higher immunomodulatory results than raw garlic. Extracts of garlic contain high concentration of organosulphur compounds, which helps in prevention of cancer of the bladder, breast, colon, lung, skin, throat, and larynx.

Numerous papers have verified the therapeutic property of *A. sativum* extract and its essential oil. The major compounds in *A. sativum* extract are alliin, allylmercaptocysteine, allicin, and S-allyl-mercapto-L-cysteine. One additional organosulphur

TABLE 15.1

List of Some Important Medicinal Plants and Their Phytochemicals against Specific Types of Cancer

Plant Name	Common name	Plant Part extract	Phytochemicals	Specific Cancer	References
Actaea racemosa	Black cohosh	Rhizome	Actein	Liver, breast, gland	Wuttke et al. (2014)
Aegle marmelos	Bael fruit	Fruit	Lupeol, skimmianine	Leukaemia, breast, liver	Baliga et al. (2013a)
Allium sativum	Garlic	Fruit	Alliin, allylmercaptocysteine, allicin	Breast, colon, gland Lymphoma, cervix	Capasso (2013)
Aloe vera	Indian aloe	Leaf	Aloesin, emodin, alexin	Anti-angiogenic activity, stomach, head, neck, leukaemia	Ahmadi (2012)
Argemone gracilenta	Prickly poppy	Complete plant	Argemonine, berberine	B cell lymphoma, leukemia	Iqbal et al. (2017)
Artemisia annua	Wormwood	Arial parts	Artemisinin	Liver and breast	Efferth (2017)
Berberis vulgaris	Barberry	Fruit	Berberine, cannabisin	Breast, colon, liver, prostate	Hoshyar et al. (2016)
Boerhavia diffusa	Punarnava	Roots	Punarnavine	Malignant melanoma	Khan et al. (2013)
Bryophyllum pinnatum	Goethe plant	Leaf	Bryophyllin	Cervical	Mahata et al. (2012)
Butea monosperma	Flame-of-the-forest	Flower	Butrin	Liver	Choedon et al. (2010)
Camellia sinensis	Tea plant	Leaf	Theabrownin, epigallocatechin gallate	Lung, brain, prostate, cervical, bladder	Luo et al. (2014)
Cannabis sativa	Hemp	Flower and leaf	Cannabinoid	Lung, pancreas, prostate, breast, colorectal	Hall et al. (2005)
Capsicum annuum	Peppers	Fruit	Luteolin, capsaicin	Colorectal	Chapa-Oliver and Mejía-Teniente (2016)
Cicer arietinum	Chickpea	Seeds	Bowman–Birk type protease inhibitor	Prostate, breast	Magee et al. (2012)
Citrus limon	Lemon	Fruit	5-hydroxy-6,7,8,30,40-pentamethoxyflavone	Colon, colorectal, buccal	Raimondo et al. (2015)
Combretum caffrum	Bushwillow tree	Fruit and bark	Combretastatins A1, A4, B1	Cervical, lung, colon	Ley et al. (2007)

(Continued)

TABLE 15.1 (CONTINUED)
List of Some Important Medicinal Plants and Their Phytochemicals against Specific Types of Cancer

Plant Name	Common name	Plant Part extract	Phytochemicals	Specific Cancer	References
Conyza canadensis	Horseweed	Roots	Conyzapyranone A, B, 3-β-Erythrodiol	Gastric	Liu et al. (2016)
Crocus sativus	Saffron	Stigma	Crocin, crocetin	Colorectal, lung	Samarghandian et al. (2010)
Croton macrobotrys	Rushfoil	Leaves	Corydine, salutaridine	Leukaemia, lung	Jain et al. (2016)
Debregeasia longifolia	Orange wild rhea	Fruit	Epicatechin, apigenin	Breast	Bo et al. (2003)
Ginkgo biloba	Maidenhair	Leaves	Kaempferol, gink	Pancreatic, breast, prostate	Zhang et al. (2008)
Glycine max	Soybean	Seeds	Genistein, Bowman–Birk Inhibitor IBB1, IBBD2	Colorectal, breast, prostate	Clemente et al. (2010)
Hibiscus mutabilis	Confederate rose	Seeds	Lectins	Breast, hepatoma	Lam and Ng (2009)
Linum usitatissimum	Flax	Roots, leaf	Cyanogenic glycosides	Breast	Szewczyk et al. (2014)
Moringa oleifera	Drumstick tree	Leaf, bark, seed	Eugenol, isopropyl isothiocynate, D-allose	Breast, pancreatic	Al-Asmari et al. (2015)
Ocimum sanctum	Basil	Leaf, aerial parts	Camphor, linalool	Lung, cervical, fibrosarcoma	Baliga et al. (2013b)
Paeonia suffruticosa	Moutan	Seeds	*Cis-, trans-*gnetin H	Gastric, breast, lung	Gao et al. (2015)
Peganum harmala	Syrian rue	Seeds	Harmine, harmaline	Leukaemia, breast	Zaker et al. (2007)
Pisum sativum	Garden pea	Seeds	Protease inhibitors rTI1B, rTI2B	Colorectal, colon	Clemente et al. (2012)
Podophyllum hexandrum	Mayapple	Rhizome, roots	Podophyllotoxin	Leukaemia, ovarian	Giri and Narasu (2000)
Malus×domestica	Apple	Bark, fruit	Quercetin, catechin	Lung, colon, breast	Madhuri and Pandey (2009)
Solanum lycopersicum	Tomato	Fruit	Alpha-solanine, lycopene	Breast	Mohsenikia et al. (2013)
Tylophora indica	Indian Ipecac	Leaf	Tylophorin, cryptopleurine	Breast	Saraswati et al. (2013)
Vaccinium macrocarpon	American cranberry	Fruit	Proanthocyanidins	Prostate	MacLean et al. (2011)
Vitis vinifera	Grape	Seed	Proanthocyanidins, procyanidins	Oral squamous	Aghbali et al. (2013)
Ziziphus jujuba	Chinese date	Fruit, seeds	*p*-Coumaroylmaslinic acid	Breast	Plastina et al. (2012)

compound derived from *A. sativum* is S-allylcysteine, which has been found to reduce the growth of tumours. In other research, allicin showed its antitumour characteristics against breast and prostate cancer, inducing programmed death (apoptosis) of cancer cells (Madhuri and Pandey 2008). Ajoene (E and Z isomers) is another important anticancer compound derived from *A. sativum* that works against leukaemia (Kaschula et al. 2011).

15.3.2 *ANNONA MURICATA*

The common name of *Annona muricata* is the soursop fruit. It is mostly found in tropical regions of South America, the Caribbean and Southeast Asia (Yajid et al. 2018). *A. muricata* belongs to the family Annonaceae (Mishra et al. 2013). The important plant parts that are commonly used as a therapeutic agent in cancer treatment are its leaf, root, bark, and fruits.

The plant parts of *A. muricata* contain several phytochemicals, such as acetogenins 1, 2, 2-hexenoic acid esters, 2-octenoic acid, β-caryophyllene, cineole, linalool, terpineol, and bullatacin, which have antitumour properties (Pieme et al. 2014). Rieser and his co-workers (1991) showed the activity of *A. muricata* seed extract, with acetogenin 1 active against the human pancreatic tumour and human lung carcinoma, whereas acetogenin 2 was active against human hepatoma carcinoma (Rieser et al. 1991).

15.3.3 *ASTRAGALUS CYTOSUS*

Commonly known as milkvetch, *A. cytosus* belongs to the family Fabaceae. A recent studies explains the effect of the related *Astragalus mongolicus* extract against COVID-19 due to the presence of phytosterols, triterpenes, saponins, isoflavonoids, etc. (Boone et al. 2020). Other studies showed the effect of *A. cytosus* extract on human lung epithelial carcinoma cell A549, mammary tumour, colon cancer, gastric cancer, and urological tumour (Tin et al. 2007).

15.3.4 *BOSWELLIA SERRATA*

The common name of *Boswellia serrata* is Indian frankincense, and it is found mostly in Asia and Africa. The exuded gum is produced from *B. serrata* plants *via* incisions made on the trunk. The gum appears like a milky resin and has several medicinal and immune modulator properties (Khajuria et al. 2008).

According to research conducted by Winking and co-workers, the resin of *Boswellia* species possesses anticancer activity, exhibiting an anti-pro-apoptotic nature in rat astrocytoma cell lines (Winking et al. 2000). Further studies showed the effect of *B. serrata* resin constituents on two important cancerous cell lines, HepG2 and HCT 116. Furthermore, there are some reports showing the effect of *Boswellia* resins on brain oedema and brain tumours. The main active constituents of *Boswellia* resin are boswellic acids, which are mainly used in cancer treatment (Roy et al. 2016).

15.3.5 *Camellia sinensis*

It is an evergreen shrub, generally recognized as the tea plant with the leaves of *C. sinensis* being utilized to produce tea. After water, the next most consumed liquid on the planet is the leaf extract of *C. sinensis* (Sharangi 2009). *C. sinensis* is a very good source of the alkaloids theophylline, theanine, caffeine, and other antioxidants. According to the National Cancer Institute, the leaves of *C. sinensis* contain highly effective antioxidants, which can ward off several types of cancer (Sharangi 2009).

C. *sinensis* extract also contains epigallocatechin, epicatechin, epigallocatechin-3, and epigallocatechin, which have various therapeutic effects against bacterial/viral infections and against cancer-causing cells (Sultan et al. 2014). These polyphenols play a significant function in cancer prevention through decreasing oxidative DNA injury in the host cells. In one of the studies conducted by Setiawan and colleagues, they found that the regular habit of drinking green tea decreased the risk of developing gastric cancer (Setiawan et al. 2001).

15.3.6 *Centella asiatica*

Centella asiatica, commonly known as pennywort, is native to the Indian subcontinent. It belongs to the family Apiaceae. The leaves or sometimes the whole plant are used for various medicinal purposes and as an immunomodulatory agent. The leaf extract of *C. asiatica* contains several flavonoids including hyperin and its various glycosides (Babu et al. 1995).

The purified extract of *C. asiatica* demonstrated action against Ehrlich tumour cell lines and Dalton's lymphoma ascites cells. Direct inhibition of DNA synthesis is the key mechanism underlying the anticancer activity of the *C. asiatica* extract. The oral consumption of *C. asiatica* leaves also provides protection against oxidative damage (Gupta and Flora, 2006).

15.3.7 *Curcuma longa*

Curcuma longa is popularly known as turmeric (Yue et al. 2010). The rhizome is the most important part of this plant and the main active ingredient present in it is known as curcumin (diferuloylmethane), a polyphenol. Other than curcumin, *C. longa* contains one other group of important constituents known as sesquiterpenoids, which also possess some important biological properties.

Curcumin has anticancer properties. It is utilized to prevent different cancers, such as blood, ovarian, gastrointestinal tract, lung, liver, skin, prostate, breast, bladder, and pancreatic cancers as well as lymphomas (Luthra and Lal 2016). Downregulating the expression of genes (encoding lysyl oxidase, NF-kappa β, epidermal growth receptors, inducible nitric oxide synthase (iNOS), cyclooxygenase, tumour necrosis factor, and matrix metallopeptidase) is the key mechanism behind the anticancer activity of curcumin.

15.3.8 PHYLLANTHUS AMARUS

P. amarus is generally identified as bhui-aamla and it belongs to the family Phyllanthaceae. The complete plant, as well as parts, such as root, shoots, and leaves, has medicinal properties. The anticancer property of *P. amarus* is due to the presence of various flavanoids, lignins, and tannins. The major phytochemicals found are gallotannins (corilagin, amariin, phyllanthusiin D, geraniin) and the lignans (phyllanthin and hypophyllanthin) (Sripanidkulchai et al. 2002).

The extract of this plant has a significant effect on reducing the tumour size in mice having Dalton's lymphoma (Rajeshkumar et al. 2002). The mechanism behind the anticancer property of *P. amarus* extract involves its ability to stimulate cell cycle arrest or by inhibiting metabolic activation of carcinogenic compounds.

15.3.9 WITHANIA SOMNIFERA

Popularly known as ashwagandha or poison gooseberry, *W. somnifera* belongs to the family Solanaceae. It is a small, perennial shrub, mainly cultivated in drier regions of India and is also found in China, Yemen, and Nepal. The roots and leaves of this plant have been traditionally used to cure and prevent several diseases (Jayaprakasam et al. 2003).

The root extract of this plant has several bioactive phytochemicals (withanolide A, withaferin A) which help in inducing apoptosis in cancerous cells. However, the synthesis or isolation of withanolides from *W. somnifera* extract is a serious limitation to their effective use in the medical field (Malik et al. 2007).

15.3.10 ZINGIBER OFFICINALE

This plant is widely known as ginger and is a member of the family Zingiberaceae. It is a herbaceous plant, commonly found in hot and humid regions of India. Traditionally, *Z. officinale* is used as medicine for the cure of a number of diseases, such as inflammatory diseases (Afzal et al. 2001). *Z. officinale* includes several bioactive phytochemicals, such as phenolic compounds (gingerol, paradol, and shogoal). These polyphenolic compounds have anti-cancer properties.

Extract of *Z. officinale* down-regulates transcriptional factors involved in the cellular proliferation of ovarian cancer cells (Nonn et al. 2007). One of the studies reported the rhizome extract of *Z. officinale* as being effective at chemosensitizing certain neoplastic cells.

15.4 PHYTOCHEMICALS USED FOR CANCER TREATMENT

15.4.1 APIGENIN

Apigenin (4′,5,7-trihydroxyflavone) is a flavone compound available mainly from *Moringa peregrina* and some other vegetables and herbs, such as chamomile, celery, and parsley. It is a yellow crystalline solid used in several therapeutic products

(Patel et al. 2007). Apigenin has specific effects in normal *versus* cancer cells in comparison with other structurally related compounds. The chemical configuration of apigenin is given below (Figure 15.2a).

Apigenin is effective against almost every form of cancer, like breast, colon, cervical, leukaemia, ovarian, prostate, skin, thyroid, neuroblastoma, and lung cancer (Patel et al. 2007). Different action mechanisms of apigenin have been identified which include anti-proliferative activity, oestrogenic/anti-oestrogenic activity, apoptosis, induction of detoxification enzymes, prevention of oxidation, and regulation of the host immune system. It has been shown to have anticancer action on human breast cancer cell lines. Apigenin showed growth inhibitory activity against breast cancer cells HER2/neu by inducing apoptosis through the phosphatidylinositol 3-kinase pathway (Way et al. 2004).

15.4.2 CURCUMIN

Curcumin (1E, 6E)-1,7-Bis (4-hydroxy-3-methoxyphenyl) hepta-1,6-diene-3,5-dione) is the major phytochemical of the popular Indian spice turmeric, *Curcuma longa*. Curcumin down-regulates different pro-inflammatory cytokines, like chemokines, tumour necrosis factor (TNF- α), interleukins (IL-1, IL-2, IL-6, IL-8, IL-12), etc. (Zhou et al. 2011). The chemical structure of curcumin is illustrated in Figure 15.2b.

Curcumin has proved to be a potential curative agent against cancer due to its property of inducing apoptosis in cancer cells without affecting normal ones. Numerous clinical trials have been completed to test its activity on tumorous cells. Kuttan and his co-workers in 1987 conducted a clinical trial and observed the reduced size of oral cancer and leukoplakia after treatment with curcumin (Kuttan et al. 1987). Curcumin also shows activity against different types of cancer, such as breast, oral, prostate, lung, multiple myeloma, colorectal, pancreatic, and neck and head squamous cell carcinoma (Gupta et al. 2013).

15.4.3 CROCETIN

Crocetin is a natural carotenoid, found in the flower of the Saffron crocus and in dehydrated stigmas of *Crocus sativus* (Gutheil et al. 2012). The structure of crocetin has 20 carbon atoms with conjugated double bonds and containing two carboxylic acid groups (**Fig. 15.2c**). Crocetin is a potential agent against skin carcinoma, hepatocellular carcinoma, colorectal cancer cells, a pancreatic cancer cell line, lung cancer, and breast cancer.

The action mechanism of crocetin includes inhibiting the synthesis of nucleic acid, enhancing the antioxidative system, which induces apoptosis and inhibits the growth factor signalling pathways (Figure 15.3). In 2013, Bathaie and his co-workers demonstrated the positive effects of crocetin on gastric adenocarcinoma and gastric cancer in rats (Bathaie et al. 2013).

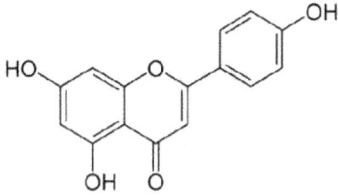

(a) Apigenin

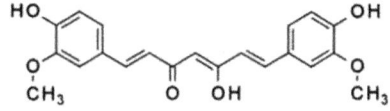

(b) Curcumin

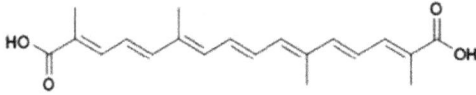

(c) Crocetin

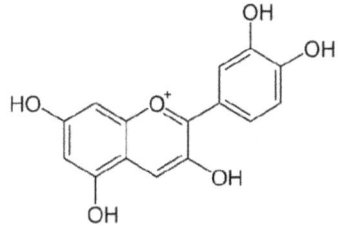

(d) Cyanidin

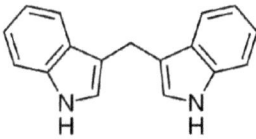

(e) Diindolylmethane

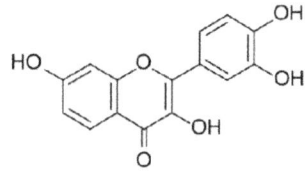

(f) Fisetin

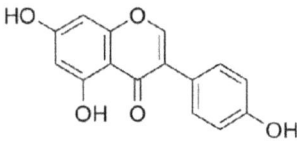

(g) Genistein

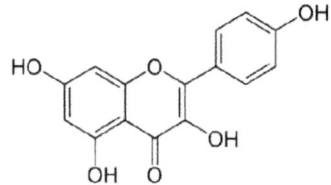

(h) Kaempferol

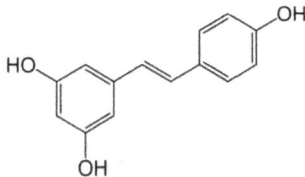

(i) Resveratrol

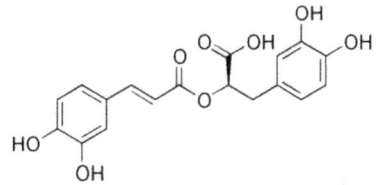

(j) Rosmarinic acid

FIGURE 15.2 Chemical structures of some important phytochemicals used against specific type of cancer.

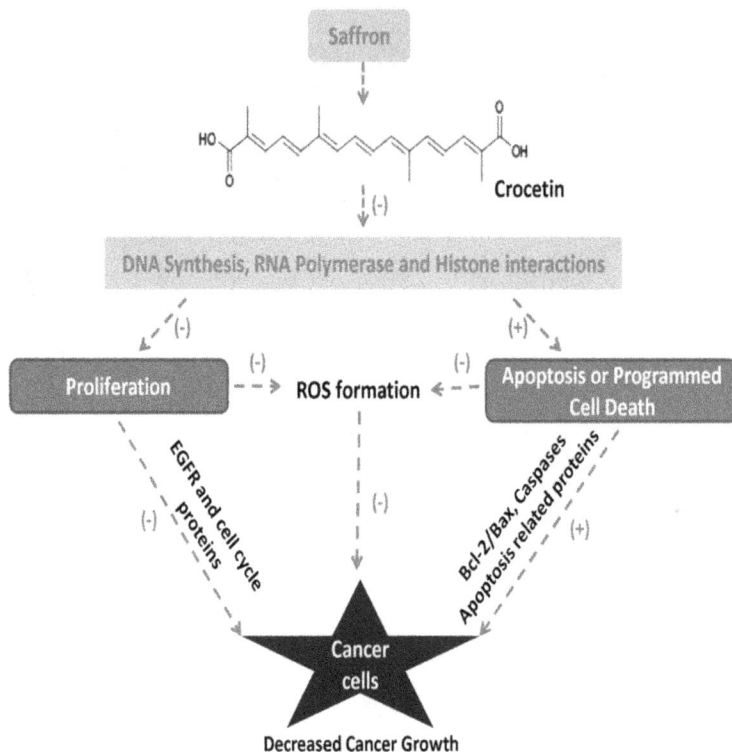

FIGURE 15.3   Possible chemopreventive mechanisms of crocetin against cancer cells.

15.4.4 CYANIDINS

Cyanidins are a group of pigments extracted from red berries, red onion, apples, plums, grapes, raspberry, blackberry, red cabbage, and cranberry. Cyanidin is a natural organic compound (an anthocyanidin) possessing radical-scavenging and anti-oxidant effects on cancer cells. The chemical structure of cyanidin is illustrated in Figure 15.2d.

Cyanidin shows activity against several cancers, such as colorectal, colon, lung, breast, leukaemia, etc. In 2010, a group of researchers concluded in their study that the cyanidin preferentially kills cancer cells with highly malignant characteristics (Cvorovic et al. 2010). Other research has demonstrated the inhibitory effect of the cyanidin glycosides (examples of anthocyanins) cyanidin-3-rutinoside and cyanidin-3-glucoside on human lung carcinoma cells.

15.4.5 DIINDOLYLMETHANE

Diindolylmethane (3,3′-methanediylbis) is a glucosinolate, produced by plant species limited to the 'cruciferous' vegetables (Brassicaceae family) such as cabbage, kale, Brussels sprouts, cauliflower, and broccoli (Hong et al. 2002). It is an analogue of indole-3-carbinol which is formed *via* condensation in the acidic medium after digestion in the stomach. Indole-3-carbinol and diindolylmethane are extremely effective in terms of anticancer effects against hormone-responsive cancers like prostate, ovarian, and breast cancers. The chemical structure of diindolylmethane is shown in (Figure 15.2e).

Some studies showed the action of diindolylmethane in human cancer cells to be by activation of the human protein p53 which results in inducing apoptosis (Ge et al. 1996). One of the other studies (Beaver et al., 2012) showed that diindolylmethane transduced signalling *via* activating transcription factors like NF-κB, Wnt, Akt, mTOR, etc. They also concluded that diindolylmethane and indole-3-carbinol had a more efficient activity to cancer at the early phases of prostate cancer.

15.4.6 FISETIN

Fisetin (2-(3,4-dihydroxyphenyl)-3,7-dihydroxychromen-4-one) is a polyphenol from the flavonoid fraction. It is mostly found in fruits and vegetables such as onion, tomato, cucumber, apple, kiwi, peach, strawberries, grape, and persimmon (Lall et al. 2015). Fisetin showed effectiveness against different cancers, such as prostate, lung, skin, colorectal, bladder, breast, leukemia, and cervical cancers. The chemical structure of fisetin is shown in Figure 15.2f.

15.4.7 GENISTEIN

Genistein (5,7-dihydroxy-3-(4-hydroxyphenyl)chromen-4-one) is an isoflavone reported from several plants such as fava beans, psoralea, lupin, kudzu, soybeans (all members of the Fabaceae), and coffee. It has been reported to have anti-angiogenic effects and may inhibit the uncontrolled cell growth associated with cancer (Yu et al. 2012). Genistein acts as a tyrosine kinase inhibitor, with a function of inhibiting DNA topoisomerase II. The chemical structure of genistein is shown in Figure 15.2g.

According to a study conducted by a group of researchers in 2008, genistein inhibits the activation of different transcription factors, such as NF-κB, STAT-3, and Akt. These transcription factors are used to sustain a homoeostatic equilibrium between its cell cycle and apoptosis (Banerjee et al. 2008). Genistein also showed activity against mammary cancer treatment. In 1995, Lamartiniere and his coworkers perform an experiment on female Sprague-Dawley rat (which had been chemically induced to express breast cancer) by pre-treating them with genistein (Lamartiniere et al. 1995). The experiment resulted in a decreased number of terminal ends and an increased number of lobular structures. Genistein was reported to be an efficient inhibitor against RTK (Receptor Tyrosine Kinase) together with EGFR (Epidermal Growth Factor Receptor)(Figure 15.4).

15.4.8 KAEMPFEROL

Kaempferol (3,5,7-trihydroxy-2-(4-hydroxyphenyl)-4*H*-chromen-4-one) is a natural polyphenol of the flavonol type isolated from a variety of fruits and vegetables, such as tomato, grapes, apples, grapefruit, tea, squash, broccoli, potato, onions, and Brussels

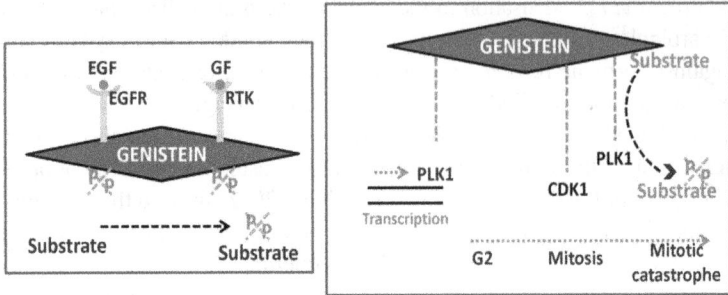

FIGURE 15.4 Mechanisms of action of genistein to exert anticancer effects.

sprouts. Numerous studies have explained the beneficial effects of dietary kaempferol in decreasing the risk of chronic diseases, particularly cancer. Kaempferol has been useful in the treatment of several cancers, like pancreatic, ovarian, colon, and lung cancer. Additionally, it is a lot less lethal to regular non-cancer cells in comparison with the usual chemotherapy drugs (Chen and Chen 2013). The chemical structure of kaempferol is shown in Figure 15.2h).

One of the studies found that the phytochemical kaempferol was useful in the treatment of ovarian cancer cells through inhibition of cancer cell proliferation and the activation of the human p53 protein. Another report illustrated that kaempferol considerably repressed cancerous pancreatic cell proliferation and significantly reduced ^{3}H-thymidine incorporation in pancreatic cancerous cell lines.

15.4.9 Resveratrol

Resveratrol (3,5,4′-trihydroxy-*trans*-stilbene) is a stilbenoid, a normal phenolic which has been reported from the skin of red grapes, blueberries, raspberries, mulberries, and peanuts. Resveratrol is effective in all three stages of cancer, i.e., initiation, promotion, and progression. Resveratrol acts by modulating the signal transduction pathways that control growth, inflammation, apoptosis, angiogenesis, and metastasis of cancerous cells (Bishayee et al. 2009). The chemical structure of resveratrol is shown in (Figure 15.2i).

Resveratrol is also involved in the treatment of cancers like, skin, breast, prostate, gastrointestinal tract, lung, etc. The anticarcinogenic activity of resveratrol is mediated through several cell signalling pathways. Other activities are also involved, such as suppression of tumor cell proliferation, cell cycle arrest, reduction of inflammation, stimulation of apoptosis, cell differentiation, and reduction of adhesion, angiogenesis, metastasis, and invasion (Shankar et al. 2007).

15.4.10 Rosmarinic Acid

Rosmarinic acid ((2*R*)-3-(3,4-dihydroxyphenyl)-2-{[(2*E*)-3-(3,4-dihydroxyphenyl) prop-2-enoyl]oxy}propanoic acid) is a common antioxidant reported from various medicinal herbs, such as rosemary, thyme, lemon balm, oregano, peppermint, and sage. Extract of rosemary plays an important role in anti-inflammation, antitumour, and antiproliferation in various *in-vitro* and *in-vivo* studies (Yesil-Celiktas et al. 2010). The chemical structure of rosmarinic acid is shown in (Figure 15.2j).

Rosmarinic acid has been shown to reduce tumour necrosis factor (TNF-α) in induced human dermal fibroblasts. It was found that treatment with rosmarinic acid considerably sensitized TNF-α and stimulated apoptosis in human leukaemia cells through repression of the nuclear transcription factor (kappa-gamma-β). Some studies reported the successful treatment of human colon carcinoma using rosmarinic acid (Xu et al. 2010).

15.5 PHYTOCHEMICAL PREPARATION

The prospective of medicinal plants as curative agents depends upon the quality and quantity of the active phytochemicals in the herbal preparation. Certain phytochemicals have been established for their anti-cancer activities. They were extracted from different plant parts using several extraction techniques. The effectiveness of phytochemicals depends upon their successful extraction and purification. A detailed scheme of phytochemical extraction, characterization, identification, and clinical trials as a cancer therapeutic agent is shown in Figure 15.5.

15.5.1 PHYTOCHEMICAL EXTRACTION

The extraction of phytochemicals from medicinal plants is the most important step in the preparation of pharmaceutical products. The extraction of phytochemicals can be done using fresh, dried, or frozen plant samples. The first step of extraction is grinding of the plant sample. Grinding is usually performed after air-drying of the plant sample and then milling and homogenization (Abascal et al. 2005).

Solvent extractions are the most frequently utilized method for isolation of plant materials due to its easy procedure, wide applicability, and high efficiency. Solvent selection is a crucial step for phytochemical extraction, because different phytochemicals have different solubility efficiencies in various solvents (Xu and Chang 2007). Solvents, such as ethyl acetate, methanol, ether, ethanol, and acetone, alone or in combination, have been used for the extraction of phytochemicals.

15.5.2 PHYTOCHEMICAL PURIFICATION

The crude extracts of plants contain a number of impurities, usually carbohydrates or lipids, which can result in very low concentrations of phenolics in the crude plant extract. To concentrate and obtain phytochemical-rich fractions before analysis, purification approaches are required. Purification can be done by several methods, such as centrifugation, filtration, chromatographic separation (column chromatography), and some other methods (solid-phase extraction, liquid-liquid partitioning, sequential extraction). In general, for the removal of lipid impurities, the crude extract is washed with non-polar solvents (Ramirez-Coronel et al. 2004), such as chloroform

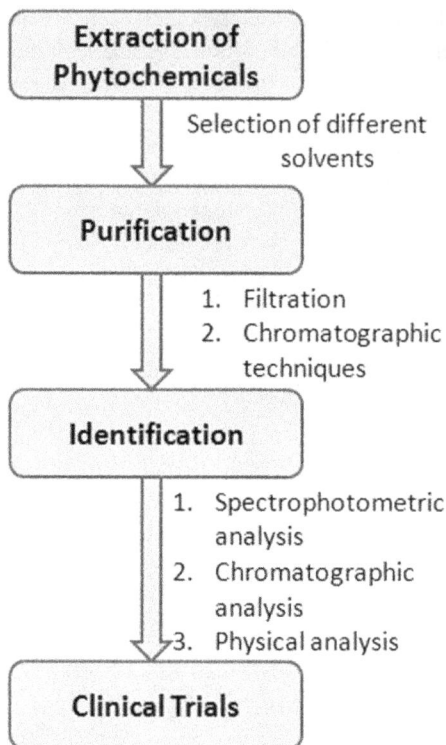

FIGURE 15.5 Detailed scheme of phytochemical preparation.

or dichloromethane (Neergheen et al. 2006), whereas, for the removal of polar non-phenolic compounds, such as organic acids and sugars, solid-phase extraction is used.

Column chromatography has been also used for the extraction of phytochemicals. Even though this process is time consuming and requires large volumes of solvent, it provides generally pure phytochemicals. Different columns used for the fractionation of phytochemicals include RP-C18 (Queiroz et al. 2005), Toyopearl (Kandil et al. 2002), LH-20 (Pedreschi and Cisneros-Zevallos, 2006) and, to a less extent, polyamide resin (Ranilla et al. 2007). Eluents used for separation include ethanol, acetone, water, or methanol, or combinations thereof. In some cases, pre-parative-scale HPLC or classical liquid–liquid extraction has also been utilized in plant extract purification (Ek et al. 2006). As a substitute for liquid chromatography, countercurrent chromatography has also been developed for fractionation of various classes of phytochemicals. The main advantage of using countercurrent chromatography is the absence of a solid matrix (Berthod et al. 1999).

15.5.3 PHYTOCHEMICAL IDENTIFICATION

The process of phytochemical identification begins with the confirmation test for biological activity of the natural extract. Then, suitable matrices are employed for the fractionation of the active extracts. Bioactivity tests are performed using several analytical techniques, such as chromatographic analysis (absorption, ion exchange, affinity, partition, High Pressure Liquid Chromatography (HPLC) and Gas Chromatography (GC), paper, etc.) (Dai and Mumper, 2010), spectrophotometric analysis (UV-Vis, MS) (Jac et al. 2006) or physical structural analysis (Fourier-transform infrared spectroscopy (FTIR), X-ray diffraction analysis (XRD), Nuclear magnetic resonance (NMR)) (Pawlowska et al. 2008) etc. These are used for the identification and separation of active fractions.

15.5.4 CLINICAL TRIALS

After identification of these phytomolecules, they must be studied to determine *in-vitro* or *in-vivo* anticancer behaviour. If an improved anticancer efficiency is achieved by the molecules, then other aspects, like pharmacokinetics, pharmacodynamics, immunogenicity, metabolic fate, biosafety and side effects, drug interactions, dose concentration, etc. must be considered for future drug design and administration.

15.6 MECHANISM OF ACTION OF PHYTOCHEMICALS ON CANCEROUS CELLS

The mechanism of action involved in cancer treatment using polyphenols is categorized in different sections. Some phytochemicals, like quercitin and resveratrol, are used for the antioxidant-mediated cancer therapy mechanism. This mechanism involves scavenging free radicals and reducing oxidative stress in cancerous cells (Childers et al. 1995). The second mechanism engaged in cancer treatment is inhibition of activity by phytochemicals. The inhibition mechanism involves reduction of cell proliferation, oncogene expression, and signal transduction pathways (Singh et al. 2006). Next is induction activity exhibited by plant extracts, such as cranberry extract in breast cancer, glutathione in colon cancer (Odom et al. 2009), quercetin in cervical cancer, etc.

Cancer therapy using phytochemicals can also be achieved by enzyme inhibition and enzyme induction mechanisms. The enzyme inhibition mechanism involves phase I enzyme, cyclooxygenase-2 inhibition, inducible nitric oxide synthase inhibition, or xanthine oxidase inhibition (Rajendran et al. 2011). The enzyme induction mechanism involves phase II enzyme induction, glutathione peroxidase induction, catalase induction, and superoxide dismutase induction (Hayes et al. 2008).

Finally, some phytochemicals show different regulation activity to treat cancerous cells. Regulation activity involves regulation of steroid hormone metabolism (Mandlekar et al. 2006), regulation of oestrogen metabolism (Clarke et al. 1996), microRNA (miRNA) regulation (Tilghman et al. 2013), or regulation of activator signal transduction pathway (Frigo et al. 2002).

15.7 CONCLUSION AND FUTURE PROSPECTS

Several conventional treatments are available for cancer therapy, but they all come with severe side effects and symptoms (kidney failure, anaemia, fertility issues, gastrointestinal disorders, etc.). The current major challenges are the increasing incidence of cancer cases, the high expense of conventional treatments, a number of limitations to the traditional remedy, and the high toxicity of current anticancer medicines. Therefore, the immediate objective is to propose and develop a substitute, eco-friendly, biocompatible and more affordable approach through a greener route. Phytochemicals obtained from medicinal plants provide a capable and valuable research field with much promise. Anticancer medicinal plants act as natural immune boosters, modulating the immune response in several disease treatments. The more eco-friendly and biocompatible nature of phytochemicals have elevated the effectiveness of these phytochemicals in cancer management. However, detailed studies are still required to gain more insights into these phytochemicals to estimate their potential functions, and their toxicological and particular genotoxic profiles against different categories of cancer.

REFERENCES

Abascal, K., Ganora, L., and E. Yarnell. 2005. The effect of freeze-drying and its implications for botanical medicine: a review. *Phytotherapy Research: An International Journal Devoted to Pharmacological and Toxicological Evaluation of Natural Product Derivatives* 19(8):655–660.

Afzal, M., Al-Hadidi, D., Menon, M., Pesek, J., and M. S. I. Dhami. 2001. Ginger: an ethnomedical, chemical and pharmacological review. *Drug Metabolism and Drug Interactions* 18(3–4):159–190.

Aghbali, A., Hosseini, S. V., Delazar, A., Gharavi, N. K., Shahneh, F. Z., Orangi, M., ... B. Baradaran. 2013. Induction of apoptosis by grape seed extract (*Vitis vinifera*) in oral squamous cell carcinoma. *Bosnian Journal of Basic Medical Sciences* 13(3):186.

Ahmadi, A. 2012. Potential prevention: Aloe vera mouthwash may reduce radiation-induced oral mucositis in head and neck cancer patients. *Chinese Journal of Integrative Medicine* 18(8):635–640.

Al-Asmari, A. K., Albalawi, S. M., Athar, M. T., Khan, A. Q., Al-Shahrani, H., and M. Islam. 2015. *Moringa oleifera* as an anti-cancer agent against breast and colorectal cancer cell lines. *PloS one* 10(8):e0135814.

Babu, T. D., Kuttan, G., and J. Padikkala. 1995. Cytotoxic and anti-tumour properties of certain taxa of Umbelliferae with special reference to *Centella asiatica* (L.) Urban. *Journal of Ethnopharmacology* 48(1):53–57.

Baliga, M. S., Jimmy, R., Thilakchand, K. R., Sunitha, V., Bhat, N. R., Saldanha, E., ... P. L. Palatty. 2013b. *Ocimum sanctum* L (Holy Basil or Tulsi) and its phytochemicals in the prevention and treatment of cancer. *Nutrition and Cancer* 65(sup1):26–35.

Baliga, M. S., Thilakchand, K. R., Rai, M. P., Rao, S., and P. Venkatesh. 2013a. *Aegle marmelos* (L.) Correa (Bael) and its phytochemicals in the treatment and prevention of cancer. *Integrative Cancer Therapies* 12(3):187–196.

Banerjee, S., Li, Y., Wang, Z., and F. H. Sarkar. 2008. Multi-targeted therapy of cancer by genistein. *Cancer Letters* 269(2):226–242.

Bathaie, S. Z., Hoshyar, R., Miri, H., and M. Sadeghizadeh. 2013. Anticancer effects of crocetin in both human adenocarcinoma gastric cancer cells and rat model of gastric cancer. *Biochemistry and Cell Biology* 91(6):397–403.

Beaver, L. M., Yu, T. W., Sokolowski, E. I., Williams, D. E., Dashwood, R. H., and Ho, E. 2012. 3,3′-Diindolylmethane, but not indole-3-carbinol, inhibits histone deacetylase activity in prostate cancer cells. *Toxicology and Applied Pharmacology* 263(3):345–351.

Berthod, A., Billardello, B., and S. Geoffroy. 1999. Polyphenols in countercurrent chromatography. An example of large scale separation. *Analusis* 27(9):750–757.

Bishayee, A. 2009. Cancer prevention and treatment with resveratrol: from rodent studies to clinical trials. *Cancer Prevention Research* 2(5):409–418.

Bo, Q., Hanqing, W., and Z. Dayuan. 2003. Investigation on the chemical constituents of *Debregeasia longifolia*. *Natural Product Research and Development* 15(1):21–23.

Boone, H. A., Medunjanin, D., and A. Sijerčić. 2020. Review on potential of phytotherapeutics in fight against COVID-19. *International Journal of Innovative Science and Research Technology* 5:481–491.

Capasso, A. 2013. Antioxidant action and therapeutic efficacy of *Allium sativum* L. *Molecules* 18(1):690–700.

Chapa-Oliver, A., and L. Mejía-Teniente. 2016. Capsaicin: from plants to a cancer-suppressing agent. *Molecules* 21(8):931.

Chen, A. Y., and Y. C. Chen. 2013. A review of the dietary flavonoid, kaempferol on human health and cancer chemoprevention. *Food Chemistry* 138(4):2099–2107.

Childers, J. M., Chu, J., Voigt, L. F., Feigl, P., Tamimi, H. K., Franklin, E. W., ... F. L. Meyskens. 1995. Chemoprevention of cervical cancer with folic acid: a phase III Southwest Oncology Group Intergroup study. *Cancer Epidemiology and Prevention Biomarkers* 4(2):155–159.

Choedon, T., Shukla, S. K., and V. Kumar. 2010. Chemopreventive and anti-cancer properties of the aqueous extract of flowers of *Butea monosperma*. *Journal of Ethnopharmacology* 129(2):208–213.

Clarke, R., Hilakivi-Clarke, L., Cho, E., James, M. R., and F. Leonessa. 1996. Estrogens, phytoestrogens, and breast cancer. In *Dietary Phytochemicals in Cancer Prevention and Treatment* (pp. 63–85). Springer, Boston, MA.

Clemente, A., Marín-Manzano, M. C., Jiménez, E., Arques, M. C., and C. Domoney. 2012. The anti-proliferative effect of TI1B, a major Bowman–Birk isoinhibitor from pea (*Pisum sativum* L.), on HT29 colon cancer cells is mediated through protease inhibition. *British Journal of Nutrition* 108(S1):S135–S144.

Clemente, A., Moreno, F. J., Marín-Manzano, M. D. C., Jiménez, E., and C. Domoney. 2010. The cytotoxic effect of Bowman–Birk isoinhibitors, IBB1 and IBBD2, from soybean (*Glycine max*) on HT29 human colorectal cancer cells is related to their intrinsic ability to inhibit serine proteases. *Molecular Nutrition and Food Research* 54(3):396–405.

Cvorovic, J., Tramer, F., Granzotto, M., Candussio, L., Decorti, G., and S. Passamonti. 2010. Oxidative stress-based cytotoxicity of delphinidin and cyanidin in colon cancer cells. *Archives of Biochemistry and Biophysics* 501(1):151–157.

Dai, J., and R. J. Mumper. 2010. Plant phenolics: extraction, analysis and their antioxidant and anticancer properties. *Molecules* 15(10):7313–7352.

Das, S., Bordoloi, R., and N. Newar. 2014. A review on immune modulatory effect of some traditional medicinal herbs. *Journal of Pharmaceutical, Chemical and Biological Sciences* 2(1):33–42.

Desai, A. G., Qazi, G. N., Ganju, R. K., El-Tamer, M., Singh, J., Saxena, A. K., ... H. K. Bhat. 2008. Medicinal plants and cancer chemoprevention. *Current Drug Metabolism* 9(7):581–591.

Douros, J., and M. Suffness. 1980. The National Cancer Institute's natural products antineoplastic development program. In *New Anticancer Drugs* (pp. 21–44). Springer, Berlin, Heidelberg.

Efferth, T. 2010. Cancer therapy with natural products and medicinal plants. *Planta Medica* 76(11):1035–1036.

Efferth, T. 2017. From ancient herb to modern drug: Artemisia annua and artemisinin for cancer therapy. In *Seminars in Cancer Biology* (Vol. 46, pp. 65–83). Academic Press.

Ek, S., Kartimo, H., Mattila, S., and A. Tolonen. 2006. Characterization of phenolic compounds from lingonberry (*Vaccinium vitis-idaea*). *Journal of Agricultural and Food Chemistry* 54(26):9834–9842.

Frigo, D. E., Duong, B. N., Melnik, L. I., Schief, L. S., Collins-Burow, B. M., Pace, D. K., …
M. E. Burow. 2002. Flavonoid phytochemicals regulate activator protein-1 signal transduction pathways in endometrial and kidney stable cell lines. *The Journal of Nutrition*
132(7):1848–1853.

Gao, Y., He, C., Ran, R., Zhang, D., Li, D., Xiao, P. G., and E. Altman. 2015. The resveratrol
oligomers, cis-and trans-gnetin H, from Paeonia suffruticosa seeds inhibit the growth
of several human cancer cell lines. *Journal of Ethnopharmacology* 169:24–33.

Ge, X., Yannai, S., Rennert, G., Gruener, N., and F. A. Fares. 1996. 3,3′-Diindolylmethane
induces apoptosis in human cancer cells. *Biochemical and Biophysical Research
Communications* 228(1):153–158.

Giri, A., and M. L. Narasu. 2000. Production of podophyllotoxin from *Podophyllum hexandrum*: a potential natural product for clinically useful anticancer drugs. *Cytotechnology*
34(1–2):17–26.

Gupta, R., and S. J. S. Flora. 2006. Effect of *Centella asiatica* on arsenic induced oxidative
stress and metal distribution in rats. *Journal of Applied Toxicology: An International
Journal* 26(3):213–222.

Gupta, S. C., Patchva, S., and B. B. Aggarwal. 2013. Therapeutic roles of curcumin: lessons
learned from clinical trials. *The AAPS Journal* 15(1):195–218.

Gutheil, G. W., Reed, G., Ray, A., Anant, S., and A. Dhar. 2012. Crocetin: an agent
derived from saffron for prevention and therapy for cancer. *Current Pharmaceutical
Biotechnology* 13(1):173–179.

Hall, W., Christie, M., and D. Currow. 2005. Cannabinoids and cancer: causation, remedia-
tion, and palliation. *The Lancet Oncology* 6(1):35–42.

Hayes, J. D., Kelleher, M. O., and I. M. Eggleston. 2008. The cancer chemopreventive actions
of phytochemicals derived from glucosinolates. *European Journal of Nutrition* 47(2)
Supplement 2:73–88.

Hong, C., Firestone, G. L., and L. F. Bjeldanes. 2002. Bcl-2 family-mediated apoptotic
effects of 3,3′-diindolylmethane (DIM) in human breast cancer cells. *Biochemical
Pharmacology* 63(6):1085–1097.

Hoshyar, R., Mahboob, Z., and A. Zarban. 2016. The antioxidant and chemical properties of *Berberis vulgaris* and its cytotoxic effect on human breast carcinoma cells.
Cytotechnology 68(4):1207–1213.

Iqbal, J., Abbasi, B. A., Mahmood, T., Kanwal, S., Ali, B., Shah, S. A., and A. T. Khalil. 2017.
Plant-derived anticancer agents: a green anticancer approach. *Asian Pacific Journal of
Tropical Biomedicine* 7(12):1129–1150.

Jac, P., Polášek, M., and M. Pospíšilová. 2006. Recent trends in the determination of polyphenols by electromigration methods. *Journal of Pharmaceutical and Biomedical
Analysis* 40(4):805–814.

Jain, S., Dwivedi, J., Jain, P. K., Satpathy, S., and A. Patra. 2016. Medicinal plants for treatment of cancer: a brief review. *Pharmacognosy Journal* 8(2): 87–102.

Jayaprakasam, B., Zhang, Y., Seeram, N. P., and M. G. Nair. 2003. Growth inhibition of
human tumor cell lines by withanolides from *Withania somnifera* leaves. *Life Sciences*
74(1):125–132.

Ji, H. F., Li, X. J., and H. Y. Zhang. 2009. Natural products and drug discovery: can thousands
of years of ancient medical knowledge lead us to new and powerful drug combinations
in the fight against cancer and dementia? *EMBO Reports* 10(3):194–200.

Kandil, F. E., Smith, M. A. L., Rogers, R. B., Pépin, M. F., Song, L. L., Pezzuto, J. M.,
and D. S. Seigler. 2002. Composition of a chemopreventive proanthocyanidin-rich
fraction from cranberry fruits responsible for the inhibition of 12-O-tetradecanoyl
phorbol-13-acetate (TPA)-induced ornithine decarboxylase (ODC) activity. *Journal of
Agricultural and Food Chemistry* 50(5):1063–1069.

Kaschula, H. C., Hunter, R., Hassan, T. H., Stellenboom, N., Cotton, J., Zhai, Q. X., and M. I. Parker. 2011. Anti-proliferative activity of synthetic ajoene analogues on cancer cell-lines. *Anti-Cancer Agents in Medicinal Chemistry* 11(3):260–266.

Khajuria, A., Gupta, A., Suden, P., Singh, S., Malik, F., Singh, J., ... G. N. Qazi. 2008. Immunomodulatory activity of biopolymeric fraction BOS 2000 from *Boswellia serrata*. *Phytotherapy Research: An International Journal Devoted to Pharmacological and Toxicological Evaluation of Natural Product Derivatives* 22(3):340–348.

Khan, M. S., Ansari, I. A., Ahmad, S., Akhter, F., Hashim, A., and A. K. Srivastava. 2013. Chemotherapeutic potential of *Boerhaavia diffusa* Linn: a review. *Journal of Applied Pharmaceutical Science* 3(01):133–139.

Khodadadi, S. 2015. Role of herbal medicine in boosting immune system. *Immunopathologia Persa* 1(1):e01. *Journal of Evidence-Based Complementary and Alternative Medicine* 22(4):982–995.

Kooti, W., Servatyari, K., Behzadifar, M., Asadi-Samani, M., Sadeghi, F., Nouri, B., and Zare Marzouni, H. (2017). Effective medicinal plant in cancer treatment, part 2: Review study. *Journal of Evidence-Based Complementary & Alternative Medicine* 22(4):982–995.

Krishnamurthi, K. 2007. 17-screening of natural products for anticancer and antidiabetic properties. *Cancer* 3(4):69–75.

Kumar, S. V., Kumar, S. P., Rupesh, D., and K. Nitin. 2011. Immunomodulatory effects of some traditional medicinal plants. *Journal of Chemical and Pharmaceutical Research* 3(1):675–684.

Kuttan, R., Sudheeran, P. C., and C. D. Josph. 1987. Turmeric and curcumin as topical agents in cancer therapy. *Tumori Journal* 73(1):29–31.

Lall, R., Syed, D., Adhami, V., Khan, M., and H. Mukhtar. 2015. Dietary polyphenols in prevention and treatment of prostate cancer. *International Journal of Molecular Sciences* 16(2):3350–3376.

Lam, S. K., and T. B. Ng. 2009. Novel galactonic acid-binding hexameric lectin from *Hibiscus mutabilis* seeds with antiproliferative and potent HIV-1 reverse transcriptase inhibitory activities. *Acta Biochimica Polonica* 56(4):649.

Lamartiniere, C. A., Moore, J., Holland, M., and S. Barnes. 1995. Neonatal genistein chemoprevents mammary cancer. *Proceedings of the Society for Experimental Biology and Medicine* 208(1):120–123.

Ley, C. D., Horsman, M. R., and P. E. Kristjansen. 2007. Early effects of combretastatin-A4 disodium phosphate on tumor perfusion and interstitial fluid pressure. *Neoplasia* 9(2):108–112.

Liu, K., Qin, Y. H., Yu, J. Y., Ma, H., and X. L. Song. 2016. 3-β-Erythrodiol isolated from *Conyza canadensis* inhibits MKN45 human gastric cancer cell proliferation by inducing apoptosis, cell cycle arrest, DNA fragmentation, ROS generation and reduces tumor weight and volume in mouse xenograft model. *Oncology Reports* 35(4):2328–2338.

Luo, K. W., Ko, C. H., Yue, G. G. L., Lee, J. K. M., Li, K. K., Lee, M., ... and C. Bik-San. 2014. Green tea (*Camellia sinensis*) extract inhibits both the metastasis and osteolytic components of mammary cancer 4T1 lesions in mice. *The Journal of Nutritional Biochemistry* 25(4):395–403.

Luthra, P. M., and N. Lal. 2016. Prospective of curcumin, a pleiotropic signalling molecule from *Curcuma longa* in the treatment of glioblastoma. *European Journal of Medicinal Chemistry* 109:23–35.

MacLean, M. A., Scott, B. E., Deziel, B. A., Nunnelley, M. C., Liberty, A. M., Gottschall-Pass, K. T., ... R. A. Hurta. 2011. North American cranberry (*Vaccinium macrocarpon*) stimulates apoptotic pathways in DU145 human prostate cancer cells in vitro. *Nutrition and Cancer* 63(1):109–120.

Madhuri, S., and G. Pandey. 2008. Some dietary agricultural plants with anticancer properties. *Plant Archives* 8(1):13–16.

Madhuri, S., and G. Pandey. 2009. Some anticancer medicinal plants of foreign origin. *Current Science* 96(6):779–783.

Magee, P. J., Owusu-Apenten, R., McCann, M. J., Gill, C. I., and I. R. Rowland. 2012. Chickpea (*Cicer arietinum*) and other plant-derived protease inhibitor concentrates inhibit breast and prostate cancer cell proliferation in vitro. *Nutrition and Cancer* 64(5):741–748.

Mahata, S., Maru, S., Shukla, S., Pandey, A., Mugesh, G., and A. C. Bharti. 2012. Anticancer property of *Bryophyllum pinnata* (Lam.) Oken. leaf on human cervical cancer cells. *BMC Complementary and Alternative Medicine* 12(1):15.

Malik, F., Kumar, A., Bhushan, S., Khan, S., Bhatia, A., Suri, K. A., ... J. Singh. 2007. Reactive oxygen species generation and mitochondrial dysfunction in the apoptotic cell death of human myeloid leukemia HL-60 cells by a dietary compound withaferin A with concomitant protection by N-acetyl cysteine. *Apoptosis* 12(11):2115–2133.

Mandlekar, S., Hong, J. L., and A. N. T. Kong. 2006. Modulation of metabolic enzymes by dietary phytochemicals: a review of mechanisms underlying beneficial versus unfavorable effects. *Current Drug Metabolism* 7(6):661–675.

McGuire, S. 2016. *World Cancer Report 2014.* Geneva, Switzerland: World Health Organization, international agency for research on cancer, WHO Press, 2015.

Mishra, S., Ahmad, S., Kumar, and B. K. Sharma. 2013. *Annona muricata* (the cancer killer): a review. *Global Journal of Pharmaceutical Research* 2(1):1613–1618.

Mohsenikia, M., Alizadeh, A. M., Khodayari, S., Khodayari, H., Karimi, A., Zamani, M., ... M. A. Mohagheghi. 2013. The protective and therapeutic effects of alpha-solanine on mice breast cancer. *European journal of Pharmacology* 718(1–3):1–9.

Neergheen, V. S., Soobrattee, M. A., Bahorun, T., and O. I. Aruoma. 2006. Characterization of the phenolic constituents in Mauritian endemic plants as determinants of their antioxidant activities in vitro. *Journal of Plant Physiology* 163(8):787–799.

Nonn, L., Duong, D., and D. M. Peehl. 2007. Chemopreventive anti-inflammatory activities of curcumin and other phytochemicals mediated by MAP kinase phosphatase-5 in prostate cells. *Carcinogenesis* 28(6):1188–1196.

Odom, R. Y., Dansby, M. Y., Rollins-Hairston, A. M., Jackson, K. M., and W. G. Kirlin. 2009. Phytochemical induction of cell cycle arrest by glutathione oxidation and reversal by N-acetylcysteine in human colon carcinoma cells. *Nutrition and Cancer* 61(3):332–339.

Patel, D., Shukla, S., and S. Gupta. 2007. Apigenin and cancer chemoprevention: progress, potential and promise. *International Journal of Oncology* 30(1):233–245.

Pawlowska, A. M., Oleszek, W., and A. Braca. 2008. Quali-quantitative analyses of flavonoids of *Morus nigra* L. and *Morus alba* L. (Moraceae) fruits. *Journal of Agricultural and Food Chemistry* 56(9):3377–3380.

Pedreschi, R., and L. Cisneros-Zevallos. 2006. Antimutagenic and antioxidant properties of phenolic fractions from Andean purple corn (*Zea mays* L.). *Journal of Agricultural and Food Chemistry* 54(13):4557–4567.

Pieme, C. A., Kumar, S. G., Dongmo, M. S., Moukette, B. M., Boyoum, F. F., Ngogang, J. Y., and A. K. Saxena. 2014. Antiproliferative activity and induction of apoptosis by *Annona muricata* (Annonaceae) extract on human cancer cells. *BMC Complementary and Alternative Medicine* 14(1):1–10.

Plastina, P., Bonofiglio, D., Vizza, D., Fazio, A., Rovito, D., Giordano, C., ... B. Gabriele. 2012. Identification of bioactive constituents of *Ziziphus jujube* fruit extracts exerting antiproliferative and apoptotic effects in human breast cancer cells. *Journal of Ethnopharmacology* 140(2):325–332.

Queiroz, E. F., Ioset, J. R., Ndjoko, K., Guntern, A., Foggin, C. M., and K. Hostettmann. 2005. On-line identification of the bioactive compounds from *Blumea gariepina* by HPLC-UV-MS and HPLC-UV-NMR, combined with HPLC-micro-fractionation.

Phytochemical Analysis: An International Journal of Plant Chemical and Biochemical Techniques 16(3):166–174.

Raimondo, S., Naselli, F., Fontana, S., Monteleone, F., Dico, A. L., Saieva, L., ... G. De Leo. 2015. Citrus limon-derived nanovesicles inhibit cancer cell proliferation and suppress CML xenograft growth by inducing TRAIL-mediated cell death. *Oncotarget* 6(23):19514.

Rajendran, P., Ho, E., Williams, D. E., and R. H. Dashwood. 2011. Dietary phytochemicals, HDAC inhibition, and DNA damage/repair defects in cancer cells. *Clinical Epigenetics* 3(1):1–23.

Rajeshkumar, N. V., Joy, K. L., Kuttan, G., Ramsewak, R. S., Nair, M. G., and R. Kuttan. 2002. Antitumour and anticarcinogenic activity of *Phyllanthus amarus* extract. *Journal of Ethnopharmacology* 81(1):17–22.

Ramirez-Coronel, M. A., Marnet, N., Kolli, V. K., Roussos, S., Guyot, S., and Augur, C. 2004. Characterization and estimation of proanthocyanidins and other phenolics in coffee pulp (*Coffea arabica*) by thiolysis - high-performance liquid chromatography. *Journal of Agricultural and Food Chemistry* 52(5):1344–1349.

Ranilla, L. G., Genovese, M. I., and F. M. Lajolo. 2007. Polyphenols and antioxidant capacity of seed coat and cotyledon from Brazilian and Peruvian bean cultivars (*Phaseolus vulgaris* L.). *Journal of Agricultural and Food Chemistry* 55(1):90–98.

Rieser, M. J., Kozlowski, J. F., Wood, K. V., and J. L. McLaughlin. 1991. Muricatacin: a simple biologically active acetogenin derivative from the seeds of *Annona muricata* (Annonaceae). *Tetrahedron Letters* 32(9):1137–1140.

Roy, N. K., Deka, A., Bordoloi, D., Mishra, S., Kumar, A. P., Sethi, G., and A. B. Kunnumakkara. 2016. The potential role of boswellic acids in cancer prevention and treatment. *Cancer Letters* 377(1):74–86.

Saklani, A., and S. K. Kutty. 2008. Plant-derived compounds in clinical trials. *Drug Discovery Today* 13(3–4):161–171.

Samarghandian, S., Boskabady, M. H., and S. Davoodi. 2010. Use of in vitro assays to assess the potential antiproliferative and cytotoxic effects of saffron (*Crocus sativus* L.) in human lung cancer cell line. *Pharmacognosy Magazine* 6(24):309.

Saraswati, S. Kanaujia, P. K., Kumar, S., Kumar, R., and A. A. Alhaider. 2013. Tylophorine, a phenanthraindolizidine alkaloid isolated from *Tylophora indica* exerts antiangiogenic and antitumor activity by targeting vascular endothelial growth factor receptor 2–mediated angiogenesis. *Molecular cancer* 12(1):82.

Sersa, G., Cemazar, M., and Z. Rudolf. 2003. Electrochemotherapy: advantages and drawbacks in treatment of cancer patients. *Cancer Therapy* 1:133–142.

Setiawan, V. W., Zhang, Z. F., Yu, G. P., Lu, Q. Y., Li, Y. L., Lu, M. L., ... C. C. Hsieh. 2001. Protective effect of green tea on the risks of chronic gastritis and stomach cancer. *International Journal of Cancer* 92(4):600–604.

Shankar, S., Singh, G., and R. K. Srivastava. 2007. Chemoprevention by resveratrol: molecular mechanisms and therapeutic potential. *Frontiers in Bioscience* 12(12):4839–4854.

Sharangi, A. B. 2009. Medicinal and therapeutic potentialities of tea (*Camellia sinensis* L.)–A review. *Food Research International* 42(5–6):529–535.

Siegel, R. L., Miller, K. D., and A. Jemal. 2019. Cancer statistics, 2019. *A Cancer Journal for Clinicians* 69(1):7–34.

Singh, A. V., Franke, A. A., Blackburn, G. L., and J. R. Zhou. 2006. Soy phytochemicals prevent orthotopic growth and metastasis of bladder cancer in mice by alterations of cancer cell proliferation and apoptosis and tumor angiogenesis. *Cancer Research* 66(3):1851–1858.

Sripanidkulchai, B., Tattawasart, U., Laupatarakasem, P., Vinitketkumneun, U., Sripanidkulchai, K., Furihata, C., and T. Matsushima. 2002. Antimutagenic and anticarcinogenic effects of *Phyllanthus amarus*. *Phytomedicine* 9(1):26–32.

Sultan, M. T., Buttxs, M. S., Qayyum, M. M. N., and H. A. R. Suleria. 2014. Immunity: plants as effective mediators. *Critical Reviews in Food Science and Nutrition* 54(10):1298–1308.

Szewczyk, M., Abarzua, S., Schlichting, A. E., Nebe, B., Piechulla, B., Briese, V., and D. U. Richter. 2014. Effects of extracts from *Linum usitatissimum* on cell vitality, proliferation and cytotoxicity in human breast cancer cell lines. *Journal of Medicinal Plants Research* 8(5):237–245.

Tilghman, S. L., Rhodes, L. V., Bratton, M. R., Carriere, P., Preyan, L. C., Boue, S. M., ... M. E. Burow. 2013. Phytoalexins, miRNAs and breast cancer: a review of phytochemical-mediated miRNA regulation in breast cancer. *Journal of Health Care for the Poor and Underserved* 24(10) Supplement:36.

Tin, M. M., Cho, C. H., Chan, K., James, A. E., and J. K. Ko. 2007. *Astragalus* saponins induce growth inhibition and apoptosis in human colon cancer cells and tumor xenograft. *Carcinogenesis* 28(6):1347–1355.

Way, T. D., Kao, M. C., and J. K. Lin. 2004. Apigenin induces apoptosis through proteasomal degradation of HER2/neu in HER2/neu-overexpressing breast cancer cells via the phosphatidylinositol 3-kinase/Akt-dependent pathway. *Journal of Biological Chemistry* 279(6):4479–4489.

Winking, M., Sarikaya, S., Rahmanian, A., Jödicke, A., and D. K. Böker. 2000. Boswellic acids inhibit glioma growth: a new treatment option? *Journal of Neuro-oncology* 46(2):97–103.

Wuttke, W., Jarry, H., Haunschild, J., Stecher, G., Schuh, M., and D. Seidlova-Wuttke. 2014. The non-estrogenic alternative for the treatment of climacteric complaints: black cohosh (*Cimicifuga* or *Actaea racemosa*). *The Journal of Steroid Biochemistry and Molecular Biology* 139:302–310.

Xu, B. J., and S. K. C. Chang. 2007. A comparative study on phenolic profiles and antioxidant activities of legumes as affected by extraction solvents. *Journal of Food Science* 72(2):S159–S166.

Xu, Y., Xu, G., Liu, L., Xu, D., and J. Liu. 2010. Anti-invasion effect of rosmarinic acid via the extracellular signal-regulated kinase and oxidation–reduction pathway in Ls174-T cells. *Journal of Cellular Biochemistry* 111(2):370–379.

Yajid, A. I., Ab Rahman, H. S., Wong, M. P. K., and W. Z. W. Zain. 2018. Potential benefits of *Annona muricata* in combating cancer: a review. *The Malaysian Journal of Medical Science* 25(1):5.

Yesil-Celiktas, O., Sevimli, C., Bedir, E., and F. Vardar-Sukan. 2010. Inhibitory effects of rosemary extracts, carnosic acid and rosmarinic acid on the growth of various human cancer cell lines. *Plant Foods for Human Nutrition* 65(2):158–163.

Yu, X., Zhu, J., Mi, M., Chen, W., Pan, Q., and M. Wei. 2012. Anti-angiogenic genistein inhibits VEGF-induced endothelial cell activation by decreasing PTK activity and MAPK activation. *Medical Oncology* 29(1):349–357.

Yue, G. G., Chan, B. C., Hon, P. M., Lee, M. Y., Fung, K. P., Leung, P. C., and C. B. Lau. 2010. Evaluation of in vitro anti-proliferative and immunomodulatory activities of compounds isolated from *Curcuma longa*. *Food and Chemical Toxicology* 48(8–9):2011–2020.

Zaker, F., Oody, A., and A. Arjmand. 2007. A study on the antitumoral and differentiation effects of *Peganum harmala* derivatives in combination with ATRA on leukaemic cells. *Archives of Pharmacal Research* 30(7):844–849.

Zhang, Y., Chen, A. Y., Li, M., Chen, C., and Q. Yao. 2008. *Ginkgo biloba* extract kaempferol inhibits cell proliferation and induces apoptosis in pancreatic cancer cells. *Journal of Surgical Research* 148(1):17–23.

Zhou, H. S., Beevers, C., and S. Huang. 2011. The targets of curcumin. *Current Drug Targets* 12(3):332–347.

16 Potential of Medicinal Plants as Immunity Booster against COVID-19

Saumya Pandey

CONTENTS

16.1 INTRODUCTION

Over the past twenty years, the world has witnessed several pandemic/epidemic viral diseases, such as Ebola virus in 2014–16, Middle East Respiratory Syndrome (MERS) in 2012, Severe Acute Respiratory Syndrome (SARS-CoV) in 2002–2003, and many more, which have represented serious issues to public health. The new contagious virus, named SARS-CoV-2 virus by ICTV (International Committee on Taxonomy of Viruses), was first reported on December 31, 2019 to the World Health Organization (WHO) office in China and was later declared as pandemic when the

DOI: 10.1201/9781003137955-16

number of COVID-19 cases outside China had increased 13-fold, involving more than 114 countries, on March 11, 2019 (Cascella et al. 2020).

According to WHO, COVID-19 has caused over one million deaths globally, with the maximum number reported from the USA(55%), followed by Europe (23%) (Sousa et al. 2020). Coronavirus disease 2019 (COVID-19), caused by the severe acute respiratory syndrome coronavirus-2 (SARS-CoV-2), is an infectious disease transmitted by direct contact, droplet, airborne, fomite, faecal-oral, bloodborne, mother-to-child, and animal-to-human (Lei et al. 2020). Since, its first appearance in late December 2019 in Wuhan (China), this disease has disrupted the living standard of billions of people, caused economic losses, and deaths globally. This disease leads to mild to severe pneumonia, septic shock, dyspnea, and multiple organ dysfunctions (MOD)/failure (Zaim et al. 2020). The fatality rates were reported to be higher among the elderly patients and the patients with pre-existing comorbidities, for example, chronic respiratory disease, hypertension, oncological disease, cardiovascular disease, and diabetes (Casmella et al. 2020).

Until now, precautionary measures to prevent community transmission and some therapeutic approaches for the treatment of infected patients such as nucleoside analogues, remdesivir, anti-inflammatory drugs, or lopinavir/ritonavir, are the best available weapons to fight against this fatal disease (Vellingiri et al. 2020). WHO has suggested several precautionary measures, such as practising social distancing, respiratory etiquettes, and hand hygiene, identification and isolation of patients at an early stage, environmental cleaning and disinfection, and conveying correct information to the public to prevent transmission of disease (WHO 2020).

Several reports suggest a higher mortality rate among patients who are immunocompromised and those with preexisting comorbidities; the factors that aid in boosting the immunity could therefore help to combat severe symptoms of COVID-19 infection (Zheng et al. 2018; Felsenstein et al. 2020). Medicinal plants have been used by mankind for thousands of years, either in a pure form or as crude extracts, to boost immunity and treat various diseases. Around 45,000 species of plants have been used in traditional medicine systems in India. The various studies have suggested that the immune-stimulating properties of medicinal plants are mainly due to the presence of a wide range of phytochemicals, such as flavonoids, lignans, terpenoids, polyphenols, carotenoids, curcumins, sulphides, phthalides, plants sterols, and saponins (Kumar et al. 2012; Benarba and Pandiella 2020). The broad range of medicinal plants possess antiviral and immune booster properties and hence can be potentially exploited for the prevention and treatment of COVID-19 infection. Recently, the Ministry of AYUSH (Ayurveda, Yoga and Naturopathy, Unani, Siddha, and Homoeopathy) of the Government of India has recommended the combined use of Kadha and Golden Milk herbal preparations for boosting the immune system against severe COVID-19 infection (Khanal et al. 2020).

16.2 SARS-CoV-2: STRUCTURAL ASSEMBLY AND MECHANISM OF ACTION IN HUMAN HOST CELL

The SARS-CoV-2, a member of family Coronaviridae, is an enveloped single-stranded RNA (ssRNA) virus containing a positive-sense RNA genome (27–32 Kb) with poly-A tail and cap structure at 3'- and 5'- ends, respectively (Chen 2020). SARS-CoV-2 is made up of four important structural proteins, namely nucleocapsid protein (N), membrane protein (M), envelope protein (E), and spike protein (S) necessary for the regulation of its structure and function (Schoeman and Fielding 2019). Based on sequence analysis, SARS-CoV-2 is classified in the genus β-coronavirus of CoVs (Cascella et al. 2020). The genome sequence of SARS-CoV-2 has shown 82% similarity with the genome of human SARS-CoV (Chan et al. 2020).

As SARS-CoV and SARS-CoV-2 share similarities between sequences of the receptor-binding domain (RBD) and the receptor-binding motif (RBM), they probably have similar mechanisms for viral infection of the human cell (Yin and Wunderink 2018; Tai et al. 2020; Zhang et al. 2020). The receptor-binding motif of SARS-CoV-2 causes the viral S protein to attach to and fuse with the ACE2 receptor of the human cell, especially in the respiratory epithelium and alveoli of the lungs (Liu et al. 2020). Attachment to the receptor subsequently activates proteases that act on the viral S protein and cleave it into two domains, S1 and S2. The S1 domain remains attached to the ACE2 receptor of the host cell whereas the S2 domain undergoes a conformational change and internalizes the membrane, followed by membrane fusion between the ACE2 receptor and the viral subunit leading to viral RNA entry into the host cell. The entry into the host cell is followed by RNA replication and cleaving and shedding of ACE2 into the extramembrane space by ADAM17 (Vellingiri et al. 2020). ACE2 shedding is possibly responsible for the increased pulmonary vascular permeability and alveolar injury observed during viral infection (Le and Clercq 2020).

16.3 MEDICINAL PLANTS AS IMMUNITY BOOSTERS AGAINST COVID-19

Medicinal plants have played a significant role in addressing global healthcare demands from ancient times because of the presence of a diverse range of secondary plant metabolites with the ability to prevent and treat infectious diseases. The traditional system of medicines, such as the Indian traditional medicinal systems (including Ayurveda, Siddha, Unani, Yoga, Naturopathy, and Homoeopathy), the traditional Chinese medicinal system, and Kampo (the traditional Japanese medicinal system), is primarily dependent upon plant, animal, and mineral products, and has been practised for centuries, if not millenia, to cure different ailments in humans (Vaidya et al. 2007; Mukherjee et al. 2017). The precise application of plant resources for particular conditions requires traditional knowledge about plants and their usage (Petrovska 2012). According to a recent WHO report, nearly 80% of the populations from underdeveloped countries still rely on traditional medicines (WHO 2019). Out of 21,000 medicinal plants listed by the WHO as having therapeutic potential, 2,500 species of plants have been reported from India (Pundarikakshudu and Kanaki 2019; Shukla et al. 2019). Despite extensive therapeutic potential, medicinal plants are still overlooked by researchers for the development of modern drugs (Yuan et al. 2016). The desired pharmacological effect needed to cure or prevent specific diseases can be obtained from phytochemicals purified as single constituents or in combination with other phytochemical compounds, as a herbal preparation (Parasuraman et al. 2014) derived from one or several plant species.

The plant-based medicines have been proved to be effective in controlling the adverse effects of infection in the case of the earlier SARS pandemic caused by SARS-CoV (Wen et al. 2011; Verma et al. 2020). As SARS-CoV2 (Coronavirus) shares homology with SARS-CoV, the medicinal plants can be recommended as a potential source to address the existing health crises (Aanouz et al. 2020; Wahedi et al. 2020). The medicinal plants have proved to be efficient in controlling and curing viral respiratory infections because they can manage the immune system by modulating inflammation and stimulating immunity.

Presently, in the absence of an established regimen against COVID-19, the whole world is facing immense uncertainty in the management of this pandemic disease. The therapeutic strategies which can be used globally against COVID-19 include: (1) an allopathic system: presently broad-spectrum antibiotics, including hydroxychloroquine, lopinavir, retinovir, and remsedivir, are used but they pose many adverse side effects; (2) vaccination: nearly 13 different vaccines (For Example: Pfizer/BioNtech, SII/Covishield, Janssen/Ad26.COV2.S, AstraZeneca/Oxford) have been administrated to large number of peoples through mass vaccination programme; (3) herd immunity: can be achieved either by vaccinating a large number of people against the disease or when a high proportion of the population contracts the disease and develops natural immunity; (4) immunity boosting: enhancing the internal power of the immune system to minimize symptoms of COVID-19 infections (Ponnam and Akondi 2020). Several natural remedies have been suggested as immune boosters from the ancient medicine systems, most importantly the use of natural herbs to strengthen the natural immunity of the individual.

Considering the present pandemic situation, the Ministry of AYUSH, India, has recommended a holistic approach for the treatment and prevention of COVID-19 that includes dietary management, symptom management, lifestyle management, and prophylactic measures to boost immunity. The cost-effective decoction known as 'Ayush Kwath', 'Ayush Kudineer', or 'Ayush Joshanda' has been recommended by AYUSH, and it comprises of five medicinal herbs, namely *Ocimum tenuiflorum*, *Cinnamomum verum*, *Piper nigrum*, *Zingiber officinale*, and *Vitis vinifera* (AYUSH 2020).

Traditional Chinese medicine system practitioners have also developed several formulae containing combinations of natural herbs based on the symptoms of COVID-19 infections (Zhao et al. 2020). Among various Chinese formulation, lung cleansing and detoxifying decoction (LCDD) is one of the clinically proven and most commonly consumed formulations, comprising twenty-one medicinal herbs, namely *Ephedra sinica*, *Cinnamomum cassia*, *Alisma plantago-aquatica*, *Atractylodes macrocephala*, *Bupleurum chinense*, *Scutellaria baicalensis*, *Pinellia ternata*, *Aster tataricus*, *Tussilago farfara*, *Iris domestica*, *Wolfiporia extensa*, and the mushroom *Polyporus umbellatus*, as well as wild ginger, Chinese yam, Korean mint, bitter orange, licorice, ansu apricot, ginger, and orange peel. The clinical trial with LCDD treatment in 1262 COVID-19 patients showed a 99.28% recovery rate; furthermore, the severity of infection did not increase in those patients with mild symptoms of infection when the treatment started (Weng 2020).

Similarly, the Government of Tamil Nadu has taken initiatives to supply the Nilavembu Kudineer Chooranam (NKC) decoction to healthcare centers to control morbidity levels during an outbreak of viral infectious diseases (Ramanathan et al., 2019). NKC is comprised of nine medicinal plants: *Andrographis paniculata, Vetiveria zizanioides, Plectranthus vettiveroides, Santalum album, Trichosanthes dioica, Cyperus rotundus, Zingiber officinale, Piper nigrum,* and *Mollugo cerviana.* NKC has shown antiviral, antipyretic, antibacterial, anti-ulcer, antioxidant, and analgesic properties, etc. (Kavinilavan et al. 2017; Jain et al. 2020). NKC also acts as an immunostimulator and an immunomodulator, thus playing important role in preventing infection symptoms by enhancing the immune system and modulating the defense response of the host (Nakkeeran et al. 2016; Kamalarajan et al. 2019).

El-Alami et al. (2020) has reported *Allium sativum, Olea europaea, Allium cepa, Zingiber officinale, Thymus maroccanus, Eucalyptus globulus, Foeniculum vulgare, Curcuma xanthorrhiza, Phoenix dactylifera, Rosmarinus officinalis, Thymus satureioides, Mentha pulegium,* and *Pimpinella anisum* to be the most widely used medicinal plants for the prevention of COVID-19 infection in Morocco. The presence of a diverse range of bioactive compounds, such as flavonoids, tannins, glycosides, lignans, carotenoids, essential oils, etc., results in positive effects on respiratory and circulatory functions. The efficiency of some selected medicinal plants in boosting the immune response of the human body to prevent COVID-19 infection is given in Table 16.1.

16.3.1 *Ocimum sanctum* L. (Tulsi, Holy Basil)

Tulsi is known as the 'Elixir of Life' and plays a significant role in boosting immunity and thus helps the human body to fight against a wide range of bacteria and viruses. It has been widely used in treating various health ailments, such as bronchitis, pyrexia, asthma, genito-urinary disorders, fever, microbial and parasitic infections, rheumatism, and anxiety because of its analgesic, antidiarrhoeal, antimicrobial, renoprotective, hepatoprotective, antipyretic, cardioprotective, antioxidant, immunomodulatory, and anti-inflammatory properties (Vasudevan et al. 1999; Cohen, 2014).

The immune-boosting property of this herb is due to the presence of various bioactive compounds, such as eugenol, cirsilineol, carnosol, ursolic acid, rosmarinic acid, apigenin, and cirsimaritin, which play a significant role in major defence mechanisms, such as suppressing NF-kB classical pathways, down-regulating interleukin-1 beta (IL-1β) and antigen-specific antibodies, up-regulating interleukin 2 (IL-2), interferon gamma (IFN-γ) and tumour necrosis factor alpha (TNF-α), enhancing Sheep Red Blood Cells agglutinin titres and haemoglobin concentration, and decreasing cyclooxygenase-2 and lipoxygenase-5 enzyme activities (Lo et al. 2002). Also, tulsi acts as an efficient immunomodulator as it aids in increasing the percentage of T helper and natural killer (NK) cells and enhances the phagocytic index and antibody titre (Mondal 2010). Mondal et al. (2011) reported an increase in the percentage of T helper cells and NK cells after four weeks in twenty-four healthy subjects given 300 mg ethanolic extract of tulsi. Also, the role of seven bioactive compounds present in tulsi has been shown to inhibit SARS-CoV replication by a molecular docking study. As SARS-CoV shares several clinical and genetic

TABLE 16.1

List of Medicinal Plants Commonly Used as Immunity Boosters to Prevent COVID-19 Infection

Common Name	Scientific Name	Parts Used	Phytoconstituents	Pharmacological Activities	References
Amla	*Emblica officinalis* Gaertn.	Fruit	Gallic acid, ellagic acid, emblicanin A, B, phyllembein, quercetin, and ascorbic acid	Anti-inflammatory, antimutagenic, immunomodulatory, analgesic, antitussive, nephron- and neuroprotective, chemopreventive, anticancer, antioxidant	Suja et al. 2009
Baheda	*Terminalia bellirica* (Gaertn.) Roxb.	Dried fruit	Tain, termilignan, thannilignan, arjungenin, belleric acid, bellericoside, cannogeno	Antiviral, anti-inflammatory, antibacterial, antifungal, antidiarrhoeal, analgesic, antimalarial, antioxidant, anticancer	Cock 2015
Bala	*Sida cordifolia* L.	Leaves	Asparagine, quinazoline, ephedrine, choline, betaine, rutin, β-sitosterol, hypaphorine, vasicinone, vasicinol	Analgesic, antispasmodic, anti-inflammatory, hypoglycaemic, hepatoprotective	Sivapalan 2015
Chandrasoor	*Lepidium sativum* L.	Leaves	Sinapic acid, sinapin, lepidine	Anti-asthmatic, anti-inflammatory, haemagglutinating	Mali et al. 2007
Clove	*Syzygium aromaticum* (L.) Merr. & L.M. Perry	Flower bud	Eugenol, thymol, cariophyllene	Anti-inflammatory, antiviral, antitumour, antibacterial, antifungal	Bownik et al. 2012
Draksa	*Vitis vinifera* L.	Fruits	flavonoids, polyphenols, anthocyanins, proanthocyanidins, procyanidines, esveratrol.	antioxidative, anti-inflammatory, antimicrobial, cardioprotective, hepatoprotective, neuroprotective	Nassiri-Asl and Hosseinzadeh 2009
Fenugreek	*Trigonella foenum-graecum* L.	Seeds and leaves	trigonolline, cholin, gentianine, diosgenin, gitogenin, yamogenin	Anti-inflammatory, antimicrobial, antidiabetic, antihyperlipidaemic, anti-obesity, anticancer, antioxidant	Yadav and Baquer 2014

(Continued)

TABLE 16.1 (CONTINUED)

List of Medicinal Plants Commonly Used as Immunity Boosters to Prevent COVID-19 Infection

Common Name	Scientific Name	Parts Used	Phytoconstituents	Pharmacological Activities	References
Kalmegh	*Andrographis paniculata* (Burm. F.) Nees.	Leaves	andrographolide, neoandrographolide, deoxyandrographolide	Immunomodulatory, antiviral, immune enhancement, antioxidant, hepatoprotective, anti-HIV	Verma et al. 2019
Kalonji	*Nigella sativa* L.	Seed	Nigellicine, nigellimine, pinene, *p*-cymene, carvene	Immunopotentiating, immunomodulatory, hypoglycaemic, anticancer, antimicrobial, anti-inflammatory, anti-ulcer	Kooti et al. 2016
Nagkesar	*Mesua ferrea* L.	Bark and root	Mesuol, mesuagin, mammeisin, 4-alkylcoumarins ferruols A and B, guttiferol, ferraxanthone, β-sitosterol.	Anti-inflammatory, immunostimulant, antioxidant, analgesic, hepatoprotective	Chahar et al. 2013
Nutmeg	*Myristica fragrans* Houtt.	Seeds	Trimyristin, myristic acid, myristicin, safrole, elimicin	Anti-inflammatory, antioxidant, anticonvulsant, analgesic, antidiabetic, antibacterial, antifungal	Asgarpanah and Kazemivash 2012
Paan	*Piper betle* L.	Leaves	Hydroxychavicol, chavibetol, estragole, eugenol, caryophyllene	Anti-inflammatory, antimicrobial, antioxidant, anticancer, antidiabetic	Madhumita et al. 2020
Sandalwood	*Santalum album* L.	Oil	α-, β-santalol, bergamotols, curcumenes, β-bisabolene	Anti-inflammatory, antiviral, antifungal, antibacterial, hepatoprotective, antipyretic, cardioprotective	Kumar et al. 2015
Satavari	*Asparagus racemosus* Willd.	Dried root	Shatavarin, asparginins, curillins, asparosides, curillosides	Anti-inflammatory, cardioprotective, antistress, antidepressant activity	Hasan et al. 2016
Wild Carrot	*Daucus maritimus* Lam.	Seeds	Daucucarotol, β-bisabolene, *trans*-β-caryophyllene, *trans*-α-asarone, β-selinene, β-bisabolene, bicyclogermacrene	Antiviral, anti-inflammatory, antidiabetic, nephroprotective, hepatoprotective, antioxidant	Al-Snafi 2017

similarities with SARS-CoV2, these bioactive compounds could significantly inhibit SARS-CoV-2 replication by blocking ACE-2 receptors (Khaerunnisa et al. 2020).

16.3.2   *PIPER NIGRUM* L. (KAALI MIRCH, BLACK PEPPER)

Also known as the 'King of Spices', *P. nigrum* contains more than 600 different bioactive compounds, such as lignans, terpenes, alkaloids, neolignans, etc. (Damanhouri et al. 2014). Due to the presence of such a vast range of phytoconstituents, it has antioxidant, analgesic, antiplatelet, immunomodulatory, antipyretic, antihypertensive, anti-asthmatic, anticarcinogenic, antispasmodic, antimicrobial, antimutagenic, antithyroid, anti-ulcer, antidepressant, hepatoprotective, and antidiarrhoeal properties (Nahak et al. 2011; Srivastava et al. 2017). The key alkaloid components, like piperine and piperamides, enhance the defence mechanism of the human body by regulating the balance between cytokines and T cells, inhibiting the expressions of GATA3, IL-4, IL-6, ILβ, I-17A, TNF-α, RORγT, and increasing the activation of macrophages and the proliferation of T and B cells (Damanhouri et al. 2014; Balkrishna et al. 2020). Furthermore, it can also inhibit mast cell activation and allergic responses, alleviate fibrotic scarring and inflammatory cell infiltration, suppress the release of histamine and antibodies IgE, anti-OVA IgG1 in serum, inhibit P glycoprotein and CYP3A4 functions, and inhibit NF-kB, CREB, ATF-2, c-Fos and PKCa/ERK pathways (Zhai et al. 2016; Bui et al. 2019).

16.3.3   *ZINGIBER OFFICINALE* ROSCOE (SUNTHI, GINGER)

Ginger belongs to the family Zingiberaceae and has potential immune-boosting and anti-inflammatory characteristics that enhance the immune responses and metabolic activities of the human body and thus provide a shield against infectious diseases. Its chemical constituents include gingerdione, 6-gingediol, germacrene, zingiberene, 6-shogaol, methyl-6-shogaol, β-sitosterol, nevirapine, etc., which play roles in the inhibition of viral replication, with β-sitosterol as the most potent inhibitor of the reverse transcriptase enzyme (Kharisma et al. 2018). Moreover, the main bioactive components of ginger, like the gingerols and shogaols, enhance fibrinolysis, inhibit pro-inflammatory cytokines (IL-1, TNF-α, IL-8), inhibit leukotriene and prostaglandin biosynthesis, and inhibit cyclooxygenase and lipoxygenase activities. A ginger preparation also inhibits the anti-influenza cytokine TNF-α, inhibits platelet aggregation and thromboxane synthetase, down-regulates expression of iNOS and COX-2 genes, and reduces the production of age-related oxidative stress markers (Habib et al. 2008; Mahluji et al. 2013).

Mahassni et al. (2019) has studied the efficacy of ginger extract in enhancing humoral immunity among male smokers and non-smokers and reported a significant increase in the IgM concentration and eosinophil count in non-smokers as compared with smokers, whereas the lymphocyte count and haemoglobin concentration in smokers were found to be higher than in non-smokers. Thus, ginger has greater potential to enhance humoral immunity in non-smokers than in smokers. Also, fresh ginger has greater effectiveness in reducing viral infection as compared with dried ginger. Bhat et al. (2010) showed that both the alcoholic extract as well as the crude extract of ginger can increase the immune response. The alcoholic extract of ginger has caused increased phagocytic activity by macrophages, whereas treatment with the crude extract has shown enhanced humoral and cell-mediated immunity in mice. The inhibitory potential of fresh ginger against the human respiratory syncytical virus was reported to be higher than that of dried ginger. Fresh ginger inhibits viral binding and internalization processes as well as stimulating mucosal cells to secrete IFN-β, thus promoting a reduction in viral infection (Srivastava et al. 2020).

16.3.4 *CINNAMOMUM VERUM* J. PRESL (DALCHINI, CINNAMON)

Cinnamon belongs to the family Lauraceae and contains various bioactive compounds, such as benzaldehyde, cuminaldehyde, cinnamaldehyde, and terpenes (Valizadeh et al. 2015). Because of its immunomodulatory and immune-boosting effects, it has been used in preventing and curing various ailments. A study showed that both high (100 mg/kg bodyweight) and low doses (10 mg/kg) can enhance the immune response, whereas the low dose increased only humoral immunity while the high dose enhances both cell-mediated as well as humoral immunity (Niphade et al. 2009). Kim et al. (2010) have demonstrated that cinnamaldehyde can inhibit the expression of phosphoinositide 3-kinase (PI3K), phosphoinositide-dependent-kinase-1 (PDK1), and nuclear factor kappa β (NF-kβ) and alleviates the host innate immune responses. Further, cinnamaldehyde brings about activation of CD29 and CD43 which, in turn, block cell migration and induce cell–cell adhesion apart from cell–fibronectin adhesion. Also, cinnamaldehyde suppresses the production of NO (nitric oxide) as well as up-regulating the pattern recognition receptors (PRRs) TLR2 and CR3 and levels of co-stimulatory molecules CD69 and CD80 expressed on the surface of cells. Chemicals such as cinnamaldehyde, cinnamophilin, etc. found in cinnamon bark have shown anti-atherosclerotic, anticoagulative, and thromboxane A2 receptor antagonist properties, preventing unnecessary platelet clumping and atherosclerotic cardiovascular diseases (Tsui et al. 2018).

The potency of cinnamon bark as an immunomodulator has been shown by its ability to down-regulate the IFN-γ expression in activated T cells with no change in IL-2 production through inhibiting the activation of p38, JNK, ERK1/2, and STAT4, but not IkBa degradation or STAT6 (Lee et al. 2011). The use of cinnamon is safe for daily dietary consumption and medicinal use.

16.3.5 *TINOSPORA CORDIFOLIA* (WILLD.) MIERS (MOONSEED, GILOE)

Giloe belongs to the family Menispermaceae and has been used in many traditional Ayurvedic medicines for therapies against several diseases, such as allergy, urinary disorder, rheumatism, leprosy, diabetes, etc. (Sonkamble and Kamble 2015). Several important bioactive compounds have been reported from parts of *Tinospora*, including steroids, glycosides, alkaloids, aliphatics, phenolics, diterpenoids, sesquiterpenoids, and flavonoids, which act as immunomodulators and support the immune system by increasing resistance of the body against various infections (Singh et al. 2003). Giloe shows antitoxic, anti-osporotic, anti-HIV, wound healing, antimicrobial, anti-allergic, antioxidant, anti-inflammatory, and antidiabetic properties (Saha and Ghosh 2012; Sharma et al. 2019). An *in-silico* study, performed using molecular docking, has demonstrated that, among the phytochemicals in *Tinospora cordifolia*, berberine can serve as a potential inhibitor in regulating 3CL^{pro} protein function, subsequently controlling viral replication (Chowdhary 2020). The herbal formulations containing a combination of giloe, tulsi, ginger, and kali mirch has been proven effective for preventing and curing COVID-19 symptoms (Srivastava et al. 2020).

16.3.6 *PANAX QUINQUEFOLIUS* L. (GINSENG)

Ginseng belongs to the family Araliaceae and has shown a broad range of biological activities including antimicrobial, antidiabetic, anti-inflammatory, anticardiovascular, antioxidative, T cell-mediated immune reaction, and anticancer properties. It also serves as an immunomodulator by playing an important role in activating natural killer cells, antagonistic reactions for immunosuppressive mediators, and triggering innate immunity (Im et al. 2016; Ratan et al. 2020). It is a source of various bioactive compounds, such as ginsenosides, polysaccharides, polyacetylenes, phytosterols, and essential oils (Wang et al. 2015). Several studies have shown the therapeutic potential of ginseng in treating diverse diseases, such as immune system disorder, neuronal disease, microbial infections, cancer, and cardiovascular disease. Ginseng has also been shown to possess protective activities against different viral infections, such as the human herpes virus, immune deficiency virus, rhinovirus, influenza virus, enterovirus, rotavirus, coxsackievirus, and norovirus (Iqbal and Rhee 2020). The pharmacological activities and stability of heat-processed ginseng have been reported to be higher than those of fresh ginseng (Im et al. 2016). The consumption of milk enriched with ginseng (150–300 ml) has been suggested because of its potential health benefit in boosting the immunity of the body (Lee et al. 2014).

16.3.7 *GLYCYRRHIZA GLABRA* L. (LICORICE, SWEET WOOD)

Licorice belongs to the family Fabaceae and exhibits a broad range of biological properties, including antimicrobial, anti-inflammatory, antioxidant anti-ulcer, antidiuretic, antidiabetic and antitussive activities (Sharma et al. 2018). Various bioactive compounds, such as glycyrrhizin, glabrin A and B, isoflavones, and glycyrrhetinic acid, are present, that have shown various pharmacological activities (Ozturk et al. 2017). Several studies have suggested the use of glycyrrhizin for the treatment of SARS infection because of its antiviral properties (Bailly et al. 2020; Chen et al. 2020).

Cinatl et al. (2003) has reported on the clinical trials of various chemical compounds present in *Glycyrrhiza* against two clinical coronavirus isolates; out of all the compounds tested, glycyrrhizin was found to be most effective in inhibiting virus replication, and was found to be effective against various viruses, including hepatitis A, B, C, varicella-zoster, HIV, herpes simplex type-1, and cytomegalovirus (Asl and

Hosseinzadeh 2008). Furthermore, the bioactive compounds glyasperin A and glyc-yrrhizic acid have been used to produce nanomembranes by electrospinning which can be used as wound dressing materials, masks, gloves and against skin infection. Glycyrrhizic acid binds to the pocket of the spike glycoprotein and prohibits the entry of the virus into the host cell, whereas glyasperin A showed higher affinity with Nsp15 endoribonuclease and affects coronavirus infection (Sinha et al. 2020).

16.3.8 *CURCUMA LONGA* L. (HALDI, TURMERIC)

Turmeric belongs to the family Zingiberaceae and its rhizome is used for medicinal purposes to treat a number of severe diseases. Turmeric has been used as a natural cleanser of the respiratory tract and has been employed for curing congestion, cough, throat infection, and bronchial asthma. It has anti-inflammatory, antiviral, antifungal, and antibacterial properties, and helps to boost the immune system to fight against infection (Zorofchian et al. 2014; Praditya et al. 2019). Curcumin, artur-merone, and zingiberene are the main bioactive constituents that show antiviral activities against a diverse range of viruses, such as dengue virus, hepatitis B virus, Zika virus (ZIKV), and chikungunya virus (Hesari et al. 2018; Nabila et al. 2020). Also, the consumption of golden milk containing one-half of a teaspoon of turmeric in 150 ml hot milk has been recommended by the Ministry of AYUSH to boost the immune system (AYUSH 2020).

16.4 IMMUNOLOGICAL RESPONSES ASSOCIATED WITH INTERACTION BETWEEN MEDICINAL PLANTS AND SARS-CoV-2

SARS-CoV-2 interacts with immune cells and subsequently affects the patient's immune system. Thus, to develop immunotherapies for COVID-19, the most crucial prerequisite is to build up a better understanding of the immunopathology of chronic lung conditions in the infected person. The immunological abnormalities evident in patients infected with COVID-19 consist of neutrophilia, increased levels of inflammatory markers in the serum, monocyte/macrophage dysfunction, and lymphopaenia, which affect CD4+ T cells, CD8+ T cells, natural killer cells, and B cells (Figure 16.1). Yang et al. (2005) reported that the ectopic expression of the SARS-CoV E protein induces T cell apoptosis and contributes to SARS-CoV-induced lymphopaenia. The interaction between BH3-like regions (Bcl-2 homology domain 3) located in the C-terminal cytosolic domain of the SARS-CoV E protein and the cellular oncogene Bcl-xL (anti-apoptotic protein) primarily causes apoptosis of T cell lymphocytes. Similar to the SARS-CoV envelope protein, conserved Bcl-2 Homology 3 (BH3)-like motifs in the C-terminal region, necessary for binding to Bcl-xl, protein has been reported in the SARS-CoV-2 envelope (E) protein (Navratil et al. 2020).

The symptoms of the disease may be associated with the functional characteristics of IgG antibodies against glycoproteins of the virus envelope. These functional

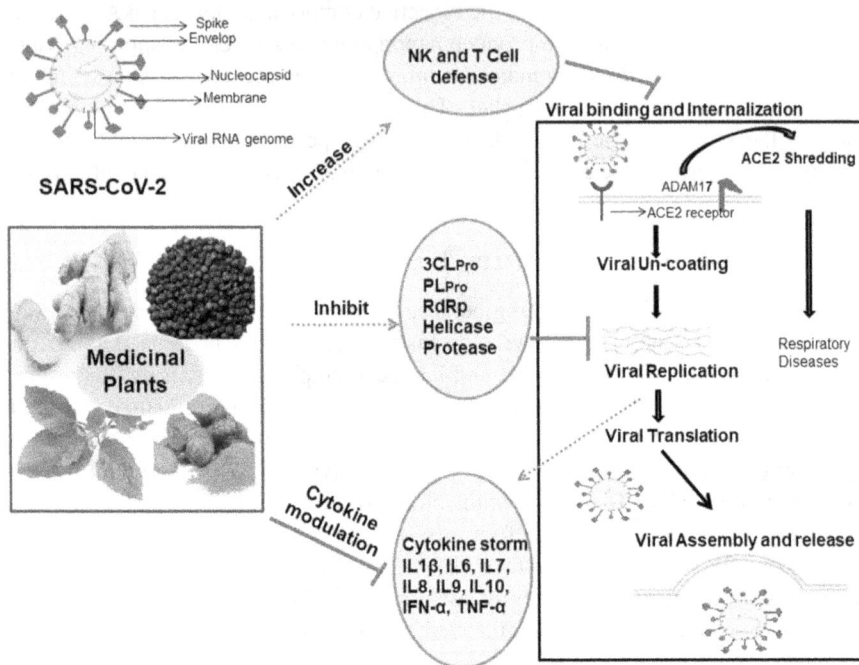

FIGURE 16.1 Immunity-boosting potential of medicinal plants against SARS-CoV-2 pathogenesis.

characteristics of IgG antibodies leads not only to neutralization of the virus and other antibody defensive functions but might also augment the immune cell infection. A study on dengue virus suggests that the undesirable action of IgG antibodies is associated with the alteration in glycosylation profile of the Fc region of IgG, leading to antibody-dependent enhancement (ADE) of virus uptake *via* macrophages, eventually causing greater secretion of pro-inflammatory cytokines and chemokines (Bournazos et al. 2020). Kruse (2020) reported that the ACE2 protein combines with the Fc domain of IgG antibodies and thus might play an important role in the treatment of COVID-19.

Several studies on medicinal plants have suggested their role in enhancing natural killer (NK) cell activity, increasing the secretions of IL-10 and INF-γ, inhibition of ATF-2, IL-4, IL-6, GATA3, down-regulation of Th-17 and Th2-related cytokines, etc. Hoffmann et al. (2020) established that the SARS-CoV-2 enters human cells *via* the ACE2 receptor. Various medicinal plants, such as *Berberis integerrima*, *Crataegus laevigata*, *Onopordum acanthium*, and *Quercus infectoria*, have shown ACE2 inhibition, of which *Quercus infectoria* was found to be the most active (94%) in terms of inhibition owing to its higher phenolic content and increased antioxidant potential (Sharifi et al. 2013).

Khanal et al. (2020) studied the AYUSH herbal preparation 'Kwath' and reported that bioactive compounds present in the formulation boost the immune system by modulating several signaling pathways such as HIF-1, p53, PI3K-Akt, MAPK, cAMP, Ras, Wnt, NF-kappa-β, IL-17, TNF, and cGMP-PKG. Similarly, *Andrographis paniculata* has been reported to suppress the enhanced level of NLRP3, CASP-1, and IL-1β molecules that play a significant role in the pathogenicity of SARS-CoV as well as in SARS-CoV-2 (Liu et al. 2020). In another study, the medicinal plant *Salacia oblonga* was found to significantly suppress the angiotensin II receptor type 1 (AT1) signal that is associated with lung damage (He et al. 2011). Thus, the immune-boosting and immunomodulatory efficacies of the medicinal plants in 'Kwath' facilitate the prevention of infection as well as ameliorating the symptoms of COVID-19 by increasing the innate immunity of an individual.

16.5   CONCLUSION

Medicinal plants with different pharmacological activities have been used for ages as herbal preparations for the treatment of viral infection and enhancement of host immune response. The outbreak of the COVID-19 disease has caused a severe threat to public health and the global economy. As the SARS-CoV-2 can escape innate immune response, an individual with weak immunity can develop a severe infection. Also, the unavailability of approved medication to date has intensified the pandemic situation. Precautionary measures against virus infection, such as social distancing, self-quarantine, respiratory etiquettes, etc., have been recommended by WHO to avoid human contact and thus minimize the risk of transmission and infection. Appropriate medicinal plants can be used as a promising resource for managing this pandemic situation owing to their capacity to boost the immune response of the human body and fight against viral infection. This pandemic situation has raised concern about the healthcare system and greater investment in research into infectious diseases is needed to avoid such pandemic situations in the future. As the pathways involved in decreasing infection load by bioactive compounds from medicinal plants are still not clearly understood, further investigation is required for effective utilization of medicinal plants in the treatment of such diseases.

REFERENCES

Aanouz, I., A. Belhassan, K. El-Khatabi, T. Lakhlifi, M. El-Ldrissi, and M. Bouachrine. 2020. Moroccan medicinal plants as inhibitors against SARS-CoV-2 main protease: Computational investigations. *Journal of Biomolecular Structure and Dynamics* 1–9.

Al-Snafi, A.E. 2017. Nutritional and therapeutic importance of Daucus carota-A. *IOSR Journal of Pharmacy* 7: 72–78.

Asgarpanah, J. and Kazemivash, N. 2012. Phytochemistry and pharmacologic properties of *Myristica fragrans* Hoyutt.: A review. *African Journal of Biotechnology* 11(65): 12787–12793.

Asl, M.N., and H. Hosseinzadeh. 2008. Review of pharmacological effects of *Glycyrrhiza* sp. and its bioactive compounds. *Phytotherapy Research: An International Journal Devoted to Pharmacological and Toxicological Evaluation of Natural Product Derivatives* 22: 709–724.

Bailly, C. and G. Vergoten. 2020. Glycyrrhizin: An alternative drug for the treatment of COVID-19 infection and the associated respiratory syndrome? *Pharmacology & Therapeutics* 214: 107618.

Balkrishna, A., S.K. Solleti, H. Singh, M. Tomer, N. Sharma, and A Varshney. 2020. Calcio-herbal formulation, Divya-Swasari-Ras, alleviates chronic inflammation and suppresses airway remodelling in mouse model of allergic asthma by modulating pro-inflammatory cytokine response. *Biomedicine & Pharmacotherapy* 126: 110063.

Benarba, B. and A. Pandiella. 2020. Medicinal plants as sources of active molecules against COVID-19. *Frontiers in Pharmacology* 11: 1189.

Bhat, J., A. Damle, P.P. Vaishnav, R. Albers, M. Joshi, and G. Banerjee. 2010. In vivo enhancement of natural killer cell activity through tea fortified with Ayurvedic herbs. *Phytotherapy Research: An International Journal Devoted to Pharmacological and Toxicological Evaluation of Natural Product Derivatives* 24: 129–135.

Bhowmik, D., K.S. Kumar, A. Yadav, S. Srivastava, S. Paswan, and A.S. Dutta. 2012. Recent trends in Indian traditional herbs Syzygium aromaticum and its health benefits. *Journal of Pharmacognosy and Phytochemistry* 1: 13–22.

Bournazos, S., A. Gupta, and J.V. Ravetch. 2020. The role of IgG Fc receptors in antibody-dependent enhancement. *Nature Reviews Immunology* 20: 633–643.

Bui, T.T., C.H. Piao, E. Hyeon, Y. Fan, T. Van-Nguyen, S.Y. Jung, D.W. Choi, S.Y. Lee, H.S. Shin, C.H. Song, and O.H. Chai. 2019. The protective role of *Piper nigrum* fruit extract in an ovalbumin-induced allergic rhinitis by targeting of NFκBp65 and STAT3 signalings. *Biomedicine & Pharmacotherapy* 109: 1915–1923.

Cascella, M., M. Rajnik, A. Cuomo, S.C. Dulebohn, and R. Di-Napoli. 2020. Features, evaluation and treatment coronavirus (COVID-19). In *Statpearls* [internet]. Treasure Island, FL: StatPearls Publishing.

Chahar, M.K., Geetha, L., Lokesh, T. and Manohara, K.P. 2013. Mesua ferrea L.: A review of the medical evidence for its phytochemistry and pharmacological actions. *African Journal of Pharmacy and Pharmacology* 7(6): 211–219.

Chan, J.F.W., K.H. Kok, Z. Zhu, H. Chu, K.K.W. To, S. Yuan, and K.Y. Yuen. 2020. Genomic characterization of the 2019 novel human-pathogenic coronavirus isolated from a patient with atypical pneumonia after visiting Wuhan. *Emerging Microbes & Infections* 9: 221–236.

Chen, J. 2020. Pathogenicity and transmissibility of 2019-nCoV—A quick overview and comparison with other emerging viruses. *Microbes and Infection* 22(2): 69–71.

Chen, L., C. Hu, M. Hood, X. Zhang, L. Zhang, J. Kan, and J. Du. 2020. A novel combination of vitamin C, curcumin and glycyrrhizic acid potentially regulates immune and inflammatory response associated with coronavirus infections: A perspective from system biology analysis. *Nutrients* 12: 1193.

Chowdhury, P. 2020. In silico investigation of phytoconstituents from Indian medicinal herb 'Tinospora cordifolia (giloy)'against SARS-CoV-2 (COVID-19) by molecular dynamics approach. *Journal of Biomolecular Structure and Dynamics* 1–18.

Cinatl, J., B. Morgenstern, G. Bauer, P. Chandra, H. Rabenau, and H.W. Doerr. 2003. Glycyrrhizin, an active component of liquorice roots, and replication of SARS-associated coronavirus. *The Lancet* 361: 2045–2046.

Cock, I.E. 2015. The medicinal properties and phytochemistry of plants of the genus *Terminalia* (Combretaceae). *Inflammopharmacology* 23: 203–229.

Cohen, M.M. 2014. Tulsi-Ocimum sanctum: A herb for all reasons. *Journal of Ayurveda and Integrative Medicine* 5: 251.

Damanhouri, Z.A., and A. Ahmad. 2014. A review on therapeutic potential of *Piper nigrum* L. Black Pepper): The king of spices. *Medicinal & Aromatic Plants* 3: 161.

El-Alami, A., A. Fatta, and A. Chait. 2020. Medicinal plants used for the prevention purposes during the covid-19 pandemic in Morocco. *Journal of Analytical Sciences and Applied Biotechnology* 2: 2–11.

Felsenstein, S., J.A. Herbert, P.S. McNamara, and C.M. Hedrich. 2020. COVID-19: Immunology and treatment options. *Clinical Immunology* 215: 108448.

Habib, S.H.M., S. Makpol, N.A.A. Hamid, S. Das, W.Z.W. Ngah, and Y.A.M. Yusof. 2008. Ginger extract (*Zingiber officinale*) has anti-cancer and anti-inflammatory effects on ethionine-induced hepatoma rats. *Clinics* 63: 807–813.

Hasan, N., N. Ahmad, S. Zohrameena, M. Khalid, and J. Akhtar. 2016. *Asparagus Racemosus*: For medicinal uses & pharmacological actions. *International Journal of Advanced Research* 4: 259–267.

He, L., Y. Qi, X. Rong, J. Jiang, Q. Yang, J. Yamahara, M. Murray, and Y. Li. 2011. The Ayurvedic medicine *Salacia oblonga* attenuates diabetic renal fibrosis in rats: Suppression of angiotensin II/AT1 signaling. *Evidence-Based Complementary and Alternative Medicine* 2011.

Hesari, A., F. Ghasemi, R. Salarinia, H. Biglari, A. Tabar Molla Hassan, V. Abdoli, and H. Mirzaei. 2018. Effects of curcumin on NF-κB, AP-1, and Wnt/β-catenin signaling pathway in hepatitis B virus infection. *Journal of Cellular Biochemistry* 119: 7898–7904.

Hoffmann, M., H. Kleine-Weber, N. Krüger, M.A. Mueller, C. Drosten, and S. Pöhlmann. 2020. The novel coronavirus 2019 (2019-nCoV) uses the SARS-coronavirus receptor ACE2 and the cellular protease TMPRSS2 for entry into target cells. *BioRxiv.*

Im, K., J. Kim, and H. Min. 2016. Ginseng, the natural effectual antiviral: Protective effects of Korean Red Ginseng against viral infection. *Journal of Ginseng Research* 40: 309–314.

Iqbal, H. and D.K. Rhee. 2020. Ginseng alleviates microbial infections of the respiratory tract: A review. *Journal of Ginseng Research* 44: 194–204.

Jain, J., A. Kumar, V. Narayanan, R.S. Ramaswamy, P. Sathiyarajeswaran, M.S. Devi, M. Kannan, and S. Sunil. 2020. Antiviral activity of ethanolic extract of Nilavembu Kudineer against dengue and chikungunya virus through in vitro evaluation. *Journal of Ayurveda and integrative medicine* 11: 329–335.

Kamalarajan, P., S. Muthuraman, M.R. Ganesh, and M.F. Valan. 2019. Phytochemical investigation of nilavembu kudineer chooranam ethyl acetate extract and its ability to reduce intracellular antioxidant levels in THP-I cells. *European Journal of Medicinal Plants* 1–13.

Kavinilavan, R., P. Mekala, M.J. Raja, M. Arthanari Eswaran, and G. Thirumalaisamy. 2017. Exploration of immunomodulatory effect of nilavembu kudineer chooranam against newcastle disease virus in backyard chicken. *Journal of Pharmacognosy and Phytochemistry* 6: 49–751.

Khaerunnisa, S., H. Kurniawan, R. Awaluddin, S. Suhartati, and S. Soetjipto. 2020. Potential inhibitor of COVID-19 main protease (Mpro) from several medicinal plant compounds by molecular docking study. *Prepr* 1–14.

Khanal, P., T. Duyu, Y.N. Dey, B.M. Patil, I. Pasha, and M. Wanjari. 2020. Network pharmacology of AYUSH recommended immune-boosting medicinal plants against COVID-19. *Journal of Ayurveda and Integrative Medicine.* https://doi.org/10.1016/j.jaim.2020.11.004.

Kharisma, V.D., L. Septiadi, and S. Syafrudin. 2018. Prediction of novel bioactive compound from Zingiber officinale as non-nucleoside reverse transcriptase inhibitors (NNRTIs) of HIV-1 through computational study. *Bioinformatics and Biomedical Research Journal* 1: 49–55.

Kim, B.H., Y.G. Lee, J. Lee, J.Y. Lee, and J.Y. Cho. 2010. Regulatory effect of cinnamaldehyde on monocyte/macrophage-mediated inflammatory responses. *Mediators of inflammation* 2010.

Kooti, W., Z. Hasanzadeh-Noohi, N. Sharafi-Ahvazi, M. Asadi-Samani, and D. Ashtary-Larky. 2016. Phytochemistry, pharmacology, and therapeutic uses of black seed (*Nigella sativa*). *Chinese Journal of Natural Medicines* 4: 732–745.

Kruse, R.L. 2020. Therapeutic strategies in an outbreak scenario to treat the novel coronavirus originating in Wuhan, China. *F1000Research* 9.

Kumar, D., V. Arya, R. Kaur, Z.A. Bhat, V.K. Gupta, and V. Kumar. 2012. A review of immunomodulators in the Indian traditional health care system. *Journal of Microbiology, Immunology and Infection* 45: 165–184.

Kumar, R., N. Anjum, and Y.C. Tripathi. 2015. Phytochemistry and pharmacology of *Santalum album* L.: A review. *World Journal of Pharmaceutical Research* 4: 1842–1876.

Lee, B.J., Y.J. Kim, D.H. Cho, N.W. Sohn, and H. Kang. 2011. Immunomodulatory effect of water extract of cinnamon on anti-CD3-induced cytokine responses and p38, JNK, ERK1/2, and STAT4 activation. *Immunopharmacology and Immunotoxicology* 33: 714–722.

Lee, J.S., H.S. Hwang, E.J. Ko, Y.N. Lee, Y.M. Kwon, M.C. Kim, and S.M. Kang. 2014. Immunomodulatory activity of red ginseng against influenza A virus infection. *Nutrients* 6: 517–529.

Lei, P., B. Fan, J. Mao, and P. Wang. 2020. Comprehensive analysis for diagnosis of novel coronavirus disease (COVID-19) infection. *The Journal of Infection* 80(6).

Li, G. and De E. Clercq. 2020. Therapeutic options for the 2019 novel coronavirus (2019-nCoV). *Nature Reviews Drug Discovery* 19: 149–150.

Liu, Z., X. Xiao, X. Wei, J. Li, J. Yang, H. Tan, J. Zhu, Q. Zhang, J. Wu, and L. Liu. 2020. Composition and divergence of coronavirus spike proteins and host ACE2 receptors predict potential intermediate hosts of SARS-CoV-2. *Journal of Medical Virology* 92: 595–601.

Lo, A.H., Y.C. Liang, S.Y. Lin-Shiau, C.T. Ho, and J.K. Lin. 2002. Carnosol, an antioxidant in rosemary, suppresses inducible nitric oxide synthase through down-regulating nuclear factor-κB in mouse macrophages. *Carcinogenesis* 23: 83–991.

Madhumita, M., P. Guha, and A. Nag. 2020. Bio-actives of betel leaf (Piper betle L.): A comprehensive review on extraction, isolation, characterization, and biological activity. *Phytotherapy Research* 34(10): 2609–2627.

Mahassni, S.H. and O.A. Bukhari. 2019. Beneficial effects of an aqueous ginger extract on the immune system cells and antibodies, hematology, and thyroid hormones in male smokers and non-smokers. *Journal of Nutrition & Intermediary Metabolism* 15: 10–17.

Mahluji, S., A. Ostadrahimi, M. Mobasseri, V.E. Attari, and L. Payahoo. 2013. Anti-inflammatory effects of Zingiber officinale in type 2 diabetic patients. *Advanced Pharmaceutical Bulletin* 3: 273.

Mali, R.G., S.G. Mahajan, and A.A. Mehta 2007. *Lepidium sativum* (Garden cress): A review of contemporary literature and medicinal properties. *Oriental Pharmacy and Experimental Medicine* 7: 331–335.

Mondal, S. 2010. *Antimicrobial and immunomodulatory effects of Tulsi (Oscimum Snctum Linn)* (Doctoral dissertation, Ph. D. Thesis, All India Institute of Medical Sciences, New Delhi, India).

Mondal, S., S. Varma, V.D. Bamola, S.N. Naik, B.R. Mirdha, M.M. Padhi, N. Mehta, and S.C. Mahapatra. 2011. Double-blinded randomized controlled trial for immunomodulatory effects of Tulsi (*Ocimum sanctum* Linn.) leaf extract on healthy volunteers. *Journal of Ethnopharmacology* 136: 452–456.

Mukherjee, P.K., R.K. Harwansh, S. Bahadur, S. Banerjee, A. Kar, J. Chanda, S. Biswas, S.M. Ahmmed, and C.K. Katiyar. 2017. Development of Ayurveda–tradition to trend. *Journal of Ethnopharmacology* 197: 10–24.

Nabila, N., N.K. Suada, D. Denis, B. Yohan, A.C. Adi, A.S. Veterini, A.L. Anindya, R.T. Sasmono, and H. Rachmawati. 2020. Antiviral action of curcumin encapsulated in nanoemulsion against four serotypes of dengue virus. *Pharmaceutical Nanotechnology* 8: 54–62.

Nahak, G. and R.K. Sahu. 2011. Phytochemical evaluation and antioxidant activity of Piper cubeba and Piper nigrum. *Journal of Applied Pharmaceutical Science* 1: 153.

Nakkeeran, C., P. Selvakumari, T. Kasthury, and R.T. Kumar. 2016. FTIR analysis on Nilavembu Kudineer Churanam and acetominaphen. *Journal of Chemical and Pharmaceutical Research* 8: 634–639.

Nassiri-Asl, M., and H. Hosseinzadeh. 2009. Review of the pharmacological effects of *Vitis vinifera* (Grape) and its bioactive compounds. *Phytotherapy Research: An International Journal Devoted to Pharmacological and Toxicological Evaluation of Natural Product Derivatives* 23: 1197–1204.

Navratil, V., L. Lionnard, S. Longhi, M. Hardwick, C. Combet, and A. Aouacheria. 2020. The severe acute respiratory syndrome coronavirus 2 (SARS-CoV-2) envelope (E) protein harbors a conserved BH3-like sequence. *bioRxiv.*

Niphade, S.R., M. Asad, G.K. Chandrakala, E. Toppo, and P. Deshmukh. 2009. Immunomodulatory activity of *Cinnamomum zeylanicum* bark. *Pharmaceutical Biology* 47: 1168–1173.

Öztürk, M., V. Altay, K.R. Hakeem, and E. Akçiçek. 2017. Pharmacological activities and phytochemical constituents. In *Liquorice* (pp. 45–72). Springer, Cham.

Parasuraman, S., G.S. Thing, and S.A. Dhanaraj. 2014. Polyherbal formulation: Concept of ayurveda. *Pharmacognosy Reviews* 8: 73.

Petrovska, B.B. 2012. Historical review of medicinal plants' usage. *Pharmacognosy Reviews* 6: 1.

Ponnam, H.B., and B.R. Akondi. 2020. AYUSH systems of medicine, a viable solution for COVID-19 amidst the uncertainty of vaccination & herd immunity-an Indian perspective. *Asian Journal of Pharmaceutical Research and Health Care* 12: 1–3.

Praditya, D., L. Kirchhoff, J. Brüning, H. Rachmawati, J. Steinmann, and E. Steinmann. 2019. Anti-infective properties of the golden spice curcumin. *Frontiers in Microbiology* 10: 912.

Pundarikakshudu, K., and N.S. Kanaki. 2019. Analysis and regulation of Traditional Indian Medicines (TIM). *Journal of AOAC International* 102: 977.

Ramanathan, M., L. Subramanian, T. Poongodi, S. Manish, E. Muneeswari, P. Pavithra, and S. Pugalendran. 2019. Formulation and evaluation of Nilavembu Kudineer capsules. *Asian Journal of Pharmaceutical Research and Development* 7: 41–45.

Ratan, Z.A., M.F. Haidere, Y.H. Hong, S.H. Park, J.O. Lee, J. Lee, and J.Y. Cho. 2020. Pharmacological potential of ginseng and its major component ginsenosides. *Journal of Ginseng Research* 45(2): 199–210.

Saha, S., and S. Ghosh. 2012. Tinospora cordifolia: One plant, many roles. *Ancient Science of Life* 31: 151.

Schoeman, D., and B.C. Fielding. 2019. Coronavirus envelope protein: Current knowledge. *Virology Journal* 16: 1–22.

Sharifi, N., E. Souri, S.A. Ziai, G. Amin, and M. Amanlou. 2013. Discovery of new angiotensin converting enzyme (ACE) inhibitors from medicinal plants to treat hypertension using an in vitro assay. *DARU Journal of Pharmaceutical Sciences* 21: 74.

Sharma, P., B.P. Dwivedee, D. Bisht, A.K. Dash, and D. Kumar. 2019. The chemical constituents and diverse pharmacological importance of Tinospora cordifolia. *Heliyon* 5: 2437.

Sharma, V., A. Katiyar, and R.C. Agrawal. 2018. Glycyrrhiza glabra: Chemistry and pharmacological activity. *Sweeteners* 87–100.

Shukla, P., S.D. Jain, A. Agrawal, and A.K. Gupta. 2019. Indian herbal plants used as anti-pyretic: A review. *International Journal of Pharmacy & Life Sciences* 10(11–12): 6406–6409.

Singh, S.S., S.C. Pandey, S. Srivastava, V.S. Gupta, B. Patro, and A.C. Ghosh. 2003. Chemistry and medicinal properties of *Tinospora cordifolia* (Guduchi). *Indian Journal of Pharmacology* 35: 83–91.

Sinha, S.K., S.K. Prasad, M.A. Islam, S.S. Gurav, R.B. Patil, N.A. AlFaris, T.S. Aldayel, N.M. AlKehayez, S.M. Wabaidur, and A. Shakya. 2020. Identification of bioactive compounds from Glycyrrhiza glabra as possible inhibitor of SARS-CoV-2 spike gly-coprotein and non-structural protein-15: A pharmacoinformatics study. *Journal of Biomolecular Structure and Dynamics* 1–15.

Sivapalan, S.R. 2015. Phytochemical study on medicinal plant–*Sida cordifolia* Linn. *International Journal of Multidisciplinary Research and Development* 2: 216–220.

Sonkamble, V.V., and L.H. Kamble. 2015. Antidiabetic potential and identification of phy-tochemicals from *Tinospora cordifolia*. *American Journal of Phytomedicine and Clinical Therapeutics* 3: 097–110.

Sousa, G.J.B., T.S. Garces, V.R.F. Cestari, R.S. Florêncio, T.M.M. Moreira, and M.L.D. Pereira. 2020. Mortality and survival of COVID-19. *Epidemiology & Infection* 148.

Srivastava, A.K., and V.K. Singh. 2017. Biological action of *Piper nigrum*-the king of spices. *European Journal of Biological Research* 7: 223–233.

Srivastava, A.K., J.P. Chaurasia, R. Khan, C. Dhand, and S. Verma. 2020. Role of medicinal plants of traditional use in recuperating devastating COVID-19 situation. *Med Aromat Plants (Los Angeles)* 9: 2167–0412.

Suja, R.S., A.M.C. Nair, S. Sujith, J. Preethy, and A.K. Deepa. 2009. Evaluation of immuno-modulatory potential of Emblica officinalis fruit pulp extract in mice. *Indian Journal of Animal Research* 43: 103–106.

Tai, W., L. He, X. Zhang, J. Pu, D. Voronin, S. Jiang, Y. Zhou, and L. Du. 2020. Characterization of the receptor-binding domain (RBD) of 2019 novel coronavirus: Implication for development of RBD protein as a viral attachment inhibitor and vaccine. *Cellular & Molecular Immunology* 17: 613–620.

The AYUSH [Internet]. https://www.ayush.gov.in. 2020. Available from: https://www.ayush.gov.in/docs/125.pdf [accessed on 10th Nov 2020].

Tsui, P.F., C.S. Lin, L.J. Ho, and J.H. Lai. 2018. Spices and atherosclerosis. *Nutrients* 10: 1724.

Vaidya, A.D., and T.P. Devasagayam. 2007. Recent advances in Indian herbal drug research guest editor: Thomas Paul Asir Devasagayam current status of herbal drugs in India: An overview. *Journal of Clinical Biochemistry and Nutrition* 41: 1–11.

Valizadeh, S., F. Katiraee, R. Mahmoudi, T. Fakheri, and K. Mardani. 2015. Biological prop-erties of Cinnamomum zeylanicum essential oil: Phytochemical component, antioxi-dant and antimicrobial activities. *International Journal of Food Safety Nutrition and Public Health* 6: 174–184.

Vasudevan, P., S. Kashyap, and S. Sharma. 1999. Bioactive botanicals from basil (*Ocimum* sp.).

Vellingiri, B., K. Jayaramayya, M. Iyer, A. Narayanasamy, V. Govindasamy, B. Giridharan, S. Ganesan, A. Venugopal, D. Venkatesan, H. Ganesan, and K. Rajagopalan. 2020. COVID-19: A promising cure for the global panic. *Science of The Total Environment* 138277.

Verma, H., M.S. Negi, B.S. Mahapatra, and A.S.J. Paul. 2019. Evaluation of an emerging medicinal crop Kalmegh [Andrographis paniculata (Burm. F.) Wall. Ex. Nees] for commercial cultivation and pharmaceutical & industrial uses: A review. *Journal of Pharmacognosy and Phytochemistry* 8: 835–848.

Verma, S., D. Twilley, T. Esmear, C.B. Oosthuizen, A.M. Reid, M. Nel, and N. Lall. 2020. Anti-SARS-CoV natural products with the potential to inhibit SARS-CoV-2 (COVID-19). *Frontiers in Pharmacology* 11: 1514.

Wahedi, H.M., S. Ahmad, and S.W. Abbasi. 2020. Stilbene-based natural compounds as promising drug candidates against COVID-19. *Journal of Biomolecular Structure and Dynamics* 1–10.

Wang, Y., H.K. Choi, J.A. Brinckmann, X. Jiang, and L. Huang. 2015. Chemical analysis of *Panax quinquefolius* (North American ginseng): A review. *Journal of Chromatography A* 1426: 1–15.

Wen, C.C., L.F. Shyur, J.T. Jan, P.H. Liang, C.J. Kuo, P. Arulselvan, J.B. Wu, S.C. Kuo, and N.S. Yang. 2011. Traditional Chinese medicine herbal extracts of *Cibotium barometz, Gentiana scabra, Dioscorea batatas, Cassia tora,* and *Taxillus chinensis* inhibit SARS-CoV replication. *Journal of Traditional and Complementary Medicine* 1: 41–50.

Weng, J.K. 2020. Plant solutions for the COVID-19 pandemic and beyond: Historical reflections and future perspectives. *Molecular Plant* 13(6): 803–807.

World Health Organization. 2019. *WHO global report on traditional and complementary medicine 2019.* World Health Organization.

World Health Organization. 2020. *Transmission of SARS-CoV-2: Implications for infection prevention precautions: Scientific brief, 09 July 2020* (No. WHO/2019-nCoV/Sci_Br ief/Transmission_modes/2020.3). World Health Organization.

Yadav, U.C., and N.Z. Baquer. 2014. Pharmacological effects of *Trigonella foenum-graecum* L. in health and disease. *Pharmaceutical Biology* 52: 243–254.

Yang, Y., Z. Xiong, S. Zhang, Y. Yan, J. Nguyen, B. Ng, H. Lu, J. Brendese, F. Yang, H. Wang, and X.F. Yang. 2005. Bcl-xL inhibits T-cell apoptosis induced by expression of SARS coronavirus E protein in the absence of growth factors. *Biochemical Journal* 392: 135–143.

Yin, Y., and R.G. Wunderink. 2018. MERS, SARS and other coronaviruses as causes of pneumonia. *Respirology* 23: 130–137.

Yuan, H., Q. Ma, L. Ye, and G. Piao. 2016. The traditional medicine and modern medicine from natural products. *Molecules* 21: 559.

Zaim, S., J.H. Chong, V. Sankaranarayanan, and A. Harky. 2020. COVID-19 and multi-organ response. *Current Problems in Cardiology* 100618.

Zhai, W.J., Z.B. Zhang, N.N. Xu, Y.F. Guo, C. Qiu, C.Y. Li, G.Z. Deng, and M.Y. Guo. 2016. Piperine plays an anti-inflammatory role in *Staphylococcus aureus* endometritis by inhibiting activation of NF-κB and MAPK pathways in mice. *Evidence-Based Complementary and Alternative Medicine* 2016.

Zhang, L., D. Lin, X. Sun, U. Curth, C. Drosten, L. Sauerhering, S. Becker, K. Rox, and R. Hilgenfeld. 2020. Crystal structure of SARS-CoV-2 main protease provides a basis for design of improved α-ketoamide inhibitors. *Science* 368: 409–412.

Zhao, Z., Y. Li, L. Zhou, X. Zhou, B. Xie, W. Zhang, and J. Sun. 2020. Prevention and treatment of COVID-19 using traditional Chinese medicine: A review. *Phytomedicine* 153308.

Zheng X.Y., X.J. Xu, W.J. Guan, and L.F. Lin. 2018. Regional, age and respiratory-secretion-specific prevalence of respiratory viruses associated with asthma exacerbation: A literature review. *Archives of Virology* 163: 845–853.

Zorofchian Moghadamtousi, S., H. A. Kadir, P. Hassandarvish, H. Tajik, S. Abubakar, and K. Zandi. 2014. A review on antibacterial, antiviral, and antifungal activity of curcumin. *BioMed Research International* 2014.

Index

Note: Locators in *italics* represent figures and **bold** indicate tables in the text.

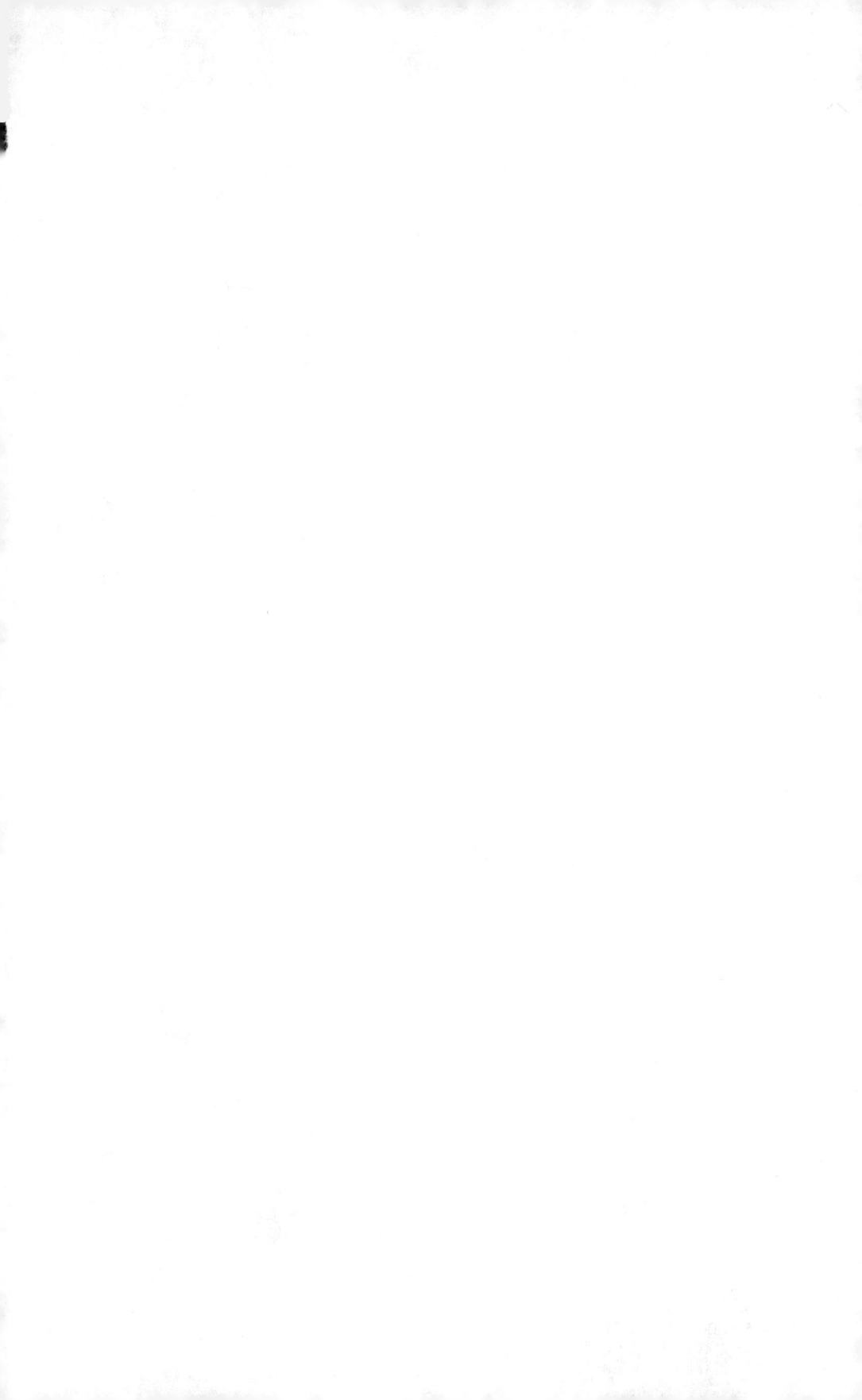

For Product Safety Concerns and Information please contact our EU
representative GPSR@taylorandfrancis.com
Taylor & Francis Verlag GmbH, Kaufingerstraße 24, 80331 München, Germany

www.ingramcontent.com/pod-product-compliance
Lightning Source LLC
Chambersburg PA
CBHW060422220326
41598CB00021BA/2263

9 781032 122243